D1711866

$110

Neuroendocrinology

Neuroendocrinology

Edited by

Charles B. Nemeroff

Professor and Chairman
Department of Psychiatry
Emory University School of Medicine
Atlanta, Georgia

CRC Press
Boca Raton   Ann Arbor   London   Tokyo

Cover: Corticotropin-releasing factor (CRF)-containing fibers in the median eminence of monkey (*Macaca fascicularis*). CRF-containing fibers are seen in the external layer of the median eminence, closely surrounding portal vessels. (Kindly provided by Dr. Björn Meister, Department of Histology and Neurobiology, Karolinska Institute, Stockholm, Sweden.)

Library of Congress Cataloging-in-Publication Data

Neuroendocrinology / editor, Charles B. Nemeroff.
  p. cm.
  Includes bibliographical references and index.
  ISBN 0-8493-8844-9
  1. Neuroendocrinology. I. Nemeroff, Charles B.
  [DNLM: 1. Behavior—physiology. 2. Neuroendocrinology. 3. Neurosecretion—physiology.
WL 102 N4945326]
QP356.4.N482 1992
612.8′042—dc20
DNLM/DLC
for Library of Congress

International Standard Book Number 0-8493-8844-9
Library of Congress Card Number 91-46098

Printed in the United States 1 2 3 4 5 6 7 8 9 0

Printed on acid-free paper

DEDICATION

To Melissa, Matthew, Amanda, and Sara-Frances

THE EDITOR

Dr. Charles B. Nemeroff was born in New York City in 1949 and was educated in the New York City Public School System. After graduating from the City College of New York in 1970, he briefly enrolled as a graduate student in evolutionary biology at the American Museum of Natural History. An interest in neuroscience, however, led him to a research assistant's position at the Neurochemistry laboratory at McLean Hospital in Belmont, Massachusetts. He simultaneously enrolled in graduate school at Northeastern University and received a Master's degree in Biology in 1973. He then relocated to North Carolina and enrolled in the Ph.D. program in Neurobiology at the University of North Carolina at Chapel Hill. His Ph.D. work, on thyrotropin-releasing hormone, was performed under the direction of a psychiatrist, Arthur J. Prange, Jr. After a year of post-doctoral training in neurochemistry, he enrolled in medical school at the University of North Carolina at Chapel Hill. His residency training in psychiatry was at both the University of North Carolina and at Duke University after which he joined the faculty of Duke University. At Duke he was Professor of Psychiatry and Pharmacology and Chief of the Division of Biological Psychiatry before relocating to Emory University School of Medicine in Atlanta, Georgia, where he currently is Professor and Chairman of the Department of Psychiatry.

Dr. Nemeroff has concentrated on the biological basis of the major neuropsychiatric disorders, including affective disorders, Alzheimer's disease, schizophrenia, and anxiety disorders. He has received numerous honors during his career, including the A. E. Bennett Neuropsychiatric Research Foundation Award in Basic Science from the Society of Biological Psychiatry (1979), the Curt P. Richter Award from the International Society of Psychoneuroendocrinology (1985), the Jordi Folch-Pi Award from the American Society for Neurochemistry (1987), the Anna Monika Foundation Award for Research in Depression (1987), the Daniel H. Efron Award from the American College of Neuropsychopharmacology (1987), the Judith Silver Memorial Young Scientist Award from the National Alliance for the Mentally Ill (1989), the Kempf Award in Psychobiology (1989), as well as the Samuel Hibbs Award (1990) from the American Psychiatric Association. He is also the recipient of a MERIT award from NIMH.

Dr. Nemeroff serves on the Clinical Biology Review Committee of NIMH and is on the editorial boards of *Synapse, Neurochemical Pathology, Psychopharmacology Bulletin, Journal of Gerontology, Regulatory Peptides, Hormones and Behavior,* and the *Journal of Neuropsychiatry and Clinical Neuroscience*, as well as co-editor-in-chief of *Critical Reviews in Neurobiology*. He has published more than 360 research reports and reviews.

But ultimately, on most days, he would rather be at the seashore with his wife, Melissa, and three children, Matthew, Amanda, and Sara-Frances, to whom this textbook is dedicated.

TABLE OF CONTENTS

1

An Introduction to Neuroendocrinology: Basic Principles and Historical Considerations

S. M. McCANN

Department of Physiology, Neuropeptide Division
The University of Texas Southwestern Medical Center at Dallas
Dallas, Texas

I. Historical Considerations

The first evidence that the pituitary gland might have a function was provided with the discovery of acromegaly by Marie in 1886, which was shown by others to be caused by eosinophilic adenomas of the anterior pituitary gland. It was not until the early 20th century that it was shown that hypophysectomy led to stunting of growth. In 1921, Evans and Long prepared aqueous extracts of the pituitary gland and showed that these would restore growth in hypophysectomized animals. The remaining pituitary hormones were discovered in the 1920s and early 1930s and the concept developed that the pituitary was the master gland and conductor of the endocrine symphony orchestra.

Frohlich (1901) described the syndrome of adiposigenital dystrophy, which was caused by tumors at the base of the brain and which frequently involved the pituitary gland. He attributed the syndrome to dysfunction of the pituitary gland. Bailey and Bremer (1921) made lesions at the base of the brain and reproduced the syndrome in dogs. Histological examination of the pituitary gland showed no abnormality and they suggested that the etiology of Frohlich's syndrome was an elimination of hypothalamic control over gonadotropin secretion rather than direct damage to the pituitary itself.

Moore and Price showed that gonadal steroids could suppress the release of gonadotropins which was the first evidence for negative feedback of target gland hormones to suppress the release of pituitary trophic hormones (Price, 1975). They believed that this action was mediated solely by a direct effect on the pituitary itself. Hohlweg (1975) observed that estrogen would evoke precocious puberty in immature rats, and postulated that this positive feedback effect of estrogen was exerted through a sex centrum in the brain, which then augmented release of gonadotropins. Even though the waxing and waning of gonadotropin secretion with the seasons had been known for many years and the ability of sexual excitement to evoke ovulation was known in rabbits, cats, and ferrets, most workers still believed that the hypothalamus had little to do with the moment-to-moment control of release of pituitary hormones.

Further evidence of hypothalamic control was provided by electrical stimulation of the hypothalamus, which induced ovulation in anesthetized rabbits. Later Harris showed that these effects could be obtained in conscious rabbits using an induction coil to stimulate the hypothalamus of the rabbits by remote control. In the early 1950s there were many experiments in which hypothalamic lesions were shown to interfere with the secretion of each and every anterior pituitary hormone, with the exception of prolactin. In the early 1940s Jacobsohn and co-workers showed that prolactin secretion was enhanced in pituitary stalk-sectioned animals that were treated with estrogen. Similarly, Desclin showed that estrogen-treated hypophysectomized animals with pituitary grafts under the kidney capsule secreted increased amounts of prolactin. Everett ran the control experiment and found that these grafts secreted excess prolactin even without estrogen treatment. Subsequent work with stalk sections and hypothalamic lesions amply confirmed that the net effect of the hypothalamus on prolactin release is inhibitory. In contrast, the net effect on the release of all the other anterior pituitary hormones is stimulatory. Additional experiments showed that adrenocorticotropic hormone (ACTH) secretion was enhanced by stimulating the hypothalamus (for references see Sawyer, 1988; McCann, 1988).

The next question was, how does the hypothalamus control the anterior pituitary gland? There was little evidence for a direct secretomotor innervation of the gland, but a possible alternate pathway was provided by the discovery of the hypophysial portal vessels by Popa and Fielding in 1930. They believed that the flow in these vessels was from the pituitary upward to the hypothalamus; however, anatomical studies by Wislocki and King led them to the conclusion that the flow had to be in the reverse direction, down from the brain to the pituitary gland. Thus it was possible to postulate that the gland was controlled by a neurohumoral mechanism involving the portal vessels. Houssay et al. observed downward flow in the living toad in 1935 and this was confirmed in the rat by Green and Harris in 1947 (see Sawyer, 1988).

Hinsey and Markee in 1933 were the first to postulate that neurohypophysial hormones might control the release of anterior pituitary hormones; however, they were not aware of the discovery of the portal vessels and postulated that these hormones would circulate through the peripheral blood to act on the anterior pituitary gland. A number of workers hypothesized during the 1930s that the control was via the newly discovered portal vessels; these workers included Brooks, Haterius, and Hinsey (see Sawyer, 1988; McCann, 1988).

Harris deserves the major credit for focusing on the possibility of neurohumoral control of the pituitary gland via release of neurohumors into the portal vessels. He began an elaborate series of experiments to test this hypothesis in the late 1940s. He first showed that following simple stalk section the portal vessels regenerate and that the regeneration of portal vessels was accompanied by a return of normal pituitary function. If the regeneration was blocked by placement of an impervious plate between the cut edges of the stalk, a permanent derangement of pituitary function ensued. The impairment in pituitary hormone secretion was the same as that in hypophysectomized rats with the pituitary grafted to a site distant from the median eminence. With Jacobsohn, Harris showed that if one hypophysectomized an animal and placed its pituitary under the median eminence so that it could be revascularized by portal vessels, there was a return of normal pituitary function (Harris, 1961). In an elaboration on this experiment, Nikitovitch-Weiner and Everett first grafted the pituitary under the kidney capsule and then later replaced it under the median eminence, which again led to a return of normal pituitary function.

These pioneering experiments of Harris and co-workers set the stage for the discovery of the releasing and inhibiting hormones. The first candidate as a releasing hormone was epinephrine. This was known to be released by stress and consequently appeared a likely candidate to mediate stress-induced ACTH secretion. A variety of experiments carried out by Long and co-workers led them to conclude that epinephrine reaching the pituitary via the systemic circulation brought about ACTH release. At about the same time Everett and Sawyer concluded that epinephrine might directly release luteinizing hormone (LH) from the pituitary gland, since they were able to induce ovulation in rabbits by direct application of the amine to the pituitary gland. Donovan and Harris claimed that this was caused by the acidity of the solutions. We found that median eminence lesions, which blocked the ACTH release by stress, also blocked the response to epinephrine. Consequently, we concluded that epinephrine acted within the brain to bring about ACTH release rather than directly on the pituitary (see McCann, 1988). Now, many years later, it is still possible that epinephrine may play a role in controlling release of pituitary hormones. There are β receptors in the gland; epinephrine can activate the release of all pituitary hormones *in vitro;* epinephrine has been found in high concentrations in portal vessels, so that it may act by this route rather than via the general circulation; the administration of β-adrenergic receptor blockers lowers plasma LH in castrate rats; and β receptors in the pituitary are altered by castration, administration of gonadal steroids, and during the estrous cycle (Petrovic et al., 1985). Therefore, Everett and Sawyer may have been correct when they postulated a direct action of the catecholamine on the pituitary to alter LH secretion. There is also evidence that it may play a physiological role in stress-induced ACTH secretion (Rivier and Vale, 1985).

The next logical step was to make extracts of the median eminence region, the area that is drained by the portal vessels, and to inject these into animals to determine if they could alter anterior pituitary function. We carried out these experiments in animals with median eminence lesions that blocked the ubiquitous stress response. Our initial experiments failed in that hypothalamic extracts produced no release of ACTH whatsoever. These lesions produced diabetes insipidus because of a deficiency of antidiuretic hormone (vasopressin). Furthermore, Verney had shown that various stresses evoked vasopressin secretion. Therefore, it occurred to us that vasopressin could be the ACTH-releasing factor and we tested Pitressin, a partially purified vasopressin preparation, in animals with median eminence lesions and found that it would release ACTH whereas oxytocin and various known transmitters such as epinephrine, norepinephrine, serotonin, substance P, etc. were without effect. Since synthetic vasopressin also released ACTH, we postulated that vasopressin might be the corticotropin-releasing factor (CRF) and that in stress it would be released into portal vessels and reach the pituitary in sufficient concentration to activate the release of ACTH. Martini independently obtained convincing evidence that vasopressin was a CRF (see Martini, 1966).

Saffran and Schally took a different approach, namely incubation of pituitaries *in vitro.* In the presence of norepinephrine they found in agreement with us that pressor pituitary extracts would increase the release of ACTH *in vitro.* However, they went on to fractionate these extracts by paper chromatography and reported that a factor different from vasopressin, which they named CRF, would also release ACTH. In the meantime, using our *in vivo* assay we were unable to find evidence for a posterior pituitary CRF other than vasopressin (see McCann, 1988).

In 1958, Royce and Sayers reported that hypothalamic extract indeed contained a CRF distinct from vasopressin using our assay, the rat with median eminence lesions. We were able to confirm this work and our failure to find the hypothalamic CRF earlier was probably related to use of a less sensitive assay at that time. Indeed, we showed that the corticotropin-releasing activity of median eminence extracts was largely accounted for by this other CRF, with vasopressin accounting for only 10 to 15% of the activity. This cleared up the controversy that had been going on for some years. The problem was that posterior pituitary extract was not suitable for purification of CRF, since nearly all of the activity in such extracts is accounted for by vasopressin. Using hypothalamic extracts, it was easy to purify CRF and to separate it from vasopressin. The view then emerged that both vasopressin and this unknown CRF were involved in the control of ACTH release (see Zimmerman, 1983; McCann, 1988).

Vasopressin has a physiological role in the control of ACTH release since there is a definite deficiency in ACTH release in animals with hereditary diabetes insipidus (McCann et al., 1966); such animals lack endogenously produced vasopressin. Another indication that vasopressin is a corticotropin-releasing factor is its direct action in stimulating ACTH release in a dose-related fashion from the pituitary incubated *in vitro* (Gillies et al., 1982). Finally, vasopressin is present in high concentrations in portal blood collected from the pituitary stalk of monkeys and rats (Fink et al., 1988); these concentrations are in the range that should stimulate ACTH release, at least under stressful conditions, at a time when vasopressin is released in large amounts.

It is now apparent that vasopressin and CRF cooperate in the control of ACTH release. Vasopressin can potentiate the action of CRF at both hypothalamic and pituitary levels (Gillies et al., 1982; McCann et al., 1982). Antiserum against CRF given intravenously largely blocks the stress response (Rivier and Vale, 1985; Ono et al., 1985b) but it can also be inhibited partially by vasopressin antiserum (Ono et al., 1985a). Furthermore, it appears that the vasopressin that reaches the pituitary comes predominantly from vasopressinergic neurons that extend to the median eminence to end in juxtaposition to portal vessels (Zimmerman, 1983). Many of the vasopressinergic neurons apparently also contain CRF, so that there may be corelease from the same terminals into portal blood (Whitnall and Gainer, 1988).

The discovery of a CRF distinct from vasopressin provoked a search for similar factors that stimulate release of other anterior pituitary hormones. In rapid succession an LH-releasing factor, follicle-stimulating hormone (FSH)-releasing factor, growth hormone-releasing factor, thyroid-stimulating hormone (TSH)-releasing factor, and prolactin-inhibiting factor were discovered. Evidence for both melanophore-stimulating hormone (MSH)-releasing and -inhibiting factors was obtained, and a growth hormone release-inhibiting factor was also described. There is some evidence for prolactin-releasing factors as well (Table 1).

An intensive effort was made to purify these new substances, to separate them from other

Table 1
History of the Peptide-Releasing and -Inhibiting Hormones

Releasing hormone	Discovery	Purified	Synthesized	Stimulates	Inhibits
Vasopressin	1954	Yes	Nonapeptide	ACTH, TSH	—
Corticotropin-releasing hormone (CRH)	1955–1959	Yes	41-aa[a] peptide	ACTH	—
LH-releasing hormone (LHRH)	1960	Yes	Decapeptide	LH, FSH	—
FSH-releasing factor (FSH-RF)	1964	Yes	No	FSH	—
Thyrotropin-releasing hormone (TRH)	1958–1962	Yes	Tripeptide	TSH, prolactin	—
Growth hormone-releasing hormone (GHRH)	1958–1964	Yes	44-aa[a] peptide	GH	—
Growth hormone-inhibiting (GHIH) (somatostatin)	1967	Yes	Tetradecapeptide	—	GH, prolactin, TSH, gastrin, glucagon, insulin
Prolactin-inhibiting factor (PIF)	1963	Yes	Yes	—	Prolactin
Prolactin-releasing factors (PRFs)					
a. Oxytocin	1981	Yes	Nonapeptide	Prolactin	—
b. VIP[b], PHI[c], AII[d], neurotensin, substance P	1978–1982	Yes	Yes	Prolactin	—
MSH-releasing factor (MRF)	1965	Yes	?	MSH	—
MSH-inhibiting factor (MIF)	1966	Yes	?	—	MSH

[a]aa, Amino acids.
[b]VIP, Vasoactive intestinal polypeptide.
[c]PHI, Peptide histidine isoleucine.
[d]AII, Angiotensin II.

active substances in hypothalamic extracts, and to determine their structure so that this could be confirmed by synthesis. Since only very small amounts of the releasing factors are present in hypothalamic tissue, this proved to be a herculean task. Apparently because of their ready access to the anterior lobe via the hypophysial portal vessels, there is no need to flood the general circulation with these releasing hormones and, therefore, no need to store large amounts in the hypothalamus. Consequently, isolation and determination of their structure required the processing of hundreds of thousands and even millions of hypothalamic fragments.

There were two keys to the elucidation of these structures. The first was the realization than neurohypophysial extracts that were commercially available were not suitable as starting material because of the small amounts of the releasing factors they contained and their high concentrations of the neurohypophysial hormones, vasopressin and oxytocin. Therefore, it was necessary to process hypothalamic tissue. The second key was the realization that truly massive numbers of fragments had to be processed because of the small quantities of the active substances present even in hypothalamic tissue (see McCann, 1988).

II. Characterization of the Releasing Hormones

A. Thyrotropin-Releasing Hormone

The first releasing factor to be characterized was thyrotropin-releasing hormone (TRH), or thyroliberin. It is a tripeptide, pyroglutamyl-histidyl-prolineamide (Table 2). The cyclic nature of the peptide caused problems in identifying the structure, but this was eventually resolved by two groups almost simultaneously in 1969 (Boler et al., 1969; Burgus et al., 1969). The synthetic hormone proved active, and this eliminated some of the doubts held at the time regarding the existence of releasing factors.

B. Luteinizing Hormone-Releasing Hormone

Luteinizing hormone-releasing factor or hormone (LHRH) was shown to be a decapeptide (Table 2) and, once again, the synthetic hormone was active (Matsuo et al., 1971). The synthetic peptide released not only LH but to a lesser extent FSH as well, which has led some to postulate that LHRH is sufficient to account for the hypothalamic stimulation of both FSH and LH release (Schally et al., 1971). Since dissociation of FSH and LH release can occur following hypothalamic lesions and stimulations and also in a variety of physiological states, an FSH-releasing factor may exist; however, this point is controversial (McCann et al., 1983). Several groups have reported partial purifications of the putative FSH-releasing factor (Lumpkin et al., 1987).

Table 2
Structure of Three Hypothalamic Hormones: Luteinizing Hormone-Releasing Hormone, Thyrotropin-Releasing Hormone, and Somatostatin

Hormone	Amino acid sequence													
	1	2	3	4	5	6	7	8	9	10	11	12	13	14
TRH	P-Glu-His-Pro-NH_2													
LHRH	P-Glu-His-Trp-Ser-Tyr-Gly-Leu-Arg-Pro-Gly-NH_2													
Somatostatin	Ala-Gly-Cys-Lys-Asn-Phe-Phe-Trp-Lys-Thr-Phe-Thr-Ser-Cys													

C. Growth Hormone Release-Inhibiting Hormone (Somatostatin)

The third hypothalamic factor to be isolated was the growth hormone release-inhibiting hormone (GHIH), a factor discovered while attempting to purify the growth hormone-releasing factor (Krulich et al., 1968, 1972). The use of monolayer cultures of pituitary cells, which are very sensitive to the inhibitory action of GHIH, led to its purification, isolation, and determination of structure (Brazeau et al., 1973). The structure of GHIH (somatostatin) is that of a tetradecapeptide (Table 2), and, in contrast to TRH and LHRH, it has no amino-terminal pyroglutamyl group. There is also a 28-amino acid form of the molecule. The relative importance of these two forms is not clear.

D. Growth Hormone-Releasing Hormone

Although intensive work had been going on for a number of years in an attempt to isolate and determine the structure of growth hormone-releasing hormone (GHRH) (see McCann, 1988), its structure was resolved only when it became apparent that GHRH could be isolated from extracts of rare extrahypothalamic tumors, which secreted it (Rivier et al., 1982; Guillemin et al., 1982). The structure of this tumor-produced GHRH is the same as that of hypothalamic GHRH. Human GHRH is a 44-amino acid peptide.

E. Corticotropin-Releasing Hormone

Probably because of its much larger size, corticotropin-releasing hormone (CRH) defied elucidation for over 20 years, after which it was determined to be a 41-amino acid peptide (Vale et al., 1981). Interestingly enough, during attempts to isolate CRH two additional brain peptides, substance P (Chang and Leeman, 1970) and neurotensin (Carraway and Leeman, 1973), were isolated from hypothalamic extracts. Thus, the structures of most of the releasing and inhibiting hormones had now been determined.

F. Hypothalamic Factors Controlling Prolactin Secretion

There is also evidence for a peptidic prolactin-inhibiting factor (PIF) and for multiple prolactin-releasing factors. Oxytocin, which is released by the suckling stimulus that also stimulates prolactin release, was proposed many years ago to be a prolactin-releasing factor. It is now clear that terminals of oxytocinergic neurons end in juxtaposition to portal vessels, that there is a high concentration of oxytocin in portal blood, and that oxytocin can stimulate the secretion of prolactin by pituitary tissue *in vitro*. Furthermore, antisera directed against oxytocin can partially inhibit the suckling-induced prolactin release. Thus it appears that oxytocin is indeed a physiologically significant prolactin-releasing factor (Samson et al., 1986). Similar evidence suggests that vasoactive intestinal polypeptide and the related peptide, peptide histidine isoleucine (PHI), may also be physiologically significant prolactin-releasing factors. Several other peptides such as angiotensin II, substance P, and neurotensin also stimulate prolactin release. Thyrotropin-releasing hormone (TRH), the first hypothalamic hormone to be synthesized, stimulates not only TSH but also prolactin release (McCann et al., 1984).

Much earlier, it was shown that dopamine could inhibit the secretion of prolactin (see MacLeod, 1976). Dopamine is found in high concentration in portal vessels, and is presumably released from terminals of the tuberoinfundibular dopaminergic tract, which ends in juxtaposition to the hypophyseal portal capillaries. Receptors for the catecholamine are found in the pituitary. Blockers of dopamine action can reverse the inhibition of prolactin release normally exercised by the hypothalamus, and it is estimated that the concentration of dopamine in portal blood may be sufficient to hold prolactin secretion in check, except when stimulated by stress or by the suckling stimulus. The elevation in prolactin that occurs under these conditions is probably related not only to withdrawal of dopaminergic inhibition but also to secretion of the various prolactin-releasing factors just described (see Neill, 1980b). A peptide PIF may also exist. In fact, the gonadotropin-releasing hormone-associated peptide (GAP), the carboxy-terminal 56-amino acid peptide of the prepro-LHRH molecule, has PIF activity both *in vitro* and *in vivo* (Nikolics and Seeburg, 1986; Yu et al., 1988). It is secreted into the portal vessels together with LHRH and may be of physiologic significance in the control of prolactin release.

G. Hypothalamic Factors Controlling Melanophore-Stimulating Hormone (MSH) Secretion

Structures of both the postulated MSH-releasing and MSH-inhibiting factors have been proposed. However, the physiologic significance of these factors is not clear and it appears that the major hypothalamic inhibitory control over MSH secretion is exercised by dopaminergic nerves in the intermediate lobe (see McCann, 1988).

III. Analogs of Releasing Hormones

With the elucidation of the structures of these releasing and inhibiting hormones, it has been possible to prepare many analogs of each of the factors. In the case of LHRH, the initial aim was to obtain inhibitory analogs that might suppress fertility. However, it was accidentally found that analogs more active than the natural compound could easily be prepared if unnatural amino acids were substituted at positions likely to be subject to proteolysis. The agonist analogs have already proven to be important clinically since the so-called super-LHRH analogs are capable of inducing ovulation in infertile women and high doses suppress gonadal steroid release. High-dose agonist analog therapy is in use to reverse precocious puberty and to suppress metastatic prostatic cancer (see McCann, 1982).

A. Multiple Actions of Releasing and Inhibiting Hormones

We have already alluded to the fact that TRH stimulates not only TSH but also prolactin release. Whether the latter action has physiologic significance remains uncertain. Similarly, LHRH has FSH-releasing activity, which has led some to abandom the name LHRH and to substitute the name gonadotropin-releasing hormone (GnRH), which is now most commonly used. Somatostatin inhibits not only growth hormone secretion but also that of most other pituitary hormones if given in sufficient dosage. It also suppresses the functions of many other systems, probably because it is distributed widely throughout the body (see below). Injected somatostatin has such an evanescent action in suppressing growth hormone release because of enzymatic degradation that it has never been shown to suppress growth. Thus, the name somatostatin is a misnomer. Recently more stable agonist analogs of the compound have been reported to suppress growth. Since the inhibitory actions of the peptide are so pervasive, it might be appropriate to change the name from somatostatin to panhibin (McCann, 1982).

B. Distribution of the Mammalian Peptides in Lower Forms

The initial clue that these hypothalamic peptides might be found in lower forms came from work on CRH, since the amphibian skin peptide sauvagine has CRH activity when tested on the pituitaries of rats. Similarly, urophysin I, a peptide obtained from the urophysis, a neurohypophysis-like organ in the caudal spinal cord of fish, has CRH activity (Vale et al., 1983). Subsequently it was shown that yeast mating factor had structural homology with the mammalian LHRH, which also induces mating in rats, and that it would even release LH from rat pituitaries, albeit with one ten-thousandth the potency of the mammalian hormone (Loumaye et al., 1982). It has previously been demonstrated that LHRH would induce mating behavior in higher forms, including mammals (Moss and McCann, 1973). Although all the evidence is not yet in, it appears that these peptides exist throughout the phylogenetic scale down to unicellular organisms. They probably have similar functions in unicellular organisms as in higher organisms. As differentiation increases as we progress up the phylogenetic scale, their localization is restricted to certain areas but their basic functions do not change. Thus, LHRH is a reproductive peptide, whereas CRH and vasopressin are stress peptides.

IV. Mechanism of Action of Releasing and Inhibiting Hormones

Peptide hormones act by combining with highly specific receptors on the cell membrane of target cells. The peptide-receptor interaction then activates one or more of the several possible pathways for induction of secretion. One pathway involves activation of adenylate cyclase with the generation of cyclic AMP. The cyclic AMP formed activates a protein kinase that may mediate most of the effects of the cyclic nucleotide on cellular function. In the case of the pituitary, it has been suggested that activation of a protein kinase by cyclic AMP results in phosphorylation of certain membrane constituents that promote exocytosis, the mechanism for secretion. The secretory granules migrate to the cell surface, fuse with the cell membrane, and the granular core containing the hormone is extruded into the extracellular space, particularly at the vascular pole of the cell. Of the various pituitary cells, it would appear that the somatotrophs utilize the cyclic AMP pathway, based on the ability of cyclic AMP to activate secretion and on its augmentation by inhibition of the breakdown of cyclic AMP by phosphodiesterase inhibitors. Similarly, the stimulatory effect of CRH on ACTH release appears to be mediated by cyclic AMP. In the gonadotrophs, the cyclic AMP system seems to play a minor role, possibly only in enhancing synthesis of LH.

Calcium plays an important part in the releasing process. Extracellular calcium is required for release of all pituitary hormones. It may also be mobilized from intracellular stores in the case of some of the hormones. For those releasing factors that operate via the cyclic AMP mechanism, a cyclic AMP-dependent protein kinase may be involved in opening calcium channels, allowing entrance of the ion, and possibly also may mobilize it from intracellular stores.

The products of arachidonic acid metabolism are active in inducing exocytosis and their relative importance varies with the pituitary cell type, just as the relative importance of cyclic AMP seems to vary with the cell type. Prostaglandins appear to be important in the release of growth hormone and ACTH, and they can activate the production of cyclic AMP. In other cells such as the gonadotrophs it appears that the leukotrienes or the epoxides play this role.

Arachidonic acid release from the cell membrane may result from a receptor-mediated activation of phospholipase C, a membrane-bound enzyme that catalyzes the hydrolysis of polyphosphoinositides into inositol triphosphate and diacylglycerol. The latter not only contains arachidonate, which is then made available to phospholipase A_2 for subsequent metabolism, but also interacts with protein kinase C, a calcium-dependent, phospholipid-activated enzyme. Protein kinase C phosphorylates several proteins that then participate in the process of hormone release. Inositol triphosphate, the other product of phospholipase C activity, mobilizes intracellular calcium from the endoplasmic reticulum.

The releasing process is far from being completely understood, but each cell type utilizes these various pathways to varying degrees. The role of guanylate cyclase and its product, cyclic GMP, is not yet clear.

The inhibiting hormones such as somatostatin act in part by inhibition of adenylate cyclase and in part also by other mechanisms, such as decreasing the availability of calcium to the cell.

If the cell membrane is depolarized by placing pituitary tissue in a high-potassium medium, release is also induced. It is not known, as yet, whether depolarization of the cell membrane actually accompanies the releasing process of normally secreting pituitary cells, but when it is artificially induced by a high potassium concentration, it probably increases calcium uptake by the cells, which then mediates the releasing process.

The means by which the secretory granules migrate to the cell surface remain an enigma. It has been postulated that this might involve microtubules or microfilaments; however, colchicine, which disrupts microtubules, not only fails to block the release of several pituitary hormones but actually augments it, suggesting the possibility that the tubules might hold the granules in the interior of the cell, and that after dissolution of the tubules the granules then migrate spontaneously to the surface, possibly because of electrostatic forces between the granule and the inside of the cell membrane.

The releasing hormones act on the cell very rapidly (within less than a minute) to either promote or inhibit release of particular pituitary hormones; however, their precise effect on the biosynthesis of these hormones has not been elucidated. With sufficient stimulation of release, synthesis is promoted, and recent evidence suggests that there is an increase in the mRNA required for the synthesis of the pituitary hormone in question. Whether this is secondary to the release process or represents another primary action of the releasing hormone on the biosynthetic process itself remains to be determined.

Specificity of action of each releasing hormone is furnished by the presence of highly specific receptors on a target cell and configurations in the releasing hormone tertiary structure that allow combination with the receptor. Presumably, wherever there is an action on a pituitary cell by a peptide there is a receptor on the surface of that cell to mediate the effect (Conn, 1989).

Isolation of cDNAs encoding most of the hypothalamic hormones as well as partial characterization of their specific genes have been accomplished in the last few years (for references see McCann, 1982; Fink, 1979; Reichlin, 1985; Conn, 1989). The structure of the mRNAs encoding CRH, somatostatin, GHRH, LHRH, and finally even TRH has been elucidated. Since TRH is a small tripeptide, it was originally thought to be synthesized by enzymatic means; however, it is also synthesized as part of a preprohormone containing many sequences of TRH throughout the molecule. It is now possible to biosynthesize these various peptides in *Escherichia coli* using expression vectors (for references see Fink et al., 1986; Reichlin, 1985).

V. Factors Affecting Responsiveness of the Adenohypophysis to Releasing and Inhibiting Hormones

The hormonal state is very important in determining the responsiveness of the adenohypophysis to the various releasing hormones. In the case of TRH, pituitary responsiveness is enhanced by removal of the thyroid and consequent loss of negative feedback by thyroxine and triiodothyronine. Conversely, responsiveness is suppressed by the administration of thyroid hormones. In fact, the negative feedback of thyroid hormone seems to take place predominantly in the pituitary gland to modulate its responsiveness to TRH (Reichlin, 1985).

It is also possible that TRH release is under inhibitory control via circulating thyroid hormones, but the evidence for this is less compelling. The mechanism by which thyroid hormones (T_3 and T_4) suppress pituitary responsiveness to TRH may involve the uptake of the thyroid hormone by receptors in the thyrotroph. Under the influence of thyroid hormone, pituitary cell mRNA synthesis is modified, stimulating synthesis of an inhibitory peptide or protein that in turn reduces the response of the cell to TRH. The evidence for this sequence is that inhibitors of DNA-directed RNA synthesis, such as actinomycin, and inhibitors of protein synthesis, such as cycloheximide, can prevent the establishment of the thyroid hormone blockade and can even reverse it after a period of time. The "lag period" is presumably the time required for the inhibitory peptide or protein to be catabolized.

In the case of CRH, there is also good evidence that adrenal steroids feed back directly at the pituitary to inhibit the response to CRH; however, this feedback also takes place at the hypothalamic level to inhibit release of CRH and vasopressin (Fink et al., 1988).

The interplay between gonadal steroids and the hypothalamic-pituitary axis is particularly complex. Following removal of the gonads and the elimination of feedback by the gonadal steroids, predominantly estrogen in the female and testosterone in the male, levels of both FSH and LH are elevated. The release of these pituitary hormones is pulsatile and occurs rhythmically. The timing of the discharge varies among species and even among individual animals within a species. In the castrate human these pulses occur hourly and are called the circhoral rhythm of LH release. This rhythm is brought about by pulsatile release of LHRH and possibly of FSH-releasing factor as well (if such a discrete factor actually exists). Following removal of negative feedback, the enhanced LHRH release increases not only the discharge of gonadotropins but also their synthesis, so that the quantities stored in the gland increase. This augmented storage is associated with an increase in responsiveness to the neurohormone. Small doses of estrogen or androgen can suppress the responsiveness to LHRH, and this occurs quickly. At least in the case of estrogen administration, it can take place within 1 hr. With long-term therapy, there is suppression not only of release of LH, but also of its synthesis, and pituitary content of gonadotropin consequently falls. This is associated with a further decline in responsiveness to LHRH, which may in part be caused by down regulation of LHRH receptors (McCann, 1982; Knobil, 1980; Yen, 1977).

In the female there are complex endocrine relationships during the menstrual cycle. Responsiveness to LHRH during the early follicular phase is minimal. Responsiveness increases as the follicular phase progresses and reaches its height at the time of the preovulatory discharge of LH. Treatment of women with estrogen has a biphasic effect on pituitary responsiveness to LHRH; the initial suppression is followed by an augmented responsiveness. Thus, estrogen secreted by the preovulatory follicles is probably responsible for the enhanced responsiveness to LHRH that occurs in the late follicular phase.

In addition, the characteristics of the preovulatory discharge of LH in response to LHRH change, the response becoming much more rapid and pulselike. This further change in responsiveness probably emanates from LHRH itself, since it can be induced by a priming injection of LHRH in the late follicular phase of the cycle. Responsiveness then declines after the ovulatory discharge (McCann, 1982; Yen, 1977).

The mechanism by which estrogen augments responsiveness to LHRH is not known. It might induce the formation of additional receptors for the neurohormone, or, alternatively, it might alter the synthesis of LH and provide a larger pool of releasable LH. Similarly, the mechanism for the self-priming action (positive feedback) of LHRH remains to be elucidated, but this could be explained by an effect on synthesis of a releasable pool of LH or, alternatively, by an effect of LHRH to induce new LHRH receptors. The ability to LHRH to upregulate its own receptors has been demonstrated (see McCann, 1982).

This remarkable increase in responsiveness to LHRH as a function of the steroid milieu undoubtedly accounts in part for the preovulatory discharge of LH, but it is believed that an enhanced release of LHRH is also involved (McCann, 1982; Fink, 1979; Neill, 1980a). This is induced once again by estrogen from the preovulatory follicle. This increased release of LHRH is probably responsible for bringing on the self-priming action of LHRH that characterizes the late preovulatory phase. Evidence for the increased release of LHRH at the preovulatory surge of LH includes the detection of increased titers of the hormone in peripheral blood in animals and humans and the observation of very high titers of LHRH in portal blood collected from the transected pituitary stalk at this stage of the cycle in animals.

It would appear, then, that the preovulatory discharge of LH is brought about by enhanced release of LHRH coupled with a marked increase in responsiveness to the neurohormone. The result is a discharge of LH far greater than that necessary to induce ovulation. Perhaps this is part of a failsafe mechanism to ensure full ovulation even when follicular development is not optimal; it might serve to prolong the reproductive life of the individual.

VI. Localization of Releasing and Inhibiting Hormones within the Brain

In order to understand the mechanisms controlling the release of the releasing factors, it is critical to know which CNS cell types synthesize and release these factors and also to know the anatomical distribution of these neurons within the brain.

The techniques of immunohistochemistry have permitted investigators to identify the neurons producing the specific releasing factors with some storage in nerve terminals in the median eminence region and pituitary stalk. Smaller amounts may actually be found in the neural lobe itself. It appears that the factors are stored in granules in axon terminals, the cell bodies of which are located at some distance from these terminals.

In the case of CRH, the hormone is located mostly in small neurons within the paraventricular nucleus, where it is frequently colocalized with other peptides, including particularly vasopressin, which as indicated above also controls ACTH release. Some CRH neurons are also located in the supraoptic nucleus, which is the major site for vasopressin neurons. These vasopressin neurons are usually of the magnocellular type and most of them project to the neural lobe, in contrast to the CRH neurons; however, the vasopressin neurons in the paraventricular nucleus project to the external layer of the median eminence, so that their vasopressin is released into the portal vessels. These neurons are probably the most important in vasopressinergic control of ACTH release; however, it is possible that vasopressin released from terminals in the neural lobe may enter the short portal vessels and also be transported to the anterior pituitary to release ACTH (Palkovits, 1988).

In the case of LHRH, the activity is found in the very regions that when stimulated release LH and when destroyed lead to deficiencies in its secretion in animals. In the human there are two populations of LHRH neurons. The first of these has cell bodies located in the medial preoptic area, immediately overlying the optic chiasm, and axons that project caudally to terminate in the median eminence. The second population of LHRH neurons has cell bodies located in the vicinity of the infundibular nucleus and relatively short axons that project to the median eminence. The axon terminals in the median eminence end in juxtaposition to hypophysial portal capillaries (Palkovits, 1988).

In the case of TRH, the perikarya are also found in the preoptic region, but another aggregation of cell bodies is found in the paraventricular nucleus. Axons project caudally from these regions and then project ventrally into the median eminence, where the bulk of the activity is stored. TRH has been found outside the hypothalamus as well and even in the spinal cord, which has raised the possibility that it may be involved in other CNS functions (Palkovits, 1988).

By immunocytochemistry, GHRH is the most restricted of the releasing factors; it is found predominantly in the arcuate nucleus and around the periphery of the ventromedial nucleus. On the other hand, somatostatin is present primarily in the paraventricular nucleus with projections to the median eminence. Extrahypothalamic projections are widespread, including the cerebral cortex. These localizations of the releasing hormones are consistent with the earlier findings from electrical stimulation and lesion studies and give the best evidence for the precise regions of the hypothalamus that are involved in controlling secretion of particular pituitary hormones (Palkovits, 1988).

VII. Putative Synaptic Transmitters Involved in Controlling the Release of Releasing Hormones

The neurons that produce releasing factors are in synaptic contact with a host of putative neurotransmitters. The hypothalamus is richly supplied with monoaminergic nerve fibers. There is a heavy input of noradrenergic fibers from neurons whose cell bodies lie in the brainstem. The distribution of these neurons has been mapped by fluorescent histochemistry. There are also terminals from epinephrine-containing neurons that end in the hypothalamus. These also appear to originate from neurons whose cell bodies are located in the brainstem.

Axons of serotonin-containing neurons whose cell bodies lie in the medial raphe nuclei project to the suprachiasmatic, anterior hypothalamic, and median eminence regions. Assays for choline acetyltransferase indicate the widespread distribution of cholinergic fibers within the hypothalamus as well. There is also an abundance of histamine that appears to be located in synaptosome-like structures, and this amine is concentrated particularly in the median eminence region, where it may also serve as a synaptic transmitter. There is evidence as well for a γ-aminobutyric acid-containing or GABAergic system that is localized partially in the infundibular nucleus with projections to the median eminence. High concentrations of GABA have been found in portal blood and GABA has a direct inhibitory action on the secretion of prolactin, raising the possibility that it may be a prolactin-inhibiting factor. Other GABAergic neurons are small interneurons localized throughout the hypothalamus, where they may well impinge on dendrites or somata of releasing hormone neurons (see McCann and Krulich, 1989).

A great deal of effort has been put into experiments in rodents and monkeys to determine the role of these possible transmitters in controlling the release of the various releasing hormones. The most extensive studies have been done on gonadotropins. It appears that there are excitatory noradrenergic synapses that may mediate not only the preovulatory release of LHRH but also the increased LHRH release that follows castration. In the case of the preovulatory release of LHRH, the synapses may be in the preoptic-anterior hypothalamic region, whereas in the case of the increased release in the castrate, the synapses may be on the other population of LHRH neurons, located in the arcuate nucleus (McCann and Krulich, 1989).

Dopamine has been postulated to both stimulate and inhibit LHRH release. The evidence is confusing, but the view held at the present time is that this catecholamine may have only a minor role (McCann and Krulich, 1989).

Serotonin, when injected into the third ventricle in castrates, can inhibit LH release; this indicates that it is an inhibitory transmitter, but other evidence suggests that it may facilitate preovulatory LH release. Histamine can stimulate LH release following its intraventricular injection in large doses. It is still not clear if this has physiologic significance (McCann and Krulich, 1989).

There is considerable evidence for a cholinergic link in gonadotropin release, since atropine can block gonadotropin release when it is administered systemically, microinjected into the third ventricle, or implanted within the hypothalamus (McCann and Krulich, 1989).

In the case of ACTH, there is considerable evidence to suggest noradrenergic control over the release of this hormone, and there is some evidence for cholinergic and serotoninergic stimulatory components as well. TRH has not been investigated extensively but may be under adrenergic control. Growth hormone release also appears to be under adrenergic control, with a simulatory α receptor and an inhibitory β receptor component, but the relative importance of dopamine and norepinephrine has yet to be clearly established (McCann and Krulich, 1989).

Prolactin is definitely under inhibitory control via dopamine. There is a tuberoinfundibular dopaminergic tract, the neurons of which have cell bodies lying in the arcuate nucleus and axons projecting to the external layer of the median eminence. Here they terminate in juxtaposition to hypophyseal portal capillaries. Dopamine agonists, such as bromocriptine, can lower plasma prolactin in hyperprolactinemic patients (McCann and Krulich, 1989).

In addition to these classical low-molecular-weight transmitters, the hypothalamus is a repository for a veritable host of neuropeptides. Not only are there the releasing and inhibiting factors just discussed, and vasopressin and oxytocin, but brain opioid peptide systems are also present. Within the hypothalamus, infundibular neurons produce proopiomelanocortin. Their axons project to other parts of the hypothalamus and other brain regions and apparently establish synaptic contacts with other cells, secreting β-endorphin, ACTH, and possibly α-MSH into the synaptic cleft. Studies using opiate receptor blockers, such as naloxone, have shown that the opioid peptides are involved in stress-induced prolactin release. The peptide involved appears to be β-endorphin, based on studies with specific antibodies against β-endorphin that block stress-induced prolactin release. β-Endorphin also appears to have a physiologically significant inhibitory role in the control of gonadotropin secretion (McCann et al., 1986).

Enkephalin and dynorphin neurons and even other classes of opioid peptides are also localized in neurons within the hypothalamus. The functional significance of these other opioid peptides remains to be clarified.

In addition to these brain peptides, many peptides that were originally thought to be localized exclusively in other organs have now been found in the brain. Among these are angiotensin II, which was first thought to be formed only in the circulation after release of renin from the juxtaglomerular apparatus of the kidney. There are angiotensin II-producing neurons within the hypothalamus and they may play a stimulatory role in controlling ACTH and prolactin secretion. The recently discovered atrial natriuretic peptide, whose main locus is the atria of the heart, has now been found within neurons in the hypothalamus and may suppress ACTH as well as vasopressin secretion (Samson, 1988).

Many gastrointestinal peptides originally thought to be localized only in the gut have been found in brain neuronal systems. An example is vasoactive intestinal polypeptide, which appears to have important roles in controlling pituitary hormone secretion by both hypothalamic and pituitary actions. As indicated above, it may be a physiologically significant prolactin-releasing factor. Cholecystokinin is also present in the brain and appears to have significance in the control of pituitary hormone secretion, as do neurotensin and substance P. Antagonists against these various peptides and antisera directed against them are being used to determine their physiological significance (McCann et al., 1986).

VIII. Short-Loop Feedback of Pituitary Hormones to Alter Their Own Release

A variety of pituitary hormones exert short-loop negative feedback actions to suppress their own release. In this case the hormone inhibits its own release without circulating through the general circulation. This is in contrast to so-called long-loop feedback of pituitary target gland hormones such as gonadal steroids (Piva et al., 1979). It was originally thought that this action might be mediated in the hypothalamus by reverse flow in portal vessels, which would deliver the pituitary hormones to the hypothalamus. There is some evidence for reverse flow under certain circumstanes, but it appears that most of the pituitary hormones may actually be produced in the brain. In the case of ACTH, it is now known that the proopiomelanocortin molecule is synthesized in neurons in the infundibular nucleus. Adrenocorticotropic hormone, a fragment of this molecule, may be secreted from cells producing proopiomelanocortin. There is also evidence that prolactin-secreting and LH-secreting neurons exist within the brain. Short-loop negative feedback has been clearly established for prolactin and growth hormone (McCann et al., 1988a). In the later case, it may be mediated not only by growth hormone itself but also by somatomedin C (insulin-like growth factor, IGF-I), either delivered via the peripheral circulation or possibly made directly in the brain. There is also considerable evidence of short-loop feedback for LH and FSH as well as ACTH (Piva et al., 1979; McCann et al., 1988). Little work has been done on TSH, but in all probability the same mechanism applies to this hormone (McCann et al., 1988a).

IX. Ultrashort-Loop Feedback of Releasing and Inhibiting Hormones to Modify Their Own Release

Ultrashort-loop feedback is an alteration in the release of a hypothalamic peptide induced by the peptide itself acting within the brain (Piva et al., 1979). It may occur as direct recurrent inhibition or via interaction with an interneuron, which in turn alters the discharge rate of the peptidergic neuron.

There is evidence from animal experiments for ultrashort-loop negative feedback of the releasing hormone neurons to inhibit their own release in the case of somatostatin, GHRH, and LHRH (McCann et al., 1986).

X. Extrapituitary Actions of Releasing Factors

The distribution of releasing factors in brain regions outside the hypothalamus (e.g., brainstem, cortex) has stimulated a search for their extrapituitary actions. As indicated earlier, TRH is found in other brain regions and even in the spinal cord; somatostatin is distributed widely throughout the nervous system and also has been found in the delta cells of the pancreatic islets of Langerhans. Since somatostatin can inhibit the release of both insulin and glucagon, it probably acts locally to control the release of these hormones from the islets.

The clearest behavioral effect of releasing factors is the induction of mating behavior by relatively low doses of LHRH in animals. The occurrence of LHRH in the preoptic area, the region of the brain that is known to be involved in mating behavior, plus the onset of this behavior shortly after the preovulatory discharge of LHRH, suggested this effect of LHRH. Indeed, LHRH induces mating behavior in many species, including primates and possibly humans. This is not caused by the gonadotropins released, since these hormones have no effect on mating behavior and since induction of the behavior is seen in the hypophysectomized rat. Further studies have shown that the effect can be obtained by microinjecting LHRH into the preoptic-anterior hypothalamic and arcuate-median eminence regions, whereas similar injections into lateral hypothalamus or cortex are ineffective. There is a latency between the injection of LHRH either into the brain or systemically and the onset of mating behavior, suggesting that some intervening steps may be involved (Moss et al., 1989).

Thyrotropin-releasing hormone has effects that indicate an arousal action of the hormone, that is, it shortens the duration of pentobarbital anesthesia. The doses required are very large; however, if the hormone is present at synaptic sites in the brain, it is conceivable that these responses to high doses could be physiological. Somatostatin, on the other hand, has been shown to depress animals. Thus the concept is emerging that the releasing factors may have important extrapituitary actions. One could even envision the possibility that they may serve as peptidic neurotransmitters and that this might be a more important role than that of governing the release of anterior pituitary hormones. There is evidence that releasing factor action in the CNS may integrate complex hormonal and neural mechanisms, for example, blood pressure and fluid control (vasopressin), stress responses (vasopressin, CRH), or reproductive processes (LHRH) (Moss et al., 1989).

Acknowledgments

This work was supported by NIH Grants HD09988 and DK10073. We wish to thank Ms. Judy Scott for typing the manuscript.

References

Bailey, P. and Bremer, F., Experimental diabetes insipidus, *Arch. Intern. Med.*, 28, 773, 1921.

Boler, J., Enzmann, F., Folkers, K., Bowers, C. Y., and Schally, A. V., The identity of chemical and hormonal properties of thyrotropin releasing hormone and pyroglutamyl-histidyl-proline amide, *Biochem. Biophys. Res. Commun.*, 37, 705, 1969.

Brazeau, P., Vale, W., Burgus, R., Ling, N., Butcher, M., Rivier, J., and Guillemin, R., Hypothalamic polypeptide that inhibits the secretion of immunoreactive pituitary growth hormone, *Science*, 179, 77, 1973.

Burgus, R., Dunn, T. F., Desiderio, D., and Guillemin, R., Structure moleculaire de facteur hypothalamique hypophysiotrope TRF d'origine ovine: mise en evidence par spectrometrie de masse de la sequence PCA-His-Pro-NH_2, *C.R. Acad. Sci. (Paris)*, 269, 1870, 1969.

Carraway, R. and Leeman, S. E., The isolation of a new hypotensive peptide, neurotensin, from bovine hypothalami, *J. Biochem.*, 248, 6854, 1973.

Chang, M. C. and Leeman, S. E., Isolation of a sialogogic peptide from bovine hypothalamic tissue and its characterization as substance P, *J. Biol. Chem.*, 245, 4784, 1970.

Conn, P. M., GnRH regulation of gonadotropin release and target cell responsiveness, in *Endocrinology*, Vol. 1, 2nd ed., DeGroot, L. J., et al., Eds., W. B. Saunders, Philadelphia, 1989, 284.

Fink, G., Feedback actions of target hormones on hypothalamus and pituitary with special reference to gonadal steroids, *Annu. Rev. Physiol.*, 41, 571, 1979.

Fink, G., Harmar, A. J., and McKerns, K. W., Eds., *Neuroendocrine Molecular Biology*, Plenum Press, New York, 1986.

Fink, G., Robinson, I. C. A. F., and Tannahill, L. A., Effects of adrenalectomy and glucocorticoids on the peptides CRF-41, AVP and oxytocin in rat hypophyseal portal blood, *J. Physiol. (London)*, 401, 329, 1988.

Frohlich, A., Ein Fall von Tumor der Hypophysis cerebri ohne Akromegalie, *Wien. Klin. Rundsch.*, 15, 883, 1901.

Gillies, G. E., Linton, E. A., and Lowry, P. J., Vasopressin and the corticoliberin complex, in *Neuroendocrinology of Vasopressin, Corticoliberin and Opiomelanocortins*, Baertschi, A. J. and Dreifuss, J. J., Eds., Academic Press, New York, 1982, 239.

Guillemin, R., Brazeau, P., Bohlen, P., Esch, F., Ling, N., and Wehrenberg, W. B., Growth hormone-releasing factor from a human pancreatic tumor that caused acromegaly, *Science*, 218, 585, 1982.

Harris, G. W., The pituitary stalk and ovulation, in *Control of Ovulation*, Vilee, C. A., Ed., Pergamon Press, Elmsford, NY, 1961, 56.

Hohlweg, W., The regulatory centers of endocrine glands in the hypothalamus, in *Pioneers in Neuroendocrinology*, Vol. 1, Meites, J., Donovan, B. T., and McCann, S. M., Eds., Plenum Press, New York, 1975, 160.

Knobil, E., Neuroendocrine control of the menstrual cycle, *Recent Prog. Horm. Res.*, 36, 53, 1980.

Krulich, L., Dhariwal, A. P. S., and McCann, S. M., Stimulatory and inhibitory effects of purified hypothalamic extracts on growth hormone release from rat pituitary *in vitro*, *Endocrinology*, 83, 783, 1968.

Krulich, L., Illner, P., Fawcett, C. P., Quijada, M., and McCann, S. M., Dual hypothalamic regulation of growth hormone secretion, in *Growth and Growth Hormone*, Pecile, A. and Muller, E., Eds., Elsevier, Amsterdam, 1972, 306.

Loumaye, E., Thorner, J., and Catt, K. J., Yeast mating pheromone activates mammalian gonadotrophs: evolutionary conservation of a reproductive hormone, *Science*, 218, 1323, 1982.

Lumpkin, M. D., Moltz, J. H., Yu, W., Samson, W. K., and McCann, S. M., Purification of FSH-releasing factor: its dissimilarity from LHRH of mammalian, avian, and piscian origin, *Brain Res. Bull.*, 18, 175, 1987.

MacLeod, R. M., Regulation of prolactin secretion, in Frontiers in *Neuroendocrinology*, Vol. 4, Martini, L. and Ganong, W. F., Eds., Raven Press, New York, 1976, 169.

Martini, L., *The Pituitary Gland*, Vol. 3, Harris, G. W. and Donovan, B., Eds., Butterworths, London, 1966, 535.

Matsuo, H., Baba, Y., Nair, R. M. G., Arimura, A., and Schally, A. V., Structure of the porcine-LH-releasing hormone. 1. The proposed amino acid sequence, *Biochem. Biophys. Res. Commun.*, 43, 1334, 1971.

McCann, S. M., Regulation of secretion of follicle-stimulating hormone and luteinizing hormone, in *Handbook of Physiology*, Vol. 4, Sect. 7, pt. 2, Greep, R. O. and Astwood, E. B., Eds., American Physiological Society, Washington, D. C., 1974, 489.

McCann, S. M., Physiology and pharmacology of LHRH and somatostatin, *Annu. Rev. Pharmacol. Toxicol.*, 22, 491, 1982.

McCann, S. M., Saga of the discovery of hypothalamic releasing and inhibiting hormones, in *Endocrinology: People and Ideas*, McCann, S. M., Eds., American Physiological Society, Baltimore, MA, 1988, 41.

McCann, S. M. and Krulich, L., Role of transmitters in control of anterior pituitary hormone release, in *Endocrinology*, Vol. 1, 2nd ed., DeGroot, L. J., et al., Eds., W. B. Saunders, Philadelphia, 1989, 117.

McCann, S. M., Antunes-Rodrigues, J., Nallar, R., and Valtin, H., Pituitary-adrenal function in the absence of vasopressin, *Endocrinology*, 79, 1058, 1966.

McCann, S. M., Lumpkin, M. D., and Samson, W. K., The role of vasopressin and oxytocin in control of anterior pituitary hormone secretion, in *Neuroendocrinology of Vasopressin, Corticoliberin and Opiomelanocortins*, Baertsche, A. J. and Dreifuss, J. J., Eds., Academic Press, London, 1982, 319.

McCann, S. M., Mizunuma, H., Samson, W. K., and Lumpkin, M. D., Differential hypothalamic control of FSH secretion: a review, *Psychoneuroendocrinology*, 8, 299, 1983.

McCann, S. M., Lumpkin, M. D., Mizunuma, H., Khorram, O., Ottlecz, A., and Samson, W. K., Peptidergic and dopaminergic control of prolactin release, *Trends Neurosci.*, 7, 127, 1984.

McCann, S. M., Samson, W. K., Aguila, M. C., Bedran de Castro, J. C., Ono, N., Lumpkin, M. D., and Khorram, O., The role of brain peptides in the control of anterior pituitary hormone secretion, in *Neuroendocrine Molecular Biology*, Fink, G., Harmar, A. J., and McKerns, K. W., Eds., Plenum Press, New York, 1986, 101.

McCann, S. M., Pan, G., Xu, R.-K. J., Martinovic, J., and Rettori, V., Modulatory hypothalamic action of ACTH on ACTH and prolactin release, in *Prolactin Gene Family and Its Receptors,* Series 819, Hushino, H., Ed., Medica International Congress Series, Amsterdam, 1988a, 211.

McCann, S. M., Samson, W. K., Ono, N., Bedran de Castro, J. C., and Petrovic, S. L., The role of peptides released during stress on gonadotropin secretion, in *Stress and Biorhythms in the Physiopathology of Reproduction,* Pancheri, A. and Zichella, L., Eds., Hemisphere Publishing Corporation, Washington, D.C., 1988b.

Moss, R. L. and McCann, S. M., Induction of mating behavior in rats by luteinizing hormone releasing factor, *Science,* 181, 177, 1973.

Moss, R. L., Dudley, C. A., and Gosnell, B. A., Behavior and the hypothalamus, in *Endocrinology,* Vol. 1, 2nd ed., DeGroot, L. J., et al., Eds., W. B. Saunders, Philadelphia, 1989, 254.

Neill, J. D., LHRH and dopamine secretion in the hypophyseal stalk blood: effects of estrogen, mating and nursing, *Front. Horm. Res.,* 6, 192, 1980a.

Neill, J. D., Neuroendocrine regulation of prolactin secretion, in *Frontiers in Neuroendocrinology,* Vol. 6, Martini, L. and Ganong, W. F., Eds., Raven Press, New York, 1980b, 129.

Nikolics, K. and Seeburg, P. H., The biosynthetic precursor of gonadotropin-releasing hormone: a multifunctional prohormone, in *Neuroendocrine Molecular Biology,* Fink, G., Harmar, A. J., and McKerns, K. W., Eds., Plenum Press, New York, 1986, 57.

Ono, N., Bedran de Castro, J. C., Khorram, O., and McCann, S. M., Role of arginine vasopressin in control of ACTH and LH release during stress, *Life Sci.,* 36, 1779, 1985a.

Ono, N., Samson, W. K., McDonald, J. K., Lumpkin, M. D., Bedran de Castro, J. C., and McCann, S. M., The effects of intravenous and intraventricular injection of antisera directed against corticotropin releasing factor (CRF) on the secretion of anterior pituitary hormones, *Proc. Natl. Acad. Sci. U.S.A.,* 82, 7787, 1985b.

Palkovits, M., in *Frontiers in Neuroendocrinology,* Vol. 10, Martini, L. and Ganong, W. L., Eds., Raven Press, New York, 1988, 1.

Petrovic, S. L., McDonald, J. K., Bedran de Castro, J. C., Snyder, G. D., and McCann, S. M., Regulation of anterior pituitary and brain beta-adrenergic receptors by ovarian steroids, *Life Sci.,* 37, 1563, 1985.

Piva, F., Motta, M., and Martini, L., Short-loop feedback of pituitary hormones to influence their own release, in *Endocrinology,* Vol. 1, DeGroot, L. J., et al., Eds., Grune & Stratton, New York, 1979, 29.

Price, D., Feedback control of gonadal and hypophyseal hormones: evolution of the concept, in *Pioneers in Neuroendocrinology,* Meites, J., Donovan, B. T., and McCann, S. M., Eds., Plenum Press, New York, 1975, 218.

Reichlin, S., Neuroendocrinology, in *Textbook of Endocrinology,* 7th ed., Wilson, J. D. and Foster, D. W., Eds., W. B. Saunders, Philadelphia, 1985, 492.

Rivier, C. and Vale, W., Role of corticotropin releasing factor, neurohypophyseal peptides and catecholamines in pituitary function, *Fed. Proc.,* 44, 189, 1985.

Rivier, J., Spiess, J., Thorner, M., and Vale, W., Characterization of a growth hormone-releasing factor from a human pancreatic islet tumor, *Nature (London),* 300, 276, 1982.

Samson, W. K., Hypothalamic actions of the atrial factors to alter hormone secretion from both the anterior and posterior pituitary, in *Biological and Molecular Aspects of Atrial Factors,* Needleman, P., Ed., Alan R. Liss, New York, 1988, 217.

Samson, W. K., Lumpkin, M. D., and McCann, S. M., Evidence of a physiological role for oxytocin in the control of prolactin secretion, *Endocrinology,* 119, 554, 1986.

Sawyer, C. H., Anterior pituitary neural control concepts, in *Endocrinology: People and Ideas,* McCann, S. M., Ed., American Physiological Society, Baltimore, MA, 1988, 23.

Schally, A. V., Arimura, A., Kastin, A. J., Matsuo, H., Baba, Y., Redding, P. W., Nair, R. M., and Debeljuk, L., Gonadotropin-releasing hormone: one polypeptide regulates secretion of luteinizing and follicle-stimulating hormones, *Science,* 173, 1036, 1971.

Vale, W. W., Spiess, J., Rivier, C., and Rivier, J., Characterization of a 41-residue ovine hypothalamic peptide that stimulates secretion of corticotropin and β-endorphin, *Science,* 213, 1394, 1981.

Vale, W. W., Rivier, C., Spiess, J., and Rivier, J., Corticotropin-releasing factor, in *Brain Peptides*, Krieger, D. T., Brownstein, M. J., and Martin, J. B., Eds., John Wiley & Sons, New York, 1983, 961.

Yen, S. S. C., Neuroendocrine aspects of the regulation of cyclic gonadotropin release in women, in *Clinical Reproductive Neuroendocrinology*, Huberno, P. O., L'Hermite, M., and Robyn, C., Eds., S. Karger, Basel, 1977, 150.

Yu, W. H., Seeburg, P. H., Nikolics, K., and McCann, S. M., Gonadotropin releasing hormone associated peptide (GAP) suppresses prolactin release without altering gonadotropin release in ovariectomized, steroid-blocked rats, *Endocrinology*, 123, 390, 1988.

Whitnall, M. H. and Gainer, H., Major pro-vasopressin-expressing and pro-vasopressin-deficient subpopulations of corticotropin-releasing hormone neurons in normal rats, *Neuroendocrinology*, 47, 176, 1988.

Zimmerman, E. A., Oxytocin, vasopressin, and neurophysins, in *Brain Peptides*, Krieger, D. T., Brownstein, M. J., and Martin, J. B., Eds., John Wiley & Sons, New York, 1983, 597.

Section I
Methods in Neuroendocrinology

Garth Bissette, Section Editor

2

Bioassay Methods

E. KEVIN HEIST AND RUSSELL E. POLAND
Department of Psychiatry
UCLA School of Medicine
Harbor-UCLA Medical Center
Torrance, California

I. Bioassays — General

A. Introduction

In his Nobel prize lecture, Dr. John Vane quoted his colleague, Dr. John Gaddum, who claimed that "the pharmacologist has been a 'jack of all trades' borrowing from physiology, biochemistry, pathology, microbiology and statistics — but he has developed one technique of his own, and that is the technique of bioassay" (Vane, 1983). Dr. Vane used bioassays extensively in his discovery of prostacyclin, for which he subsequently was awarded the Nobel prize. Many of the bioassay techniques used by Dr. Vane in his experiments date back several decades, with bioassay methodology itself dating back even further (Dale, 1912; Elliott, 1912; Stewart and Rogoff, 1919; Gaddum, 1959). Before the development of radioimmunoassay and radioreceptor assay procedures, pharmacologists and endocrinologists had few tools other than intact biological systems in which to perform their experiments, and bioassays were used extensively. As other techniques were developed, scientists increasingly viewed the bioassay as "dated" and abandoned it in order to jump on the bandwagon of newer and simpler methodologies. However, those who continued experimentation with bioassays have brought about great improvements in the technique in recent years. For this reason and others discussed below, bioassays are currently experiencing a resurgence in popularity, as this technique is unique in many respects and has provided solutions to many scientific questions that have proven problematic using more "modern" methodologies.

This chapter will focus on bioassays that are currently in use and the insights that scientists have gained through the application of this methodology. Particular attention will be given to the use of bioassays in conjunction with radioimmunoassays (RIA), radioreceptor assays (RRA), and gene cloning. The number of hormones and other substances that have been analyzed by bioassay is prohibitively large to allow for all or even most to be considered within the confines of a single chapter. Therefore, three hormones, adrenocorticotropic hormone (ACTH), parathyroid hormone (PTH), and interleukin-6 (IL-6), have been selected for detailed consideration in this chapter because their respective bioassays are representative of the theoretical and practical issues surrounding the use of bioassays and because bioassays have yielded especially interesting results on the respective physiological roles of these hormones. The reader is referred elsewhere for detailed discussions of the principles and mathematics of bioassay (Chayen, 1980; Finney, 1952; Gaddum, 1953; Goldstein, et al., 1974).

B. The Definition of a Bioassay

Bioassays measure the functional response of an organism, target organ, tissue, or group of cells to an analyte, irrespective of whether the properities of the material being assayed are known or unknown. The discovery of most of the known hormones was made possible through the use of one or more bioassays. Such a discovery usually begins with the observation that a biological compound (often the extract of an endocrine gland) exerts a measurable effect when administered to a biological system. Although the purpose of most bioassays is to quantify the concentration of a hormone or other analyte, other purposes are also possible, including a comparison of the effects of different hormones on a biological system and a comparison of the effects of a single hormone on different biological systems (Bangham, 1983). As shown in Figure 1, bioassays can be performed on a spectrum of biological systems, including live animals, target organs, segments or sections of target organs, and dissociated target cells. In part, the particular hormone to be measured and the function to be quantified will dictate which of these systems is best suited for a particular experiment.

Hormones generally produce a multitude of responses, any one of which can be quantified by bioassay analysis. Thus, for example, a bioassay for PTH can involve the phosphaturic effect of the hormone, its hypercalcemic effect, or more subtle intracellular effects such as cAMP generation in target cells. All things being equal, it is generally advisable to select the effect to be quantified that is most representative of the function of interest (Robertson et al., 1987). In the example with PTH, a scientist attempting to correlate plasma PTH with change in bone density would be likely to choose the PTH bioassay that quantifies PTH-induced hypercalcemia or its associated cAMP response rather than PTH-induced phosphaturia. All bioassays are not equal in terms of sensitivity, precision, requirement for technical equipment, and sample through-put, however, and it is quite likely that one or more of these factors will determine which bioassay will ultimately be chosen to measure PTH.

As mentioned, bioassays are based on the functional effect that a hormone exerts on a biological system. In contrast, RIAs are based on the binding of antigenic determinants by specific antibodies that were raised against the hormone (or hapten) of interest. As a result, bioassays measure the ability of a given sample to produce a hormone-like effect while RIAs measure the concentration of antigenic determinants in a sample, whether or not those determinants are contained within biologically active regions of the molecule. If an RIA is performed in which the antibodies are derived from antiserum, then the antigenic determinants to which the antibodies bind and the affinity of binding can vary from one antiserum preparation to the next. In contrast, a monoclonal antibody preparation has a constant, reliable specificity and affinity for antigenic determinants. However, regardless of whether polyclonal

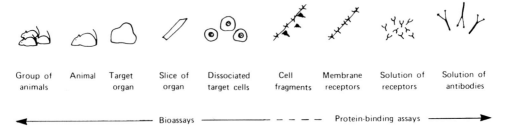

| Group of animals | Animal | Target organ | Slice of organ | Dissociated target cells | Cell fragments | Membrane receptors | Solution of receptors | Solution of antibodies |

◀─────────────── Bioassays ─────────── ─ ─ ─ ─ Protein-binding assays ─────────▶

Figure 1. The spectrum of assay techniques, ranging from *in vivo* bioassays to immunoassays. (Reprinted with permission from Bangham, D. R., in *Cytochemical Bioassays; Techniques and Clinical Applications,* Chayen, J. and Bitensky, L., Eds., Marcel Dekker, New York, 1983, 7.)

or monoclonal antibodies are used, the RIA measures only antigenic determinants and hence is an analytical assay while the bioassay is a functional assay.

Another analytical assay that is somewhat newer than the RIA is the radioreceptor assay (RRA). The RRA is, like the RIA, a binding assay, but it utilizes receptors derived from biological tissues to measure hormone concentrations (Ferkany, 1987). The RRA is similar to the bioassay in that it is based on a real biological system (a receptor) rather than an antibody, but it is, like the RIA, an analytical rather than a functional assay. Only the physical binding of molecules to receptors is quantified by RRA, and the physiological effects resulting from this binding, which are the basis for bioassay measurements, usually cannot be determined by receptor-binding analysis (Robertson et al., 1987).

C. The Role of Bioassays

Before comparing the usefulness of various types of assays in modern neuroendocrinology, it is necessary to discuss what the characteristics of any good assay are, whether the assay in question is a bioassay or not. The most important characteristics for an assay to possess are the following (Robertson et al., 1987):

1. The assay should be specific for the hormone and physiologic function of interest.
2. The assay should have good precision over a large working range, both within the assay and between assays.
3. The assay should be capable of high through-put and should not require the use of highly specialized equipment.
4. The assay should be sensitive enough to detect the hormone of interest in normal and subnormal concentrations in plasma, preferably without the need for extraction.

The classical *in vivo* bioassays, which were utilized primarily before the development of the RIA, could generally fulfill the first three criteria, but not the fourth. Without the sensitivity to measure even normal plasma concentrations of most hormones, these bioassays were quite restrictive in their use. When RIAs were introduced, many scientists hoped and believed that these assays would completely replace the generally more tedious bioassays. In contrast to most bioassays available at the time, RIAs were generally very precise, simple, and much more sensitive. Normal and subnormal concentrations of many hormones could be analyzed by RIA without extracting the hormone from plasma or tissue. During the years immediately following the development of the RIA, there was also a widespread belief that this type of assay was more accurate than the bioassay because it measured the mass concentration of a hormone rather than the much "less tangible" activity of the hormone (Bangham, 1983).

During the 1960s and 1970s, the belief that data derived from RIA were "better" than results obtained by bioassay, coupled with the ease and sensitivity of RIA, caused many endocrinologists and pharmacologists to abandon use of the bioassay. However, in experiments on a wide variety of hormones, it has become increasingly clear that results obtained by RIA are inconsistent with respect to the physiological status of many subjects. These results uncovered a fundamental shortcoming of RIA-derived data; that is, the number of antigenic determinants which a sample contains is not necessarily representative of the number of active hormone molecules in the sample (Chayen and Bitensky, 1983). Several factors may account for this. The most critical of these is that degradation products of a hormone that have lost all biological activity will retain immunoreactivity as long as the antigenic determinants to which the antibodies bind remain intact. As a result of this, the biological half-life of most hormones is considerably shorter than the immunological half-life (Ambler et al., 1982; Robertson et al., 1987). Another factor that may contribute to this discrepancy is the existence of biologically inactive precursor forms of the hormone that are also immunoreactive and are sometimes found in very high concentrations in the blood of patients with various illnesses, including certain types of cancer (Robertson et al., 1987). For these reasons, the concentration of a hormone in plasma as measured by RIA is often considerably higher than the concentration as measured by bioassay.

Although receptor-binding assays may be somewhat more specific than immunoassays, they also lack the functional component provided by the bioassay. RRAs measure only the affinity of binding of molecules to receptors and not the biochemical and physiological effects that this binding induces. At first, this distinction may seem unimportant in relation to assay specificity. However, simple binding of a molecule to a receptor does not ensure that the full functional effect linked to that receptor will be activated. RRAs (usually) cannot distinguish whether the molecules that bind to a receptor are agonists or antagonists, and also cannot distinguish different forms of a hormone that may bind to receptors with similar affinity but produce somewhat different functional effects. A further complication in interpreting the results of receptor-binding studies is the possibility that the binding of hormones to receptors may be transient while the response to the binding is cumulative over time (Bangham, 1983). In such a circumstance, RRA analysis will provide information only on the transient binding of the hormone to the receptor, while analysis by bioassay can more accurately portray the cumulative nature of the physiological response to that binding.

RIAs and RRAs are not the only assays with specificity problems; bioassays may also, under certain conditions, give misleading results. Compounds that are not related structurally to a hormone but are able to mimic the effects of the hormone are likely to be measured by bioassay. These substances are not measured by RIA, however, and their biological activity is not blocked by hormone-specific antibodies. For example, in some patients with malignancy-induced hypercalcemia, it is believed that a protein is present that exerts the same functional effect on bone resorption as PTH, yet bear no structural similarity with the molecule. In this situation, RIA analysis correctly measures the concentration of PTH in plasma while bioassay yields a falsely high value for plasma PTH (Strewler et al., 1983). However, bioassay does correctly predict the PTH-like effect of hypercalcemia, and thus the bioassay result is accurate from a physiological viewpoint even though it is inaccurate from an analytical viewpoint, since it is measuring more than just "true" PTH. Thus, depending on the question being asked, bioassay results, as with results obtained using other methodologies, can be correct or incorrect.

As stated previously, one of the initial shortcomings of the bioassay was its low sensitivity, which prevented it from measuring normal and subnormal levels of most hormones in unextracted plasma. Were this still the case, then RIAs and RRAs, with their relatively high degree of sensitivity, would remain the method of choice for most experiments despite their specificity problems. In recent years, however, bioassay techniques have been improved to the degree that they can now be used to measure physiological levels of most hormones in plasma. One very specialized bioassay technique that has been developed, the cytochemical bioassay, is approximately 1,000 times more sensitive than the equivalent RIA (Chayen and Bitensky, 1983). Although the cytochemical bioassay technique requires the use of specialized equipment and is somewhat difficult to perform, it is the only means of analysis available for measurement of extremely low concentrations of hormone and/or very small sample volumes. When the high degree of sensitivity of the cytochemical bioassay is not required for an experiment, other *in vitro* bioassays are available for many hormones that can measure normal hormone concentrations in plasma and generally require less technical equipment and expertise than does the cytochemical assay.

It is necessary to have a very sensitive and specific assay procedure in order to develop hormone standards against which other hormone preparations and samples can be measured. Realizing the specificity problems associated with RIAs, the World Health Organization (WHO, 1969) recommended that bioassays be run in parallel with RIAs in order to determine standards for hormones. By 1975, the WHO Expert Committee on Biological Standardization (ECBS) found that a "limitation on the use of immunoassays for evaluating hormonal bioactivity is that the methods measure a composite of antigenic activity, which is not necessarily related to the bioactivity of the hormone" (WHO, 1975). This position of the WHO ECBS on the usefulness of bioassays in biological standardization was further strengthened in 1982, when it was decided that hormone preparations to be used for standardization should consist of "the natural and unaltered material that showed the highest potency in a classical *in vivo* assay system generally recognized by the scientific community as defining that hormone" (WHO, 1982).

Another area in which the high degree of specificity of the bioassay is useful is gene cloning and expression. When a gene is isolated and cloned into an expression vector, it is often difficult to determine whether the protein that is produced is a complete and unaltered copy of the protein of interest. When the protein is a hormone or other biologically active substance, a bioassay can provide a simple and effective means of making this determination. In contrast, RIA is ineffective because it measures only the presence of an antigenic determinant usually consisting of a very small section of the protein. Consequently, it would be likely to identify truncated proteins, incompletely glycosylated proteins, and other biologically inactive proteins as mature, correctly expressed proteins. Because such small factors as the extent of glycosylation of pituitary glycoprotein hormones can greatly affect their biological activity (Robertson et al., 1987), the bioassay is an essential procedure for determining whether or not the product of a cloned gene is a correctly expressed copy of the protein of interest.

D. Bioassay Methods

The first bioassays were *in vivo* experiments in which the purified extract from a tissue was administered to a living organism, and the biological effect was measured and compared to a control. These experiments had the advantages of technical simplicity and the ability to analyze hormone effects in intact organisms. Furthermore, this type of assay had the unique capacity to account for hormone metabolism and measure the long-term effects of a hormone and its metabolites on an organism (Bangham, 1983). Unfortunately, these experiments had poor sensitivity such that they generally could not measure normal levels of hormones in plasma, and also contained a large degree of between-animal variability that made the results from these assays difficult to interpret (Chayen et al., 1976). Although *in vivo* assays are still commonly used for many purposes by clinical endocrinologists and pharmacologists, actual hormone measurements are now generally performed using *in vitro* techniques.

In vitro bioassays may be performed on a wide variety of systems, including complete organs, segments or sections of organs, or dispersed cells from target organs. The "superfusion" technique pioneered by Vane consisted of excising a segment of tissue, often smooth muscle from the intestinal tract of an organism, and then bathing it with a stream of nutrient-rich fluid, commonly whole blood. This stream of fluid was momentarily interrupted to allow for administration of a test substance, and then the stream was allowed to continue. The physiological effects exerted by the test substance, such as vascular bed dilation caused by prostacyclin, could then be quantified (Vane, 1983).

In the case of both tissue assays and most dispersed cell assays, new animals must be sacrificed for each experiment. This is somewhat problematic in that animals must be continuously available in order to perform these assays, and using new animals for each experiment creates between-animal variability. Dispersed cells to be used for bioassay analysis are generally maintained in a nonproliferative state in order to maintain complete differentiation and full physiological function. It has been discovered that when chick cell cultures are allowed to proliferate, the cultures will eventually consist primarily of fibroblasts, which do not retain the biological functions of mature myocardial cells and hence are useless for bioassay (Chayen, 1980). Work is currently being performed to develop continuous cultures that will retain the physiological function of the cells. One example is the FRTL-5 cell line, which is a strain of rat thyroid follicular cells that can be used to measure thyroid-stimulating hormone (TSH) concentrations by accumulation of intracellular cAMP in response to TSH agonists. These cells can be maintained in a continuously proliferating culture in a partially differentiated state and retain the ability to quantify TSH by the cAMP bioassay (Bidey et al., 1984). Devolopment of continuous cultures such as the FRTL-5 cell line will make bioassays simpler and more cost effective as well as increasing their precision by eliminating between-animal variability. However, the possibility that the specificity of the response changes over time should not be overlooked.

One bioassay technique that warrants special consideration is the cytochemical bioassay. This type of bioassay is perhaps the most sensitive of all assays, often as much as 1,000 times more sensitive than the corresponding immunoassay. The cytochemical bioassay is an *in vitro* assay that involves the precipitation of a colored reaction product. This colored product is then measured by microspectrometry and microdensitometry (Chayen, 1980). Two types of cytochemical bioassays have been developed, the cytochemical segment assay and the cytochemical section assay. The major disadvantages inherent to the cytochemical segment bioassay are the requirement for extremely specialized equipment and the low sample through-put of the assay. The cytochemical section assay allows for much higher through-put than the segment assay, but the need for specialized equipment remains.

The procedure for the cyotochemical segment bioassay involves cutting the target organ into several segments, reacting each segment with the sample or standard of interest, and then freezing the segments in a cryostat. A thin section is then sliced from each segment, exposed to a reagent that forms a colored precipitate based on a hormone-dependent intracellular reaction, and analyzed by microspectrometry and microdensitometry (Chayen, 1980). One of the major disadvantages of the cytochemical segment bioassay is that the number of segments that can be obtained from each animal is usually only 8 or 10 at the most. Because at least four of these segments must be used in constructing a standard curve, the number of samples that can be analyzed for each animal used is generally very small. In order to overcome this shortcoming, the cytochemical section bioassay was developed. The section bioassay is very similar to the segment assay except that the standard or sample is not applied to the tissue until after it has been sectioned (Chayen et al., 1976). Because the number of sections that can be sliced from a single animal generally numbers in the hundreds, the section assay allows for a much higher sample through-put than the segment assay and greatly expands the usefulness of the cytochemical bioassay.

The general methods of data analysis are the same for all bioassays, regardless of what particular bioassay technique is used. A standard curve is formed that plots measured biological activity vs. hormone concentration. Unknown samples are analyzed by measuring their biological activity in the same assay from which the standard curve was obtained and interpolating hormone concentration from the curve. It is advisable to check for parallelism by comparing different concentrations of standard preparation (i.e., the standard curve) with different concentrations of the analyte. The two dose-response curves should be parallel (i.e., have the same slope). If the curves are not parallel, then it is likely that the analyte is not identical to the standard, and any results obtained from such an assay might be invalid

(Chayen, 1980). However, the nonparallelism of a biological response to an unknown sample might indicate that important and biologically active substances are present that are different than the reference material to which the response is being compared. In fact, nonparallelism is found with the cytochemical bioassay of ACTH with a 1:50 dilution of plasma but not with a 1:1000 dilution (Reader et al., 1982), suggesting that other bioactive material might be present in plasma that is not measurable at high dilution (Poland et al., 1989). Other important qualities of assays, in general, and bioassays, in particular, are precision (reproducibility of results), accuracy (correctness of results), and low variability, both intraassay and interassay. The sensitivity needed will depend on the concentration of analyte in the samples to be measured and may dictate which particular bioassay method is chosen.

II. Specific Bioassays

In order to illustrate some of the advantages and disadvantages of bioassay procedures, the bioassay methodology for three hormones, adrenocorticotropic hormone (ACTH), parathyroid hormone (PTH), and interleukin-6 (IL-6) will be discussed.

A. Adrenocorticotropic Hormone (ACTH)

ACTH is a 39-amino acid hormone that is secreted from the anterior pituitary gland and which has its primary effect on the control of the secretion of glucococorticoids from the adrenal cortex (Guyton, 1986). Amino acids 1 to 24 (N terminal) are needed for biological activity of the molecule, while amino acids 25 to 39 (C terminal) are not required for bioactivity and are somewhat species specific. As a result of this, antibodies that are produced against foreign ACTH usually recognize sites on the C-terminal rather than the N-terminal end of the molecule. There are also a wide variety of bioassays that have been developed to measure ACTH. The first bioassays were *in vivo* procedures that measured the ascorbic acid depletion in the adrenal glands of hypophysectomized rats in response to administration of ACTH. As with most *in vivo* assays, these bioassays were not sufficiently sensitive to measure ACTH levels in plasma and were also subject to considerable between-animal variability (Sayers et al., 1948).

In vitro bioassays for ACTH were later developed that were somewhat more sensitive than the *in vivo* assays. One *in vitro* ACTH assay utilizes cAMP accumulation in adrenal cells as a means of determining ACTH concentration (Sayers and Beall, 1973). Other *in vitro* ACTH assays measure ACTH indirectly via its steroidogenic effect on dispersed adrenal cells. The quantity of corticosteroids produced (the functional effect being measured by the assay) then is determined either by fluorometric means (Lowry et al., 1973) or by RIA (Poland et al., 1989). Hypophysectomy of animals prior to excision of the adrenal glands was found to increase the sensitivity of the both the cAMP assay and the corticosteroid assay (Sayers and Beall, 1973). Even with hypophysectomy, however, these assays are not sufficiently sensitive to measure normal and subnormal plasma levels of ACTH without extraction.

A cytochemical segment bioassay for ACTH was subsequently developed. This method is significantly more sensitive than the corresponding RIA and could easily measure plasma levels of ACTH without extraction (Chayen et al., 1972). This assay quantifies ACTH-induced ascorbate depletion in adrenal segments by microdensitometric analysis of prussian blue (ferric ferrocyanide) formation (Chayen et al., 1976). High concentrations of ACTH lead to low levels of ascorbate in the adrenal segments and correspondingly low levels of prussian blue. This cytochemical segment assay is sensitive to 5.0 fg/ml, but had low through-put

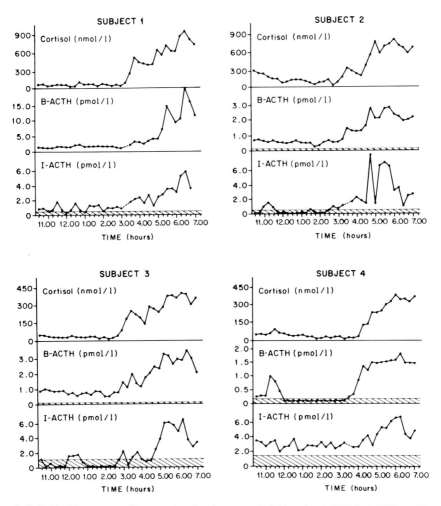

Figure 2. Individual hormone profiles over time for plasma cortisol, bioactive ACTH (B-ACTH), and immuno-reactive ACTH (I-ACTH). Hatched areas represent the lower limit of sensitivity of each assay at the 95% confidence level. (Note: The scales for cortisol and ACTH are different for some subjects.) (Reprinted with permission from Poland, R. E., Hanada, K., and Rubin, R. T., *Acta Endocrinol.*, 121, 857, 1989.)

(Chayen et al., 1974). A cytochemical section assay was developed shortly thereafter that retained the sensitivity and accuracy of the segment assay but allowed for much higher through-put (Alaghband-Zadeh, 1974).

The values obtained for ACTH by bioassay are often quite different from the values obtained by RIA. Generally, the RIA values are higher than bioassay values. In order to be measurable by bioassay, early studies required subjects to have elevated ACTH concentrations. One such study used Cushing's patients and metapyrone-treated normal subjects to obtain these high levels of ACTH. This study found the ratio of immunoactive to bioactive (I/B) ACTH ranged from 1.6 for Cushing's patients to 2.8 for metapyrone-treated normals (Matsuyama et al., 1972). Recent work with a sensitized isolated adrenal bioassay for ACTH allowed measurement of normal nocturnal levels of plasma ACTH in eight normal subjects. As shown in Figures 2 and 3, nocturnal bioactive ACTH concentrations correlate much more strongly ($r = +0.93$) with plasma cortisol than do immunoactive ACTH concentrations ($r = +0.69$) (Poland et al., 1989). In six of the eight subjects, the I/B ACTH is >1. However, in two

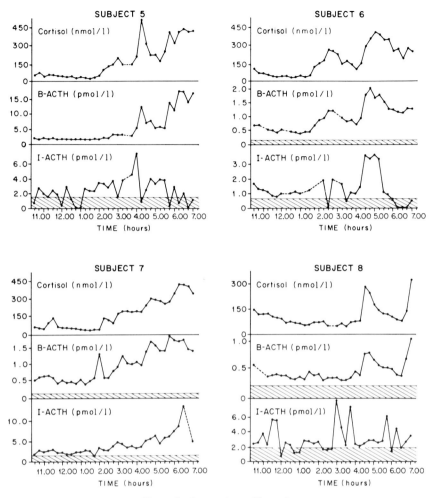

Figure 3. See caption to Figure 2.

subjects the ratios are <1. The consistently higher within-subject correlations beween bioactive ACTH and cortisol compared to immunoactive ACTH and cortisol, coupled with the observation that two of the subjects showed considerably higher bioactive ACTH concentrations, suggests that there might be substances in plasma with ACTH bioactivity that are not ACTH, or at least not measured by RIA (Poland et al., 1989).

In the insulin hypoglycemia test (IHT), insulin is administered to subjects and an ACTH peak occurs 45 to 60 min later (Fleisher et al., 1974). The I/B ACTH at baseline is 1.67, which temporarily decreases to 0.93 after administration of insulin, but then gradually increases to 3.0 (approximately twice baseline) 90 min after insulin injection (Goverde et al., 1989). The investigators suggest that much of the ACTH being measured by RIA is actually degradation products. During the rise of ACTH immediately after insulin administration, the majority of ACTH in the blood is newly secreted hormone and very little of it has been in the bloodstream long enough for it to be degraded. Consequently, most of the immunoreactive ACTH is intact, bioactive $ACTH_{1-39}$, and the I/B ratio is lower than baseline. After 90 min, most of the ACTH in the bloodstream has been there for a relatively long time and has been subject to degradation. Thus, most of the ACTH at 90 min is partially degraded and is immunoreactive but not bioactive, producing an I/B ratio above baseline (Goverde et al., 1989).

Other experiments have also supported the theory that much of the immunoactive ACTH is actually degradation products. Both *in vivo* and *in vitro*, bioactive ACTH has been found to disappear more quickly than immunoactive ACTH. The addition of the enzyme inhibitor trasylol to plasma slows the disappearance of both bioactive and immunoactive ACTH, suggesting that ACTH degradation occurs by an enzymatic process (Besser et al., 1971). Furthermore, immunoactive ACTH as measured by N-terminal antibodies disappears more quickly than ACTH as measured by C-terminal antibodies (Besser et al., 1971). This suggests that the N terminal of ACTH is degraded first, a finding later confirmed by a study that demonstrated that $ACTH_{1-39}$ is quickly degraded with a $T_{1/2}$ of approximately 2.5 min to its major metabolite, $ACTH_{3-39}$. $ACTH_{3-39}$ retains full C-terminal immunoactivity and some N-terminal immunoactivity, yet possesses only 3.6% of the steroidogenic potency of $ACTH_{1-39}$ (Ambler et al., 1982). Separation of native ACTH from its fragments by high-performance liquid chromatography indicated that $ACTH_{1-39}$ contributed to ACTH immunoactivity to only a minor extent (Schöneshöfer and Fenner, 1981).

Another study that demonstrates a large dissociation between immunoactive ACTH and bioactive ACTH concerns the discovery of "big ACTH". Big ACTH has been identified in pituitary and tumor extracts as well as in the plasma of patients with Addison's disease, Cushing's disease, Nelson's syndrome, and normal patients with artificially stimulated ACTH secretion. The molecule is significantly larger and more acidic than $ACTH_{1-39}$ (Yalow and Berson, 1973). The bioactivity of big ACTH is less than 4% of $ACTH_{1-39}$, yet the immunoactivity of the two molecules is comparable. After digestion by the proteolytic enzyme trypsin, big ACTH is degraded to $ACTH_{1-39}$ and acquires full bioactivity as well as retaining full immunoactivity (Gewirtz et al., 1974). This suggests that big ACTH is a precursor of $ACTH_{1-39}$. This hormone is secreted both by tumors that lack the posttranslational processing machinery found in the secretory cells of the anterior pituitary, and by normal secretory cells when their production is stimulated to the point that they cannot fully process all of the precursor hormone molecules prior to secretion, as also might be the case in subjects with a major depression (Kathol et al., 1989).

Clearly, bioassays provide a more accurate assessment of a functional ACTH molecule than do immunoassays. Considering the short *in vivo* half-life of $ACTH_{1-39}$, one might wonder if most of the bioactive ACTH in a sample is degraded before it can be assayed. If this were the case, the bioassay would yield an accurate measurement of $ACTH_{1-39}$ concentration at the time the assay was performed, but would greatly underestimate the concentration of $ACTH_{1-39}$ that was present at the time the blood sample was drawn. However, bioactive ACTH has been found to have a much longer half-life *in vitro* than *in vivo*. ACTH retains full bioactivity for at least 1 hr in heparinized blood and 2 hr in plasma at 22°C and is also unaffected by two cycles of freezing and thawing (Lambert et al., 1985). Thus, if reasonable care is taken with blood samples, the ACTH concentration as measured by bioassay is likely to be a very accurate representation of the $ACTH_{1-39}$ concentration that existed in the subject at the time the blood was drawn. If it is necessary to subject plasma samples to room temperature for more than 2 hr or to freeze them more than two times, it has been suggested that trasylol be added to the samples to inhibit enzymatic degradation, provided that trasylol does not interfere with the particular bioassay being used. In this regard, we have found that trasylol does affect the isolated adrenal cell response to ACTH (Poland et al., 1989).

B. Parathyroid Hormone (PTH)

PTH is a hormone secreted from the parathyroid gland and whose major effects include bone resorption and phosphate excretion from the kidneys. PTH is first synthesized as a 155-

amino acid preprohormone. This pre-PTH is cleaved first to a prohormone and finally to the 84-amino acid mature PTH prior to secretion (Guyton, 1986). The N-terminal fragment (PTH$_{1-34}$) retains full biological activity, while removal of the first amino acid from PTH renders the hormone completely biologically inactive (Chayen, 1980).

There are several bioassay methods available to measure PTH concentrations. *In vivo* PTH bioassays generally rely on PTH-induced hypercalcemia (Parsons et al., 1973). These assays are sensitive to nanogram levels of PTH (Nissenson et al., 1981) and hence lack the sensitivity required to measure normal plasma levels of bioactive PTH, which average 10 pg/ml (Chambers et al., 1978). A more sensitive bioassay involves quantification of PTH-induced cAMP accumulation in renal cortical plasma membranes and is capable of measuring picogram levels of PTH (Nissenson et al., 1981). In order to compensate for basal cAMP levels, this assay is generally performed for each serum sample both in the presence and absence of PTH inhibitor, and the difference in response is used to calculate PTH concentrations (Seshadri et al., 1985).

The most sensitive bioassay method available to measure PTH is the cytochemical bioassay. This assay measures PTH-induced glucose-6-phosphate (G6P) dehydrogenase activity by means of a colored formazan precipitate that can be analyzed by microdensitometry (Chambers et al., 1978). This cytochemical bioassay is sensitive to femtogram concentrations of PTH, and thus can easily quantify normal and suppressed plasma PTH levels (Nissenson et al., 1981).

PTH is a relatively labile compound in whole blood and, to a lesser degree, in plasma, so blood samples that are to be analyzed for PTH content should be processed expeditiously. Bioactive PTH is stable in plasma for 90 min at 4°C. More than 95% of PTH bioactivity is lost from whole blood stored for 30 min at 4°C, and 85% of PTH bioactivity is lost from plasma stored for 30 min at room temperature (Kent and Zanelli, 1983). Thus, blood samples should be immediately centrifuged, and the resulting plasma should be snap frozen in order to retain full PTH bioactivity.

Receptor-binding studies with PTH demonstrate a very high correlation to bioassay results. Only PTH, PTH fragments, and PTH analogs that are bioactive are able to bind to PTH receptors; PTH fragments that are biologically inactive show no affinity for PTH receptors (Segre et al., 1979). Analogs of PTH$_{1-34}$ have been synthesized that demonstrate significantly greater bioactivity than natural PTH (Rosenblatt and Potts, 1977). Based on a cAMP bioassay for PTH, the relative biological potencies of such analogs have been found to correlate strongly with the binding affinity of each to PTH receptors. Similarly, the *in vitro* inhibitory potency of synthetic PTH antagonists correlates strongly with receptor-binding affinity (Segre et al., 1979).

Correlations between immunoactive and bioactive PTH concentrations are lower than correlations between RRA and bioassay values. PTH concentrations determined by RIA are in the range of hundreds of picograms per milliliter, while the concentrations determined by bioassay are approximately 10 pg/ml (Chambers et al., 1978). These results can be explained by the finding that the C-terminal end of PTH has a much longer half life than the N-terminal end. The predominant circulating forms of PTH contain the middle and C-terminals, and these fragments are measured by most immunoassays as if they are PTH, despite the fact that they are biologically inactive (Segre et al., 1974). Because C-terminal PTH fragments have a relatively long half-life *in vivo*, PTH measurements based on C terminal-directed antiserum correlate well with long-term PTH abnormalities such as hyperparathyroidism and hypoparathyroidism. In contrast, PTH measurements based on N-terminal antiserum correlate well with bioactive PTH levels and reflect acute changes in PTH secretion (Arnaud et al., 1974).

Large discrepancies between bioactive and immunoactive PTH have been found in patients with certain diseases. In a case of malignancy-associated hypercalcemia (MAH), a protein was found to be secreted by renal carcinoma cells that produced hypercalcemia. When renal carcinoma cells from this patient were grown in nude mice, the mice also exhibited hypercalcemia. The protein secreted by these cells possessed significant PTH-like bioactivity based on a cAMP bioassay that could be effectively blocked by a PTH antagonist. However, this protein is not PTH_{1-84}; it is larger than PTH_{1-84} as determined by gel-filtration column chromatography and was not detected by a variety of PTH antisera (Strewler et al., 1983). Similar results have been attained with the use of the cytochemical bioassay for PTH. A protein secreted by cells of a metastatic bronchial carcinoid from a patient with MAH demonstrated significant bioactivity based on the cytochemical assay but also was not detected by PTH antibodies (Loveridge et al., 1985).

Another disease that further illustrates the discrepancy between immunoactive and bioactive PTH measurements is type I pseudohypoparathyroidism (PSPI). PSPI is a form of hypoparathyroidism associated with secondary hyperparathyroidism, in which target organs do not respond to PTH. These patients have typical symptoms of hypoparathyroidism, including short stature, a round face, and mental retardation. Immunoactive PTH levels in these patients are elevated considerably, while bioactive PTH concentrations are in the low to normal range (Loveridge et al., 1982). Administration of intravenous calcium to normal subjects tends to decrease both immunoactive and bioactive PTH, while administration of intravenous calcium to PSPI patients lowers immunoactive PTH but does not affect bioactive PTH (Loveridge et al., 1986a). This suggests that a PTH inhibitor is present that prevents PTH from acting at target organs and whose secretion is, like PTH itself, inversely related to blood calcium concentration. The finding that plasma from PSPI patients exhibits abnormally low recovery of PTH, while plasma from former PSPI patients who have undergone parathyroidectomy exhibits normal PTH recovery, suggests that this inhibitor is secreted from the parathyroid gland (Loveridge et al., 1982). Further experimentation succeeded in isolating this protein by gel-permeation chromatography and demonstrating that it is in fact an inhibitor of PTH bioactivity (Loveridge et al., 1986b).

These results demonstrate two very interesting cases of dissociation of PTH bioactivity from immunoactivity. In both MAH and PSPI, RIA correctly determined the PTH concentrations while results from the bioassay gave excessively high PTH values in the case of MAH, and excessively low values in the case of PSPI. However, the RIA results were completely inconsistent with clinical symptomology. In patients with MAH, it appears that RIA is unable to measure the protein that is secreted from tumor cells but which acts on PTH target cells. Similarly, in patients with PSPI, the RIA is unable to measure the PTH inhibitor. Thus, although the results from RIA are analytically correct regarding the actual concentration of PTH in these patients as compared to normal subjects, the RIA results alone are essentially useless from a clinical standpoint. The bioassay results, although incorrect from an analytical perspective, do correctly predict the physiological state of patients with these diseases.

C. Interleukin-6 (IL-6)

IL-6 is one of a number of B cell proliferation factors that are essential for the immune response. Several names have been designated for IL-6, including HGF, 26-kDa protein, and BSF-2; only recently has it been demonstrated that these molecules all represent the same compound (Brakenhoff et al., 1987). The humoral response to a foreign antigen is the proliferation and maturation of B lymphocytes to antibody-secreting cells. The binding of antigen molecules to the antibodies on B cells is necessary for B cell proliferation and maturation, but must be accompanied by proliferation factors for the correct B cell response to occur (Melchers and Andersson, 1986). Although many of the B cell proliferation factors that have been discovered are derived from lymphocytes, IL-6 is produced by monocytes. It has been postulated that dependence on IL-6 for B cell growth is a mechanism to prevent uncontrolled B cell proliferation (Aarden et al., 1987). The pathway for B cell proliferation and maturation is shown in Figure 4.

The only method that currently exists to measure B cell proliferation factors such as IL-6 is bioassay.* The IL-6 bioassay measures cell proliferation based on [³H]thymidine incorporation by B lymphocytes that are maintained on microtiter plates (Du Bois et al., 1974). Early IL-6 assays utilized B13.29, a B cell hybridoma cell line that is dependent on IL-6 for proliferation (Lansdorp et al., 1986). By subjecting B13.29 cell cultures to very low concentrations of IL-6, the subclone B9 cell line was isolated, which is extremely sensitive to the presence of IL-6 and whose use has increased the sensitivity of the IL-6 bioassay by four- to eightfold. The sensitivity of the B9 cell line allows for measurement of IL-6 production by single cells, and was used to demonstrate that IL-6 is secreted by monocytes (Aarden et al., 1987). Figure 5 shows a comparison of the sensitivities of the hybridoma cell lines B13.29 and B9 to IL-6 as measured by [³H] thymidine incorporation.

When a cloned gene is expressed, it is necessary to determine whether or not the recombinant gene product is a functional protein with the same properties as the natural

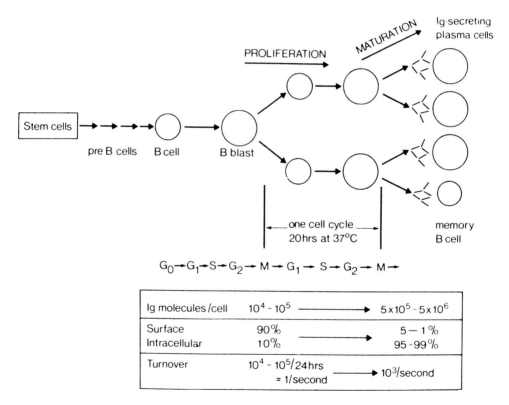

Figure 4. Different stages of the B cell cycle showing development from stem cells to IG-secreting plasma cells and memory B cells. IL-6 stimulates the proliferation stage of development. (Reprinted with permission from Melchers, F. and Andersson, J., *Annu. Rev. Immunol.*, 4, 13, 1986.)

---

* Note added in proof. Since this chapter was written, a radioimmunoassay and an ELISA for IL-6 have become available.

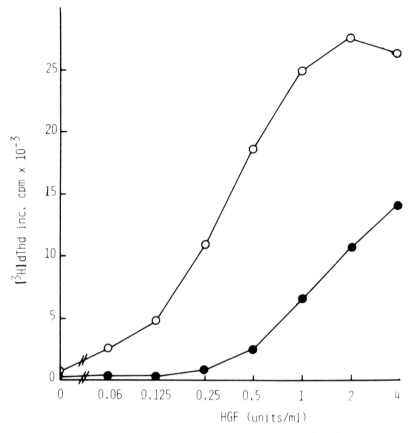

Figure 5. Sensitivity of the B13.29 line and its variant B9. A standard preparation of IL-6 was titrated in the IL-6 bioassay using either the wild-type B13.29 cell line (solid circles) or its subclone B9 (open circles). (Reprinted with permission from Aarden, L. A., De Groot, E. R., Schaap, O. L., and Lansdorp, P. M., *Eur. J. Immunol.*, 17, 1411, 1987.)

protein. The bioassay is a very effective way to make this determination and, in the case of B cell proliferation factors, it is the only way to do this. In one study, human monocyte poly(A⁺) RNA was used to make cDNA for the IL-6 gene, and this gene was expressed in *Escherichia coli* with the pUC9 expression vector. The B9 bioassay was then used to demonstrate that the expressed protein was active IL-6 (Brakenhoff et al., 1987). Without the bioassay, it would have been impossible to determine whether or not mature IL-6 was expressed by these cells.

Subsequent work with the IL-6 bioassay has demonstrated a synergistic effect between IL-6 and IL-1. As measured by [³H] thymidine incorporation, the combination of IL-6 and IL-1 increases the rate of B-cell proliferation by 20-fold compared to the effects of either hormone alone. Furthermore, it was discovered that IL-6 induces T cell proliferation at a rate comparable to that produced by IL-2 and greater than that produced by IL-4, cell proliferation factors that are normally associated with T cell growth. This effect exerted by IL-6 on T cells is also synergized by IL-1 (Van Snick et al., 1988).

It should be noted that with the use of bioassay methodology, studies investigating immune-hormonal interactions have been made possible. For example, it has been shown that IL-6 is produced by bone osteoblasts *in vitro* and the production of bioassayable IL-6 is stimulated by PTH. This effect is not influenced by calcitonin but it is antagonized by the synthetic glucocorticoid dexamethasone (Feyen et al., 1989). Furthermore, it has been found that neuroendocrine activity is influenced by various components of the immune system and vice versa (Bateman et al., 1989), as demonstrated by the stimulation of the hypothalamo-pituitary-adrenocortical (HPA) axis by IL-6, an effect exerted via hypothalamic corticotropin-releasing factor (CRF) secretion (Naitoh et al., 1988). Thus, the traditional boundaries between these two physiologic systems have become less distinct. Although it is impossible to predict what new insights will be made in the future regarding the roles of IL-6 and other factors of the immune system, it appears certain that bioassay techniques will continue to be an integral part not only of neuroendocrinologic research in general, but with research efforts designed to unravel the complex web of interactions between immunological function and neuroendocrine activity.

III. Conclusion

It is not the intention of this chapter to underrate the importance of nonbiological assay methods in modern neuroendocrine research. On the contrary, methods such as RIA and RRA have had profound effects on the field in past decades and will doubtlessly continue to do so for decades to come. Rather, this chapter is intended to focus attention on the expanding role of bioassay techniques in neuroendocrinology. The insensitive and relatively imprecise "classical" *in vivo* bioassays have been largely replaced by *in vitro* methods that are, in many instances, significantly more sensitive than comparable immunologic and receptor-binding techniques. Bioassays are extremely effective for evaluating products of gene expression because they can discriminate between correctly expressed, functional proteins and proteins that are incompletely or incorrectly expressed and hence nonfunctional. Some circulating factors (see footnote on page 33) can be measured only by bioassay. For other hormones such as ACTH and PTH, which can be measured by immunoassay, RRA, and by bioassay, the functional effects that are measured by bioassay are often found to correlate more strongly with the physiological status of an organism than do values obtained using more analytical techniques. Frequently, this results from the presence of hormone degradation products that are immunoactive but not bioactive. Under certain pathophysiologic conditions, the presence of hormone inhibitors and the effects of bioactive substances that are not immunoactive further dissociate RIA from bioassay results. Regarding how this information should be interpreted by scientists, perhaps the most prudent advice is offered by the World Health Organization, which suggests that bioassays be run in parallel with immunoassays (WHO, 1969). This allows for determination of which type of assay yields results that are most consistent with physiologic symptoms. If significant dissociations are discovered between bioassay and RIA results for a particular clinical condition, this information itself should be useful in furthering our understanding of the disease process. As frequently occurs in science, we seem to have come full circle. It would appear that, for good reason, bioassays are here to stay.

Acknowledgments

This work was supported in part by National Institute of Mental Health (NIMH) Grants MH34471 (to R.E.P.), NIMH Research Scientist Development Award MH00534 (to R.E.P.), and by National Institutes of Health General Clinical Research Center Grant RR00425.

References

Aarden, L. A., De Groot, E. R., Schaap, O. L., and Lansdorp, P. M., Production of hybridoma growth factor by human monocytes, *Eur. J. Immunol.,* 17, 1411, 1987.

Alaghband-Zadeh, J., Development of a section-bioassay for the routine assay of corticotrophin, *Ann. Clin. Biochem.,* 11, 43, 1974.

Ambler, L. Bennett, H. P. J., Hudson, A. M., and McMartin, C., Fate of human corticotrophin immediately after intravenous administration to the rat, *J. Endocrinol.,* 93, 287, 1982.

Arnaud, C. D., Goldsmith, R. S., Bordier, P. J., and Sizemore, G. W., Influence of immunoheterogeneity of circulating parathyroid hormone on results of radioimmunoassays of serum in man, *Am. J. Med.,* 56, 785, 1974.

Bangham, D. R., What's in a bioassay?, in *Cytochemical Bioassays; Techniques and Clinical Applications,* Chayen, J. and Bitensky, L., Eds., Marcel Dekker, New York, 1983, 7.

Bateman, A., Singh, A., Kral, T., and Solomon, S., The immune-hypothalamic-pituitary-adrenal axis, *Endocrinol. Rev.,* 10, 92, 1989.

Besser, G. M., Orth, D. N., Nicholson, W. E., Byyny, R. L., Abe, K., and Woodham, J. P., Dissociation of the disappearance of bioactive and radioimmunoactive ACTH from plasma in man, *J. Clin. Endocrinol.,* 32, 595, 1971.

Bidey, S. P., Chiovato, L., Day, A., Turmaine, M., Gould, R. P., Ekins, R. P., and Marshall, N. J., Evaluation of the rat thyroid cell strain FRTL-5 as an in-vitro bioassay system for thyrotropin, *J. Endocrinol.,* 101, 269, 1984.

Bitensky, L. and Chayen, J., The cytochemical bioassay, in *Cytochemical Bioassays; Techniques and Clinical Applications,* Chayen, J. and Bitensky, L., Eds., Marcel Dekker, New York, 1983, 143.

Brakenhoff, J. P. J., De Groot, E. R., Evers, R. F., Pannekoek, H., and Aarden, L. A., Molecular cloning and expression of hybridoma growth factor in *Escherichia coli, J. Immunol.,* 139, 4116, 1987.

Chambers, D. J., Dunham, J., Zanelli, J. M., Parsons, J. A., Bitensky, L., and Chayen, J., A sensitive bioassay of parathyroid hormone in plasma, *Clin. Endocrinol.,* 9, 375, 1978.

Chayen, J., *The Cytochemical Bioassay of Polypeptide Hormones,* Springer-Verlag, Berlin, 1980, 1.

Chayen, J. and Bitensky, L., General introduction to cytochemical bioassays, in *Cytochemical Bioassays; Techniques and Clinical Applications,* Chayen, J. and Bitensky, L., Eds., Marcel Dekker, New York, 1983, 1

Chayen, J., Loveridge, N., and Daly, J. R., A sensitive bioassay for adrenocorticotrophic hormone in human plasma, *Clin. Endocrinol.,* 1, 219, 1972.

Chayen, J., Bitensky, L., Chambers, D. J., Loveridge, N., and Daly, J. R., Studies on the mechanism of cytochemical bioassays, *Clin. Endocrinol.,* 3, 349, 1974.

Chayen, J., Daly, J. R., Loveridge, N., and Bitensky, L., The cytochemical bioassay of hormones, *Recent Prog. Horm. Res.,* 32, 33, 1976.

Dale, H. H., The anaphylactic reaction of plain muscle in the guinea-pig, *J. Pharmacol. Exp. Ther.,* 4, 167, 1912.

Du Bois, R., Meinsez, A., Bierhorst-Eijlander, A., Groenewoud, M., Schellekens, P. T. A., and Eijsvoogel, V. P., The use of microtiter plates in mixed lymphocyte cultures, *Tissue Antigens,* 4, 458, 1974.

Elliott, T. R., The control of the suprarenal glands by the splanchnic nerves, *J. Physiol.,* 44, 374, 1912.

Ferkany, J. W., The radioreceptor assay: a simple, sensitive and rapid analytical procedure, *Life Sci.,* 41, 881, 1987.

Feyen, J. H. M., Elford, P., Di Padova, F. E., and Trechsel, U., Interleukin-6 is produced by bone and modulated by parathyroid hormone, *J. Bone Min. Res.,* 4, 633, 1989.

Finney, D. J., *Statistical Method in Biological Assay,* Hafner Press, New York, 1952.

Fleisher, M. R., Glass, D., Bitensky, L., Chayen, J., and Daly, J. R., Plasma corticotrophin levels during insulin-hypoglycaemia: comparison of radioimmunoassay and cytochemical bioassay, *Clin. Endocrinol.,* 3, 203, 1974.

Gaddum, J. H., Simplified mathematics for bioassays, *J. Pharmaceut. Pharm.,* 5, 345, 1953.

Gaddum, J. H., Bioassay procedures, *Pharmacol. Rev.,* 11, 241, 1959.

Gewirtz, G., Schneider, B., Krieger, D. T., and Yalow, R. S., Big ACTH: conversion to biologically active ACTH by trypsin, *J. Clin. Endocrinol. Metab.*, 38, 227, 1974.

Goldstein, A., Aronow, L., Kalman, S. M., *Principles of Drug Action,* John Wiley & Sons, New York, 729, 1974.

Goverde, H. J. M., Gerard, J. P., and Smals, A. G. H., The bioactivity of immunoreactive adrenocorticotrophin in human blood is dependent on the secretory state of the pituitary gland, *Clin. Endocrinol.*, 31, 255, 1989.

Guyton, A. C., *Textbook of Medical Physiology,* 7th ed., W. B. Saunders, Philadelphia, 1986, 909.

Kathol, R. G., Jaeckle, R. S., Lopez, J. F., and Meller, W. H., Pathophysiology of HPA axis abnormalities in patients with major depression: an update, *Am. J. Psychiat.*, 146, 311, 1989.

Kent, G. N. and Zanelli, J. M., Parathyroid hormone, in *Cytochemical Bioassays; Techniques and Clinical Applications,* Chayen, J. and Bitensky, L., Eds, Marcel Dekker, New York, 1983, 255.

Lambert, A., Frost, J., and Robertson, W. R., Preliminary experiences with a bioassay for adrenocorticotrophin (ACTH) in unextracted human plasma using dispersed guinea-pig adrenal cells, *Clin. Endocrinol.*, 21, 33, 1984.

Lambert, A., Frost, J., Ratcliffe, W. A., and Robertson, W. R., On the stability in vitro of bioactive human adrenocorticotrophin in blood and plasma, *Clin. Endocrinol.*, 23, 253, 1985.

Lansdorp, P.M., Aarden, L.A., Calafat, J. and Zeiljemaker, W.P. (1986) A growth-factor dependent B-cell hybridoma. Curr. Top. Microbio. Immunol. 132:105.

Loveridge, N., The techniques of cytochemical bioassays, in *Cytochemical Bioassays; Techniques and Clinical Applications,* Chayen, J. and Bitensky, L., Eds., Marcel Dekker, New York, 1983, 45.

Loveridge, N., Fischer, J. A., Nagant De Deuxchaisnes, C., Dambacher, M. A., Tschopp, F., Werder, E., Devogelaer, J. P., De Meyer, R., Bitensky, L., and Chayen, J., Inhibition of cytochemical bioactivity of parathyroid hormone by plasma in pseudohypoparathyroidism type I, *J. Clin. Endocrinol. Metab.*, 54, 1274, 1982.

Loveridge, N., Kent, G. N., Heath, D. A., and Jones, E. L., Parathyroid hormone-like bioactivity in a patient with severe osteitis fibrosa cystica due to malignancy: renotropic actions of a tumour extract as assessed by cytochemical bioassay, *Clin. Endocrinol.*, 22, 135, 1985.

Loveridge, N., Fischer, J. A., Devogelaer, J. P., and Nagant De Deuxchaisnes, C., Suppression of parathyroid hormone inhibitory activity of plasma in pseudohypoparathyroidism type I by IV calcium, *Clin. Endocrinol.*, 24, 549, 1986a.

Loveridge, N., Tschopp, F., Born, W., Devogelaer, J. P., Nagant De Deuxchaisnes, C., and Fischer, J. A., Separation of inhibitory activity from biologically active parathyroid hormone in patients with pseudohypoparathyroidism type I, *Biochem. Biophys. Acta*, 889, 117, 1986b.

Lowry, P. J., McMartin, C., and Peters, J., Properties of a simplified bioassay for adrenocorticotrophic activity using the steroidogenic response of isolated adrenal cells, *J. Endocrinol.*, 59, 43, 1973.

Matsuyama, H., Harada, G., Ruhmann-Wennhold, A., Nelson, D. H., and West, C. D., A comparison of bioassay and radioimmunoassay for plasma corticotropin in man, *J. Clin. Endocrinol.*, 34, 713, 1972.

Melchers, F. and Andersson, J., Factors controlling the B-cell cycle, *Annu. Rev. Immunol.*, 4, 13, 1986.

Naitoh, Y., Fukata, J., Tominaga, R., Nakai, Y., Tami, S., Mori, K., and Imura, H., Interleukin-6 stimulates the secretion of adrenocorticotropic hormone in conscious freely moving rats, *Biochem. Biophys. Res. Commun.*, 155, 1459, 1988.

Nissenson, R. A., Abbott, S. R., Teitelbaum, A. P., Clark, O. H., and Arnaud, C. D., Endogenous biologically active human parathyroid hormone: measurement by a guanyl nucleotide-amplified renal adenylate cyclase assay, *J. Clin. Endocrinol. Metab.*, 52, 840, 1981.

Parsons, J. A., Reit, B., and Robinson, C. J., A bioassay for parathyroid hormone using chicks, *Endocrinology*, 92, 454, 1973.

Poland, R. E., Hanada, K., and Rubin, R. T., Relationship of nocturnal plasma bioactive and immunoactive ACTH concentrations to cortisol secretion in normal men, *Acta Endocrinol.*, 121, 857, 1989.

Reader, S. C. J, Daly, J. R., and Robertson, W. R., Effect of human plasma on the bioactivity of adrenocorticotropin, *J Endocrinol.*, 92, 449, 1982.

Robertson, W. R., Lambert, A., and Loveridge, N., The role of modern bioassays in clinical endocrinology, *Clin. Endocrinol.,* 27, 259, 1987.

Rosenblatt, M. and Potts, J. T., Design and synthesis of parathyroid hormone analogues of enhanced biological activity, *Endocrinol. Res. Commun.,* 4, 115, 1977.

Sayers, G. and Beall, R. J., Isolated adrenal cortex cells: hypersensitivity to adrenocorticotropic hormone after hypophysectomy, *Science,* 179, 1330, 1973.

Sayers, M. A., Sayers, G., and Woodbury, L. A., The assay of adrenocorticotrophic hormone by the adrenal ascorbic acid-depletion method, *Endocrinology,* 42, 379, 1948.

Schöneshöfer, M. and Fenner, A., ACTH immunoreactivities predominating in normal human plasma are not attributable to the human ACTH 1-39 molecule, *Biochem. Biophys. Res. Commun.,* 102, 476, 1981.

Segre, G. V., Niall, H. D., Habener, J. F., and Potts, J. T., Metabolism of parathyroid hormone, physiologic and clinical significance, *Am. J. Med.,* 56, 774, 1974.

Segre, G. V., Rosenblatt, M., Reiner, B. L., Mahaffey, J. E., and Potts, J. T., Characterization of parathyroid hormone receptors in canine renal cortical plasma membranes using a radioiodinated sulfur-free hormone analogue, *J. Biol. Chem.,* 254, 6980, 1979.

Seshadri, M. S., Chan, Y. L., Wilkinson, M. R., Mason, R. S., and Posen, S., Some problems associated with adenylate cyclase bioassays for parathyroid hormone, *Clin. Sci.,* 68, 311, 1985.

Stewart G. N. and Rogoff, J. M., The action of drugs upon output of epinephrine from the adrenals, *J. Pharmacol.,* 13, 95, 1919.

Strewler, G. J., Williams, R. D., and Nissenson, R. A., Human renal carcinoma cells produce hypercalcemia in the nude mouse and a novel protein recognized by parathyroid hormone receptors, *J. Clin. Invest.,* 71, 769, 1983.

Vane, J. R., Adventures and excursions in bioassay: the stepping stones to prostacyclin, *Br. J. Pharmacol.,* 79, 821, 1983.

Van Snick, J., Vink, A., Uyttenhove, C., Houssiau, F., and Coulie, P., B and T cell responses induced by interleukin-6, *Curr. Top. Microbiol. Immunol.,* 141, 181, 1988.

White, A., Smith, H., Hoadley, M., Dobson, S. H., and Ratcliffe, J. G., Clinical evaluation of a two-site immunoradiometric assay for adrenocorticotrophin in unextracted human plasma using monoclonal antibodies, *Clin. Endocrinol.,* 26, 41, 1987.

WHO Expert Committee on Biological Standardization, 21st Report, WHO Technical Report Series, No. 413, 1969.

WHO Expert Committee on Biological Standardization, 26th Report, WHO Technical Report Series, No. 565, 1975.

WHO Expert Committee on Biological Standardization, 32nd Report, WHO Technical Report Series, No. 673, 1982.

Yalow, R. S. and Berson, S. A., Characteristics of "big ACTH" in human plasma and pituitary extracts, *J. Clin. Endocrinol. Metab.,* 36, 415, 1973.

3

Radioimmunoassay Methods

GARTH BISSETTE AND JAMES C. RITCHIE
Department of Psychiatry
Duke University Medical Center
Durham, North Carolina

I. Introduction

Radioimmunoassays (RIAs) are one of several types of binding assays that have proven invaluable in the investigation of biological mechanisms. Other variations of binding assays include enzyme-linked immunoassays (ELISAs), immunoradiometric assays (IRMAs), and receptor-binding assays, to name just a few. These assays are popular because the specificity of the binding agent allows one to measure the ligand of choice from a mixture of different substances. This is precisely what is required when examining biological fluids and tissues that usually contain a wide array of substances. The ligand to be measured is often at very low concentrations, but present methodology can quantitate femtomolar (10^{-5} M) concentrations of substances routinely and attomolar (10^{-8} M) concentrations are resolvable under optimum conditions. As this range represents only a few thousand molecules, the sensitivity of these assays is quite impressive.

The discovery of neuropeptide transmitters and releasing factors at picomolar to femtomolar concentrations has pushed the development of sensitive and specific radioimmunoassays to near their practical limit. As with most state-of-the-art techniques, however, a certain amount of diligence and rigor is required of those who would effectively employ these methods. This chapter will discuss some of the areas where such skills are crucial to the successful use of binding assays. Although most of the parameters to be discussed display wide ranges of activity in various assays, some general tenets can be made. However, almost all of the generalizations presented here have significant exceptions. As an in-depth treatment of this subject is beyond the scope of this chapter, some general reference works are suggested for both initiates and veterans who wish a more detailed treatise. For the general principles and the operation of RIAs and other binding assays, Chard's book (1982) on laboratory techniques is easy to read and loaded with helpful hints. Although now somewhat dated, one of the best "cookbook" compendiums of specific methodology for various RIAs used in hormone measurement is found in Jaffe and Behrman's *Methods of Hormone Radioimmunoassay* (1979). There are several other useful texts devoted to binding assays currently available as well, but the two mentioned above are a good place to start. Additionally, the recent review by Gosling (1990) is suggested for those readers wishing an overview of the developments in immunoassay methodology during the last 10 years.

The radioimmunoassy technique was developed by Berson and Yalow in 1960, while investigating insulin metabolism, for which Dr. Yalow shared the Nobel Prize in 1977. Since that time this measurement technique has been continually refined, altered, and improved upon to such an extent that in several of its most recent incarnations it might be unrecognizable to its original creators. Development of this technique revolutionized the study of endocrinology and made possible the direct quantitation of minute (10^{-2} to 10^{-5} M) amounts of endogenous and nonendogenous substances in complex biological matrices. This method could truly be considered the "molecular biology" of the 1960s.

RIA technique requires three components: a specific binding substance, a "tagged" analog of the substance to be measured (i.e., a "tagged" ligand), and a precise method of separating tagged ligand that is bound to the binding substance from that which is not bound. Additionally, the matrix in which the assay is performed exerts a large influence on its outcome. Factors such as pH, temperature, ionic strength, incubation time, and other ligands or enzymes in solution all impact on the successful use of this technique.

The binding substance most typically employed in RIA is the antibody, but membrane-bound receptors or circulating binding proteins may also be used. The binding component is usually used in solution but can be bound to a polystyrene bead, an enzyme, or be dried as a coating on the wells of a plastic plate or test tube. The endogenous ligand to be measured is presented to the binder along with a known amount of tagged ligand and a competition for binding sites on the binder results. Conditions are usually manipulated so that the amount of ligand bound allows for the greatest sensitivity of the assay. The amount of tagged ligand bound must then be separated from the unbound tagged ligand, and for this a variety of physicochemical techniques are in use. A radioactive molecule incorporated into the ligand is the most common way of quantifying the amount of "cold" or unlabeled endogenous ligand. The binder can also be labeled, resulting in an immunoradiometric assay (IRMA). By comparing the displacement of the radioactive ligand with known amounts of purified ligand, a standard curve can be constructed that allows extrapolation of the amount of unknown endogenous or "cold" ligand in the biological sample being analyzed.

For standard RIAs the relationship between the amount of tagged ligand bound and the endogenous ligand concentration is inverse and sigmoidal. This has resulted in the development of a wide variety of techniques for data analysis of these assays. The most commonly used today is the log-logit method developed by Rodbard (1974). This method clearly delineates the linear portion of the standard curve (thus setting the usable limits of the assay) as well as controls for the changing activity of the tagged ligand and binder solutions between assays. This method has gained such wide acceptance that it is now routinely included in the software packages available on most gamma and scintillation counters. However, the log-logit method is not perfect and represents a compromise between the computing power available in most laboratories and the exact numerical relationship between bound ligand and endogenous ligand concentration. Methods of immunoassay data analysis continue to be developed and improved as evidenced by the recent introduction of several polynomial curve-fit programs.

The RIA technique in general produces assays with very low within-assay variance (intra-assay variation). Typically this runs between 1 and 5% for most well-characterized assays. Between-assay variance (inter-assay variation) can be the real Achilles' heel of this technique, however. Every effort should be made to keep interassay variance below 10% for the useful range of the standard curve. It cannot be overemphasized that RIAs change with time. Solutions and radioactive tracers change constantly. Incubation temperatures and durations change slightly with each assay. Sample matrix and technicians change over time. Two (nonexclusive) approaches are used to minimize and control assay variations in RIAs. The first is rather straightforward and is simply to run, wherever possible, all the specimens from one study or experiment in a single RIA run. Obviously, if only a single assay run is used in a given experiment the question of interassay variance is moot. Unfortunately, most studies continue over prolonged time spans, and so this is not always possible. Thus, a second system of assay quality control has been developed to track and minimize both intraassay and interassay variance. The system consists of strict monitoring of the standard curve parameters: slope, y intercept, and the 80, 50, and 20% binding points. Monitoring these parameters ensures that a similar standard curve is used for every assay. After several runs, confidence intervals can be constructed for each of these parameters and the subsequent standard curves can be easily evaluated. Additionally, the use of quality control specimens is highly recommended as a part of overall assay quality assurance. These specimens are simply samples of appropriate concentration (usually low, medium, and high) that have been evaluated some time previously and are then included in every subsequent assay run as though they were unknowns. Using the approach stated above for the standard curve, albeit with somewhat different statistical calculations, means and confidence intervals can be readily established for each quality control specimen. In this manner the investigator has an immediate readout as to whether a particular run meets or exceeds the expected variance (both intra- and inter-) for that assay. Plotting these parameters for each assay (although it does nothing inherently to minimize intraassay variation) does seem to improve both intra- and interassay variance simply by making everyone in the laboratory aware of their existence. Additionally, this approach allows one to determine the concentrations in an unknown sample with a measured level of confidence. Using the quality control method outlined above, although cumbersome, is highly recommended as it removes most of the guesswork from the proverbial question, "Is the assay okay?".

While on the subject of assay quality assurance, mention must be made of the other types of controls that are routinely run in assays in our laboratories. These controls are used not so much to help in assay quality assurance, but rather to help evaluate problems when things go awry. The first of these is the nonspecific binding control (NSB). This set of tubes contains everything except binder. For polyclonal antisera, the binder should be replaced with an appropriate dilution of nonimmune sera. For monoclonal antibodies it may be enough to use assay buffer, although an antibody-stripped ascites fluid or appropriately diluted tissue culture fluid is more appropriate. This control is helpful in evaluating the "stickiness" of the tagged ligand for glassware, pipettors, buffer components, etc. It can be especially useful in evaluating homemade trace-labeled ligands and idiotypic binding. We also include an antibody "excess" control (Ab_x) in most of our assays. This control is basically a zero-point tube to which an excess amount of primary antibody is added, usually a 10-fold excess. The Ab_x is helpful in determining the immunoreactivity of the trace-labeled ligand over time, as well as any variations in the assay matrix (i.e., new buffer lots, changes in pH, fresh working dilutions of primary antibody, etc.). Finally, we also advocate the use of total count (TC) controls. These tubes simply contain trace-labeled ligand. They are useful in evaluating whether dilutions of the tracer were made correctly and, if constant dilutions of tracer are made over its lifetime, reflect the detectable activity remaining as the tracer ages. We realize that it is not necessary to include the total counts for assay calculations, but we find that it is a useful control nonetheless.

The sensitivity and accuracy of binding assays are affected by the concentrations of reagents and buffers, incubation times, pH, and temperature as well as the physiochemical characteristics of the binding substance. When beginning to characterize a new assay, ideally all of these parameters should be altered, one at a time, to see if the manipulation enhances or detracts from the performance of the assay. In practice, the prejudices based on previous experiences often determine which initial conditions are tried. An empirical approach is mandatory and can be gradually explored by comparing the performance of a sample with one or another reagent missing with the performance given by the "complete" system. The necessity of occasionally testing the various parameters cannot be overemphasized.

II. Binding Substances

As stated previously, the most commonly used binder in RIAs today is an antibody (either polyclonal or monoclonal). It should be noted, however, that binding proteins or membrane-bound receptors may work just as well. Indeed, some would argue that concentrations of a ligand determined in an assay utilizing the natural receptor for that ligand are more physiologically relevant (approaching a bioassay) than those determined using a highly specific antibody. The importance of this argument rests on the ligand involved and the form it may take in the organism. The pros and cons of this problem with regard to the atrial natriuretic peptides has recently been reported (Capper et al., 1990). The use of a naturally occurring transport or binding protein also has some advantages. It is naturally abundant, modestly specific, and readily available. The prime disadvantage of these binders is their rather low specificity compared to antibodies. If, however, the compound to be measured is in high concentration compared to other reactive compounds, use of the natural binding protein as a binder may be advisable. In fact, one of the author's (J.C.R.) laboratory has used such a method for over 15 years to quantitate total glucocorticoids in rat, human, monkey, and bovine plasma (Murphy, 1967).

It is hoped that the above discussion serves to impress the reader that selection of the appropriate binder is of primary importance in developing a successful RIA. The binder ultimately determines both the specificity and the sensitivity of the assay. The sensitivity of the assay is directly related to the K_A (affinity constant) of the antibody for its ligand.

It is in the above regard that the use of monoclonal antibodies must be considered. A discussion of the production of monoclonal antibodies is beyond the scope of this chapter. For our purposes it is sufficient to know that monoclonal antibodies are produced by a single clone of immunoglobulin-manufacturing cells. Each clone thus produces a single type of immunoglobulin. For example, one clone may express an antibody with immunity toward the peptide adrenocorticotropic hormone $(ACTH)_{1-8}$ while another might produce an antibody against $ACTH_{15-22}$, and so on. As can be seen, this system has the capability to produce antibodies of extremely high specificity. For reasons not completely understood, however, monoclonal antibodies in general seem to have a reduced affinity for their ligands when compared to antisera produced by more traditional polyclonal methods. This lower affinity and its subsequent lowering in assay sensitivity has been one of the primary reasons for the slow conversion of more traditional RIAs to those employing monoclonal antibodies. It has also led directly to the development of the two-site immunoradiometric assay (IRMA). This assay system, which is ideal for the direct measurement of large ligands, is run in the antibody excess condition, thus virtually eliminating the need for high-affinity antibodies. Briefly, the system can be described as follows: a "capture" antibody of known specificity is immobilized on a solid support. This antibody may be either polyclonal or monoclonal, although a monoclonal is inherently preferred. A large excess of this immobilized capture antibody is then incubated with the sample containing the ligand of interest. A second tagged antibody of different specificity is then incubated with the sample. Since the second antibody can attach only where ligand is present and all of the ligand is now bound to the capture antibody, due to the original antibody excess condition, a signal is generated for each molecule of ligand. This assay system has been used successfully to directly quantitate growth hormone, thyroid-stimulating hormone, and ACTH in plasma.

It is important to keep in mind that specificity is a relative term in immunoassays. As described above, antibodies can now be produced that react with only a small portion of a natural ligand (for example, $ACTH_{1-6}$). In fact, *most* antibodies react with only a small portion of their antigen at the combining site. Thus, it is important to remember that an RIA is

Table 1

Amino Acid Sequence of Neurotensin, Neurotensin Fragments, and Xenopsin

Compound	Amino acid sequence													K_{aff}^{a}
	1	2	3	4	5	6	7	8	9	10	11	12	13	
NT_{1-13}	pGlu	Leu	Tyr	Glu	Asn	Lys	Pro	Arg	Arg	Pro	Tyr	Ile	Leu-OH	8.3×10^{9}
NT_{1-6}	pGlu	Leu	Tyr	Glu	Asn	Lys-OH								$\lll 1.2 \times 10^{8}$
NT_{1-8}	pGlu	Leu	Tyr	Glu	Asn	Lys	Pro	Arg-OH						5.0×10^{9}
NT_{1-10}	pGlu	Leu	Tyr	Glu	Asn	Lys	Pro	Arg	Arg	Pro-OH				6.6×10^{9}
NT_{8-13}								Arg	Arg	Pro	Tyr	Ile	Leu-OH	$\lll 1.2 \times 10^{8}$
NT_{9-13}									Arg	Pro	Tyr	Ile	Leu-OH	$\lll 1.2 \times 10^{8}$
Xenopsin						pGlu	Gly	Lys	Arg	Pro	Trp	Ile	Leu-OH	$\lll 1.2 \times 10^{8}$

[a]The K_{aff} value is the reciprocal of the concentration of NT that gives 50% binding to a fixed concentration of primary antiserum and is expressed as liters per mole.

generally not specific for a whole molecule, but rather some portion of that molecule. This is especially germain when considering the measurement of neuropeptides as they may exist in various forms throughout the organism depending on posttranslational processing, differential release of processed peptides, or catalysis. Any characterization of an RIA should, therefore, test the cross-reactivities of similar ligand species in the assay system. If fragments or substituted analogs are available, one may be able to determine the precise amino acid sequence necessary for recognition. An example of this is found in Bissette et al. (1984) for neurotensin (Table 1). Using available fragments and amino acid-substituted analogs, we were able to establish that our antiserum recognized the midportion sequences Lys-Pro-Arg. This allowed testing of other ligands with this sequence and the demonstration that they were not immunoreactive, probably due to tertiary structural differences. Cross-reactivities should also be determined for other ligands likely to be encountered in the specimens even though no direct structural similarity is evident. It is also true, for the above reasons, that binding of a ligand to an antibody cannot be used as positive proof of the identity of the ligand. Other methods [molecular sieving, electrophoresis, high-performance liquid chromatography (HPLC), etc.] must be used to confirm absolutely the identity of such a bound ligand. Additionally, the reader is cautioned that parallelism of dilutions of an unknown cannot be used as conclusive proof of identity for a ligand in an RIA. Whereas nonparallelism is indicative of nonidentity, parallelism by itself proves nothing (Balfe, 1987).

The primary advantages of RIA continue to be its adaptability and the ease with which it can be brought to bear to measure new ligands. Any new ligand that can somehow be made antigenic can theoretically be measured by this technique. The production of polyclonal antisera and monoclonal antibodies is virtually a routine practice in many laboratories today. The following discussion, although not comprehensive, is meant to outline the procedures and pitfalls inherent in these processes. Because the affinity of an antibody for a ligand is determined by the inherent characteristics of the antibody, the amount of antiserum needed to bind a portion of the available ligand varies among different antibody populations. As both monoclonal and polyclonal antisera are originally produced in individual animals, usually several attempts must be made before a good response is obtained. This means several animals must be immunized in the production of polyclonal antisera and several mouse spleen cell lines must be characterized when producing monoclonal antibodies. Notwithstanding a certain amount of luck, several procedures are available that increase the likelihood of success in producing antisera. Foremost of these is the purity and antigenicity of the target ligand or hapten. Obviously, impurities run the risk of being antigenic themselves with subsequent dilutions of the immune response. Additionally, unless performing one's own synthesis it is important to know the company that supplies the antigen. One research group recently reported on the purity of tachykinin peptides from various sources (Brown et al., 1986). They found a disturbing number of inadequacies in quality control. Purification may be improved by recrystallization or chromatography. If the molecular weight of the hapten is less than 10,000 daltons, it will probably not be antigenic enough alone to stimulate a robust immune response. The immune response usually is improved by increasing the size of the antigen, and this is best achieved by conjugation with a larger molecule. Thyroglobulin and hemocyanin, as well as chains of amino acids (polyglutamate), are some of the most popular conjugates for small haptens with limited antigenicity. The hapten is covalently coupled to the carrier by mild chemical reactions. The reaction chosen may allow particular aspects of the hapten to be preferentially oriented for production of antisera with site-directed specificity. Several types of conjugation reactions may be successfully employed, including carbodiimide, glutaraldehyde, diisocyanate, etc. The choice of the reaction is determined by which aspect of the hapten one wants to present to the immune system. For example, if one wants a C-terminally directed antisera, adding succinic acid groups to the carrier molecule and esterification of the carboxylic acid groups on the hapten should allow the C-terminus of the hapten to be presented to the immune system when using the carbodiimide reactions, which couple amino groups of the hapten to carboxyl groups of the carrier via a peptide bond. Depending on the size of the target hapten, even 10 to 20% incorporation of the hapten with the carrier molecule may be sufficient for a good immune response. Incorporation of a small amount of radioactive tracer ligand allows one to easily determine the amount of hapten association with the carrier. The carrier-hapten conjugate is referred to as the immunogen and can be injected into the laboratory animal to produce the polyclonal antibodies or, for monoclonals, the stem cells sought. The species chosen depends on the amount of antisera one needs. For smaller amounts of antisera and limited budgets guinea pigs or rabbits are often used, whereas amounts of antisera sufficient for affinity column use must be produced in sheep or goats or, for monoclonal antibodies, grown in cultures. The dose of immunogen varies with the size of the species, but from 100 μg to 1 mg seems to be the ideal range for rabbit-sized animals. The initial immunogen injection should be given in multiple small volumes (20 to 50 μl) in peripheral tissues with good lymphatic drainage. Freund's adjuvant is usually used for the initial immunization to ensure a robust immune response. For production of monoclonal antibodies this is usually all that is needed. An adequate sample of preimmune serum should also be drawn with which to compare later titers. For polyclonal antisera the titer of antisera should be checked every 1 to 2 weeks and the animal is usually boosted with less than half the initial dose of immunogen after the initial titer begins to drop, or at 4 to 6 weeks if no response is seen to the initial immunization. If the titer does not increase further after the third boost, the animal is usually exsanguinated. Multiple boosts run the risk of drift in specificity. The serum should be tested for titer and specificity at each bleed. Titer is determined as the dilution required to bind a particular portion of the trace ligand presented. The most sensitive RIAs usually use antisera dilutions between 10^3 and 10^5. Assay sensitivity is determined by the amount of tracer bound relative to the endogenous ligand being measured. It is usually defined as the apparent concentration reflected on the standard curve of the mean tracer counts minus two standard deviations when no endogenous ligand is present (i.e., at the zero standard binding point). Most RIAs attempt to use an antisera titer that will bind between 15 and 35% of the trace in the assay tube with no endogenous ligand present. The IC_{50} is the concentration of cold ligand that will displace 50% of the trace bound by a known amount of antisera. This parameter is usually not changeable with normal variations in assay conditions and can be used to normalize assays run with standard curves that have deviated from the benchmark. The IC_{50} of an antiserum should be close to the amount of endogenous ligand encountered in practice, as this is the area of the curve that has the highest precision, due to the relatively large number of counts separating standards on either side of the assay midpoint.

One other point regarding antibodies for RIA must be mentioned. In the last year it has become possible to produce designer antibodies by molecular biology techniques. Using the genome for the constant portion of the IgG molecule researchers have been able to insert customized genes for different variable regions and thus produce functional IgG molecules straight from culture. If this system works at its stated potential it may some day do away with the use of laboratory animals for antibody production as well as the necessity to use ultrapure antigens and their subsequent conjugation into an immunogen. Thus it might be possible, by this technique, to produce an unlimited supply of an ultraspecific, high-affinity antibody directed against virtually any ligand.

III. Tagged Ligands

Radioactive tracers can use a variety of isotopes. The requirements of radioimmunoassay make the use of long-lived, slowly decaying isotopes such as ^{14}C or ^{3}H difficult, although assays using these isotopes are commonly used to measure steroids, etc. ^{125}I is ideally suited, as its relatively short half-life (60 days) and its emission of penetrating gamma radiation allow production of a tracer that can be used for weeks to months. Additionally, direct measurement of decay products can be made. Much higher resolution is possible when using radioactivity as the "tag" than is presently possible with enzyme-linked photometric assays. While many iodinated ligands are available commercially, most laboratories find that substantial quantities of tracer are more economically prepared in the lab. This has the advantage of allowing the use of freshly prepared trace ligand and use of the best immunoreactive fractions of the purified tracer ligand. While there are several published methods of incorporating a radioactive molecule into a ligand, the most commonly employed methods for proteins are the chloramine-T method initially described by Bolton, Hunter, and Greenwood and the equally effective, but more gentle, lactoperoxidase method. Both of these methods generate the ^{125}I-labeled cation, which is electrophilically substituted into the aromatic ring of tyrosyl or histidyl moieties. If these are not present on the native ligand or if they occur in a region that is recognized by the antisera, substituted molecules that incorporate a tyrosyl addition to the N terminus (Tyr^{0}) or first amino acid position (Tyr^{1}) are usually commercially available. Volumes of reagents must be kept to the minimum necessary to assure complete mixing of components. Reaction times for chloramine-T run from 10 to 30 s and are usually stopped by addition of reducing agents, while lactoperoxidase is usually reacted for several minutes and terminated by dilution. Separation of unreacted iodine and unreacted peptide from iodinated peptide is achieved by gel filtration, ion-exchange column chromatography, or HPLC. The use of HPLC requires dedicating the equipment for this purpose, as it will be contaminated by ^{125}I. Since each tyrosine can hold two iodine molecules, separation of mono- from diiodinated ligand may be necessary for maximum assay performance. Most methods to achieve this take advantage of the pK changes that iodination of the tyrosyl residues elicits. Although different peptides can vary extensively, most monoiodinated tyrosines have a pK of 8.5 while diiodinated tyrosines have a pK of 7.0. Thus ion-exchange separations employ a pH above 9.0 to retain both iodinated forms on the column, with a drop of pH to around 8.0 to elute the perferred monoiodinated fraction. When first establishing the required parameters for each peptide, gradient elution is used, but once the specific conditions are registered, stepwise or isocratic elution may give superior results. Once purified, tracer should be stabilized by addition of albumen or other "buffer" proteins and diluted to around two times the initial working concentrations. This minimizes emission degradation of the tracer and allows use across at least a half-life interval. Each fraction with high radioactivity should initially be characterized for immunoreactivity; assessing binding to several concentrations of primary antiserum. Once the fraction of iodinated ligand with the highest immunoreactivity is determined and the titer of primary antiserum that gives the desired signal strength (usually from 15 to 35% of radioactivity added to the assay tube) is resolved, the measurement of unknown samples and the construction of a standard curve are possible.

Sensitivity in RIA is partially related to the specific activity of the tracer employed. In general, the higher the specific activity (i.e., activity per mole of ligand) of the tagged ligand the more sensitive the assay. This would seem intuitive in that a larger signal [i.e., higher counts per million (cpms)] would be generated given the same competition between "cold" and tagged ligand. In practice, however, high specific activity tracers are usually less immunoreactive and undergo much more radiolysis than do lower specific activity tagged ligands. Thus, an empirical approach in selecting initially which tracer fraction to use in the assay is fully justified. This is also one of the reasons γ-emitting tracers are preferred over their β-decaying analogs, since tritiated and ^{14}C tracers generally lack high specific activity.

The amount of time that the endogenous ligand and trace is exposed to the primary antiserum can substantially affect the performance of an assay. Equilibrium assays allow the endogenous ligand and tracer to compete for binding sites after simultaneous addition to the primary antiserum and are most often employed when maximal sensitivity is not required. The incubation of endogenous ligand with the primary antiserum for a period of time before addition of trace and relatively rapid addition of second antibody to terminate the reaction is designated a displacement or saturation assay and usually possesses greater sensitivity than an equilibrium assay. It is important to use the same design and time intervals when characterizing trace ligands as are used in the actual assay. If tracer is characterized under equilibrium conditions and the assay is performed with displacement intervals, the amount of binding expected based on the characterization assay will be significantly reduced under displacement conditions. While the optional time intervals vary from assay to assay, diminishing returns are apparent after around 5 days, so most assays are performed under this time period. A typical equilibrium assay will have tracer and endogenous ligand compete for 24 hr before addition of second antibody for another 24 hr and separation of bound from free radioactivity on the third day. A typical displacement assay permits endogenous ligand to bind to the primary antisera for 12 to 24 hr preceding the addition of trace and incubation for 6 to 8 hr followed by second antibody for another 2- to 24-hr incubation. The optimization of the above time intervals is best determined by experimentally deriving the affinity constants (K_A) for each of the involved ligands, using self-displacement assays. Once the K_A values for each ligand and its concentration in the assay are known, it is relatively easy to choose the optimum incubation time for each reaction to achieve equilibrium or linearity. This information is also helpful to know since most tagged ligands do not possess exactly the same affinity for the antibody as do their untagged analogs.

Currently, immunoassays employing radioactive tracers are the most sensitive methods for quantitating most endogenous ligands. Many other tagging strategies have been proposed and attempted. None, however, has been able to match the radioactive tag for ease of labeling and sensitivity. Recently, enhanced chemiluminescence assays using europium chelates as tags have begun to appear. These assays are said to be more sensitive than comparable RIAs. Sensitivities of 0.001 IU/ml have been reported for human thyroid-stimulating hormone (TSH). Additionally, one company (Pharmacia, Inc., Uppsala, Sweden) has made the tag available for in-house assay development. Only time will tell whether this new label approaches or exceeds the usefulness of the radioactive tag. For now, radioactive-tagged ligands remain the ligands of choice for assays of highest sensitivity.

IV. Separation Strategies

Separation of bound radioactive ligand from free, unbound trace is accomplished by a variety of physicochemical methods. While talc or charcoal precipitation gives adequate sensitivity for substances in picomolar or greater concentrations, the use of a second, species-specific antiserum or staphylococcyl membranes is preferred when maximum sensitivity is required. Using this technique a second antibody, directed against the IgG of the species in which the primary antibody was produced, is incubated with the products of the primary RIA reaction and a fixed amount of normal, non-immune serum homologous with the primary antibody. The precipitate produced by this second reaction contains, among other things, tagged ligand bound to the primary antibody. Virtually no free tagged ligand is precipitated by this method. This results in a clean separation of bound from free ligand. The precipitate is centrifuged to the bottom of the tube and the supernatant, containing the free tagged ligand, is decanted or aspirated away. The precipitate can then be quantitated in a radioactivity counter.

When using a second antibody method, the amount of second antibody should be titrated to concentrations that precipitate maximal amounts of primary antibody-trace complex. Because binding is sensitive to temperature, all manipulations should take place in a thermally stable environment, usually at 4°C. Additionally, the amount of added non-immune serum should be kept to a minimum to limit nonspecific interactions. The timing of the addition of this serum is a subject of much debate and may be assay specific. Some researchers prefer to add this as buffer component at the initiation of the assay. Others prefer to add it directly before the addition of second antibody. Either approach may work and theoretically neither has any particular advantage. If the normal, non-immune serum is added as a buffer component, however, it does save one pipetting step.

Separation of bound and free ligand has been one of the major drawbacks in using β particle-emitting tracers (i.e., ^{3}H or ^{14}C). Pellets produced by the second antibody precipitation method cannot be counted directly in a scintillation counter, as they are insoluble in most scintillants. Thus, to use these tracers investigators must either resolubilize the precipitate containing the bound ligand or count the free portion of the reaction. Resolubilization is messy and time consuming and counting of the free component of the assay is inherently less accurate. Thus, wherever possible, γ-emitting tracers have been used. Within the last year, Amersham, Inc. has introduced several scintillation proximity reagents to overcome this problem. These reagents consist of a second antibody covalently linked to a large microsphere that contains an immobilized scintillant. The primary antibody-ligand complex is captured by the second antibody and held in close proximity to the scintillant. Counting is thus accomplished without the addition of an organic-based scintillation cocktail. This approach holds great potential for expanding the kinds of tagged ligands that can be routinely used and therefore the number of compounds that can be quantitated by RIA.

Another strategy for the separation of bound from free ligand is solid-phase technology. This approach solves the problem of getting a clean separation by immobilizing either the primary or the second antibody onto a solid surface (most often on a bead or the wall of a test tube). Unbound reactants are then simply washed away and the bead or tube counted. Of the two approaches, immobilization of the primary antibody is preferred, as it eliminates the use of a second costly reagent and a second incubation. Several methods are available to accomplish this binding; however, the use of the biotin-avidin complex seems to be preferred due to its ease and high avidity. Regardless of which method is used, one must be careful to ensure a uniform coating of the solid-phase surface with the antibody. Fluctuations in the amount of antibody immobilized may have disastrous consequences for the assay. Most commercially available RIAs today employ solid-phase technology to one extent or another.

V. Standard Curves and Matrix Effects

The standard curve is usually prepared using pure synthetic ligand or ligand fragments that are contained in the immunoreactive sequence of the compound being measured. Because most proteins and peptides are usually prepared as lyophilized extracts that can contain up to 20% water by weight, the amount of substance weighed out may not truly represent the amount of immunoreactive ligand present. If water content is known, correction can be made, otherwise one must depend on the accuracy of the source company in supplying the amount in the container that is specified on the label. Variations among batches of standards can be detected if one has a good idea of the IC_{50} of the antiserum and can be calculated using displacement of tracer by cold ligand in a series of standard curves. This procedure should also be performed with a synthetic ligand of one lot number with as great a purity and with as much analytic information as is commercially available. A single dilution of this reference standard should be prepared and aliquoted into separate, nonabsorptive tubes in amounts needed for one standard curve and kept deep frozen. Usually a minimum of 30 separate standard curves employing at least 10 separate batches of tracer should be used in calculating the IC_{50}. Once this is known it is usually possible to use less stringently characterized standard preparations that may be much more economical.

There are two schools of thought regarding construction of standard curves. Many laboratories successfully employ serial dilution of an initially concentrated (mg/ml) solution. The danger is that an initial error is often magnified greatly as one proceeds through the series of dilutions. The alternative, diluting an initial concentration to very high volumes to give the small concentrations needed for the sensitive end of the curve, also has caveats. These include the difficulty of thoroughly mixing small additions to large volumes, leading to sampling errors, and the increased amount of standard required with the associated expense. As many synthetic peptides, e.g., corticotropin-releasing factor (CRF), cost as much as $400/mg, such cost considerations may not be trivial. Volumes of less than 5 µl are difficult to measure accurately and are quite irreproducible below 0.5 µl. With concentration and great care serial dilutions can be quite reproducible and the interassay variance can be held within 10%. This is adequate for most applications across significant periods of time. When measuring small biological samples with marginal amounts of endogenous ligand and when preparing standard solutions with low (picogram) concentrations, nonspecific absorption to surfaces can often be a significant limitation to preparation of reproducible solutions. Coating with gelatin or albumin or siliconizing glass surfaces is often necessary when making such dilute solutions, along with rapid preparation and use to minimize time for absorption. Nonspecific absorption is also a problem for the antiserum when used in dilutions above 1:5000. Experience has taught us to begin adding primary antiserum to the high-concentration end of the standard curve for the first volume of antiserum used in the dispenser. On refilling the dispenser, any nonspecific binding has already occupied the binding sites and the amount of antiserum delivered to the critical reference or zero-concentration tube is representative of what will be applied to the rest of the unknown sample tubes. These precautions greatly increase both the reliability and reproducibility of a series of RIAs.

Every effort should be made to have the matrix in which the standards are dissolved mimic as closely as possible the samples that are being analyzed. Matrix effects have been shown to be extremely important in RIA. Often these effects have been responsible for errors of one order of magnitude in calculated ligand concentrations. It is not simply enough to dissolve standards in a physiologic buffer solution and compare unknowns (often in complex biologic matrices) with them. Ideally, the normal biologic matrix devoid of the compound of interest is the perfect vehicle in which to prepare standards. The "stripped" matrix can be prepared either by physical stripping with chemically inert agents (i.e., charcoal, glass beads, etc.) or if the compound of interest is labile by simply incubating the matrix for several days at physiologic temperatures. Both approaches have their advantages and drawbacks. Physical stripping often alters the matrix and physiologic stripping often does not completely eliminate the endogenous ligand. Both methods have been used successfully with various ligands, however.

Often the matrix is not available in sufficient quantity to undergo the stripping process. This is especially true for many of the matrices of interest to neuroscientists. Cerebrospinal fluid (CSF) and brain homogenates are not normally available in large quantities. For this type of specimen the approach is to construct a purely synthetic matrix that duplicates the naturally occurring one. Thus one can find several references to synthetic CSF in the neuropeptide RIA literature. This approach, though a compromise to some extent, has proven quite successful, but is inherently limited to the less complex biologic matrices.

Matrix effects sometimes are so complex that they are not easily overcome. When the compound of interest exists at very low concentrations or is very labile and is in an extremely complex biologic matrix, accurate determination often cannot be made using a direct RIA. Where this occurs (as often happens with the measurement of peptides in plasma), extraction of the compound of interest may be the only option. Many extraction methods are available, depending on the compounds of interest (e.g., siliac acid, phase separation, extraction cartridges), and we will not attempt their elucidation in any detail. Suffice it to say that any extraction method must be specific, must not damage the ligand, must allow for determination of extraction efficiency, or must be performed on standards as well as samples (otherwise another level of matrix problems might be encountered). Although cumbersome, extracted RIAs often provide the most accurate determinations of ligand concentrations.

VI. Conclusion

RIA is currently *the* most accurate and cost-effective method of quantifying many compounds (both endogenous and exogenous). While demanding total concentration during a few critical phases, these assays can be made to perform with the accuracy required to measure picogram amounts routinely and subpicogram amounts under optimum conditions. Because of their unique properties, RIA will remain one of the primary methods to quantify biological substances into the foreseeable future.

References

Balfe, A., Parallelism of dilution curves in radioimmunoassay, *Clin. Chem.*, 33, No. 12, 2320, 1987.

Bissette, G., Richardson, C., Kizer, J. S., and Nemeroff, C. B., Ontogeny of brain neurotensin in the rat: a radioimmunoassay study, *J. Neurochem.*, 43, 283, 1984.

Bolton, A. E. and Hunter, A. M., The labeling of proteins of high specific radioactivities by conjugation to a ^{125}I-containing acylating agent, *Biochem. J.*, 133, 529, 1973.

Brown, J. R., Hunter, J. C., Jordan, C. C., Tyers, M. B., Ward, P., and Whittington, A. R., Problems with peptides — all that glitters is not gold, *Trends Neurosci.*, 9, 100, 1986.

Bryant, M. G., Radioactive labelling, in *Radioimmunoassay of Gut Regulatory Peptides,* Bloom, S. R. and Long, R. G., Eds., Praeger, New York, 1982, 21.

Capper, S. J., Smith, S. W., Spensley, C. A., Whateley, J. G., Specificities compared for a radioreceptor assay and a radioimmunoassay of atrial natriuretic peptide, *Clin. Chem.,* 36, No. 4, 656, 1990.

Carraway, R. E., Neurotensin and related substances, in *Methods of Hormone Radioimmunoassay,* Jaffe, B. M. and Behrman, H. R., Eds., Academic Press, New York, 1979, 139.

Chard, T., *An Introduction to Radioimmunoassay and Related Techniques,* Work, T. S. and Work, E., Eds., Elsevier Biomedical Press, Amsterdam, 1982.

Gosling, J. P., A decade of development in immunoassay methodology, *Clin. Chem.,* 36, No. 8, 1408, 1990.

Hunter, W. M. and Greenwood, F. C., Preparation of iodine-131 labeled human growth hormone of high specific activity, *Nature (London),* 194, 495, 1962.

Jaffe, M. J. and Behrman, H. R., *Methods of Hormone Radioimmunoassay,* Academic Press, New York, 1979.

Murphy, B. E. P., Some studies on the protein-binding of steroids and their application to the routine micro and ultramicro measurement of various steroids in body fluids by competitive protein-binding radioassay, *J. Clin. Endocrinol.,* 27, 973, 1967.

Rodbard, D., Statistical quality control and routine date processing for radioimmunoassays and immunoradiometric assays, *Clin. Chem.,* 20, No. 10, 1255, 1974.

Yalow, R. S. and Berson, S. A., Immunoassay of endogenous plasma insulin in man, *J. Clin. Invest.,* 39, 1157, 1960.

4

Electrochemical Detection: Applications in Neuroendocrinology

CLINTON D. KILTS
Departments of Psychiatry and Pharmacology
Duke University Medical Center
Durham, North Carolina

The field of neuroendocrinology focuses on the regulation of endocrine systems by the central nervous system (CNS). In the CNS the hypothalamus is regarded as the center for integrating the complex influence of neurotransmitters on the synthesis and release of hormones or their releasing factors. Such neurotransmitters convey the distinct information from forebrain, midbrain, and hindbrain regions and function as important elements in the feedback regulation of endocrine systems and the influence of hormones on the function of the CNS. The anatomical and functional organization of neurotransmitter-containing neurons of the hypothalamus has been an area of intense investigation in the last 20 years. The findings obtained have defined the relationship between neural and endocrine systems and have come far in identifying the substrates of the effects of drugs and of the pathophysiology of hormonal systems.

The tools and techniques that have led this field are many and diverse. The elegant application of immunocytochemistry by Swanson and colleagues (e.g., Swanson et al., 1981) has defined the origin, course, and termination of hypothalamic cells that contain releasing factors or hormones. Radioimmunoassays of releasing factors and hormones (see Chapter 3) have been instrumental in profiling the rhythms characteristic of their release, probing the neurotransmitters responsible for their regulation and defining their neurochemical anatomy. This chapter will review the past and present impact of high-performance liquid chromatography (HPLC), particularly in its combination with electrochemical (EC) detection, on the field of neuroendocrinology. The combination of HPLC and EC is ideally suited to the separation and detection of relatively low molecular weight electroactive neurochemicals such as catecholamines and indoleamines and their metabolites, although other neurotransmitters as well as neuropeptides are amenable to quantitative assay by HPLC-EC. Before discussing specific applications of HPLC-EC to neuroendocrinology, a general discussion of the mechanisms mediating HPLC separation and EC detection is prudent.

I. Fundamental Theories of Operation of HPLC and EC

A. HPLC Separation

The force behind the immense separation power of HPLC is the resin, which is packed under positive pressure into rigid columns, typically stainless steel, of varying internal diameter and length. Resins are grouped into two general categories. Normal-phase resins consist of microparticulate silica differing in shape (usually spherical or irregular) and diameter (usually 3, 5, or 10 μm). Mobile phases used in normal-phase HPLC provide a medium for delivery of analytes for interaction with the resin and are typically mixtures of organic solvents such as methanol, acetonitrile, and tetrahydrofuran. In principle, analytes are separated by their relative affinity for the siloxyl groups of the resin, with the most polar analytes eluting last. The poor electroconductivity of the mobile phases renders normal-phase HPLC an incompatible combination with EC detection.

The second category, bonded-phase resins, consists of a large family of distinct functionalities bonded via silyl ether linkages to microparticulate silica of differing shape and diameter. While some bonded phases, such as cyano and amino groups, exhibit properties of normal-phase resins, the most commonly used functionalities are alkyl hydrocarbons of varying numbers of carbon atoms. Methyl and octyl groups are often used, while octyldecyl-bonded silica represents the most commonly employed bonded-phase resin for neurobiological research. For the nonpolar bonded phases, the most nonpolar analytes elute last. This reverse order of elution compared to normal-phase HPLC led to the description of alkyl hydrocarbon bonded-phase HPLC as reverse-phase HPLC. Additional bonded phases include cyano-, phenyl-, or protein A-bonded silica, the latter of particular use in the purification of immunoglobulins used for radioimmunoassays. Mobile phases used in alkyl hydrocarbon bonded-phase HPLC play a more dynamic role in analyte retention and separation compared to normal-phase resins and are typically aqueous buffers to which modifiers are added.

Using octyldecyl (C_{18})-bonded silica as an example, the following illustrates the dynamic contribution of the mobile phase to the relative retention and separation of analytes. This contribution represents the source of the remarkable power of separation of this form of HPLC. Relevant physicochemical properties of analytes include the net hydrophobicity, ionogenic characteristics, and nature of the charge for ionogenic analytes. The relevant properties of the mobile phase include the buffered pH (relative to the pK_a values of the analytes of interest), the type and amount of miscible organic solvents, and the presence of ion-pairing reagents of a fixed charge. For a hydrophobic analyte, the aqueous character of the mobile phase exerts a driving force that extrudes the analyte toward the nonpolar bonded C_{18} groups and thus increases its retention time. This force is decreased nonselectively by the addition to the mobile phase of organic solvents (modifiers) that enhance the affinity of the analyte for the mobile phase and thus decrease its retention time. The degree of ionization of ionogenic analytes (and hence their polarity) can often be adjusted by changes in mobile-phase pH relative to their pK_a values. This strategy can be particularly useful in chromatographically resolving analytes of differing acid-base properties (Kilts et al., 1981), in suppressing the ionization of functionalities such as carboxylate anions (e.g., DOPA; Kilts and Anderson, 1987), and in increasing analyte ionization to promote the interaction with ion-pairing reagents. The addition to mobile phases of ion-pairing reagents such as the alkylsulfonates and quaternary tetraalkylammonium compounds has proven to be an effective means for increasing the HPLC retention of positively and negatively charged analytes, respectively (Moyer and Jiang, 1978). The increase in HPLC retention presumably results from the chromatography of more nonpolar analyte-ion pair reagent complexes and the dynamic ion-exchange properties of the resin imparted by the intercalation of the hydrophobic alkyl functionalities of the ion pair reagent within the C_{18} groups of the resin. The crown ethers represent additional, valuable complexing reagents that, due to their cavity dimensions, limit complex formation to particular analyte properties (Nakagawa et al., 1983; Kilts et al., 1984).

B. EC Detection

Few, if any, analytical techniques have had the impact on the field of neurochemistry that the combination of HPLC and EC detection has had. HPLC-EC has essentially placed the sensitivity and specificity of gas chromatography/mass spectrometry (GC/MS) into the hands of many neurochemists for a fraction of the cost and instrumentation complexity.

In principle, EC detectors measure the minute (nanoampere) currents generated by electrons resulting from electrochemical reactions (oxidation or reduction) at electrodes maintained at fixed potentials (amperometry). These amperometric EC detectors for HPLC have been largely of two designs, which differ primarily in their electrode surface area and hence percentage of eluting analyte that is electrolyzed (low in conventional amperometric and high in coulometric electrodes). The functions of both types of EC detectors are indirectly or directly based on Faraday's law and are of a three-electrode design consisting of a working, reference, and current sensing electrode. While claims of superior sensitivity of analyte detection have been made for coulometric detectors, practical experience indicates that both types of detectors offer comparable levels of detection. The advantage of coulometric electrodes having a high efficiency of electrolysis resides in their use in series-configured multiple-electrode EC detectors; low-efficiency electrodes may be effectively used in parallel configurations with the signal from one electrode subtracted from that of the other (Kilts et al., 1992). High-efficiency electrolysis detectors permit significant improvements in assay specificity by the simultaneous application of oxidative and reductive potentials or different oxidative potentials to each of the working electrodes. In such applications, the reductive/oxidative EC reactions in many instances unique to the analyte of interest are exploited by applying potentials yielding maximal reactions in either an oxidation-reduction or reduction-oxidation mode (e.g., Hall et al., 1988). The distinction between analytes in ease of EC oxidation may also be exploited by using a lower potential applied to an upstream electrode to minimize signals detected at the downstream monitored electrode to simplify chromatograms (e.g., Kilpatrick et al., 1986). Both techniques of multiple-electrode EC detection enhance assay specificity by optimizing the conditions of detection for the specific EC properties of an analyte or class of analytes.

II. Applications of HPLC-EC to Neuroendocrinology

This section will focus on the applications of HPLC-EC to the "neuro" aspects of the field of neuroendocrinology. The mechanisms of operation of HPLC and EC detection discussed in the previous section will be integrated into specific applications focusing on the neurochemical anatomy of neurotransmitter systems in the rat hypothalamus and on the determination of the dynamics of such systems. The hypothalamus is not a homogeneous structure but rather represents an aggregate of biochemically, cytologically, hodologically, and functionally distinct nuclei or areas (Saper, 1990; Figure 1). Meaningful study of the functional roles of neurotransmitters in the hypothalamus must be conducted at a corresponding level of anatomical resolution.

A. Neurochemical Anatomy of the Rat Hypothalamus

The sensitivity and specificity of the combination of HPLC and EC detection are well suited to the task of mapping the quantitative distribution of neurotransmitters in the rat hypothalamus. Of the classical neurotransmitters the catecholamines norepinephrine, epineph-

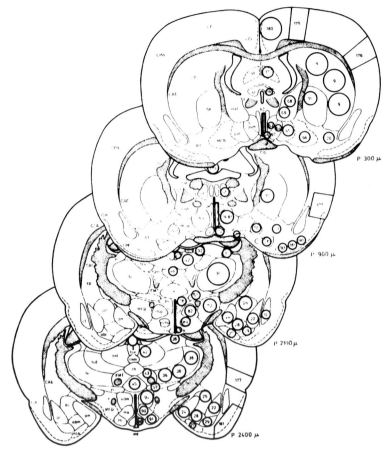

Figure 1. Schematic illustration of the component nuclei and areas of the hypothalamus of the rat visualized in the coronal plane. The selected sections were reorganized from the atlas of Palkovits (1980) in an anterior to posterior (distance posterior to bregma indicated in micrometers in lower right of each section) format. Relevant abbreviations are as follow: pom, medial preoptic nucleus; pol, lateral preoptic nucleus; nsc, suprachiasmatic nucleus; nso, supraoptic nucleus; npe, periventricular nucleus; nha, anterior hypothalamic nucleus; na, arcuate nucleus; npv, paraventricular nucleus; me, median eminence; ndm, dorsomedial nucleus; ac, central amygdaloid nucleus.

rine, and dopamine are thought to play the most significant role in the hypothalamus in regulating pituitary-endocrine target organ function (Axelrod and Reisine, 1984). The distribution of norepinephrine, epinephrine, and dopamine in the component nuclei of the rat hypothalamus is illustrated in Table 1. Catecholamine concentrations in selected nonhypothalamic nuclei are included for comparison. Hypothalamic nuclei or areas were micropunch dissected from frozen, 300-μm thick coronal sections of the rat brain (Palkovits, 1973). The vicinyl diols of the catechol ring were utilized in their solid-phase extraction using aluminum oxide and EC detection. On-line trace-enrichment HPLC on a short cation-exchange enrichment column (Kilts et al., 1984; Kilts and Anderson, 1987) prior to assay by HPLC-EC was employed to purify and enrich the samples. This technique (diagramatically outlined in Figure 2) eliminates negatively charged or uncharged compounds and was designed and incorporated to address the axiom (my own) that in HPLC-EC (and other) assays, the challenge often lies not in detecting what you want to detect, but in not detecting what you don't want to detect. Typical chromatograms of catecholamines in the micropunch-dissected medial and central nuclei of the rat

Table 1
Catecholamine Distribution in the Rat Hypothalamus[a]

Nuclei or area	Norepinephrine	Epinephrine	Dopamine
Arcuate	21.5 ± 0.80	0.73 ± 0.06	11.4 ± 1.9
Median eminence	21.5 ± 1.3	1.6 ± 0.11	78.4 ± 7.7
Paraventricular			
Parvocellular	52.2 ± 4.1	3.1 ± 0.27	4.8 ± 0.6
Magnocellular	22.3 ± 2.6	0.91 ± 0.11	2.4 ± 0.3
Periventricular	26.3 ± 2.5	0.78 ± 0.06	3.4 ± 0.51
Dorsomedial	33.9 ± 2.7	0.90 ± 0.06	1.6 ± 0.21
Ventromedial	12.9 ± 0.90	0.27 ± 0.02	1.7 ± 0.10
Medial preoptic	23.8 ± 2.2	0.98 ± 0.18	3.4 ± 0.68
Lateral preoptic	16.3 ± 2.1	nd[b]	1.7 ± 0.18
Anterior	10.0 ± 0.79	nd	1.6 ± 0.07
Lateral	14.7 ± 1.0	0.46 ± 0.03	0.63 ± 0.10
Supraoptic	13.0 ± 1.1	0.23 ± 0.03	1.4 ± 0.08
Suprachiasmatic	14.5 ± 2.1	0.41 ± 0.04	2.2 ± 0.21
Central amygdaloid	6.7 ± 0.39	0.17 ± 0.04	20.2 ± 1.6
Bed nucleus of the stria terminalis (infracommissural)	67.4 ± 3.4	0.35 ± 0.40	1.9 ± 0.18
Locus coeruleus	20.6 ± 1.3	0.13 ± 0.01	2.5 ± 0.59

[a]Values represent the mean ± SEM of four to eight determinations expressed as nanograms catecholamine per milligram protein.
[b]nd, Not detectable (<10 pg/sample).

amygdaloid complex obtained by on-line trace-enrichment HPLC-EC are illustrated in Figure 3.

The results of this mapping study indicate a rich innervation of the hypothalamus by norepinephrine-containing neurons, with the density varying widely between its component nuclei. The density is highest in the parvocellular subdivision of the paraventricular nucleus. Although quantitatively minor in comparison to norepinephrine, epinephrine is present in detectable concentrations in the hypothalamic nuclei, with the highest concentrations present in the parvocellular subdivision of the paraventricular nucleus. The localization of norepinephrine and epinephrine in the parvocellular subdivision of the paraventricular hypothalamic nucleus is concordant with the density of noradrenergic and adrenergic fibers innervating this hypothalamic subnucleus as defined by immunocytochemical techniques (Moore and Card, 1984; Hokfelt et al., 1984) and the important functional roles played by these neurotransmitters in the regulation of corticotropin-releasing factor (CRF)-containing cells in this hypothalamic subnucleus (Szafarczyk et al., 1987). The localization of dopamine in the arcuate nucleus and especially the median eminence reflects the localization of the cell bodies and terminals of the tuberoinfundibular dopamine system, which regulates the synthesis and secretion of prolactin by the anterior pituitary (Moore, 1987). If, indeed, the anatomical distribution of catecholamines in the rat hypothalamus reflects their functional organization (as suggested by the examples discussed above), then these results reinforce the concept that a given catecholamine exerts a focal, nuclei-variable influence on the endocrine and other functions (e.g., clock) of the hypothalamus.

B. Dynamics of Epinephrine-Containing Neurons Innervating Discrete Hypothalamic Nuclei: Focal Role in Regulation of the HPA Axis

The following is an example of the utility of HPLC-EC as a means of examining the

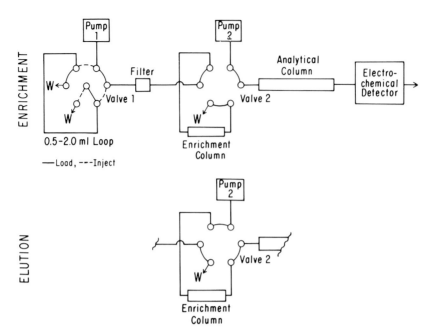

Figure 2. Schematic diagram of the orientation of the components of an on-line trace-enrichment HPLC-EC system and the direction of flow of both mobile phases during catecholamine enrichment and back elution. W, Waste reservoirs.

dynamics and functional role of a neurotransmitter, in this case epinephrine, in mediating at a hypothalamic level the regulation of a neuroendocrine axis. Although a quantitatively minor catecholamine, epinephrine-containing neurons innervating the paraventricular hypothalamic nuclei originating from medullary cell bodies may be a major determinant of the activity of CRF-containing neurons in the parvocellular subdivision of the paraventricular nucleus. Evidence in support of this contention includes anatomical evidence indicating that phenylethanolamine-*N*-methyltransferase (PNMT)-immunopositive (adrenergic) nerve terminals make direct synaptic contacts with the dense CRF-immunopositive cells in this hypothalamic subnucleus (Swanson et al., 1981; Liposits et al., 1986) and functional/pharmacological evidence indicating that the microinjection of epinephrine into the cerebral ventricles or the vicinity of the paraventricular nucleus results in a robust increase in the plasma concentration of ACTH (Szafarczyk et al., 1987). In an attempt to more clearly define a causal relationship between the adrenergic innervation of the paraventricular hypothalamic nucleus and the activity of CRF-containing neurons emanating from the paraventricular nucleus, the firing rate of epinephrine-containing neurons was biochemically estimated under conditions of increased and decreased activity of the CRF-containing neurons. The paraventricular nucleus was micropunch dissected from animals sacrificed 90 min following administration of the PNMT inhibitor LY 134046 (Fuller et al., 1981). The epinephrine content was determined by on-line trace-enrichment HPLC-EC detection (Kilts and Anderson, 1987).

The administration of LY 134046 induced a monoexponential decline in the concentration of epinephrine in the paraventricular nucleus (Figure 4). The fractional rate constant (k) of epinephrine depletion (turnover rate) calculated from the slope of the data illustrated in Figure 4 was -0.278 hr^{-1}. This value indicates that this population of epinephrine-containing neurons has an estimated firing rate that is slower than that of the majority of mesotelencephalic dopamine neurons and similar to that of noradrenergic neurons (Kilts and Anderson, 1987).

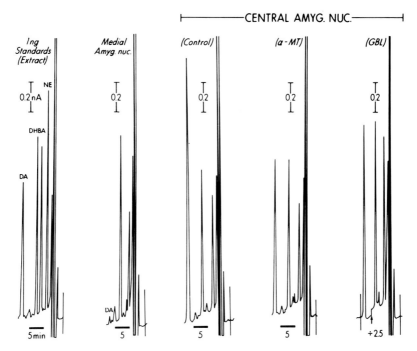

Figure 3. Chromatograms of a calibration curve point and extracts of the micropunch-dissected medial and central amygdaloid nuclei generated by on-line trace-enrichment HPLC-EC assays. The effects of tyrosine hydroxylase inhibition by α-methyltyrosine (α-MT) and the anesthetic γ-butyrolactone (GBL) are illustrated.

Disinhibition of CRF-containing neurons in the paraventricular nucleus 48 hr following bilateral adrenalectomy was associated with a significant increase in the extent of LY 134046-induced depletion of epinephrine in the paraventricular hypothalamic nucleus (Figure 5). This effect of adrenalectomy was completely reversed by the subcutaneous implantation of corticosterone pellets at the time of surgery. These results indicate a covarying activity of epinephrine neurons innervating the paraventricular nucleus and its emanating CRF-containing cells, though it is unclear from this experiment whether epinephrine neurons drive CRF cells or vice versa.

A second experiment also utilizing HPLC-EC and PNMT inhibition examined the estimated activity of epinephrine neurons innervating the paraventricular nucleus under the opposite state of hypothalamus-pituitary-adrenocorticotropin (HPA) axis activity — the inhibition induced by administration of dexamethasone. In contrast to the first experiment, which was conducted between 0930 and 1130 hr, the second experiment was performed between 1700 and 1900 hr, when HPA axis activity attains a maximum in its circadian rhythm (De Boer and Van der Gugten, 1987). Two findings of this experiment are noteworthy. First, the extent of the LY 134046-induced depletion of epinephrine in the paraventricular nucleus observed in the late afternoon was greater than that observed in the morning (Figure 5). These results

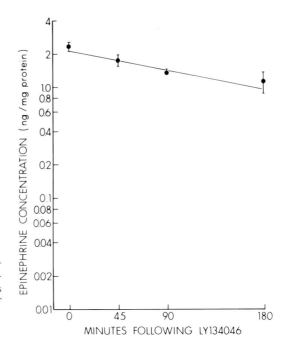

Figure 4. Semilogarithmic plot of the concentration of epinephrine in the parvocellular subdivision of the paraventricular hypothalamic nucleus vs. time following administration of the PNMT inhibitor LY 134046.

indicate that the activity of adrenergic neurons innervating the paraventricular nucleus fluctuates with the physiological rhythm of the HPA axis. Second, in contrast to the effect of adrenalectomy, the dexamethasone-induced inhibition of the HPA axis was associated with a *decrease* in the extent of LY 134046-induced depletion of epinephrine in the paraventricular nucleus.

Collectively, these data support an intimate functional relationship between the adrenergic innervation of the parvocellular subdivision of the paraventricular nucleus of the hypothalamus and the CRF-containing neurons that emanate from this subnucleus and represent the apex of the HPA regulatory cascade. These findings also indicate that these adrenergic neurons exert a *facilitory* influence on the activity of CRF-containing cells. It is important to note that this combination of HPLC-EC and PNMT inhibition affords an understanding of the focal relationship between epinephrine-containing and CRF-containing neurons in the paraventricular hypothalamic nucleus that cannot be probed by approaches such as receptor pharmacology, *in vivo* voltammetry, or microdialysis and thus illustrates an invaluable contribution of HPLC-EC to neuroendocrinology.

C. Dynamics of Hypothalamic Noradrenergic and Adrenergic Neurons: Microdialysis/HPLC-EC

The promise and ability of intracerebral microdialysis to determine the neuronal release of neurotransmitters is inextricably linked to the use of HPLC-EC to quantitate catecholamines and other neurotransmitters in the dialysates. Several recent reports have studied the dynamics of noradrenergic and adrenergic neurons in the hypothalamus using microdialysis/HPLC-EC. Routledge and Marsden (1987) examined the basal and experimentally altered concentrations of epinephrine and norepinephrine in the extracellular fluid of the posterior hypothalamus. Using HPLC-EC assays of dialysates, these authors demonstrated that PNMT inhibition and electrical stimulation of the medullary C_1 adrenergic cell bodies resulted in significant decreases and increases, respectively, in the extracellular concentration of epinephrine. The

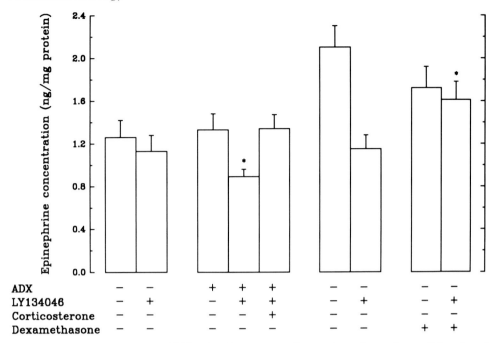

Figure 5. Effects of adrenalectomy (ADX) and corticosterone supplementation or dexamethasone (0.1 mg/kg, sc) administration (150 min prior to sacrifice) on the LY 134046-induced decrease in the epinephrine concentration of the paraventricular hypothalamic nucleus.

extracellular hypothalamic concentration of norepinephrine was unaffected by either manipulation. These results suggest that the adrenergic innervation of a large area of the hypothalamus of unknown boundaries subserves neurotransmitter functions distinct from that of noradrenergic neurons, although neuroendocrine regulatory functions were not the focus of this study.

The intracerebral microdialysis of extracellular hypothalamic norepinephrine was also examined by Tanaka and co-workers (1990). Various stressors increased the dialysate concentrations of norepinephrine determined by HPLC-EC. Although neuroendocrine function was also not a focus of this study, the results of both studies support the ability of HPLC-EC to reliably quantitate the low (nanomolar) concentrations of norepinephrine or epinephrine in the extracellular fluid of the hypothalamus sampled by intracerebral microdialysis. Although limited by the uncertain volume of brain sampled and the lengthy time of integration of response, the powerful combination of intracerebral microdialysis and HPLC-EC will prove to be of increasing value in probing the neural regulation of endocrine systems.

III. Summary

The techniques of HPLC separation and EC detection have made remarkable contributions to the field of neurobiology and our evolving understanding of the neuronal regulation of endocrine systems. The principles of operation of HPLC and EC detection described in this chapter are also evolving technologies that will have greater roles and impact in future studies of neuroendocrine function and dysfunction. HPLC-EC has had limited utility in the study of hypothalamic releasing factors and hormones relative to RIA techniques, but future progress in the formation of electrochemically active derivatives may add powerful approaches to the profiling of the products of posttranslational processing of prepropeptides that mediate or regulate hormone secretion. HPLC-EC will remain the unrivaled approach in terms of sensitivity, specificity, and simplicity of operation to the definition of the distribution and physiology of hypothalamic neurotransmitters that are organized into populations of neurons projecting to discrete focal fields of projection.

Acknowledgment

The invaluable contributions to this work of Carl Anderson, Karen Johnson, and Mary Kolodny are gratefully acknowledged.

References

Axelrod, J. and Reisine, T. D., Stress hormones: their interaction and regulation, *Science*, 224, 452, 1984.

De Boer, S. F. and Van der Gugten, J., Daily variations in plasma noradrenaline, adrenaline and corticosterone concentrations in rats, *Physiol. Behav.*, 40, 323, 1987.

Fuller, R. W., Hemrick-Luecke, S., Toomey, R. E., Horng, J.-S., Ruffolo, R. R., and Molloy, B. B., Properties of 8,9-dichloro-2,3,4,5-tetrahydro-1*H*-2-benzazepine, an inhibitor of norepinephrine *N*-methyltransferase, *Biochem. Pharmacol.*, 30, 1345, 1981.

Hall, M. E., Hoffer, B. J., and Gerhardt, G. A., Rapid and sensitive determination of catecholamines in small tissue samples by high performance liquid chromatography coupled with dual-electrode coulometric electrochemical detection, *LC-GC*, 7, 258, 1988.

Hokfelt, T., Johansson, O., and Goldstein, M., Central catecholamine neurons as revealed by immunohistochemistry with special reference to adrenaline neurons, in *Handbook of Chemical Neuroanatomy*, Vol. 2. (Part I, Classical transmitters in the CNS), Björklund, A. and Hökfelt, T., Eds., Elsevier, Amsterdam, 1984, 157.

Kilpatrick, I. C., Jones, M. W., and Phillipson, O. T., A semiautomated analysis method for catecholamines, indoleamines, and some prominent metabolites in microdissected regions of the nervous system: an isocratic HPLC technique employing coulometric detection and minimal sample preparation, *J. Neurochem.*, 46, 1865, 1986.

Kilts, C. D., Breese, G. R., and Mailman, R. B., Simultaneous quantification of dopamine, 5-hydroxytryptamine and four metabolically related compounds by means of reversed-phase high-performance liquid chromatography with electrochemical detection, *J. Chromatogr.*, 225, 347, 1981.

Kilts, C. D., Gooch, M. D., and Knopes, K. D., Quantitation of plasma catecholamines by on-line trace enrichment high performance liquid chromatography with electrochemical detection, *J. Neurosci. Methods*, 11, 257, 1984.

Kilts, C. D. and Anderson, C. M., Mesoamygdaloid dopamine neurons: differential rates of dopamine turnover in discrete amygdaloid nuclei of the rat brain, *Brain Res.*, 416, 402, 1987.

Kilts, C. D., Grobin, A. C., Scibilia, R. J., and Weiss, J. M., Effect of a footshock stress paradigm on the estimated activity of norepinephrine-containing neurons in the rat brain: lack of effect on noradrenergic neurons innervating the amygdaloid complex, *Neurosci. Lett.*, in press, 1992.

Liposits, Zs., Phelix, C., and Paull, W. K., Adrenergic innervation of corticotropin releasing factor (CRF)-synthesizing neurons in the hypothalamic paraventricular nucleus of the rat, *Histochemistry*, 84, 201, 1986.

Moore, K. E., Hypothalamic dopaminergic neuronal systems, in *Psychopharmacology: The Third Generation of Progress*, Meltzer, H. Y., Ed., Raven Press, New York, 1987, 127.

Moore, R. Y. and Card, J. P., Noradrenaline-containing neuron systems, in *Handbook of Chemical Neuroanatomy*, Vol. 2, (Part I), Classical Neurotransmitters in the CNS), Björklund, A. and Card, J. P., Eds., Elsevier, Amsterdam, 1984, 123.

Moyer, T. P. and Jiang, N.-S., Optimized isocratic conditions for analysis of catecholamines by high-performance reversed-phase paired-ion chromatography with amperometric detection, *J. Chromatogr.*, 153, 365, 1978.

Nakagawa, T., Shibukawa, A., and Uno, T., Liquid chromatography with crown ether-containing mobile phases. III. Retention of catecholamines and related compounds in reversed-phase high-performance liquid chromatography, *J. Chromatogr.*, 254, 27, 1983.

Palkovits, M., Isolated removal of hypothalamic or other brain nuclei of the rat, Brain Res., 59, 449, 1973.

Palkovits, M., *Guide and Map for the Isolated Removal of Individual Cell Groups from the Rat Brain*, Akademiai Kiado, Budapest, 1980.

Routledge, C. and Marsden, C. A., Adrenaline in the CNS: *In vivo* evidence for a functional pathway innervating the hypothalamus, *Neuropharmacology*, 26, 823, 1987.

Saper, C. B., Hypothalamus, in The Human Nervous System, Paxinos, G., Ed., Academic Press, San Diego, 1990.

Swanson, L. W., Sawchenko, P. E., Berod, A., Hartman, B. K., Helle, K. B., and Vanorden, D. E., An immunohistochemical study of the organization of catecholaminergic cells and terminal fields in the paraventricular and supraoptic nuclei of the hypothalamus, *J. Comp. Neurol.*, 196, 271, 1981.

Szafarczyk, A., Malaval, F., Laurent, A., Gibaud, R., and Assenmacher, I., Further evidence for a central stimulatory action of catecholamines on adrenocorticotropin release in the rat, *Endocrinology*, 121, 883, 1987.

Tanaka, T., Yokoo, H., Tsuda, A., and Tanaka, M., Stress induced hypothalamic noradrenaline release studied by intracerebral dialysis method, Neurosciences, 16, 293, 1990.

5

Receptor Binding Theory and Techniques

DIMITRI E. GRIGORIADIS AND ERROL B. DE SOUZA
The DuPont Merck Pharmaceutical Co.
Central Nervous System Diseases Research
Wilmington, Delaware

I. General Concepts

A. Historical Perspectives

The concept of a receptor was first proposed in the early 20th century by Langley (1906) based on the effects of nicotine and curare on muscle contraction, and by Paul Ehrlich based on studies of antibodies. Both realized that in order for drugs or antibodies to exert specific effects, they first had to interact with a receptive substance, or a receptor. Subsequently, it was discovered that receptors were specific cellular components that recognize and interact with specific ligands, including hormones, growth factors, neurotransmitters, antibodies, and drugs, to transmit stimuli. The study of receptors and receptor systems has since spiraled and many different systems have now been identified and fully characterized.

The investigations of Ariens and colleagues (Ariens et al., 1964; Ariens and Beld, 1977) led to the concept of the evolutionary relationship and commonalities between receptor systems and enzyme interactions. In both systems, there is a common first step of a ligand binding to a receptor, which is then followed by some biochemical reaction. The distinction was presented between the *affinity* with which the drug binds to the receptor and the particular *effect* than it induces. Therefore the complete study of a receptor system cannot end with the characterization of the receptor protein alone, but must include the effector system to which the receptor is coupled. This effector system can either be an enzyme such as adenylate cyclase, a hormone secretory system such as prolactin, ion channels such as sodium, calcium, or potassium, or a brain metabolic pathway such as glucose metabolism. In all cases, the binding of a specific agonist to the receptor activates the effector system (either in a positive or negative manner) and thus initiates a response. The antagonist of a particular system is a compound that will block the action of the agonist (either in a competitive or noncompetitive manner) without having any effect on its own. Hence the analogy between the regulatory enzyme function and a receptor system is realized.

B. Receptor-Binding Theory

General receptor-binding theory was first described using classical pharmacological terminology relating the *response* of a particular system with the agonist *concentration* (Ariens et al., 1964). Since it was accepted that in order for a ligand to be active it must first "bind", models were generated that would focus on the binding of a ligand with its specific receptor. The resulting dose-response curves in their simplest form were based on the law of mass action and could be described using the following equation:

$$H + R \underset{k_{-1}}{\overset{k_{+1}}{\rightleftharpoons}} RH \rightarrow RESPONSE$$

where H represents the hormone or drug, R represents the receptor, and k_{+1} and k_{-1} represent the forward and reverse reaction rate constants, respectively. The function k_{-1}/k_{+1} equals the equilibrium dissociation constant (K_D) between a ligand and its receptor in a simple bimolecular interaction. These relationships will be partially derived in the following equations. The simplest form of the equation assumes that all the receptors in this particular system are identical, will bind the ligand independently of each other, and that only one ligand can bind to one receptor. Thus, if one now had a labeled ligand or hormone as described in the previous section, (H*), the equation that represents an actual bimolecular interaction between a receptor and a drug or hormone would be

$$H^* + R \underset{k_{-1}}{\overset{k_{+1}}{\rightleftharpoons}} H^*R \rightarrow RESPONSE \tag{1}$$

We can describe the above relationship by two equations such that

$$\frac{d(H^*R)}{dt} = k_{+1}(H^*)(R) \quad \text{and} \quad -\frac{d(H^*R)}{dt} = k_{-1}(H^*R)$$

Based on the above relationship, then, at equilibrium (when the forward rate of the reaction equals the reverse rate)

$$\frac{d(H^*R)}{dt} = -\frac{d(H^*R)}{dt}$$

Therefore

$$\frac{k_{-1}}{k_{+1}} = K_D = \frac{(H^*)(R)}{(H^*R)} \tag{2}$$

where K_D now represents the equilibrium dissociation constant of the hormone and the receptor. There are two parameters of interest in Equation 2, namely, the K_D (the dissociation constant or affinity of the ligand for the receptor) and R (the total number of specific receptors in a given unit of tissue). Under the conditions generally used in binding assays, however, only two parameters can be measured directly — the free concentration of labeled hormone (H*) and the amount of radiolabeled hormone specifically bound to the receptor (H*R). The *total* number of receptors present in a tissue cannot usually be measured directly but can be estimated indirectly in the following manner. If we represent the total number of receptors by R_T, then the total number of receptors in a tissue is equal to the number of labeled receptors (H*R) plus unlabeled receptors (R). Thus

$$R_T = (H^*R) + R$$

or

$$R = R_T - (H^*R) \tag{3}$$

Since R_T represents the maximum number of receptors in the tissue, it is equivalent to $(H*R)_{max}$ only if all the receptors in the tissue could be bound and labeled. By substituting for R in Equation 2, the affinity or K_D of a ligand for its receptor can be described as

$$K_D = \frac{(H^*)[R_T - (H^*R)]}{(H^*R)} \tag{4}$$

By rearranging the above equation, we can approximate the number of receptors that can be bound at a given ligand concentration if we know the affinity (K_D) of the ligand for the receptor. Thus

$$\frac{(H^*R)}{(H^*R)_{max}} = \frac{1}{[1 + (K_D^* / H^*)]} \tag{5}$$

where the function $(H*R)/(H*R)_{max}$ now represents the fraction of the total number of receptors labeled at a given radioligand concentration, or the *fractional occupancy*. When a radioligand is used at a concentration equal to its dissociation constant (i.e., $H^* = K_D$) then 50% of the receptor population will be labeled. It follows also that at very low radioligand concentrations, that is, when $H^* \ll K_D$, the value of K_D/H^* approaches zero and the fractional occupancy is extremely low. Conversely, at very high radioligand concentrations, when $H^* \gg K_D$, the fractional occupancy approaches 100%. These models are the basis for all receptor binding when a single radioligand molecule is assumed to bind to a single receptor molecule. It is important to note at this point that any radiolabeled compound will be observed to bind to any given tissue. The difficulty is in determining the fraction of radioligand that is specifically bound to the receptor protein of interest. Pharmacologically, there are certain definitions and criteria that can differentiate between the binding of a radioligand to a *bona fide* receptor and the binding that is to drug "acceptor" sites. These will be described in the following sections.

C. Definition of a Receptor

Receptors for endogenous substances such as neurotransmitters, as well as those for exogenous compounds such as drugs, are comprised of two major components, the recognition or binding site at the cell surface and the intracellular effector component that converts the recognized information into cellular function. The dual function of receptors, that is, to first recognize the hormone or transmitter with high affinity and specificity and to translate the recognition process into altered cellular function through second messenger-mediated processes, differentiates receptors from other binding sites that may subserve other cellular functions such as transport of nutrients, uptake of neurotransmitters into terminals, passage of transmitters through channels, or altered enzyme activity. These latter binding sites have been termed *acceptors*.

D. Criteria for Identification of a Receptor

Certain basic criteria must be met in order to define a binding site as a receptor. These criteria include saturability, stereospecificity, distribution, and pharmacological profile and are outlined in Table 1. The definitions of these criteria have been described in complete detail elsewhere (Burt, 1985). For the purposes of this chapter, a brief description will follow. One of the first determinations for a receptor relates to the use of increasing concentrations of a radiolabeled compound and the observation that the specific binding of the radioligand eventually plateaus. This is termed *saturability*; that is, there is a finite number of receptors in a given tissue that have the ability to bind this particular ligand. The ligand should also exhibit high affinity for the binding site or at least demonstrate an affinity for the receptor related to its physiological concentration. For example, the dopamine D_2 receptor in the anterior pituitary has an affinity for dopamine of approximately 10 nM, which coincides extremely well with the measured concentration of dopamine in the hypophyseal portal circulation. For the most part, when dealing with hormones or transmitters, especially neurotransmitters, the affinity of the respective receptors is relatively high (nanomolar range). Since most neurotransmitters and hormones act in a reversible manner, it follows that the ligand should bind in a reversible manner and, furthermore, the recognition site should bind to the ligand and lose the binding at rates parallel to the production and loss of physiological effects of the ligand. Since (as described above) the receptor contains specific active points of attachment for the ligand, ligands must bind to receptors in a stereospecific manner. Thus, if one stereoisomer of a ligand can bind to a recognition site with high affinity and saturability, then its enantiomer should not bind to that same binding site with equal affinity. In general, one optical isomer is 100 to 1000 times more potent than the other isomer. The term *stereoselectivity* thus simply indicates a preference of a receptor for one optical isomer. The term *stereospecificity* is reserved for those cases where all of the activity resides in one enantiomer or stereoisomer.

Distribution of a receptor is another major criterion for identifying a binding site as a *bona fide* receptor. In other words, the binding site must be present in tissues or cells that are known to produce a certain function related to that particular receptor system. Furthermore, there should be an absence of the binding site in those tissues or cells demonstrated not to have the physiological effect. Probably the single most important criterion for the characterization of a binding site as a receptor is the pharmacological rank order profile of related compounds. This is sometimes referred to as the "fingerprint" of a receptor. Briefly, compounds that are related to the transmitter or hormone should be able to bind to the receptor with relatively high affinity and those compounds unrelated to the hormone should not be able to interact with the protein. A classic example of the power of this fingerprint for receptors is demonstrated in the adrenergic system. For β-adrenergic receptors, the order of potencies for activity is (–)isoproterenol > (–)epinephrine > (–)norepinephrine. In a related family of receptors, the α-adrenergic receptors have the pharmacological profile of potencies of (–)epinephrine > (–)norepinephrine > (–)isoproterenol. This alteration of potencies differentiates these two receptors in terms of binding ability and physiological effect. For both adrenergic receptors, dopamine, serotonin, and related monoamines are not potent, as they represent different families of monoamine receptors. Finally, other criteria used in strengthening the definition of binding sites as receptors include tissue linearity (i.e., increasing specific binding with increasing receptor concentration), temperature dependence (i.e., the receptor protein should be heat labile and

Table 1

Criteria Used for Defining a Binding Site as a Receptor

1.	Saturability
2.	Stereospecificity
3.	Pharmacological profile
4.	Distribution
5.	Heat lability, kinetics, functional correlates

demonstrate inability to bind following temperatures in excess of 50°C), and pH and ion sensitivity (i.e., binding should occur at or close to the physiologically relevant pH and ion concentrations). Thus, if all these criteria are met, there is a very high probability that the protein being considered is a fucntional receptor. Following the detailed binding profile outlined, however, it must still be demonstrated that the receptor protein can be linked to some physiological function that can be correlated to the binding characteristics.

II. Techniques Used in the Study of Receptor Systems

A. Radioligand Binding Methods for Studying Receptors

1. Homogenate-Binding Studies

Detailed strategies for the identification, characterization, and quantification of receptors in membrane homogenates have been described for many receptor systems, each one with its own set of particular conditions that have been painstakingly established to satisfy all the criteria outlined in Section I. A summary of these various techniques is given in Table 2. This section will introduce a very basic strategy used in the labeling of receptors from a variety of tissues in a homogenate form and describe how these studies can be used to fulfill the criteria listed above. The radioligand must be of high enough specific activity in order that it will still be detectable in the low picomolar to nanomolar range once it is bound to the receptor. It has been calculated that a minimum specific activity of 5 Ci/mmol is sufficient for most receptor systems (Seeman, 1985). The most common or popular isotopes used today are tritium (^{3}H) and iodine (^{125}I). Once the ligand has been radiolabeled to a sufficient specific activity, the binding of the ligand to tissue homogenates is performed as follows. The tissue preparation for binding studies is unique for the receptor system under study. The conditions for binding (protein concentration, pH, temperature, and buffer ingredients) all must be worked out prior to the actual analysis of binding data. Tissues from discrete brain areas (for neurotransmitters), endocrine organs (for hormones), or other tissues are homogenized to yield a membrane suspension and are incubated under optimal conditions (time, temperature, pH, ion content) with the radioligand that is specific for a given receptor. Nonspecific binding is measured in a parallel set of tubes that contain an excess (100 nM to 10 µM) of unlabeled drug that has a high specificity for the receptor of interest. The radiolabeled receptor in the membrane can then be separated from the free, unbound radiolabel by a variety of techniques including filtration, centrifugation, precipitation, and so on. The details for the determination of the optimal binding parameters as well as all of the separation techniques are beyond the scope of this chapter but are detailed elsewhere (Enna, 1982; Levitsky, 1985; Bennett and Yamamura, 1985).

In general, there are two types of binding experiments, the saturation or Scatchard type

Table 2

Techniques Used to Study Neurotransmitter Receptors

1.		Radioligand methods for receptor characterization
	a.	Reversible radioligand binding to receptors in homogenates
	b.	Irreversible affinity labeling of receptors
	c.	*In vitro* receptor autoradiography
	d.	*In vivo* receptor autoradiography
	e.	Positron emission tomography
2.		Neurotransmitter-mediated changes in second messenger activity
3.		Immunocytochemistry using antibodies for receptors
4.		*In situ* hybridization histochemistry using probes for receptor mRNA and cDNA

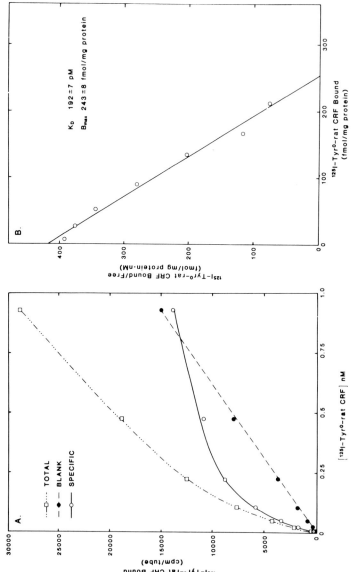

Figure 1. Binding of ^{125}I-Tyr^0-rat/human CRF to rat brain homogenates. The binding of ^{125}I-Tyr^0-rat/human CRF to rat olfactory bulb membranes as a function of increasing ligand concentration. (A) Direct plot of the data showing the total amount of ^{125}I-Tyr^0-rat/human CRF bound, the amount of ^{125}I-Tyr^0-rat/human CRF bound in the presence of 1 μM unlabeled ovine CRF (blank) and specific (total minus blank) binding. (B) Scatchard plot of ^{125}I-Tyr^0-rat/human CRF specific binding. (Reproduced with permission from De Souza, E. B., *J. Neurosci.* 7, 88, 1987.)

and the competition type. In the saturation experiment, increasing concentrations of radiola-beled ligand are incubated (usually in triplicate) under specific conditions with membrane homogenates. A parallel set of tubes is incubated with radioligand plus membranes along with a 1000-fold excess of unlabeled drug. The latter set of tubes allows the assessment of radioligand binding to nonspecific attachment sites. The difference in the amount of radioligand remaining between these two sets of tubes defines the specific binding from which one can determine the binding parameters, such as the dissociation constant or affinity (K_D) and the maximal density of binding sites (B_{max}). An example of this type of radioligand binding experiment is demonstrated in Figure 1 using the radioligand [^{125}I]Tyr^0-rat corticotropin-releasing factor ([^{125}I]Tyr^0-rat CRF). Rat brain membranes were homogenized in buffer and incubated with increasing concentrations of [^{125}I]Tyr^0-rat CRF in the absence (total binding) or presence (nonspecific binding) of 1 μM unlabeled ovine CRF. The amount of specific binding of the radioligand in the brain was determined by subtracting the amount of bound radioligand in the total and nonspecific tubes. The line generated by plotting specifically bound [^{125}I]Tyr^0-rat CRF in relation to the concentration of added radioligand (i.e., free [^{125}I]Tyr^0-rat CRF) will reach a plateau when the amount of specifically bound receptors reaches the B_{max} (see Figure 1A). Figure 1B demonstrates the Scatchard transformation of the same data shown in Figure 1A. This linear transformation offers a simple extrapolation of the K_D value (which is equivalent to the negative inverse of the slope) and the B_{max} (which is the x-axis intercept). These graphical methods provide quick estimates of the binding parameters and are generally used to obtain initial estimates of the K_D and B_{max} prior to more detailed analytical methods, which will be described in the following section.

The second type of binding experiment is the competition type, where only a single concentration of radioligand is incubated in tubes along with the membrane homogenates as well as increasing concentrations of unlabeled or "cold" drug. In this type of experiment, one can determine the affinities of various compounds (K_i values) for a receptor type based on the ability of these compounds to compete for a known concentration of radioligand. The pharma-cological profile described in earlier sections is defined using the competition type of experi-ment. As an example, Figure 2 shows a number of peptides that are potent in inhibiting the binding of [^{125}I]Tyr^0-r/h CRF to rat brain membranes. The fingerprint of a receptor described above is evident in this figure from the progressively rightward shift of the apparent affinities of these peptides. The peptides that are potent inhibitors of the radioligand (i.e., it takes less competing drug to inhibit the binding) have K_i values that are low (i.e., on the left side of the graph). Compounds that are less potent or not potent at all at this receptor system, such as vasoactive intestinal peptide (VIP) or arginine vasopressin (AVP), are unable to inhibit the binding of [^{125}I]Tyr^0-rat CRF to CRF receptors (see Figure 2). Both types of experiment can be analyzed using the same bimolecular models described above. In order to fully define a receptor system, both types of experiments need to be included in the methodology. The relative ease of this technique, using the two types of binding experiments outlined, lends itself well to the studying of the kinetic characteristics, pharmacological specificity, and modulation of receptors *in vitro* as well as following *in vivo* treatments.

2. Analysis of Binding Data

The analysis of radioligand binding data has taken a great leap forward since the introduc-tion of microcomputers to the everyday laboratory. Prior to computer-assisted analysis of radioligand-binding data, all results were analyzed almost exclusively by various graphical methods. Although graphical methods offer simple methods of analysis, a transformation of the data (usually to a linear form) was generally required prior to estimation of the parameters. It is obvious, however, that the most accurate determination of radioligand-binding parameters

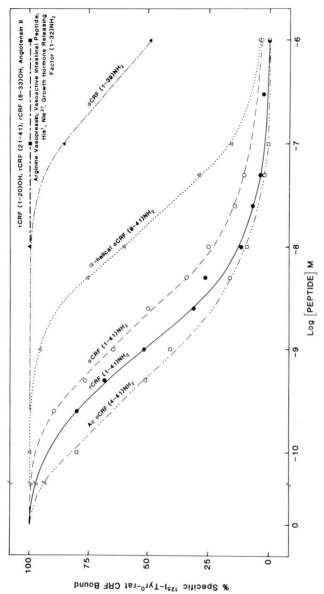

Figure 2. Pharmacological profile of CRF receptors in brain. Characterization of the pharmacological specificity of ^{125}I-Tyr^0-rat/human CRF binding in rat olfactory membranes. Crude mitochondrial/synaptosomal preparations were incubated in the presence of 0.1 nM ^{125}I-Tyr^0-rat/human CRF and varying concentrations of CRF-related and -unrelated peptides. Nonspecific binding was determined in the presence of 1 μM unlabeled ovine CRF. (Reproduced with permission from De Souza, E. B., *J. Neurosci.*, 7, 88, 1987.)

such as the K_D and B_{max} should be estimated from the raw data as defined by the experimental protocol rather than by a mathematical transformation of the analytical method. It is not the purpose of this chapter to compare all of the available programs for the analysis of binding data but to introduce the power of computer-assisted analysis in the determination of the binding parameters for the interactions of various ligands with their receptors. One of the most popular programs available for the analysis of ligand-binding data is named LIGAND (Munson and Rodbard, 1980). This program uses the theorems described in the above sections based on the thermodynamic and kinetic laws of mass action and provides estimates of the binding parameters (K_D, B_{max}), and nonspecific binding for any number of ligands reacting simultaneously with any number of receptors. The program does make a few assumptions about the binding characteristics, include the following: (1) multiple ligands can bind simultaneously to multiple sites; (2) the binding reaction being analyzed is under equilibrium conditions; (3) the binding is bimolecular and reversible, and (4) there is total and true separation of bound ligand from free ligand. Binding curves can be fit to single- or multisite models using the "extra-sum-of-squares" principle to allow the user to decide statistically and objectively whether a fit to a more complex model is justified and differs from a fit to a simpler method. That is, it tests whether the increase in the "goodness-of-fit" (based on least-squares analysis, or the minimum sum of the squared distances from each data point to the fitted line) for a model with more parameters is significantly better than would be predicted by chance alone. The extra-sum-of-squares principle can be simply described as follows:

$$F = \frac{(SS1 - SS2)/(df1 - df2)}{SS2/df2} \tag{6}$$

where SS1 and SS2 are the residual sum of squares of the deviations of the points to the fitted curve and df1 and df2 are the associated degrees of freedom (number of data points minus the number of estimated parameters) for the original and the more complex models, respectively. The calculated F ratio is then compared to the tabulated value for the F statistic with $(df1 - df2)$ and df2 degrees of freedom. The more complex model then is chosen only if the F ratio exceeds the tabulated value.

The general numerical method for n ligands binding to m classes of binding sites was first proposed by Feldman (Feldman, 1972; Feldman et al., 1972) and was enhanced by Munson and Rodbard in the program called LIGAND to include parameters for nonspecific binding as well as correction factors to allow comparison of data accounting for the variation in protein concentration from day to day. The advantage of this method is that it fits the raw experimental data in an untransformed coordinate system where errors are more likely to be normally distributed and uncorrelated with the independent variable. Curves from several experiments can also be considered and analyzed simultaneously, thus improving the reliability of the data analysis and hence the validity of the final results and interpretations. As an example, a single curve generated from competition data will be analyzed by increasingly complex models to demonstrate the goodness-of-fit principle on the estimated parameters. [³H]Spiperone, a dopaminergic D$_2$ receptor antagonist, was incubated at a concentration of 100 pM with increasing concentrations of the dopaminergic agonist (±)-2-amino-6,7-dihydroxy-1,2,3,4-tetrahydronaphthalene (ADTN) (Grigoriadis and Seeman, 1985). In Figure 3A, the data were fit using the program LIGAND to the most simple single-site model. The parameters estimated were only the affinity of the agonist and the level of nonspecific binding. The fit of the line, and hence the estimates of the parameters, were significantly different from the observed data points at the $p < 0.01$ level. Figure 3B shows the same data set now fit to a two-site model and the fit compared to that of the single-site model. Again, the estimated parameters (the line) and

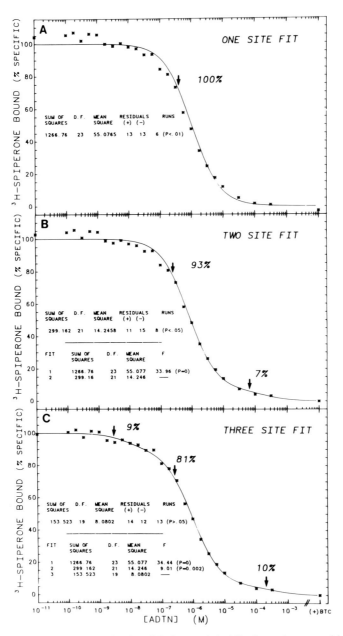

Figure 3. Use of LIGAND for the determination of the best statistical fit of complex competition data. Analysis of data by LIGAND illustrates successive fits of increasingly complex models to describe the same set of data. The data are from a [^{3}H]spiperone vs. ADTN competition curve and have been analyzed for (A) one, (B) two, and (C) three independent sites, respectively. Each panel contains information regarding the goodness of fit as well as a statistical comparison of the various fits. As indicated, these parameters (insets) provided the statistical justification for progression to more complex models. Arrows denote the estimated affinity values and the proportions of sites present for each determination. (Reproduced with permission from Grigoriadis, D. E. and Seeman, P., *J. Neurochem.*, 44, p. 1925, 1985.)

the data points were significantly different from each other; however, this time the level of significance was reduced to the $p < 0.05$ level. Furthermore, the F value of 33.96 demonstrates that the second fit (Figure 3B) is more favorable than the first (Figure 3A) even though it does not quite approximate the data itself. Figure 3C shows the same data set now fit to three independent sites. The fit of the line (hence the estimated parameters) is now highly significant, and the line now approximates the data at the $p > 0.05$ level. The conclusion, therefore, is that the data represent a binding of the agonist to three independent classes of sites, since in using this model there was no significant difference between the raw data and the fitted parameters. Furthermore, the F value indicated that the three-site model chosen was significantly better than the two-site model at a level of significance of $p < 0.002$ (see Figure 3). At this point, it must be stressed that the power of computer analysis rests solely on the precision of the raw data. If too much emphasis is placed on a single binding experiment or a poorly designed experiment, the computer-generated results can lead to extremely erroneous interpretations and conclusions.

3. Affinity Labeling of Receptors

Affinity labeling was introduced approximately in the 1960s for enzymes (Baker et al., 1967) and antibody-combining sites (Wofsy et al., 1962). Both the theoretical and practical applications of affinity labels were established primarily from work done on antibody-binding sites (Lenard and Singer, 1966; Good et al., 1967; Fenton and Singer, 1971). Affinity labels are generally small molecules that combine specifically and reversibly with the binding site of the receptor under investigation. Unlike conventional labels, the affinity label contains a reactive group that is able to form a covalent bond with a suitably oriented nucleophilic amino acid within the active site of the protein. The use of a radiolabeled form of an affinity reagent can therefore greatly expedite the identification of the ligand-binding subunit of intact receptors and their derivatized fragments. In general, affinity reagents must have the following require-ments: the reagent must have affinity for the receptor greater than 100 pM, it must have high selectivity for the receptor protein, and there must exist a nucleophilic center located within or in close proximity to the binding site. The limitation of this technique is that since any nucleophilic site can act as an acceptor, the nonspecific binding to proteins is usually higher.

Despite these shortcomings, chemical affinity probes have been successfully employed for the molecular characterization of membrane receptors. One of the first reported cases where affinity labeling of a membrane-bound receptor had been successfully employed was the work of Karlin and co-workers (Karlin et al., 1971; Reiter et al., 1972), who used 4-(M-maleimido)-α-benzyltrimethylammonium iodide (MBTA) to specifically alkylate the acetyl-choline receptor in eel electroplax. Specificity of the ligand was demonstrated by protection with reversible and irreversible inhibitors, as well as by specific oxidation of the reduced receptor with the affinity oxidizing reagent dithiobischoline, prior to alkylation with MBTA. A single and specifically labeled component of apparent molecular weight 42,000 Da was then identified by sodium dodecyl sulfate (SDS)-gel electrophoresis (for review see Changeaux et al., 1984). Many ligands since then have been modified to incorporate an active and functional alkylating group for the purpose of irreversible labeling of receptor proteins.

If a specific ligand cannot be modified to incorporate an active group, various bifunctional cross-linking reagents are currently commercially available that act as functional "bridges" between the ligand probe and the receptor for which it has high affinity. These molecules are simple in structure and may contain either chemically or photoactive derivatives on two ends. Disuccinimidyl suberate (DSS) is an example of an irreversible amine-reactive homobifunctional cross-linker. This reagent has been widely used for the elucidation of the structural and biochemical characteristics of various peptidergic systems. For example, studies have been reported using DSS to functionally couple human [^{125}I]somatotropin (Caamano et al., 1983), [^{125}I]angiotensin II (Petruzzelli et al., 1985), vasoactive intestinal peptide (Wood and O'Dorisio, 1985), and atrial natriuretic factor (Vandelen et al., 1985) to their respective receptors. In addition, DSS has recently been used to characterize the CRF receptor in a variety of species and tissues, including bovine anterior pituitary (Nishimura et al., 1987; Grigoriadis and De Souza, 1989a), AtT-20 mouse pituitary tumor cells (Rosendale et al., 1987), bovine, porcine, rat, and monkey anterior and neurointermediate pituitary (Grigoriadis and De Souza, 1989a), as well as in rat, monkey, and human brain (Grigoriadis and De Souza, 1988). The affinity cross-linking of [^{125}I]oCRF to membrane homogenates permitted elucidation of the microheterogeneity of CRF receptors in the various tissues. Affinity cross-linked CRF receptors were found to differ in molecular weights in pituitary and brain from a variety of species as defined by SDS-polyacrylamide gel electrophoresis followed by autoradiography (Grigoriadis and De Souza, 1988). Figure 4 is an example of brain and pituitary homogenates that have been radiolabeled with [^{125}I]oCRF, affinity cross-linked using the reagent DSS, and electrophoresed on SDS-polyacrylamide gels. The difference in the molecular weights of the cross-linked CRF receptor in the two tissues is evident and can be quantified. The differences in the molecular weight were subsequently found to be due to differential glycosylation of these proteins in the two tissues and thus represented posttranslational modification of these proteins depending on the tissue type (Grigoriadis and De Souza, 1989b).

B. Receptor-Mapping Techniques

1. General Principles of Receptor Mapping

The fundamental advantages of microscopic receptor mapping are increased anatomical

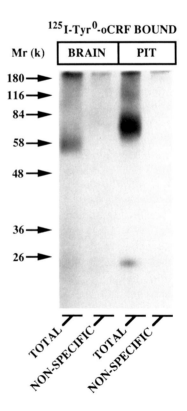

Figure 4. Affinity cross-linking of ^{125}I-oCRF to brain and pituitary membranes. Membranes from rat frontal cortex (BRAIN) and anterior pituitary (PIT) were homogenized, incubated with [^{125}I]oCRF, cross-linked using the reagent DSS, and electrophoresed on SDS-polyacrylamide gels. Covalent incorporation of the radioligand followed by autoradiography of SDS-polyacrylamide gels revealed that the apparent molecular weight of the CRF receptor in brain was 58,000 Da while the CRF-binding protein in the anterior pituitary was 75,000 Da. Nonspecific binding was defined in the presence of 1 μM unlabeled rat/human CRF (NON-SPECIFIC).

resolution and greatly increased sensitivity of measurement when compared to the biochemical approaches described in the previous sections. The reason for the increased sensitivity of this technique is based on the fact that one can detect radiolabel binding to microscopically discrete areas of tissue sections. With this method, receptor densities can be localized to areas of the brain that cannot be obtained even by microdissection techniques. The increase in the sensitivity of this technique can be orders of magnitude greater than that found in biochemical studies. Thus receptor mapping will be useful in any situation that requires receptor measurement in small regions or where the overall quantities of receptors (but not necessarily the densities) are low.

In general, there are two important principles that one must keep in mind when carrying out receptor-mapping experiments. The first is the selective or preferential labeling of receptors. The development of large numbers of radioactive ligands and the availability of extensive pharmacological studies on many receptors using primarily radioligand-binding homogenates (see above) have provided the foundation on which to precisely define the receptor type in question. The second principle is the selection of appropriate methods of visualization. This is a key factor in the mapping of receptors on tissue sections since the radiolabeled receptors are not visualized directly. Rather, the bound radioligand is processed quickly to reduce the opportunity of the bound ligand to diffuse away from its original binding site and then exposed to film to produce an image of its binding pattern on the section. These autoradiograms can then be analyzed for the labeling pattern. The methods for the identification, localization, characterization, and quantification of receptors by autoradiography is beyond the scope of this chapter; however, these have been expertly reviewed (Kuhar 1981, 1985; Kuhar et al., 1986). There are two main approaches in the study of receptors by autoradiographic techniques: *in vitro* labeling procedures and *in vivo* labeling procedures. These two methods will be briefly described in the following sections.

2. In Vitro *Labeling Autoradiography*

In *in vitro* labeling autoradiography, slide-mounted unfixed tissue sections that have been cut from fresh frozen tissues are incubated with a radiolabeled compound to equilibrium under very controlled conditions (Rotter et al., 1979; Young and Kuhar, 1979). Following receptor labeling, the slide-mounted tissue sections are rinsed in order to decrease the amount of nonspecific adsorption of the radioligand and improve the ratio of specific to nonspecific binding. Once the slide-mounted tissue sections have been prepared such that selective receptor labeling has occurred, autoradiograms can be generated, usually by apposing the labeled slide-mounted sections directly to emulsion-coated coverslips (Young and Kuhar, 1979; Kuhar, 1985), or tritium-sensitive Ultrofilm (Amersham) or X-ray film (Palacios et al., 1981; Kuhar, 1985). Both emulsion-coated coverslips or films can be developed by standard development methods following the appropriate time of exposure to the sections. The exposure time required will vary for each receptor system and is directly related to the specific activity of the ligand used, the total number of receptors present in the area of interest, and the efficiency of the label. Exposure times can be varied to allow for the maximum resolution of the binding of the radioligand to the receptor while keeping the overall background exposure low. In this way, localization of receptors can be made to even microscopically discrete areas of tissues.

3. In Vivo *Labeling Autoradiography*

Detailed strategies for carrying out the *in vivo* labeling of receptors and some examples of these *in vivo* receptor-binding studies have been described in detail (Kuhar, 1981, 1985; Kuhar et al., 1986). The term *in vivo receptor labeling* applies to the procedure in which receptors are labeled in intact living animals following systemic administration of the radioligand. If the ligand has a very high affinity for the receptor, only tracer amounts of the drug need to be injected into the animal. Thus, after a short time, the drug is carried systemically to the target tissue, where it can bind to specific receptors. The remaining unbound drug is removed from the tissues by the normal excretory pathways. The key to the success of *in vivo* labeling of receptors lies in the affinity of the radioligand being used. The ligand must have high enough affinity for the receptor such that proximity to the receptor causes retention of the drug in the vicinity of the receptor molecule prior to its being excreted. Again, following a previously determined time following injection of the radiolabel, the animal is sacrificed and tissues are dissected, sectioned, and apposed to either coverslips or film as described in the previous section. The procedure for generation of autoradiograms from these sections is now identical to that described above for *in vitro* autoradiographic labeling techniques.

4. Imaging Receptors In Vivo: *Positron-Emission Tomography Scanning Techniques*

Recent developments have utilized positron-emitting ligands to image and quantify neurotransmitter receptor distributions in living humans using emission tomographic techniques (Wagner et al., 1983; Wong et al., 1984; Frost et al., 1985). *In vivo* labeling autoradiography (described above) has been an important first step in the development of positron-emission tomography (PET) scanning images of receptors because of the feasibility of labeling certain neurotransmitter receptors *in vivo*. PET is a technique whereby a computerized image of the labeling pattern can be generated from the distribution of binding of the positron-emitting compounds. In this technique, a ligand containing a radioactive isotope that decays by emitting a positron (positive electron) is injected into an animal or human. If the ligand is suitable, then receptors in the tissue (usually the brain) will be preferentially labeled. Emitted positrons will immediately combine with an electron and the two are mutually annihilated. The annihilation event results in the release of two γ rays that leave the site in very nearly opposite directions, pass through the tissue, and hit a circular array of γ detectors outside the subject. These signals are quantified and transformed by computer into a reconstructed image of the spatial distribution of the radioactivity. The great advantage of this approach is that it is a noninvasive method whereby receptors can be visualized and quantified in living animals.

5. Uses of Receptor Mapping

Some of the uses of receptor mapping are summarized in Table 3. Receptor maps provide powerful insights into the mechanisms of drug action by identifying those brain regions that contain the receptors and thus those areas that will be affected by drug administration. For example, administration of opiate drugs causes a variety of physiological effects, including analgesia, pupillary constriction, respiratory depression, and suppression of various visceral reflexes. Perhaps the only way this wide range of physiological action can be fully understood is to associate the various physiological effects with receptors involved in different neuronal circuits that may mediate these effects (Kuhar, 1981). In other words, identifying the neuronal circuits that contain these receptors and which will be affected by drug administration may provide an understanding of how these drugs produce their effects. Receptor mapping is also a valuable adjunct to neurotransmitter mapping. Receptor maps help to complete our view of the biochemical organization of the brain. For example, studies on CRF receptors (De Souza et al., 1984, 1985) have shown that these receptors are found in many regions of the brain where endogenous CRF-containing neurons have been identified. Figure 5 is an example of an autoradiogram from rat brain demonstrating the discrete areas of the rat brain where CRF receptors are localized. The power of this technique for the localization of receptors in an anatomical environment represents an important tool in the characterization of receptor

Table 3
Uses of Receptor-Mapping Techniques

1. Mechanisms of drug action
2. Complementation of neurotransmitter histochemical maps
3. Target sites for different experiments
4. Neuropathology

systems. Specifically, in rodents, CRF cell bodies are contained in laminae II and III of the neocortex with projections to laminae I and IV (Swanson et al., 1983b), areas that have high densities of receptors (De Souza et al., 1984, 1985). This lamination of CRF receptors within the cerebral cortex can be discerned in Figure 5. Other uses of receptor maps include providing needed data for a variety of different types of experiments, such as locating targets for experiments involving direct drug injections into discrete tissue areas. A major use of receptor maps involves identifying changes in receptors in neuropathological conditions as well as in neuropsychiatric disorders. Although the uses of receptor-mapping techniques are many and diverse, there are distinct advantages and limitations that must be addressed when comparing various receptor-mapping techniques.

6. Advantages and Limitations of In Vitro and In Vivo Receptor-Mapping Techniques

In vitro labeling procedures have many advantages over *in vivo* labeling procedures. The *in vitro* labeling procedures provides greater specificity and efficiency. Inhibitors can be added to prevent metabolism of the labeled ligand, and ligands that will not cross the blood-brain barrier during *in vivo* procedures (e.g., peptides) can easily be used. Various receptor distributions can be easily compared since it is possible to use different ligands on sequential tissue sections. This approach has the advantage of being low in cost since whole-body doses of radioactive drug do not have to be used in order to label the relatively small numbers of specific receptors. It is also possible to carry out these types of studies on human post-mortem tissues. An additional advantage of *in vitro* labeling is that one can quite precisely define the receptor subtype by performing parallel standard biochemical assays. However, in spite of all the advantages of *in vitro* receptor labeling, *in vivo* receptor labeling can still offer useful information about a particular receptor system. Perhaps the main advantage of *in vivo* labeling is that receptors can be labeled and subsequently imaged using a variety of noninvasive techniques such as PET. The disadvantages of *in vivo* labeling using PET scanning are that it is expensive to perform and requires a large team of trained technicians along with a complicated technology. For example, a cyclotron is required to produce the very short-lived radioisotopes used in PET scanning and nuclear chemists are required to rapidly incorporate these short half-life isotopes into receptor-specific ligands. Another difficulty, compared to *in vitro* autoradiographic methods, is that the resolution of PET scans is not very high; a resolution unit is on the average approximately 1 cm^3. Nevertheless, despite some of these limitations PET scanning represents a great potential for the study of receptors *in vivo*.

In vitro autoradiography with all of its advantages still has some significant limitations. Although one can use ligands with lower affinity than are necessary for *in vivo* labeling autoradiography, low-affinity sites are still not easily identified. If the dissociation rate of the ligand is relatively high, then there will be a significant diffusion of the radioligand away from the receptor site during the wash period required to reduce nonspecific binding. Another limitation rests with the preparation of the tissue samples. Since tissues must be first dissected, then quick frozen before sectioning, this process can produce morphological defects in the sections and receptors themselves may be destroyed. Finally, it must also be remembered that

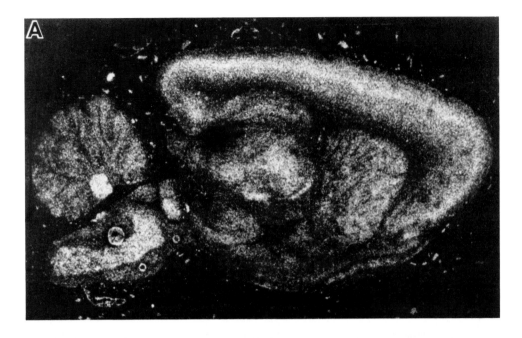

Figure 5. Autoradiographic localization of CRF receptors in rat brain. Autoradiographic distribution of CRF receptor-binding sites in rat brain labeled with Nle^{21}, ^{125}I-Tyr^{32}-oCRF. (A and B) Dark-field photomicrographs (^{3}H-Ultrofilm) showing the distribution of autoradiographic grains in sagittal sections of rat brain. In dark-field illumination the autoradiographic grains (i.e., binding sites) appear as white spots and the tissue is not visible. Thus the brightest areas have the highest concentration of binding sites. (A) shows the "total" binding and (B) shows the binding in the presence of 1 μM unlabeled Nle^{21}, Tyr^{32}-oCRF (nonspecific binding). Bar = 2 mm. (Reproduced with permission from De Souza, E. B., Insel, T. R., Perrin, M. H., Rivier, J. E., Vale, W. W., and Kuhar, M. J., *J. Neurosci.*, 5, 3189, 1985.)

the techniques of both *in vivo* and *in vitro* autoradiography described in this chapter are primarily light microscopic in nature and still lack the ultrastructural resolution necessary for a complete picture of the distribution of receptors at the level of the membrane.

C. Additional Receptor Methodological Approaches

1. Receptor-Mediated Changes in Second Messenger Activity

Neurotransmitter receptors affect synaptic transmission through the effects of second messenger systems. For example, neurotransmitters can act by stimulating or inhibiting the formation of cAMP, stimulating the hydrolysis of phosphotidylinositol, and/or altering the flux of ions such as sodium, calcium, chloride, or potassium across their respective ionophores. As discussed in Section I, receptors are differentiated from acceptors by having binding sites associated with second messenger effector mechanisms. Thus the measurement of neurotransmitter receptor-mediated changes in second messenger activity provides a good index of not only the binding site but also of the interaction between the binding site and its effector complex. Taken together these parameters provide information on the whole functional receptor system. The details and full descriptions of the methodologies for the measurement of receptor-mediated changes in second messenger activity can be found in a number of reviews (Birnbaumer et al., 1985; Abdel-Latif, 1986).

2. Immunocytochemistry Using Antibodies for Receptors

The availability of antibodies for receptors provides an important alternative to the localization of receptors using immunocytochemistry. In addition, immunoneutralization of the receptors using antibodies would provide insights into functions mediated by the receptors. The antibodies could be used to localize receptors at the light microscopic level using fluorescent markers. In addition, for light or electron microscopy an enzymatic reaction product can be deposited locally. For example, a commonly employed enzyme is peroxidase, which is linked to the receptor via an antibody bridge. For electron microscopy, electron-dense labels can be attached to the antibodies: ferritin, hemocyanase, or colloidal gold are commonly used labels. Important successes have been made in localizing neurotransmitters in brain, including nicotinic cholinergic receptors (Lentz and Chester, 1977; Swanson et al., 1983a), dopamine receptors (Goldsmith et al., 1979), β-adrenergic receptors (Strader et al., 1982), delta-opiate receptors (Carr et al., 1987), and the γ-aminobutyric acid (GABA)/benzodiazepine receptor complex (Richards et al., 1986, 1987). In the absence of antibodies to the receptor proteins themselves, anti-idiotypic antibodies can be raised to compounds known to bind to receptors and used as immunohistochemical agents. This has been demonstrated using autoantiidiotypic acetylcholine antibodies to localize acetylcholine receptors in locust brain (Vieillemaringe et al., 1987) and a vasopressin antiidiotypic antibody to localize AVP receptors in the magnocellular neurons of the supraoptic and paraventricular nuclei (Knigge et al., 1987). Immunohistochemical techniques have the distinct advantage over autoradiographic techniques in that autoradiograms do not need to be generated. These labels can be visualized directly at the light microscopic level and thus the receptors to which these probes are attached can be visualized directly. Also, these techniques may be useful under experimental conditions where tissue morphology is better preserved. An important advantage of immunocytochemical studies is that cell bodies containing receptors are clearly delineated (Swanson et al., 1983a; Richards et al., 1986, 1987), whereas this is not always the case with autoradiography. Finally, ultrastructural techniques with antibodies would have better electron microscopic resolution than those with autoradiography (see Barnard, 1979). A major disadvantage to immunohisto-chemical approaches to receptor characterization is that the data are not as easily quantifiable as compared to autoradiographic methods.

3. Molecular Biological Approaches to Study Receptors

Major advances have been made in recent years in the development of molecular biologi-cal tools in the study of receptors. The use of gene cloning techniques to identify the structures of protein macromolecules that comprise receptors for neurotransmitters are currently being used. For example, genes for the various subunits of the nicotinic cholinergic receptor (Mishina et al., 1984) and the β-adrenergic receptor (Dixon et al., 1986) have been cloned. Very recently, the gene for the binding subunit of the dopamine D_2 receptor has also been identified and cloned (Bunzow et al., 1988). Furthermore, it seems that some of these receptors are beginning to fall into categories of "gene families" based on some of their sequence homologies to each other. These families are thought to be related through the domains that are involved in receptor coupling to guanine nucleotide regulatory proteins. In parallel to these studies, rapid advances have been made in the use of molecular biological probes to quantify and localize messenger RNA levels using Northern blot analysis and *in situ* hybridization histochemical techniques, respectively. The application of these techniques to quantify and localize message levels for cloned receptors will provide new insights into the synthesis rates of receptors as well as the turnover of these receptor macromolecules. Nicotinic receptor mRNA was detected in high concentrations in rat hypothalamus, hippocampus, habenula, cerebellum, and adrenal gland using Northern blot analysis and *in situ* hybridization tech-niques (Boulter et al., 1986; Goldman et al., 1986). The use of molecular biological techniques to study receptors in combination with "traditional" radioligand-binding techniques would allow us to better define the mechanisms (synthesis and/or degradation) underlying changes in receptors following experimental manipulations, drug treatments, or as a result of disease.

References

Abdel-Latif, A. A., Calcium-mobilizing receptors, polyphosphoinositides and the generation of second messengers, *Pharmacol. Rev.*, 38, 227, 1986.

Ariens, E. J. and Beld, A. J., The receptor concept in evolution, *Biochem. Pharmacol.*, 26, 913, 1977.

Ariens, E. J., Simonis, A. M., and Van Rossum, J. M., The relationship between stimulus and effect, in *Molecular Pharmacology, The Mode of Actions of Biologically Active Compounds*, Vol. 1, Ariens, E. J., Ed., Academic Press, New York, 1964, 401.

Baker, B. R., Lee, W. W., Tong, E., and Ross, O., Potential anticancer agents LXVI. Nonclassical antimetabolites III. 4(Iodoacetamido)-salicylic acid, an exoalkylating irreversible inhibitor of glutamic dehydrogenase, *J. Am. Chem. Soc.*, 83, 3713, 1967.

Barnard, E. A., Visualization and counting of receptors at the light and electron microscopic levels, in *The Receptor*, Vol. 1 (General principles and procedures), O'Bried, R. D., Ed., Plenum Press, New York, 1979, 247.

Bennett, J. P., Jr. and Yamamura, H. I., Neurotransmitter, hormone and receptor binding, in *Neuro-transmitter Receptor Binding*, 2nd ed., Yamamura, H. I., Enna, S. E., and Kuhar, M. J., Eds., Raven Press, New York, 1985, 61.

Birnbaumer, L., Codina, J., Mattera, R., Cerione, R., Hildebrandt, J., Sunyer, T., Rojas, F., Caron, M., Lefkowitz, R., and Iyengar, R., Structural basis of adenylate cyclase stimulation and inhibition by distinct guanine nucleotide regulatory proteins, in *Molecular Mechanisms of Transmembrane Signalling*, Cohen, P. and Houslay, M., Eds., Elsevier, Amsterdam, 1985, 131.

Boulter, J., Evans, K., Goldman, D., Martin, G., Treco, D., Heinemann, S., and Patrick, J., Isolation of a cDNA clone encoding for a possible neural nicotinic acetylcholine receptor α-subunit, *Nature (London)*, 319, 368, 1986.

Bunzow, J. R., Van Tol, H. H., Grandy, D. K., Albert, P., Salon, J., Christie, M., Machida, C. A., Neve, K. A., and Civelli, O., Cloning and expression of a rat D_2 dopamine receptor cDNA, *Nature (London)*, 336, 783, 1988.

Burt, D. R., Criteria for receptor identification, in *Neurotransmitter Receptor Binding*, 2nd ed., Yamamura, H. I., Enna, S. E., and Kuhar, M. J., Eds., Raven Press, New York, 1985, 41.

Caamano, C. A., Fernandez, H. N., and Paladini, A. C., Specificity of covalently stabilized complexes of ^{125}I-labeled human somatotropin and components of the lactogenic binding sites of rat liver, *Biochem. Biophys. Res. Commun.*, 115, 29, 1983.

Carr, D. J., DeCosta, B., Jacobson, A. E., Bost, K. L., Rice, K. C., and Blalock, J. E., Immunoaffinity-purified opiate receptor specifically binds the delta-class opiate receptor ligand, *cis*-(+)-3-methylfentanylisothiocyanate, SUPERFIT, *FEBS Lett.*, 224(2), 272, 1987.

Changeaux, J. P., Devillers-Thiery, A., and Chemouilli, P., Acetylcholine receptor. An allosteric protein, *Science*, 225, 1335, 1984.

De Souza, E. B., Corticotropin-releasing factor receptors in the rat central nervous system: characterization and regional distribution, *J. Neurosci.*, 7, 88, 1987.

De Souza, E. B., Perrin, M. H., Insel, T. R., Rivier, J. E., Vale, W. W., and Kuhar, M. J., Corticotropin-releasing factor receptors in rat forebrain: autoradiographic identification, *Science*, 224, 1449, 1984.

De Souza, E. B., Insel, T. R., Perrin, M. H., Rivier, J. E., Vale, W. W., and Kuhar, M. J., Corticotropin-releasing factor receptors are widely distributed within the rat central nervous system: an autoradiographic study, *J. Neurosci.*, 5, 3189, 1985.

Dixon, R. A. F., Kobilka, B. K., Strader, D. J., Benovic, J. L., Dohlman, H. G., Frielle, T., Bolanowski, M. A., Bennett, C. D., Rands, E., Diehl, R. E., Mumford, R. A., Slater, E. E., Sigal, I. S., Caron, M. G., Lefkowitz, R. J., and Strader, C. D., Cloning of the gene and cDNA for mammalian β-adrenergic receptor and homology with rhodopsin, *Nature (London)*, 321, 75, 1986.

Enna, S. J., Radioreceptor assays for neurotransmitters and drugs, in *Handbook of Psychopharmacology*, Vol. 15, Iversen, L. L., Iversen, S. D., and Snyder, S. H., Eds., Plenum Press, New York, 1982, 75.

Feldman, H. A., Mathematical theory of complex ligand-binding systems at equilibrium: some methods for parameter fitting, *Anal. Biochem.*, 48, 317, 1972.

Feldman, H. A., Rodbard, D., and Levine, D., Mathematical theory of cross-reactive radioimmunoassay and ligand binding systems at equilibrium, *Anal. Biochem.*, 45, 530, 1972.

Fenton, J. W., II and Singer, S. J., Affinity labeling of antibodies to the *p*-azophenyltrimethylammonium hapten, and a comparison of affinity labeled antibodies of two different specificities, *Biochemistry*, 10, 1429, 1971.

Frost, J. J., Wagner, H. N., Dannals, R. F., Ravert, H. T., Links, J. M., Wilson, A. A., Burns, H. D., Wong, D. F., McPhearson, R. W., Rosenbaum, A. E., Kuhar, M. J., and Snyder, S. H., Imaging opiate receptors in the human brain by positron tomography, *J. Comput. Tomogr.*, 9, 231, 1985.

Goldman, D., Simmins, D., Swanson, L. W., Patrick, J., and Heinemann, S., Mapping of brain areas expressing RNA homologous to two different acetylcholine receptor α-subunit cDNAs, *Proc. Natl. Acad. Sci. U.S.A.*, 83, 4076, 1986.

Goldsmith, P. C., Cronin, M. J., and Weiner, R. I., Dopamine receptor sites in the anterior pituitary, *J. Histochem. Cytochem.*, 27, 1205, 1979.

Good, A. H., Traylor, P. S., and Singer, S. J., Affinity labeling of the active sites of rabbit anti-2,4-dinitrophenyl antibodies with *m*-nitrobenzenediazonium fluoroborate, *Biochemistry*, 6, 873, 1967.

Grigoriadis, D. E. and De Souza, E. B., The brain corticotropin-releasing factor (CRF) receptor is of lower apparent molecular weight than the CRF receptor in anterior pituitary, *J. Biol. Chem.*, 263, 10927, 1988.

Grigoriadis, D. E. and De Souza, E. B., Corticotropin-releasing factor (CRF) receptors in intermediate lobe of the pituitary: biochemical characterization and autoradiographic localization, *Peptides*, 10, 179, 1989a.

Grigoriadis, D. E. and De Souza, E. B., Heterogeneity between brain and pituitary corticotropin-releasing factor (CRF) receptors is due to differential glycosylation, *Endocrinology*, 125(4), 1877, 1989b.

Grigoriadis, D. E. and Seeman, P., Complete conversion of brain D_2 dopamine receptors from the high- to the low-affinity state for dopamine agonists, using sodium ions and guanine nucleotide, *J. Neurochem.*, 44, 1925, 1985.

Karlin, A., Prives, J., Deal, W., and Winnik, M., Affinity labeling of the acetylcholine receptor in the electroplax, *J. Mol. Biol.*, 61, 175, 1971.

Knigge, K. M., Piekut, D. T., Berlove, D. J., Junig, J. T., and Melrose, P. A., Staining of magnocellular neurons of the supraoptic and paraventricular nuclei with vasopressin anti-idiotype antibody: a potential method for receptor immunocytochemistry, *Brain Res.*, 338(1), 69, 1987.

Kuhar, M. J., Autoradiographic localization of drug and neurotransmitter receptors in the brain, *Trends Neurosci.*, 4, 60, 1981.

Kuhar, M. J., Receptor localization with the microscope, in *Neurotransmitter Receptor Binding*, Yamamura, H. I., Enna, S. J., and Kuhar, M. J., Eds., Raven Press, New York, 1985, 153.

Kuhar, M. J., De Souza, E. B., and Unnerstall, J. R., Neurotransmitter receptor mapping by autoradiography and other methods, *Annu. Rev. Neurosci.*, 9, 27, 1986.

Langley, J. N., On the reactions of cells and nerve endings to certain poisons, in regards to the reaction of striated muscle to nicotine and curare, *J. Physiol.*, 33, 374, 1906.

Lenard, J. and Singer, S. J., Specificity of affinity labeling of anti-DNP molecule antibodies, *Immunocytochemistry*, 3, 51, 1966.

Lentz, T. L. and Chester, J., Localization of acetylcholine receptors in central synapses, J. Cell Biol., 75, 258, 1977.

Levitsky, A., *Receptors: A Quantitative Approach,* Benjamin/Cummings, Menlo Park, CA, 1985.

Mishina, M., Kurosaki, T., Tobimatsu, T., Morimoto, Y., Noda, M., Yamamoto, T., Terao, M., Lindstrom, J., Takahashi, T., Kuno, M., and Numa, S., Expression of functional acetylcholine receptor from cloned cDNA's, *Nature (London)*, 307, 604, 1984.

Munson, P. J. and Rodbard, D., LIGAND: a versatile approach for characterization of ligand binding systems, *Anal. Biochem.*, 107, 220, 1980.

Nishimura, E., Billestrup, N., Perrin, M. H., and Vale, W., Identification and characterization of a pituitary corticotropin-releasing factor binding protein by chemical cross-linking, *J. Biol. Chem.*, 262, 12893, 1987.

Palacios, J. M., Niehoff, D. L., and Kuhar, M. J., Receptor autoradiography with tritium-sensitive film: potential for computerized densitometry, *Neurosci. Lett.*, 24, 111, 1981.

Petruzzelli, L., Herrera, R., Garcia-Arenas, R., and Rosen, O. M., Acquisition of insulin-dependent protein tyrosine kinase activity during *Drosophila* embryogenesis, *J. Biol. Chem.*, 260, 16072, 1985.

Reiter, M. J., Cowburn, D. A., Prives, J. M., and Karlin, A., Affinity labeling of the acetylcholine receptor in the electroplax. Electrophoretic separation in sodium dodecyl sulfate, *Proc. Natl. Acad. Sci. U.S.A.*, 69, 1168, 1972.

Richards, J. G., Mohler, H., and Haefely, W., Mapping benzodiazepine receptors in the CNS by radiohistochemistry and immunohistochemistry, in *Neurology and Neurobiology*, Vol. 16 (Neurohistochemistry, modern methods and applications), Panula, P., Paivarinta, H., and Soinila, S., Eds., Alan R. Liss, New York, 1986, 629.

Richards, J. G., Schoch, P., Haring, P., Takacs, B., and Mohler, H., Resolving $GABA_A$/benzodiazepine receptors: cellular and subcellular localization in the CNS with monoclonal antibodies, *J. Neurosci.*, 7(6), 1866, 1987.

Rosendale, B. E., Jarrett, D. B., and Robinson, A. G., Identification of a corticotropin-releasing factor-binding protein in the plasma membrane of AtT-20 mouse pituitary tumor cells and its regulation by dexamethasone, *Endocrinology*, 120, 2357, 1987.

Rotter, A., Birdsall, N. J. M., Burgen, A. S. V., Field, P. M., Hulme, E. C., and Raisman, G., Muscarinic receptors in the central nervous system of the rat. I. Technique for autoradiographic localization of the binding of [^{3}H]-propylbenzilylcholine mustard and its distribution in the forebrain, *Brain Res. Rev.*, 41, 1, 1979.

Seeman, P., Drug receptors, in *Principles of Medical Pharmacology*, Kalant, H., Roschlau, W. H. E., and Sellers, E. M., Eds., University of Toronto Press, Toronto, 1985.

Strader, C. D., Pickel, V. M., Joh, T. H., Strohsacker, M. W., Shorr, R. G. L., Lefkowitz, R. J., and Caron, M. G., Antibodies to the β-adrenergic receptor: functional characterization and receptor immunolocalization in brain, *Soc. Neurosci. Abstr.*, 8, 526, 1982.

Swanson, L. W., Lindstrom, J., Tzartos, S., Schmued, L. C., O'Leary, D. D. M., and Cowan, W. M., Immunohistochemical localization of monoclonal antibodies to the nicotinic acetylcholine receptor in chick midbrain, *Proc. Natl. Acad. Sci. U.S.A.*, 80, 4532, 1983a.

Swanson, L. W., Sawchenko, P. E., Rivier, J., and Vale, W. W., Organization of ovine corticotropin-releasing factor immunoreactive cells and fibers in the rat brain: an immunohistochemical study, *Neuroendocrinology*, 36, 165, 1983b.

Vandelen, R. L., Arcur, K. E., and Napier, M. A., Identification of a receptor for atrial natriuretic factor in rabbit aorta membranes by affinity cross-linking, *J. Biol. Chem.*, 260, 10889, 1985.

Vieillemaringe, J., Souan, M. L., Grandier-Vazeilles, X., and Geffard, M., Immunocytochemical localization of acetylcholine receptors in locust brain using auto-anti-idiotypic acetylcholine antibodies, *Neurosci. Lett.*, 79(1–2), 59, 1987.

Wagner, H. N., Burns, H. D., Dannals, R. F., Wong, D. F., Langstrom, B., Duelfer, T., Frost, J. J., Ravert, H. T., Links, J. M., Rosenbloom, S. B., Lukas, S. E., Kramer, A. V., and Kuhar, M. J., Imaging dopamine receptors in the human brain by positron tomography, *Science*, 221, 1264, 1983.

Wofsy, L., Metzger, H., and Singer, S. J., Affinity labeling: a general method for labeling the active sites of antibody and enzyme molecules, *Biochemistry*, 1, 1031, 1962.

Wong, D. F., Wagner, H. N., Jr., Dannals, R. F., Links, J. M., Frost, J. J., Ravert, H. T., Wilson, A. A., Rosenbaum, A. E., Gjedde, A., Douglas, K. H., Petronis, J. D., Folstein, M. F., Toung, J. K. T., Burns, H. D., and Kuhar, M. J., Effects of age on dopamine and serotonin receptors measured by positron tomography in the living human brain, *Science*, 226, 1393, 1984.

Wood, C. L. and O'Dorisio, M. S., Covalent cross-linking of vasoactive intestinal polypeptide to its receptors on intact human lymphoblasts, *J. Biol. Chem.*, 260, 1243, 1985.

Young, W. S., II, and Kuhar, M. J., A new method for receptor autoradiography: ^{3}H-opioid labeling in mounted tissue sections, *Brain Res.*, 179, 255, 1979.

Section II
Anatomical Neuroendocrinology

Tomas Hökfelt, Section Editor

6

The Organization of Monoaminergic Neurons in the Hypothalamus in Relation to Neuroendocrine Integration

BARRY J. EVERITT
Department of Anatomy
University of Cambridge
Cambridge, England

AND

BJÖRN MEISTER AND TOMAS HÖKFELT
Department of Histology and Neurobiology
Karolinska Institute
Stockholm, Sweden

I. Introduction

Monoaminergic neurons have been implicated in neuroendocrine control mechanisms partly on the basis of the observations, using the Falck-Hillarp fluorescence technique (Falck et al., 1962), showing that the hypothalamus is especially rich in noradrenaline-, dopamine- and 5-hydroxytryptamine (5-HT)-containing fibers and terminals and also that a group of dopaminergic cell bodies, located in the arcuate nucleus, is the origin of a rich terminal plexus in the external layer of the median eminence (Dahlström and Fuxe, 1964; Fuxe, 1964, 1965; Fuxe and Hökfelt, 1966, 1969; Fuxe et al., 1985; Björklund et al., 1973; Hökfelt, 1973; Moore and Bloom, 1978, 1979; Azmitia, 1978; Steinbusch, 1981; Descarries and Beaudet, 1978; Ungerstedt, 1971). Since these initial observations, and as several of the chapters in this volume show, many pharmacological and neurochemical experiments have amply confirmed the impact of altering monoaminergic activity on the secretion of the majority of hypothalamic and/or anterior pituitary hormones (see also Lightman and Everitt, 1986a). The advent of immunocytochemistry has allowed clarification of the innervation of the hypothalamus by monoaminergic neurons, mainly through visualization of the intraneuronal enzymes involved in amine synthesis (see Figure 1; Hökfelt et al., 1973, 1976, 1984a,b; Björklund and Lindvall, 1984; Swanson and Hartman, 1975; Jaeger et al., 1984; Fuxe et al., 1978). In addition, new elements of the monoaminergic systems innervating the hypothalamus, in particular the adrenaline-containing neurons (Hökfelt et al., 1974, 1984a; Ruggiero et al., 1985), have also been revealed by these techniques, whereas it had not been possible to identify them using earlier methods. Perhaps even more important is that these immunocytochemical procedures have also allowed visualization of the neuronal systems containing the hypothalamic release and release-inhibiting hormones themselves (see Barry et al., 1985; Ceccatelli et al., 1989; Hökfelt et al., 1986, 1987; Hoffman et al., 1982; Jennes et al., 1982; Khatachurian et al., 1985;

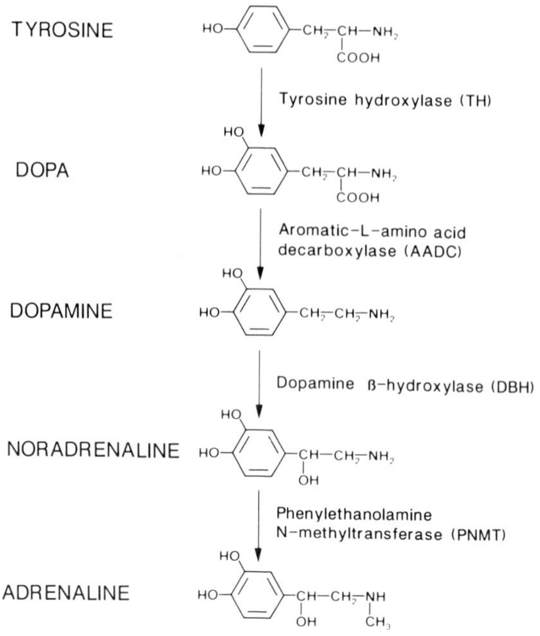

TYROSINE

Tyrosine hydroxylase (TH)

DOPA

Aromatic–L–amino acid decarboxylase (AADC)

DOPAMINE

Dopamine β–hydroxylase (DBH)

NORADRENALINE

Phenylethanolamine N–methyltransferase (PNMT)

ADRENALINE

Figure 1. Summary of the pathway and enzymes involved in the synthesis of catecholamines.

Swanson et al., 1983). Thus, the relationships between monoaminergic systems and hypothalamic peptidergic systems have become much clearer, sometimes at the ultrastructural level, such that synaptic contacts have been demonstrated between monoaminergic and peptidergic neurons, thereby indicating the neuroanatomical basis for the endocrine consequences of aminergic drug treatments (see below).

It is the purpose of this chapter to review the distribution of noradrenergic, adrenergic, dopaminergic, and serotoninergic neurons in the hypothalamus, focusing on those structures that are important in neuroendocrine control mechanisms in order to provide a basis for the functional data reviewed elsewhere in this volume. This has been the subject of a number of reviews during the past 20 or so years and the reader is referred to them in order to gain different perspectives (Ajika, 1980; Grant and Stumpf, 1974; Fuxe and Hökfelt, 1969; Hökfelt and Fuxe, 1972; Hökfelt et al., 1978, 1984; Lightman and Everitt, 1986a; McCann and Ojeda, 1976; Neill, 1980; Sawchenko and Swanson, 1982; Sawyer et al., 1978; Swanson et al., 1981, 1986).

II. Noradrenergic and Adrenergic Innervation of the Hypothalamus

Immunocytochemical analysis of the patterns of tyrosine hydroxylase (TH), dopamine β-hydroxylase (DBH), and phenylethanolamine-N-methyltransferase (PNMT) immunoreactivities (IR) has been used differentially to demonstrate dopamine-, noradrenaline-, and adrenaline-containing neurons in the central nervous system (see Figure 1). Used in conjunction with retrograde tracing and lesion studies, it has been demonstrated that the noradrenergic innervation of the hypothalamus arises mainly from cell groups A1, A2 in the medulla oblongata, and A6 in the pons, whereas the adrenergic innervation arises from cell groups C1, C2, and C3, situated mainly in the medulla (Swanson, 1987; Chan-Palay et al., 1984; Swanson et al., 1981; Sawchenko and Swanson, 1982; see Figures 2 through 5). The locus coeruleus (A6; see Figure 4) gives rise to the most restricted noradrenergic projection, innervating primarily the periventricular

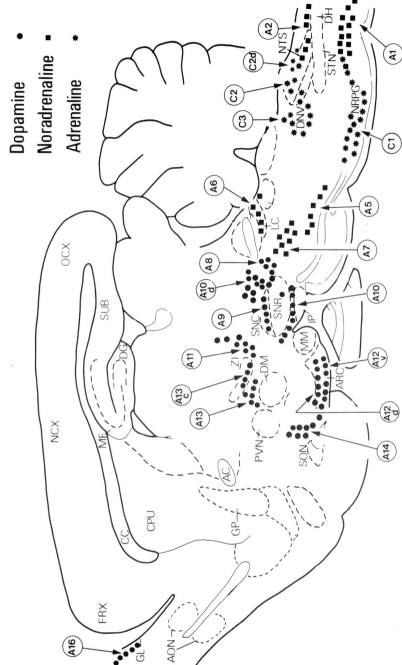

Figure 2. Schematic representation of the distribution of catecholamine cell groups in the rat brain. A1 to A7 represent noradrenaline cell groups. A8 to A16 dopamine cell groups, and C1 to C3 adrenaline cell groups. Nomenclature according to Dahlström and Fuxe (1964) and Hökfelt et al. (1984b). AC, anterior commissure; AON, anterior olfactory nucleus; ARC, arcuate nucleus; CC, corpus callosum; CPU, caudate-putamen; DG, dentate gyrus; DM, dorsomedial hypothalamic nucleus; DNB, dorsal motor nucleus of vagus; FRX, frontal cortex; GL, glomerular layer of the olfactory bulb; GP, globus pallidus; IP, interpeduncular nucleus; LC, locus ceruleus; MM, medial mamillary nucleus; NCX, neocortex; NRP, nucleus reticularis paragigantocellularis; NTS, nucleus tractus solitarii; OCX, occipital cortex; PVN, hypothalamic paraventricular nucleus; SNC, substantia nigra, pars compacta; SNR, substantia nigra, pars reticulata; SON, supraoptic nucleus; SUB, subiculum; ZI, zona incerta.

Dopamine ●
Noradrenaline ■
Adrenaline ✻

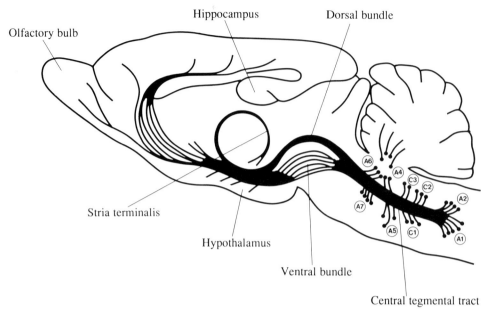

Figure 3. Schematic drawing illustrating the projections from catecholamine cell groups in the medulla oblongata and pons. Redrawn from Ungerstedt (1971) and Everitt and Hökfelt (1989).

nucleus throughout the rostrocaudal extent of the hypothalamus, including the periventricular domains of the paraventricular and arcuate nuclei, as well as the preoptic area (Sawchenko and Swanson, 1982). The subset of A6 neurons innervating this region of the hypothalamus appears preferentially to contain neuropeptide Y (NPY) as a cotransmitter (Holets et al., 1988). Many hypothalamic nuclei receive a relatively rich noradrenergic innervation, including the medial preoptic, suprachiasmatic, supraoptic (SON), paraventricular (PVN, magnocellular and parvocellular parts), arcuate, ventromedial, and dorsomedial nuclei, as well as the retrochiasmatic area (Hökfelt et al., 1984b; Chan-Palay et al., 1984; Swanson, 1987). In general, the A1 cell group is the major site of origin of these projections, but the A2 cell group provides important components of the noradrenergic innervation of some structures, such as parts of the PVN (Sawchenko and Swanson, 1982; Swanson, 1987).

Although less extensively studied, it is clear that a number of these structures also receive a rich adrenergic innervation, especially the medial and dorsal parvocellular PVN, the medial preoptic area, periventricular nucleus, parts of the arcuate nucleus, and also the dorsomedial nucleus (Hökfelt et al., 1984a; Swanson, 1987). While cell group C1 seems to be the main origin of these projections, neurons in the C2 and C3 cell groups have also been shown to be retrogradely labeled following injections of fluorescent tracers into various of these nuclei, but especially the PVN (Sawchenko and Swanson, 1982; Swanson, 1987). Large numbers of the noradrenaline neurons and almost all of the adrenaline neurons innervating the hypothalamus also contain NPY (Everitt et al., 1984; Everitt and Hökfelt, 1989; Hökfelt et al., 1986; Swanson, 1987; see below and Figure 6).

A. Magnocellular Neurosecretory Neurons

The most detailed analysis of hypothalamic noradrenaline-containing terminals has focused on the PVN and SON (Sawchenko and Swanson, 1982; Swanson et al., 1981; Swanson, 1987; see Figure 7). Within the SON and magnocellular parts of the PVN, the dense noradren-

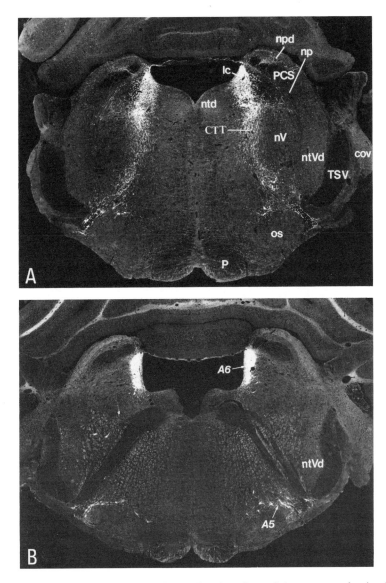

Figure 4 (A,B). Immunofluorescence photomicrographs of sections of the rat pons after incubation with antiserum to tyrosine hydroxylase (TH), showing cell groups A5 and A6 (locus ceruleus). Fibres forming the central tegmental tract (CTT) are clearly seen in A.

ergic innervation is largely confined to the region of the vasopressin neurons (e.g., in the ventral part of the SON and central part of the PVN) and arises mainly from cell group A1 (Figures 7 and 8). Oxytocin neuron domains of these nuclei are very weakly innervated by noradrenergic neurons. Few PNMT-IR nerve terminals are found in these locations, indicating only a minor adrenergic control of vasopressin neuronal activity. The relatively rich plexus of NPY-containing terminals in the same regions of the SON and PVN (Figure 8) probably also largely arises from the A1 cell group, since about half of the dopamine β-hydroxylase-IR (DBH-IR) neurons in this area also contain the peptide (Everitt and Hökfelt, 1989; Swanson, 1987). This pattern of innervation of neurosecretory vasopressin (AVP) neurons by A1

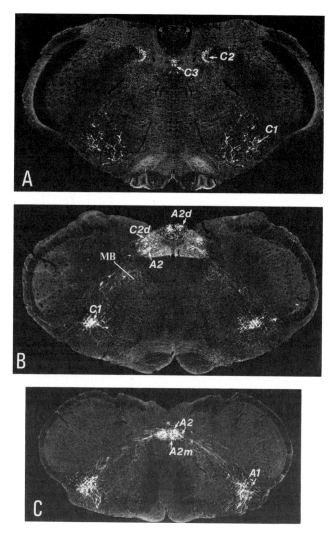

Figure 5 (A–C). Immunofluorescence photomicrographs of sections of the rat medulla oblongata after incubation with antiserum to tyrosine hydroxylase (TH), showing cell groups A1, A2, C1, C2, and C3.

noradrenergic neurons clearly indicates an important role for noradrenergic transmission in the regulation of AVP secretion and this has been confirmed in a variety of functional studies (Lightman et al., 1983, 1984). The connections of the A1 cell group in the ventrolateral medulla indicate the sort of physiological situation in which this noradrenergic control might be important. It receives a rich projection from the nucleus of the solitary tract (NTS), which is an important relay for primary visceral afferent information arriving via cranial nerves X, IX, and VII (Sawchenko and Swanson, 1982; Swanson and Mogenson, 1981). Thus it might be predicted, for example, that the AVP response to hypovolemia-induced hypotension might be compromised by lesions of the noradrenergic afferents to the PVN/SON, since the relay of such information via the NTS will be interrupted; this has been shown to be the case (Lightman and Everitt, 1986b). Experiments on the effects of NPY on magnocellular neurosecretory function have yielded equivocal results and only high dosages of NPY or APP applied to the region of vasopressin-containing neurons in the SON are effective, and tend to increase the

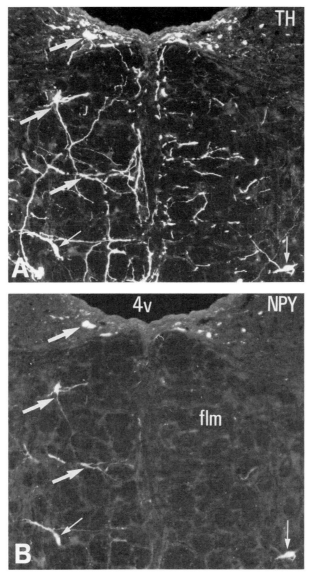

Figure 6 (A–C). Immunofluorescence photomicrographs of sections of the C1 region in the rat medulla oblongata showing colocalization of tyrosine hydroxylase (TH) (A) and neuropeptide Y (NPY) (B) in a double-labeled section.

firing of such neurons, thereby mimicking the effects of noradrenaline (Day et al., 1985). However, when given together with noradrenaline, the peptide appears to antagonize the effects of the catecholamine (Day et al., 1985).

The rate-limiting enzyme in the synthesis of catecholamines, tyrosine hydroxylase, has been demonstrated in magnocellular neurons of the SON and PVN (Swanson et al., 1981; Chan-Palay et al., 1984; Hökfelt et al., 1984; Van den Pol et al., 1984; Li et al., 1988; Spencer et al., 1985). Increased production of TH is observed in the diabetes insipidus rat of the Brattleboro strain (vasopressin deficient) (Kiss and Mezey, 1986; Meister et al., 1990a), after administration of hyperosmotic stimuli (Figure 9; Kiss and Mezey, 1986; Young et al., 1987;

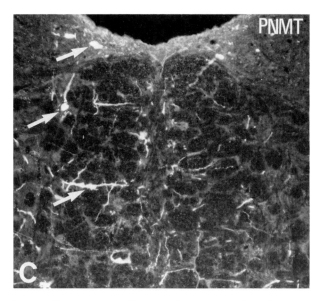

Figure 6 (A—C)(continued). (C) represents an adjacent section incubated with antiserum to phenylethanolamine-
N-methyltransferase (PNMT). Note that cells indicated by large arrow contain all three immunoreactivities. Thin
arrows point to cells showing TH- and NPY-immunoreactivity. flm = fasciculus longitudinalis medialis, 4v =
fourth ventricle.

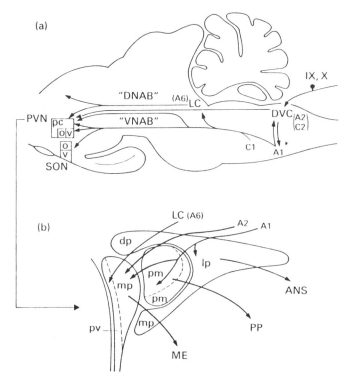

Figure 7. Afferent and efferent connections of the paraventricular and supraoptic nuclei in the rat, with emphasis
on ascending catecholaminergic neurons. (Redrawn from Lightman and Everitt, 1986a after the original work of
Sawchenko and Swanson, 1982).

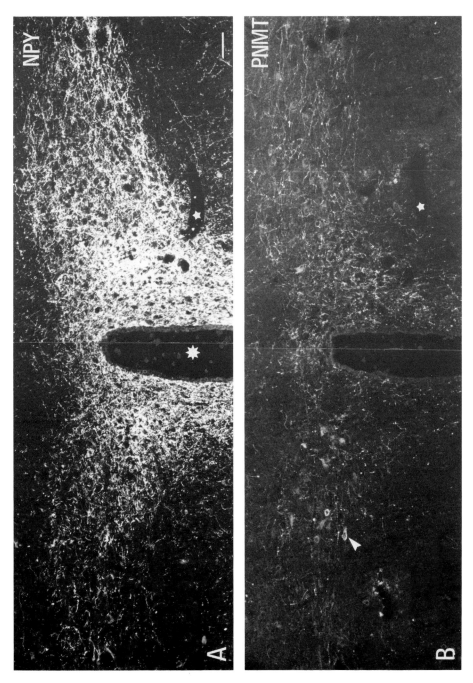

Figure 8 (A–D). Immunofluorescence photomicrographs of sections of the hypothalamic paraventricular nucleus (PVN) after incubation with antisera to neuropeptide Y (NPY) (A), phenylethanolamine-*N*-methyltransferase (PNMT) (B), dopamine β-hydroxylase (DBH).

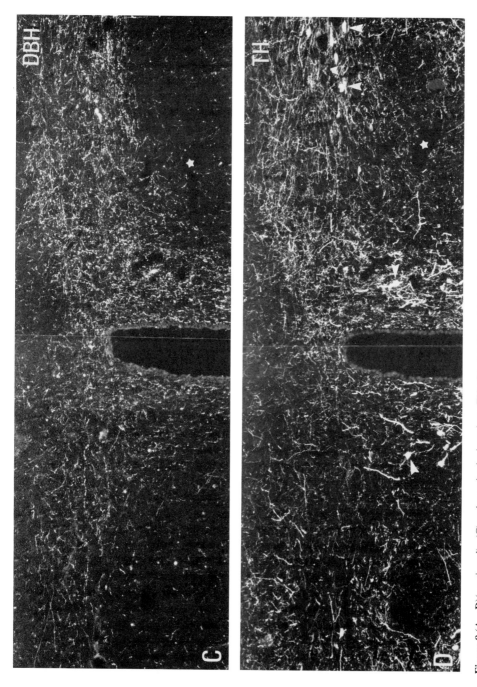

Figure 8 (A—D)(continued). (C) and tyrosine hydroxylase (TH) (D). A unilateral lesion has been made in the rostral brain stem. On the control side (right hand side), fibers containing NPY-, PNMT-, DBH-, and TH-immunoreactivity can be seen in the parvo- and magnocellular parts of the PVN. On the lesioned side (left hand side), there is a marked decrease in the number of immunoreactive fibers, indicating a common, brainstem source of the peptide- and the catecholamine-containing neurons. (Palkovits, Mezey, Skirboll, and Hökfelt, unpublished.)

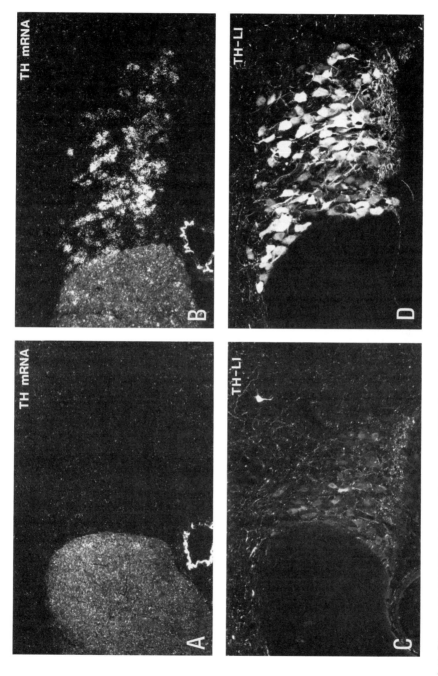

Figure 9 (A–D). Dark-field (A,B) and immunofluorescence (C,D) photomicrographs of sections of the supraoptic nucleus showing tyrosine hydroxylase (TH) mRNA, as visualized with *in situ* hybridization and TH-immunoreactivity, as demonstrated with immunohistochemistry. In control rats (A,C), virtually no TH mRNA or TH-containing cells can be observed, whereas administration of a hyperosmotic stimulus (2% saline in the drinking water, B,D) induces the appearance of many cells containing TH mRNA and TH-immunoreactivity (compare A with B and C with D).

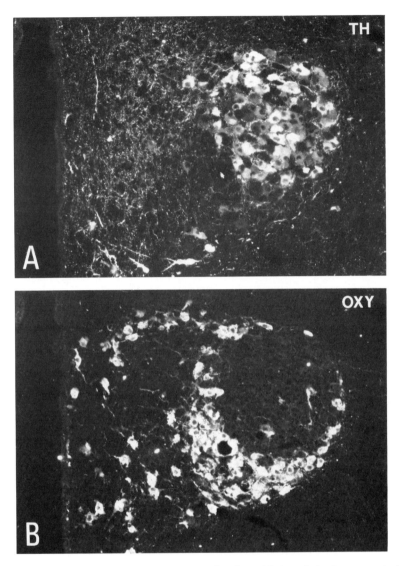

Figure 10 (A–D). Immunofluorescence photomicrographs of sections of the hypothalamic paraventricular nucleus (PVN) (A,B) and supraoptic nucleus (SON) (C,D) after incubation with antisera to tyrosine hydroxylase (TH) (A,C), oxytocin (OXY) (B) and vasopressin (VP) (D). A and B as well as C and D represent double-labelled sections. (A,B) After salt loading (2% saline in the drinking water for two weeks), several TH-immunoreactive cell bodies are seen in the central part of the PVN, whereas OXY-immunoreactive cell bodies are observed in the peripheral part of the PVN. There is no evidence for colocalization.

Meister et al., 1990a,b), or after transections that disrupt afferents from the lower brainstem to the SON and PVN (Kiss and Mezey, 1986). The enzyme is exclusively located in the vasopressin-containing subpopulation of magnocellular neurons, which also contains the peptides galanin (GAL), dynorphin, and Leu-enkephalin (Figure 10; Meister et al., 1990a). Although both TH immunoreactivity and TH mRNA have been demonstrated in magnocellular neurons, no aromatic L-amino acid decarboxylase (AADC), dopamine immunoreactivity, or dopamine histofluorescence has been detected in the SON or magnocellular PVN (see Meister

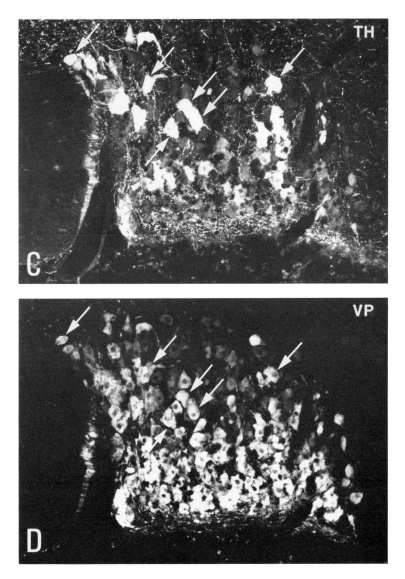

Figure 10 (A—D)(continued). (C,D) TH-positive cell bodies are seen in all parts of the SON, and many of the TH-immunoreactive cells also contain VP (see arrows).

et al., 1990a), and this has raised the question as to what extent these neurons produce dopamine itself. A similar situation exists in the arcuate nucleus (see below).

B. Parvocellular Neurosecretory Neurons

The medial and dorsal subdivisions of the parvocellular PVN, which are rich in peptide-containing neurosecretory neurons (including CRF, TRH, enkephalin, VIP), receive a prominent noradrenergic innervation that arises predominantly from the A2 cell group in the NTS and also a dense adrenergic innervation arising from the C1, C2, and C3 cell groups (Hökfelt et al., 1984b; Sawchenko and Swanson, 1982; Swanson, 1987). The adrenergic neurons almost all contain NPY (Figure 6) and this is consistent, therefore, with the dense NPY-IR terminal plexus found in the medial PVN (Everitt and Hökfelt, 1989; Everitt et al., 1984). However, not all the NPY terminals in the PVN arise from this site, since the NPY-IR neurons found in the medial arcuate nucleus apparently project to these regions of the PVN (Bai et al., 1985). The C1 adrenergic neurons, like the A1 noradrenergic neurons, receive projections from the NTS, indicating that these may also relay visceral afferent influences on the secretion of neuropeptides into the portal circulation (Sawchenko and Swanson, 1982; Swanson, 1987). The involvement of noradrenergic mechanisms in the control of the secretory activity of the parvocellular PVN has been studied most extensively in the context of CRF secretion, especially since there is great overlap between adrenergic and noradrenergic fibers/terminals and CRF-IR neurons in the parvocellular PVN (Cunningham and Sawchenko, 1988; Cunningham et al., 1990). Synaptic contacts between catecholamine-containing nerve terminals and CRF-containing parvocellular PVN neurons have been observed at the ultrastructural level (Liposits et al., 1986a,b). However, the picture is not a very clear one. Infusion of noradrenaline, adrenaline, or NPY directly into the PVN of rats all result in increased corticosterone secretion (Härfstrand, 1987; Leibowitz, 1988; Leibowitz et al., 1988, 1989). Similarly, lesions of the ventral noradrenergic pathway impair the corticosterone response to swimming and footshock stress (Selden et al., 1990, and in press). It has also been demonstrated that individually subeffective doses of adrenaline and NPY, when coinfused into the PVN, result in a corticosterone response obtained only with substantially higher doses of each alone (Everitt and Martensz, unpublished observations), indicating that cotransmission of the amine and peptide may be of functional importance in this system. However, there is much that remains to be established concerning the relative importance of noradrenergic and adrenergic effects on CRF secretion, especially whether or not both systems mediate stress responses of the hypothalamo-pituitary-adrenal axis, or whether they have separable functions. It has been demonstrated that the population of CRF neurons in the PVN also contains other neuropeptides, including neurotensin (NT), TRH, VIP, and enkephalin (Ceccatelli et al., 1989), and that these may respond differentially to stressors as well as to the feedback effects of corticosterone (Swanson et al., 1986). It may be important to investigate the patterns of peptide immunoreactivities or gene expression in these neurons in response to noradrenergic, adrenergic, or NPY manipulations of the PVN in order to understand better the contributions of each to the regulation of their secretory activity.

Many TRH neurons are found in the medial parvocellular PVN, medial to the major group of CRF neurons (see Lechan & Toni, this volume). There is some anatomical evidence of direct regulation of their secretory activity by noradrenergic and/or adrenergic afferents, since DBH- and PNMT-containing terminals have been observed in direct contact with identified TRH neurons (Shioda et al., 1986; Liposits et al., 1987). In addition, NPY-containing terminals also appear to make direct contact with TRH neurons in the PVN. Pharmacological studies have clearly indicated stimulatory noradrenergic and adrenergic influences on TRH neurons (Lechan and Toni, this volume), although it is as yet unclear whether NPY affects TRH secretion, either directly or by modulating noradrenaline or adrenaline release within the PVN.

The periventricular preoptic area, including the medial preoptic nucleus, receives a moderate noradrenergic and adrenergic innervation, as revealed by immunocytochemical localization of DBH- and PNMT-containing fibers and terminals (Chan-Palay et al., 1984; Simerly and Swanson, 1986; Simerly et al., 1986; Swanson, 1987). Throughout this area and up into the medial septum, LHRH-IR neurons are found (Barry et al., 1985; Hoffman this volume) and there is some evidence of direct synaptic contacts between catecholamine-containing (TH-IR) and LHRH neurons (Hoffman et al., 1982; Jennes et al., 1982). There is pharmacological evidence of catecholaminergic influences on LHRH secretion (Coen and Coombs, 1983; Coen and Gallo, 1986; Sawyer et al., 1978), but the sites of action and identity of the catecholamine involved remain uncertain. Both noradrenaline and adrenaline, when given intraventricularly, stimulate LH secretion in ovariectomized, steroid-primed rats (Krieg and Sawyer, 1976; Gallo and Drouva, 1979; Condon et al., 1986), whereas inhibition of noradrenaline and, more specifically, adrenaline synthesis prevents both the preovulatory LH surge and estrogen-induced LH release (Adler et al., 1983; Coen and Coombs, 1983; Martensz et al., 1990). Experiments involving lesions of the noradrenergic innervation of the hypothalamus using 6-hydroxydopamine have provided less convincing evidence of an important role for noradrenergic mechanisms in regulating LHRH secretion (Hancke and Wuttke, 1977, 1979; Hansen et al., 1980, 1981; Martensz et al., 1990; Nicholson et al., 1978). However, there is a substantial body of evidence indicating that preoptic adrenergic and, to a lesser extent, noradrenergic neurons mediate opioid peptide influences on LH secretion. Thus, naloxone-induced LH secretion in male rats is prevented by treatments that reduce preoptic area adrenaline, but not noradrenaline, concentrations (Kalra, 1981; Kalra and Crowley, 1982; Kalra and Kalra, 1984; Martensz et al., 1990; Miller et al., 1985; Van Vugt et al., 1981). Although the preoptic area has been shown to be one important site at which these interactions between adrenaline/noradrenaline and opioid peptides occur (Kalra, 1981; Kalra and Simpkins, 1981; Martensz et al., 1990), there are also data to suggest an additional site of interaction in the mediobasal hypothalamus (Kalra, 1981). The preponderance of data indicates a presynaptic modulation of catecholamine release by opioid, presumably preopiomelanocortin (β-endorphin)-containing, neurons (Martensz et al., 1990; Kalra, 1981), but there is little ultrastructural evidence indicating that such an interaction occurs in either the preoptic area or mediobasal hypothalamus.

Little can be said with certainty about the influence of noradrenergic and adrenergic terminal plex uses in the periventricular preoptic/anterior hypothalamic areas on the secretory activity of somatostatin-containing neurons there, which have clearly been demonstrated to give rise to the major somatostatin terminals in the external layer of the median eminence (Ishikawa et al., 1987; Kawano and Daikoku, 1988; see Meister and Hökfelt, this volume).

While not a site at which neurosecretory neurons are found, the *suprachiasmatic nucleus* is clearly important in a neuroendocrine setting because light-entrained circadian rhythms of hormone secretion are determined by the activity of this structure (Hastings and Herbert, 1986). In monoaminergic terms, the nucleus is prominent because of its exceptionally rich 5-HT innervation (see below), but it also receives a relatively rich noradrenergic innervation, especially in its external part. These noradrenergic afferents enter the nucleus via the supraoptic decussation, but their precise origin has not been determined (Chan-Palay et al., 1984; Swanson, 1987). There are few functional data to date on the role of this noradrenergic innervation of the suprachiasmatic nucleus.

The *ventromedial nucleus* is generally devoid of catecholamine-containing terminals, but the nucleus is surrounded by a moderately dense adrenergic plexus (see Figure 11), while the capsule of the nucleus appears, from biochemical experiments, to receive a noradrenergic innervation arriving via the so-called ventral noradrenergic bundle (see Chan-Palay et al., 1984 for discussion). However, immunocytochemical analysis has indicated that the capsular parts of the ventromedial nucleus are devoid of DBH-IR terminals and fibers (Chan-Palay et al., 1984). It is in the region of the capsule of the ventromedial nucleus that GRH-containing, as well as TH-containing, neurons are found (Meister et al., 1986; see Meister & Hökfelt, this volume). It is not clear, however, as to whether these neurons are contacted by catecholamine neurons originating in the brainstem.

The *arcuate nucleus* is of central importance in neuroendocrine control mechanisms and has long been known to contain a population of dopaminergic neurons projecting to the external layer of the median eminence where the amine is secreted (Fuxe and Hökfelt, 1966,

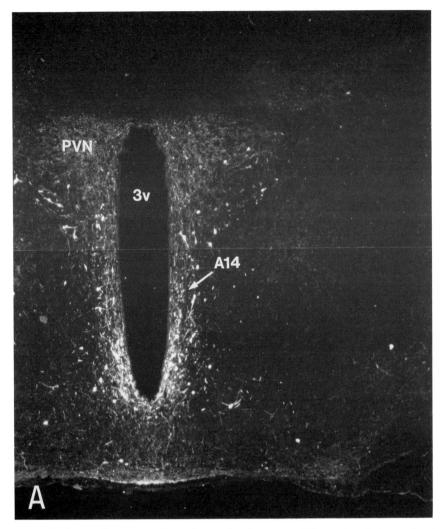

Figure 11 (A,B). Immunofluorescence photomicrographs of sections of the rat hypothalamus showing the distribution of tyrosine hydroxylase-immunoreactive cell bodies. Dopamine-containing cell groups A12, A13 and A14 are depicted. d = dorsal, ME = median eminence, PVN = paraventricular nucleus, v = ventral, VMN = ventromedial nucleus, 3v = third ventricle.

1969; Lechan et al., 1982; Van den Pol and Cassidy, 1982). However, this nucleus also receives a noradrenergic projection arising from the A1 cell group and an adrenergic projection arising from the C1 cell group (see Chan-Palay et al., 1984; Swanson, 1987). There are many TH-IR fibers and terminals within the nucleus that probably also represent local aborizations of the arcuate dopaminergic neurons themselves. The putative role of noradrenergic and adrenergic afferents in regulating the secretion of dopamine, GRH, and other hormones from arcuate neurons, either by direct effects within the nucleus or via terminal interactions in the external layer of the median eminence, is unclear and will be discussed further below in the context of the arcuate dopaminergic neurons themselves.

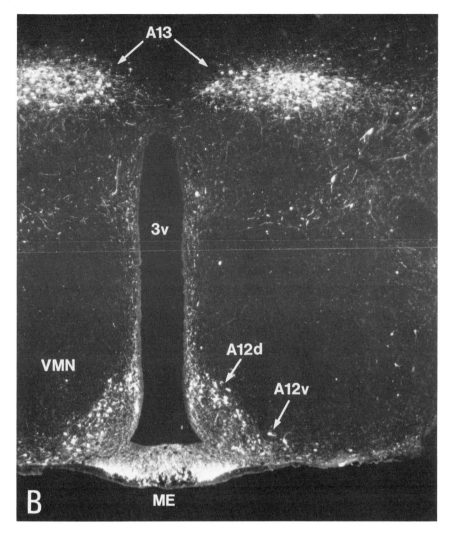

Figure 11 (A,B) (continued).

III. Dopaminergic Neurons in the Hypothalamus

Dopamine has for many years been implicated in the control of both hypothalamic and pituitary hormone secretion, largely through pharmacological experiments and the demonstration of the tuberoinfundibular dopaminergic system (Fuxe and Hökfelt, 1966, 1969). The importance in the regulation of prolactin secretion of dopamine secreted from the terminals of these arcuate neurons into the portal vessels running through the palisade zone of the external layer of the median eminence is beyond doubt (MacLeod and Lehmeyer, 1974; McNeilly, 1986; Neill, 1980). However, the importance of synaptic or paracrine influences of dopamine in the median eminence on the secretion of hypothalamic releasing hormones from parvocellular neuron terminals into the portal vessels in the median eminence (Hökfelt, 1968), as well as the functional importance of effects of the catecholamine on ependymal elements in the mediobasal hypothalamus (see below), is still unclear. Other complexities in understanding neuroendocrine functions of dopamine must also be considered. In addition to arcuate (A12) dopaminergic neurons, there are numbers of additional intrinsic, hypothalamic cell groups possibly of dopaminergic nature: A15 in the dorsal preoptic area, under the anterior commissure as well as above the optic chiasm, these being "joined" in the dorsoventral direction by cell group A14 in the periventricular nucleus, which expands into the paraventricular nucleus; A13 and A11 — not strictly in the hypothalamus, but in the overlying zona incerta with their axons running *inter alia* to the preoptic/anterior hypothalamic area (see Figure 11; Björklund et al., 1975, 1979, 1984; Hökfelt et al., 1984b; Jacobowitz and Palkovits, 1974; Kizer et al., 1976b; Kawano and Daikoku, 1987; Lindvall and Björklund, 1978; Moore and Bloom, 1978). In general, the projections and functions of these intrahypothalamic cell groups are poorly understood.

Of particular interest the recent demonstration of multiple and complex patterns of peptide, amine, and amino acid coexistence in the dopaminergic neurons of the arcuate nucleus (Everitt et al., 1986; Meister and Hökfelt, 1988; Meister et al., 1989a). This formerly simple group of dopaminergic neurosecretory neurons involved in the regulation of prolactin secretion from the anterior pituitary is now a most complex neuroendocrine structure that appears to elaborate a large array of amine, amino acid, and peptide chemical messengers that may be secreted into the portal vessels or act as hypothalamic neurotransmitters/cotransmitters, or both. The functions of this small, yet complex nucleus are only beginning to be understood.

A. The Arcuate Nucleus

The arcuate nucleus is generally subdivided into three main parts: dorsomedial, ventrolateral, and ventromedial (Fuxe et al., 1985; Meister and Hökfelt, 1988; Meister et al., 1989a). The dorsomedial part contains smaller TH-immunoreactive (IR) neurons, the ventrolateral part larger TH-IR neurons, and the ventromedial part does not contain TH-IR neurons (Figures 12 and 13), but has a substantial population of NPY-IR and somatostatin-IR neurons. Until recently, it has been generally assumed that all TH-IR neurons in the arcuate nucleus synthesize, transport, and release dopamine into the portal vessels. However, this assumption must now seriously be questioned. It has always been apparent that the dorsomedial cells, besides being smaller, are chemically different from ventrolateral cells, being more strongly fluorescent when TH-like immunoreactivity (LI) is examined using fluorescent markers (Everitt et al., 1986; Meister and Hökfelt, 1988; Meister et al., 1989a). But the ventrolateral group of neurons, while clearly containing TH IR and TH mRNA (Meister et al., unpublished results), does not appear to contain aromatic L-amino acid decarboxylase (AADC), the enzyme that converts L-dopa to dopamine (Figure 14, Jaeger et al., 1984; Okamura et al., 1988a), or dopamine-LI, or formaldehyde-induced fluorescence of the native catecholamine (Meister et al., 1988). Thus, there is considerable doubt as to the dopaminergic nature of these neurons. One possibility is that they synthesize and secrete not dopamine, but L-dopa, which may then be decarboxylated to dopamine by AADC known to be present in blood vessel walls (Bertler et al., 1964; Constantinidis et al., 1969), such that the catecholamine can travel in portal blood to act on the anterior pituitary. It has recently been demonstrated that some of these neurons do indeed contain L-dopa-LI (Okamura et al., 1988), although it is unclear whether this represents an end, or an intermediate, product. Determining the nature of the active catecholamine chemical messenger released by the ventrolateral arcuate TH-IR neurons is an important goal of future research since, if they are shown to secrete L-dopa, rather than dopamine, a new principle of neuroendocrine control must be considered.

This issue aside, there is an additional level of complexity in the chemical signal released

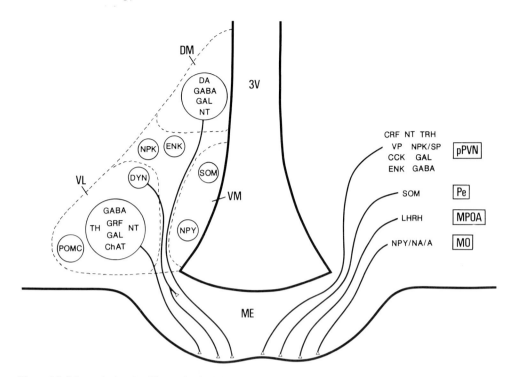

Figure 12. Schematic drawing illustrating both the distribution of neuroactive compounds in different parts of the arcuate nucleus and also afferents to the median eminence. Anatomical abbreviations: DM = dorsomedial; MO = medulla oblongata; MPOA = medial preoptic area; Pe = periventricular (hypothalamic) nucleus; pPVN = parvocellular (hypothalamic) paraventricular nucleus; VM = ventromedial; VL = ventrolateral; and 3V = third ventricle. Abbreviations for transmitters and peptides: A = adrenaline; CCK = cholecystokinin; ChAT = choline acetyltransferase; CRF = corticotropin-releasing factor; DA = dopamine; DYN = dynorphin; ENK = enkephalin; GABA = gamma-aminobutyric acid; GAL = galanin; GRF = growth hormone-releasing factor; NA = noradrenaline; NPK = neuropeptide K; NPY = neuropeptide Y; NT = neurotensin; POMC = proopiomelanocortin; SOM = somatostatin; SP = substance P; TH = tyrosine hydroxylase; TRH = thyroptropin-releasing hormone and VP = vasopressin. From Meister et al., 1989.

from arcuate TH-IR neurons and this is the result of the demonstration of complex patterns of coexistence (Figure 12). Thus, the dorsomedial TH-IR (dopaminergic) neurons have been shown to contain glutamic acid decarboxylase (GAD)-H, neurotensin (NT) and, to a somewhat lesser extent, dynorphin (DYN), galanin (GAL)-LI, and Leu-enkephalin-LI (see Figure 12; Everitt et al., 1984, 1986; Hökfelt et al., 1986, 1987; Ibata et al., 1983; Meister et al., 1988, 1989).

The situation is perhaps even more bewildering in the ventrolateral group of TH-IR neurons. Here, an extremely large proportion of the neurons also contain choline acetyltransferase (ChAT)-, GAD-, NT-, growth hormone-releasing hormone (GRH) and GAL-LI, while a rather small population of the TH-IR neurons contain Met-enkephalin and dynorphin-LI (see Figure 12; Everitt et al., 1984, 1986; Hökfelt et al., 1986, 1987; Melander et al., 1986; Meister et al., 1986, 1988, 1989).

Using a thin section (3 to 5 µm) technique coupled with direct double immunostaining, it has been confirmed that TH-containing terminals and fibers in the external layer of the median eminence in the region of the portal capillaries do, in fact, also contain GAD-LI. Furthermore, NT-, GAL-, and GRH-, but not somatostatin-LI, have been shown to colocalize with GAD (Meister and Hökfelt, 1988). This indicates that the population of neurosecretory neurons in

106 Barry J. Everitt, Björn Meister, and Tomas Hökfelt

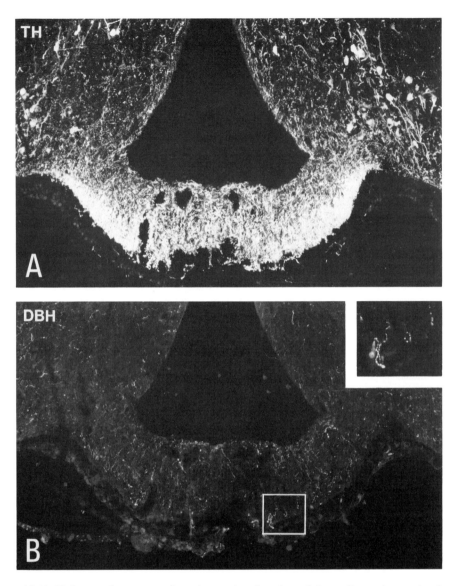

Figure 13 (A–C). Immunofluorescence photomicrographs of sections of the median eminence showing the distribution of tyrosine hydroxylase (TH)-, dopamine β-hydroxylase (DBH)-, and neuropeptide Y (NPY)-immunoreactive fibers. (A) TH-immunoreactive fibers are distributed in the entire median eminence, with the highest density in the lateral palisade zone of the external layer. Several TH-positive cell bodies are seen in the arcuate nucleus. (B) Only single DBH-immunoreactive fibers are seen in the median eminence (see inset as indicated by square).

the dorsomedial and ventrolateral arcuate nucleus do give rise to terminals in the neurosecretory zone that both contain and presumably release a number of chemical messengers. These data are clearly consistent with the view that these subgroups of arcuate neurons may secrete into the portal vessels, in addition to dopamine itself, GABA, NT, GRH, GAL, and, presumably, acetylcholine, enkephalin, and dynorphin and that this potentially complex mixture of chemical messengers may, singly or together, influence the activity of a variety of hormone-producing cell types in the adenohypophysis (see Everitt et al., 1986).

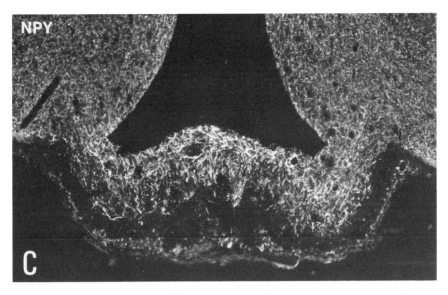

Figure 13 (A—C)(continued). (C) Many NPY-immunoreactive fibers are distributed in the median eminence, predominantly in the internal layer. Note also dense innervation of the arcuate nucleus by NPY-immunoreactive fibers.

In some instances, peptide immunoreactivities in terminals and fibers in the external layer of the median eminence could have a number of origins — for example, NT, GAL, and GRH neurons are also present, in varying numbers, in the parvocellular paraventricular nucleus (Ceccatelli et al., 1989; Swanson et al., 1986). In the case of NT, experiments with monosodium glutamate-induced lesions of the ventrolateral arcuate nucleus clearly indicate that the median eminence terminals and fibers containing this peptide arise exclusively from the ventrolateral arcuate and not at all from the dorsomedial arcuate or medial paraventricular nuclei (Meister et al., 1989a). In addition, the great majority of these NT neurons also contain TH-IR (but probably not dopamine), acetylcholine, GAL, GABA, and GRH (see Figure 12). In the case of GAL, similar lesion experiments indicate that the paraventricular neurons may also contribute to GAL-IR fibers and terminals in the median eminence, but that the great majority arise in the ventrolateral arcuate nucleus and, like NT neurons, they usually contain TH-LI, acetylcholine, and GRH (Meister et al., 1989a; see Figure 12). Monosodium glutamate-induced lesions of the ventrolateral arcuate nucleus also revealed that, similar to GAL, the vast majority of GRH-IR terminals and fibers in the external layer arise primarily from this site, but that some may derive from the small number of GRH-IR neurons in the paraventricular nucleus (Meister et al., 1989a). Again, these GRH neurons usually contain a rich array of additional messengers, including TH-LI, acetylcholine, NT, and GAL (see Figure 12). The majority of the Met-enkephalin-IR fibers in the external layer, by contrast, appear mostly to originate in the parvocellular paraventricular nucleus and not the arcuate nucleus (Meister et al., 1989a). Dynorphin-IR fibers, like proopiomelanocortin-containing fibers, are rarely seen in the external layer (Everitt et al., 1986).

Another, special feature of the arcuate nucleus in terms of its dopaminergic neurons concerns the demonstration of DARPP-32 [a dopamine- and cyclic adenosine-3′,5′-monophosphate (cAMP)-regulated phosphoprotein of m.w. 32 kDa] immunoreactivity in the specialized ependymal tanycytes, which are found in the floor of the third ventricle and also in the median eminence (Figure 15; Ouimet et al., 1984; Meister et al., 1988b; Everitt et al., 1986).

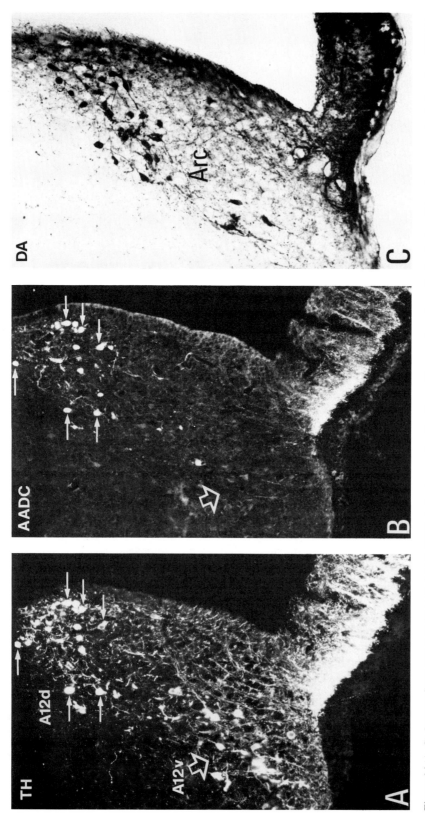

Figure 14 (A–C). Immunofluorescence (A,B) and bright-field (C) photomicrographs of sections of the arcuate nucleus after incubation with antisera to tyrosine hydroxylase (TH) (A), aromatic L-amino acid decarboxylase (AADC) (B) and dopamine (DA) (C). Cells in the dorsal part of the arcuate nucleus (A12d) contain TH-, AADC- and DA-immunoreactivity, whereas cells in the ventral part (A12v) only exhibit TH-immunoreactivity. For further discussion see text.

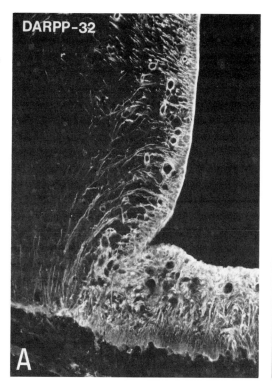
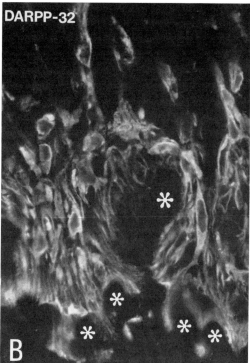

Figure 15 (A–D). Immunofluorescence photomicrographs of sections of the arcuate nucleus-median eminence complex after incubation with antisera to DARPP-32 (A,B), tyrosine hydroxylase (TH) (C) and LHRH (D). (A,B) DARPP-32-containing tanycytes are seen lining the floor and lateral walls of the third ventricle, sending processes through the arcuate nucleus, and down towards the median eminence. At high magnification (B), tanycyte cell bodies and processes are seen close to portal capillaries (asterisks).

These cells have processes that extend through the arcuate nucleus and median eminence to end, along with neurosecretory terminals, in association with the primary portal capillaries in the external layer (see Flament-Durand and Brion, 1985 and Figure 15). The importance of DARPP-32 in the brain is related to the fact that it is found in dopaminoceptive cells that contain the D_1 receptor and it has been suggested to function as a third messenger mediating the actions of dopamine (see Hemmings et al., 1987). It has been demonstrated that binding of dopamine to D_1 receptors in neurons is followed by phosphorylation of DARPP-32, increased cAMP formation, and stimulation of a cAMP-dependent protein kinase (see Hemmings et al., 1987). Combined immunocytochemistry of DARPP-32 with TH and LHRH (Meister et al., 1988b) has revealed a specially close relationship between the tanycyte end feet, which surround the portal capillaries, and nerve terminals containing both TH-IR (derived from arcuate neurons) and LHRH-IR (derived from LHRH neurons in the medial preoptic area and septum). At the ultrastructural level, a combination of pre- (TH and DARPP-32) and post (LHRH)-embedding immunocytochemistry has clarified the relationship between these different cellular and chemical entities (Figure 16). There are direct contacts between TH-IR nerve terminals and DARPP-32-IR tanycytes, while the tanycytes themselves cover the surface zone of the median eminence, appearing to engulf the LHRH terminals, thereby restricting their access to the fenestrated portal capillaries (Figure 16; Meister et al., 1988b).

These anatomical observations clearly suggest the basis for a functional relationship between D_1 dopamine receptor-mediated events involving the tanycytes and the secretion of LHRH into the portal vessels. It is generally accepted that dopaminergic drugs decrease LHRH

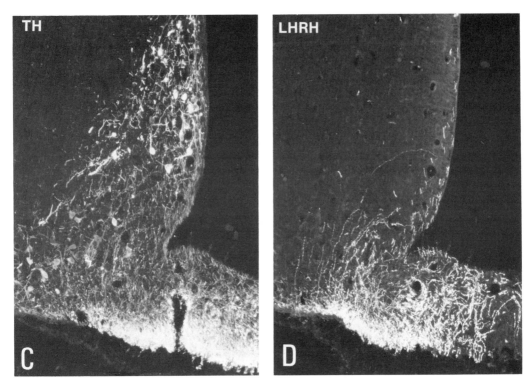

Figure 15 (A–D) (continued).   Note close relation to TH- (C) and LHRH (D)-containing neurons.

and LH secretion (see Everitt and Keverne, 1986). It has been suggested that at least part of the mechanism underlying dopaminergic regulation of LHRH secretion might involve the tanycytes (Everitt et al., 1986; Meister et al., 1988b). Thus, dopaminergic activation of the tanycytes may support the envelopment of the portal capillaries by the swollen end feet, thus preventing access of the LHRH-containing terminals, thereby limiting secretion (Figure 17). Decreased dopaminergic activity or dopamine receptor blockade, on the other hand, may be followed by retraction of the end-feet processes of the tanycytes and access of the LHRH terminals to the secretory zone of the capillaries (Figure 17). Related processes, namely glial movements in association with different functional states involving vasopressin and oxytocin secretion, have been observed to occur in the SON and in the posterior pituitary (Hatton, 1988; Hatton et al., 1984).

Dopamine-containing nerve fibers and terminals have been demonstrated in the *posterior pituitary* by means of formaldehyde histofluorescence (Baumgarten et al., 1972; Björklund et al., 1973). Later immunohistochemical studies have identified THH in fibers of the neurointermediate lobe (Figure 18; Stoeckel et al., 1985; Vuillez et al., 1987; Meister and Hökfelt, 1988). Pituicytes of the neurohypophysis may be targets for pituitary dopamine, since DARPP-32 has been demonstrated in these cells (Figure 18; Meister et al., 1989b). In support of this proposal, it has been demonstrated that the selective D_1 dopamine receptor agonist, SKF 38393, stimulates protein phosphorylation in the neurohypophysis (Treiman and Greengard, 1985). Dehydration has been shown to increase dopamine concentrations in the posterior pituitary (Alper et al., 1980; Racke et al., 1986) as well as alter the shape of pituicytes (Hatton et al., 1984). Thus, dopamine and DARPP-32 may be involved in these regulatory mechanisms.

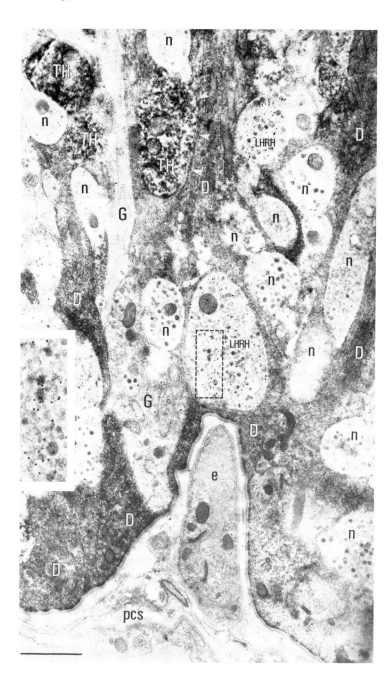

Figure 16. Electron microscopic photograph of a section of the external layer of the median eminence after pre-embedding staining with antisera to tyrosine hydroxylase (TH) and DARPP-32 (D) giving rise to a dark reaction product localized to nerve endings (TH- positive terminal contains secretory vesicles) and tanycytes (DARPP-32; without vesicles). In a second step, post-embedding staining with LHRH-antiserum has been performed. LHRH-containing nerve endings have been visualized with gold particles (see inset as indicated by rectangle). It can be seen that TH-containing nerve endings are in close appoposition with DARPP-32 containing tanycytes (arrows). DARPP-32-containing tanycytes may limit the accessibility of LHRH-containing nerve endings to the pericapillary space (pcs). G represent another glial element not stained with DARPP-32 antiserum. e = endothelial cell and n = nerve ending. (From Meister, B. et al., *Neuroscience*, 27, 607—622, 1988b. With permission.)

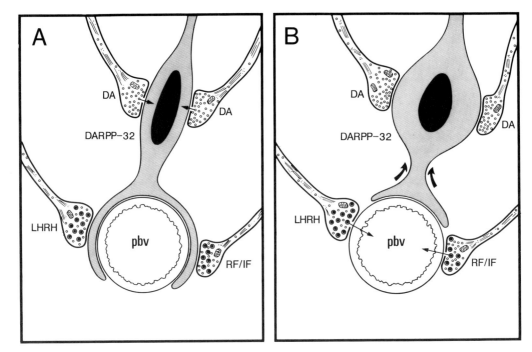

Figure 17 (A,B). Schematic drawing illustrating the hypothetical role of tanycytes in the median eminence. (A) Tanycytes, containing the dopamine- and cAMP-regulated phosphoprotein DARPP-32, have end feet that surround the portal blood vessels (pbv). Dopaminergic nerve endings (DA) control the dynamic state of the tanycyte by releasing dopamine. The tanycyte processes prevent nerve endings containing LHRH or some other releasing factor (RF) or inhibiting factor (IF) from having free access to the pericapillary space. (B) When the dopaminergic inhibition is reduced, the tanycyte contracts, leading to retraction of the end feet around the portal vessels. Following retraction, nerve endings in the external layer of the median eminence gain closer access to the pericapillary space and so facilitate their secretory products into the portal blood vessels. For further information, see text.

Functional Consequences of Coexistence in Arcuate Neurons

The role of peptide and amine secretory products released from the terminals of arcuate neurons in the regulation of anterior pituitary function is well known and reviewed elsewhere in this volume. The major issue raised by the observation of multiple messenger coexistence in these neurons and their terminals in the median eminence concerns the neurosecretory impact of complex messages that are the consequence of corelease. In addition, it will be important to understand the conditions under which one, or another, or combinations of these messengers are synthesized and/or released. This is a subject that has only begun to be studied relatively recently.

Using cultured pituitary cells, the effects on GRH-stimulated GH secretion of putative cotransmitters have been investigated (Meister and Hulting, 1987). Dopamine, for example, reduced GRH-stimulated GH secretion, as did GAL. Combining dopamine and galanin in the incubation medium resulted in almost total inhibition of GH secretion in response to GRH (Meister and Hulting, 1987). These data are in general agreement with a range of studies showing inhibitory effects of dopamine and its agonists on GH secretion. It seems that, within GRH neurons, there resides the chemical mechanism that not only stimulates, but can then limit, the stimulation of GH secretion from anterior pituitary somatotropes. This again emphasizes the importance of defining the conditions under which is released each component of the complex chemical message residing in such neurons in the arcuate nucleus.

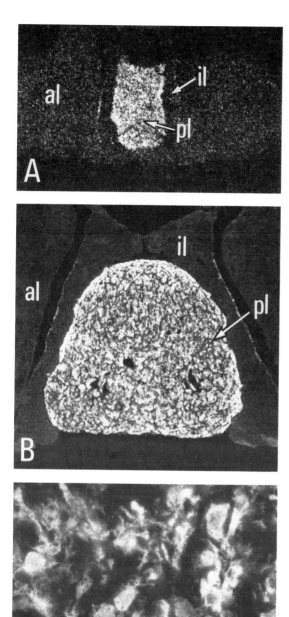

Figure 18 (A–C). Immunofluorescence photomicrographs of sections of the pituitary gland showing DARPP-32 mRNA (A) and DARPP-32-like immunoreactivity (B) located in the posterior lobe (pl). At higher magnification (C), it is seen that DARPP-like immunoreactivity is distributed in the cytoplasm of pituicytes. al = anterior lobe and il = intermediate lobe.

B. Other Hypothalamic Dopaminergic Cell Groups

As indicated above, little is known of the projections and functions of the other dopaminergic neuronal cell groups within the hypothalamus and zona incerta. The dopamine-containing nerve fibers in the neurointermediate lobe of the pituitary arise from the anterior hypothalamus, as originally shown by Björklund et al. (1973) using electrolytic lesions. Subsequent

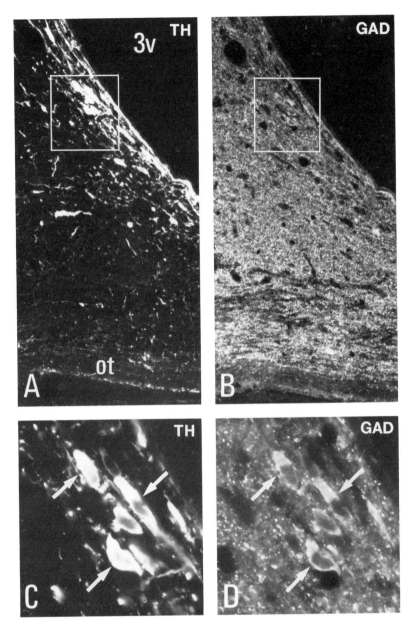

Figure 19 (A–H). Immunofluorescence photomicrographs to sections of the anterior hypothalamic periventricular nucleus (A14 area) (A to D), pituitary (E,F) and median eminence (G,H) after double-labelling with antisera to tyrosine hydroxylase (TH) (A,C,E,G) and glutamic acid decarboxylase (GAD) (B,D,F,H). Cell bodies located in the periventricular area contain both TH- and GAD-like immunoreactivity (see high magnifications (C,D) as indicated by squares in A and B). Fiber varicosities in both the neural lobe (nl) and intermediate lobe (nl) as well as in the external layer of the median eminence colocalize TH- and GAD-like immunoreactivity (see arrows).

tracing studies have shown that there is dense labeling in the anterior periventricular area (A14 cell group) after injection of tracer into the posterior lobe (Kawano and Daikoku, 1987). A large proportion of the TH-IR cell bodies in the A14 cell group as well as fibers in the neurointermediate lobe cocontain GAD and GABA-IR (Figure 19) (Stoeckel et al., 1985;

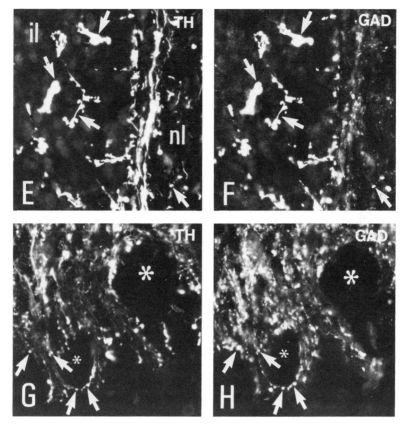

Figure 19 (A–H). (continued)

Vuillez et al., 1987; Meister and Hökfelt, 1988). It seems reasonable to suggest that the TH-IR neurons in the paraventricular and periventricular nuclei might interact with neurosecretory neurons in these areas (e.g., CRF, TRH, and somatostatin neurons) as well as contribute to dopaminergic projections to the external layer of the median eminence. This has not unequivocally been demonstrated. Several studies have indicated that the TH-IR neurons in the zona incerta project to the medial preoptic/anterior hypothalamic areas (Lindvall and Björklund, 1978) and influence both LHRH neurosecretory activity as well as testosterone-dependent patterns of copulatory behavior in male rats (see Everitt, 1978; Everitt et al., 1983). Elucidation of the functions of these hypothalamic dopaminergic systems awaits further experimentation.

IV. 5-Hydroxytryptaminergic Innervation of the Hypothalamus

The mesencephalic dorsal and median raphe nuclei represent the major source of 5-hydroxytryptamine (5-HT)-containing neurons innervating the hypothalamus, as indicated by 5-HT immunocytochemistry in combination with anterograde or retrograde tracing studies, as well as lesions (Figures 20 and 21; Azmitia, 1978, 1987; Azmitia and Segal, 1978; Calas et al., 1974; Everitt et al., 1975; Fuxe and Jonsson, 1974; Parent et al., 1981; Steinbusch, 1981; Steinbusch et al., 1981; Swanson, 1987). It is not entirely clear whether these two nuclei have overlapping, or separate, terminal domains within the hypothalamus, although it appears at

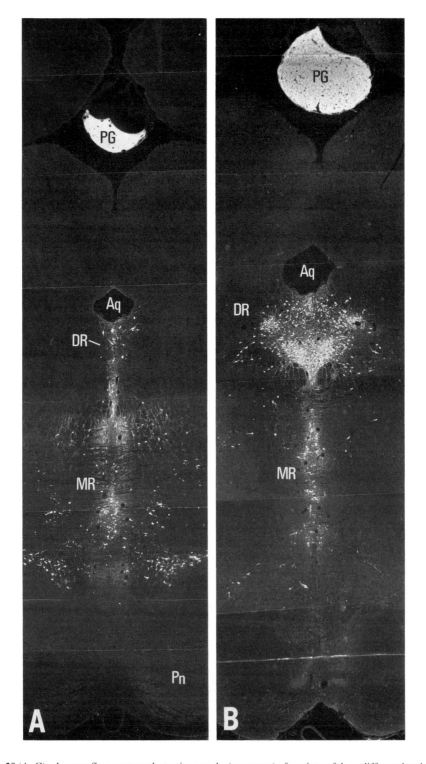

Figure 20 (A–C). Immunofluorescence photomicrographs (montages) of sections of three different levels of the midbrain to demonstrate the dorsal (DR) and median (MR) raphe nuclei after incubation with antiserum to 5-hydroxytryptamine (5-HT). Aq = aqueduct, PG = pineal gland, and Pn = pontine nuclei.

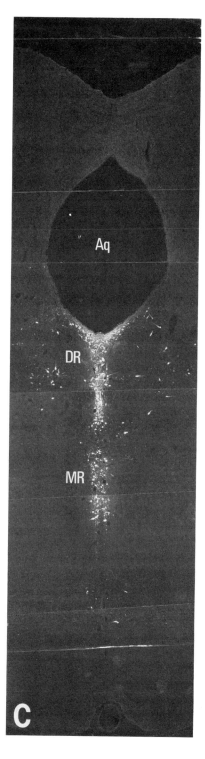

Figure 20 (A–C) (continued).

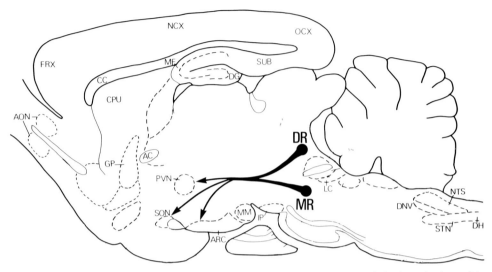

Figure 21. Schematic drawing of the rat brain (sagittal section) illustrating the hypothalamic projections of the dorsal (DR) and median (MR) raphe nuclei. Abbreviations as for Figure 2, except: SUB = subiculum; DG = dentate gyrus; AON = accessory olfactory nucleus.

present that some areas, such as the anterior periventricular nucleus, receive afferents only from the dorsal raphe, while other areas, such as the paraventricular and arcuate nuclei, receive afferents from both nuclei (Azmitia and Segal, 1978). Most hypothalamic nuclei receive a moderate innervation, but the suprachiasmatic nucleus alone stands out as a structure having a very dense 5-HT-containing terminal plexus (see Steinbusch, 1981). There is some discrepancy between neurochemical and anatomical data regarding the 5-HT innervation of the arcuate nucleus. Neurochemical measurements and also formaldehyde-induced fluorescence methods suggest it has a substantial innervation (Saavedra et al., 1975; Kent and Sladek, 1978), whereas 5-HT immunocytochemistry reveals few isolated fibers in the nucleus (Steinbusch and Nieuwenhuys, 1981). This may reflect the detection of non-5-HT indolamines by the chemical and formaldehyde-induced fluorescence techniques that are not demonstrated by 5-HT immunocytochemistry (Steinbusch and Nieuwenhuys, 1981). Some 5-HT-containing fibers are seen in the external layer of the median eminence, especially in the lateral parts, with more being seen at rostral, rather than caudal, levels, while serotonin-IR fibers are also seen in the posterior lobe of the pituitary, especially near the border with the intermediate lobe (Steinbusch and Nieuwenhuys, 1981). However, again there is some discrepancy with neurochemical and formaldehyde-induced fluorescence data, since appreciable amounts of 5-HT are also found in the anterior and intermediate lobes using these techniques (Saavedra et al., 1975; Kent and Sladek, 1978). A small group of 5-HT-containing neurons has also been demonstrated within the dorsomedial nucleus following pretreatment with nialimide and L-tryptophan, but it is unclear whether these neurons project within, or outside, the hypothalamus (Steinbusch, 1981).

Drugs interfering with 5-HT synthesis, release, or receptor function have a wide range of neuroendocrine effects, including alterations in cortisol, GH, prolactin, and LHRH secretion (Arendash and Gallo, 1978; Coen and MacKinnon, 1976; Gillies and Lowry, 1986; Quabbe, 1986; McNeilly, 1986; Everitt and Keverne, 1986; see also chapters in this volume). The neuroanatomical loci at which these effects of serotoninergic drugs are mediated have not generally been elucidated. At least some of these neuroendocrine effects may reflect interactions between the drugs and circadian control mechanisms residing within the *suprachiasmatic nucleus.* Indeed, 5-HT-depletions of this nucleus clearly disrupt the circadian regulation of corticosterone secretion (see Hastings and Herbert, 1986; Honma et al., 1979). It seems unlikely, however, that all endocrine responses induced by serotoninergic drugs reflect modulation of the circadian system, effects on GH and prolactin secretion being particularly rapid and likely to represent direct effects of such drugs on GRH neurons and hypothalamic prolactin releasing, or release-inhibiting hormone-containing neurons (see this volume; Quabbe, 1986; McNeilly, 1986).

The 5-HT neurons innervating the *medial preoptic area* and adjacent *medial septum* have been studied in some detail in connection with the LHRH-IR neurons found in this region. The light microscopic data clearly indicate that 5-HT-IR and LHRH-IR neurons make close, putatively synaptic, contacts, thus providing some evidence of a neuroanatomical basis for 5-HT-dependent mechanisms affecting the hypothalamo-pituitary-gonadal axis (Jennes et al., 1982; Kiss and Halasz, 1985). There is also marked overlap between LHRH- and 5-HT-containing elements in the organum vasculosum of the lamina terminalis. However, the precise functional importance of serotonin in regulating LHRH release in males and females is unresolved. Manipulations of 5-HT within the preoptic area also have quite marked effects on the expression of some elements of the sexual response repertoire, such as lordosis in female rats (Everitt, 1978; Everitt et al., 1975; Luine et al., 1982), and this has been suggested to represent an interaction with hormone-dependent components of the neural systems underlying sexual behavior (see Everitt, 1978).

However, it is clear from the experimental literature that the importance in hypothalamic hormone secretion of serotoninergic systems innervating hypophysiotropic areas of the hypothalamus is poorly understood. There are many conflicting reports concerning the direction of change in hormone secretion following 5-HT transmission-enhancing or -inhibiting treatments; for example, 5-HT, or its direct and indirect agonists, has been reported to have no effect, to increase, and to decrease CRF secretion (Gillies and Lowry, 1986). Similar controversy surrounds effects of serotonin on episodic growth hormone secretion and the growth hormone response to insulin-induced hypoglycemia (Quabbe, 1986). Few studies have examined the effects of manipulating 5-HT transmission directly within the relevant hypothalamic areas and the picture is likely to remain confused until such studies are undertaken.

V. Summary

Brainstem noradrenergic, adrenergic, and serotoninergic neurons have long been known to project to neuroendocrine domains of the hypothalamus and these systems represent the neuroanatomical basis of many drug effects on hypothalamic hormone secretion. The populations of tyrosine hydroxylase-immunoreactive neurons in the arcuate nucleus have for many years been the focus of neuroendocrine experiments, but following the initial demonstration of their importance in regulating prolactin secretion via the secretion of dopamine into the portal vessels, their neuroendocrine complexity has increased considerably. The impact of chemical messenger coexistence and corelease on the regulation of anterior pituitary function has only recently begun to be investigated and is as yet poorly understood. Clearly this is an important area for future research.

VI. Acknowledgments

This study was supported by grants from the Swedish Medical Research Council (04X-2887), Tore Nilsons, Stiftelse and Stiftelsen Sigurd, and Elsa Goljes Minne.

References

Adler, B. A., Johnson, M. D., Lynch, C. O., and Crowley, W. R., Evidence that norepinephrine and epinephrine systems mediate stimulatory effects of ovarian hormones on luteinizing hormone and luteinizing hormone-releasing hormone, *Endocrinology*, 113, 1431, 1983.

Ajika, K., Relationship between catecholaminergic neurons and hypothalamic hormone-containing neurons in the hypothalamus, in *Frontiers in Neuroendocrinology*, Vol. 6, Martini, L. and Ganong, W. F., Eds., Raven Press, New York, 1980.

Alper, R. H., Demarest, K. T., and Moore, K. E., Dehydration selectively increases dopamine synthesis in tuberohypophyseal dopaminergic neurons, *Neuroendocrinology*, 32, 112, 1980.

Arendash, G. W. and Gallo, R. V., Serotonin involvement in the inhibition of episodic luteinizing hormone release during the electrical stimulation of the midbrain dorsal raphe nucleus in ovariectomized rats, *Endocrinology*, 102, 1199, 1978.

Arnauld, E., Grino, M., Cayton, B., and Renaud, L. P., Contrasting actions of amino acids, acetylcholine, noradrenaline and leucine enkephalin on the excitability of supraoptic vasopressin-secreting neurons, *Neuroendocrinology*, 36, 187, 1983.

Azmitia, E. C., The serotonin-producing neurons of the midbrain median and dorsal raphe nuclei, in *Handbook of Psychophrenology*, Vol. 9, Iversen, L. C., Iversen, S. D., and Snyder, S. H., Eds., Plenum Press, New York, 1978, 233.

Azmitia, E. C., The CNS serotonergic system: progression toward a collaborative organization, in *Psychopharmacology: The Third Generation of Progress*, Meltzer, H. Y., Ed., Raven Press, New York, 1987, 61.

Azmitia, E. C. and Segal, M., An autoradiographic analysis of the differential ascending projections of the dorsal and median raphe nuclei in the rat, *J. Comp. Neurol.*, 179, 641, 1978.

Bai, F. L., Yamano, M., Shiotani, Y., Emson, P., Smith, A. D., Powell, J. F., and Tohyama, M., An arcuato-paraventricular and dorsomedial hypothalamic neuropeptide Y-containing system which lacks noradrenaline in the rat, *Brain Res.*, 331, 172, 1985.

Barry, J., Hoffman, G. E., and Wray, S., LHRH-containing systems, in *Handbook of Chemical Neuroanatomy*, Vol. 4, *GABA and Neuropeptides in the CNS*, Part 1, Björklund, A. and Hökfelt, T., Eds., Elsevier, Amsterdam, 1985, 166.

Baumgarten, H. G., Björklund, A., Holstein, A. F., and Nobin, A., Organization and ultrastructural identification of the catecholamine nerve terminals in the neural lobe and pars intermedia of the rat pituitary, *Z. Zellforsch.*, 126, 483, 1972.

Bertles, A., Falck, B., and Rosengren, E., The direct demonstration of a banner mechanism in the brain capillaries, *Acta Pharmacol.*, 20, 317—321, 1964.

Björklund, A. and Lindvall, O., Dopamine-containing systems in the CNS, in *Handbook of Chemical Neuroanatomy*, Vol. 2 (Part 1, Classical transmitters in the CNS), Björklund, A. and Hökfelt, T., Eds., Elsevier, Amsterdam, 1984, 55.

Björklund, A. and Nobin, A., Fluorescence histochemical and microspectrofluorometric mapping of dopamine and noradrenaline cell groups in the rat diencephalon, *Brain Res.*, 51, 193, 1973.

Björklund, A. and Skagerberg, G., Evidence for a major spinal cord projection from the diencephalic A11 dopamine cell group in the rat using transmitter specific fluorescent retrograde tracing, *Brain Res.*, 177, 170, 1979.

Björklund, A., Moore, R. Y., Nobin, A., and Stenevi, U., The organization of tubero-hypophyseal and reticulo-infundibular catecholamine neuron system in the rat brain, *Brain Res.*, 51, 171, 1973.

Björklund, A., Lindvall, O., and Nobin, A., Evidence of an incerto-hypothalamic dopamine neurone system in the rat, *Brain Res.*, 89, 29, 1975.

Calas, A., Alonso, G., Arnauld, E., and Vincent, J. O., Demonstration of indolaminergic fibres in the median eminence of the duck, rat and monkey, *Nature (London)*, 250, 241, 1974.

Ceccatelli, S., Eriksson, M., and Hökfelt, T., Distribution and coexistence of CRF-, neurotensin-, enkephalin-, cholecystokinin-, galanin- and VIP/PHI-like peptides in the parvocellular part of the paraventricular nucleus, *Neuroendocrinology*, 49, 309, 1989.

Chan-Palay, V., Zaborszky, L., Köhler, C., Goldstein, M., and Palay, S. L., Distribution of tyrosine-hydroxylase-immunoreactive neurons in the hypothalamus of rats, *J. Comp. Neurol.*, 227, 467, 1984.

Coen, C. W. and Coombs, M. C., Effects of manipulating catecholamines on the incidence of the preovulatory surge of the luteinizing hormone and ovulation in the rat: evidence for a necessary involvement of hypothalamic adrenaline in the normal or 'midnight' surge, *Neuroscience*, 10, 187, 1983.

Coen, C. W. and Gallo, R. V., Effects of various inhibitors of phenylethanolamine *N*-methyltransferase on pulsatile release of LH in ovariectomized rats, *J. Endocrinol.*, 111, 51, 1986.

Coen, C. W. and MacKinnon, P. C. B., Serotonin involvement in oestrogen-induced luteinizing hormone release in ovariectomized rats, *J. Endocrinol.*, 71, 49P, 1976.

Condon, T. P., Handa, R. J., Gorski, R. A., Sawyer, C. H., and Whitmoyer, D. I., Ovarian steroid modulation of norepinephrine action on luteinizing hormone release, *Neuroendocrinology*, 43, 550, 1986.

Constantinidis, J., de la Torre, J. C., Tissot, R., and Geissbuhler, F., La barriere capillaire pour la dopa dans le cerveau et les differents organes. *Psychopharmacologia*, 15, 75, 1969.

Cunningham, E. T. and Sawchenko, P. E., Anatomical specificity of noradrenergic inputs to the paraventricular and supraoptic nuclei of the rat hypothalamus, *J. Comp. Neurol.*, 274, 60, 1988.

Cunningham, E. T., Bohn, M. C., and Sawchenko, P. E., Organization of adrenergic inputs to the paraventricular and supraoptic nuclei of the hypothalamus in the rat, *J. Comp. Neurol.*, 292, 651, 1990.

Dahlström, A. and Fuxe, K., Evidence for the existence of monoamine containing neurons in the central nervous system. I. Demonstration of monoamines in cell bodies of brain stem neurons, *Acta. Physiol. Scand.*, 62 (Suppl. 232), 1, (1964).

Day, T. A., Jhamandas, J. H., and Renaud, L. P., Comparison between the actions of avian pancreatic polypeptide, neuropeptide Y and norepinephrine on the excitability of rat supraoptic vasopressin neurons, *Neurosci. Lett.*, 62, 181, 1985.

Descarries, L. and Beaudet, A., The serotonin innervation of adult rat hypothalamus, in *Cell Biology of Hypothalamic Neurosecretion,* Vol. 80, Vincent, J. D. and Kordon, C., Eds., Coll. Internat. C.N.R.L., 1978, 135.

Everitt, B. J., A neuroanatomical approach to the study of monoamines and sexual behaviour, in *Biological Determinants of Sexual Behaviour,* Hutchison, J. B., Ed., John Wiley & Sons, New York, 1978, 555.

Everitt, B. J. and Keverne, E. B., The neuroendocrinology of reproduction, in *Neuroendocrinology*, Lightman, S. L. and Everitt, B. J., Eds., Blackwell Scientific, Oxford, 1986, 472.

Everitt, B. J. and Hökfelt, T., The coexistence of neuropeptide Y with other peptides and amines in the central nervous system, in *Proc. Nobel Symposium on NPY,* Pergamon Press, Oxford, 1989, 61.

Everitt, B. J., Fuxe, K., and Jonsson, G., The effects of 5,7-dihydroxytryptamine lesions of ascending 5-hydroxytryptamine pathways on the sexual and aggressive behaviour of female rats, *J. Pharmacol. (Paris),* 6, 25, 1975.

Everitt, B. J., Herbert, J., and Keverne, E. B., The neuroendocrine anatomy of the limbic system: a discussion with special reference to steroid responsive neurons, neuropeptides and monoaminergic systems. Reprinted from *Progress in Anatomy,* Vol. 3, Navaratnam, V. and Harrison, R. J., Eds., Cambridge University Press, London, 1983.

Everitt, B. J., Hökfelt, T., Terenius, L., Tatemoto, K., Mutt, V., and Goldstein, M., Differential co-existence of neuropeptide Y (NPY)-like immunoreactivity with catecholamines in the central nervous system of the rat, *Neuroscience*, 11, 443, 1984a.

Everitt, B. J., Hökfelt, T., Wu, J.-Y., and Goldstein, M., Coexistence of tyrosine hydroxylase gamma aminobutyric acid-like immunoreactivities in neurons of the arcuate nucleus, *Neuroendocrinology*, 39, 189, 1984b.

Everitt, B. J., Meister, B., Hökfelt, T., Melander, T., Terenius, L., Rökaeus, A., Theodorsson-Norheim, E., Dockray, G., Edwardson, J., Cuello, C., Elde, R., Goldstein, M., Hemmings, H., Ouimet, C., Walaas, I., Greengard, P., Vale, W., Weber, E., and Wu, J.-Y., The hypothalamic arcuate nucleus-median eminence complex: immunohistochemistry of transmitters, peptides and DARPP-32 with special reference to coexistence in dopamine neurons, *Brain Res. Rev.*, 11, 97, 1986.

Falck, B., Hillarp, N. A., Thieme, G., and Torp, A., Fluorescence of catecholamines and related compounds with formaldehyde, *J. Histochem. Cytochem.*, 10, 348, 1962.

Flament-Durand, J. and Brion, J. P., Tanycytes: morphology and functions, a review, *Int. Rev. Cytol.*, 96, 121, 1985.

Fuxe, K., Cellular localization of monoamines in the median eminence and infundibular stem of some mammals, *Z. Zellforsch.*, 61, 719, 1964.

Fuxe, K., Evidence for the existence of monoamine neurons in the central nervous system. IV. Distribution of monoamine nerve terminals in the central nervous system, *Acta Physiol. Scand.*, 64 (Suppl. 247), 37, 1965.

Fuxe, K. and Hökfelt, T., Further evidence for the existence of tubero-infundibular dopamine neurons, *Acta Physiol. Scand.*, 66, 245, 1966.

Fuxe, K. and Hökfelt, T., Catecholamines in the hypothalamus and in the pituitary gland, in *Frontiers in Neuroendocrinology*, Ganong, W. F. and Martini, L., Eds., Academic Press, New York, 1969, 47.

Fuxe, K. and Jonsson, G., Further mapping of central 5-hydroxytryptamine neurons: studies with the neurotoxic dihydroxytryptamine, in *Advances in Biochemical Psychopharmacology*, Vol. 10, Costa, E., Gessa, G. L., and Sandler, M., Eds., Raven Press, New York, 1974.

Fuxe, K., Hökfelt, T., Agnati, L. F., Johanson, O., Goldstein, M., Perez de la Mora, M., Possani, L., Tapia, R., Tern, L., and Palacios, R., Mapping out central catecholamine neurons: immunohisto-chemical studies on catecholamine-synthesizing enzymes, in *Psychopharmacology: A Generation of Progress*, Lipton, M. A., DiMascio, A., and Killam, K. F., Eds., Raven Press, New York, 1978, 67.

Fuxe, K., Agnati, L., Kalia, M., Goldstein, M., Andersson, K., and Härfstrand, A., Dopaminergic systems in the brain and pituitary, in *The Dopaminergic System*, Fluckiger, E., Müller, E. E., and Thorner, M. O., Eds., Springer-Verlag, Berlin, 1985, 11.

Gallo, R. V. and Drouva, S. V., Effects of intraventricular infusion of catecholamines on luteinizing hormone release in ovariectomized and ovariectomized, steroid-primed rats, *Neuroendocrinology*, 29, 149, 1979.

Gillies, G. E. and Lowry, P. J., Adrenal function, in *Neuroendocrinology*, Lightman, S. L. and Everitt, B. J., Eds., Blackwell Scientific Publications, London, 1986, 360—388.

Grant, L. D. and Stumpf, W. E., Hormone uptake sites in relation to CNS biogenic amine systems, in *Anatomical Neuroendocrinology*, Int. Conf. Neurobiology of CNS-Hormone Interactions, University of North Carolina Press, Chapel Hill, 1974, 445.

Hancke, J. L. and Wuttke, W., Effect of lesions of the ventral noradrenergic bundle or the medial preoptic area on preovulatory LH release in rats, *Exp. Brain Res.*, 35, 127, 1977.

Hancke, J. L. and Wuttke, W., Effect of chemical lesions of the ventral noradrenergic bundle or of medial preoptic area on preovulatory LH release in rats, *Brain Res.*, 35, 127, 1979.

Hansen, S., Stansfield, S. J., Everitt, B. J., The role of ventral bundle noradrenergic neurones in sensory components of sexual behaviour and coitus-induced pseudopregnancy, *Nature (London)*, 286, 152, 1980.

Hansen, S., Stanfield, S. J., and Everitt, B. J., The effects of lesions of lateral tegmental noradrenergic neurons on components of sexual behavior and pseudopregnancy in female rats, *Neuroscience*, 6, 1105, 1981.

Härfstrand, A., Brain neuropeptide-Y mechanisms: basic aspects and involvement in cardiovascular and neuroendocrine regulation, *Acta Physiol. Scand.*, 131 (Suppl. 565), 1, 1987.

Hastings, M. H. and Herbert, J., Endocrine rhythms, in *Neuroendocrinology*, Lightman, S. L. and Everitt, B. J., Eds., Blackwell Scientific, Oxford, 1986, 49.

Hatton, G. I., Pituicyte control of posterior pituitary secretion, in *Neuroendocrine Control of the Hypothalamo-Pituitary System*, Imura, H., Eds., Karger, Basel, 1988, 201.

Hatton, G. I., Perlmutter, L. S., Salm, A. K., and Tweedle, C. D., Dynamic neuronal-glial interactions in hypothalamus and pituitary: implications for control of hormone synthesis and release, *Peptides*, 5, 121, 1984.

Hemmings, H. C., Jr., Nairn, A. C., Aswad, D. W., and Greengard, P., DARPP-32, a dopamine- and adenosine 3':5'-monophosphate-regulated phosphoprotein enriched in dopamine-innervated brain regions. II. Purification and characterization of the phosphoprotein from bovine caudate nucleus, *J. Neurosci.*, 4, 99, 1984.

Hemmings, H. C., Jr., Walaas, S. I., Ouimet, C. C., and Greengard, P., Dopaminergic regulation of protein phosphorylation in the striatum: DARPP-32, *Trends Neurosci.*, 10, 77, 1987.

Hoffman, G. E., Wray, S., and Goldstein, M., Relationship of catecholamines and LHRH: light microscopic study, *Brain Res. Bull.*, 9, 417, 1982.

Holets, V. R., Hökfelt, T., Rökaeus, A., Terenius, L., and Goldstein, M., Locus coeruleus neurons in the rat containing neuropeptide-Y, tyrosine hydroxylase or galanin and their efferent projections to the spinal cord, cerebral cortex and hypothalamus, *Neuroscience*, 24, 893, 1988.

Hökfelt, T., Possible site of action of dopamine in the hypothalamic pituitary control, *Acta Physiol. Scand.*, 89, 606, 1973.

Hökfelt, T., Fuxe, K., Goldstein, M., and Johansson, O., Immunohistochemical evidence for the existence of adrenaline neurons in the rat brain, *Brain Res.*, 66, 235, 1974.

Hökfelt, T., Johansson, O., Fuxe, K., Goldstein, M., and Park, D., Immunohistochemical studies on the localization and distribution of monoamine neuron systems in the rat brain. 1. Tyrosine hydroxylase in the mes- and diencephalon, *Med. Biol.*, 54, 427, 1976.

Hökfelt, T., Elde, R., Fuxe, K., Johansson, O., Ljungdahl, Å., Goldstein, M., Luft, R., Efendic, S., Wilsson, G., Terenius, L., Ganten, D., Jeffcoate, S. L., Rehfeld, J., Said, S., Perez de la Mora, M., Possani, L., Tapia, R., Teran, L., and Palacios, R., Aminergic and peptidergic pathways in the nervous system with special reference to the hypothalamus, in *The Hypothalamus*, Reichlin, S., Baldessarini, R. J., and Martin, J. B., Eds., Raven Press, New York, 1978, 69.

Hökfelt, T., Johansson, O., and Goldstein, M., Central catecholamine neurons as revealed by immunohistochemistry with special reference to adrenaline neurons, in *Handbook of Chemical Neuroanatomy*, Vol. 2 (Part 1, Classical transmitters in the CNS), Björklund, A. and Hökfelt, T., Eds., Elsevier, Amsterdam, 1984a, 157.

Hökfelt, T., Mårtensson, R., Björklund, A., and Kleinau, S., Distributional maps of tyrosine hydroxylase-immunoreactive neurons in the rat brain, in *Handbook of Chemical Neuroanatomy*, Vol. 2, (Part 1, Classical transmitters in the CNS), Björklund, A. and Hökfelt, T., Eds., Elsevier, Amsterdam, 1984b, 277.

Hökfelt, T., Everitt, B., Meister, B., Melander, T., Schalling, M., Johansson, O., Lundberg, J. M., Hulting, A.-L., Werner, S., Cuello, C., Hemmings, H., Ouimet, C., Walaas, I., Greengard, P., and Goldstein, M., Neurons with multiple messengers with special reference to neuroendocrine systems, *Recent Prog. Horm. Res.*, 42, 1, 1986.

Hökfelt, T., Meister, B., Everitt, B. J., Staines, W., Melander, T., Schalling, M., Mutt, V., Hulting, A.-L., Werner, S., Bartfai, T., Nordström, O., Fahrenkrug, J., and Goldstein, M., Chemical neuroanatomy of the hypothalamic-pituitary axis: focus on multiple messenger systems, in *Integrative Neuroendocrinology: Molecular, Cellular and Clinical Aspects*, Geoffrey Harris Memorial Lecture at 1st Inst. Congr. Neuroendocrinology, McCann, S. and Weiner, R. I., Eds., S. Karger, Basel, 1987, 1.

Honma, K.-I., Watanabe, K., and Hiroshige, T., Effects of PCPA and 5,6-DHT on the free-running rhythms of locomotor activity and plasma corticosterone in the rat exposed to continuous light, *Brain Res.*, 169, 531, 1979.

Ibata, T., Fukui, K., Okamura, H., Kawakami, T., Tanaka, M., Obata, H. L., Tsuto, T., Terubayashi, H., Yanaihara, C., and Yanaihara, N., Coexistence of dopamine and neurotensin in hypothalamic arcuate and periventricular neurons, *Brain Res.*, 269, 177, 1983.

Ishikawa, K., Taniguchi, Y., Kurosumi, K., Suzuki, M., and Shinoda, M., Immunohistochemical identification of somatostatin-containing neurons projecting to the median eminence of the rat, *Endocrinology*, 121, 94, 1987.

Jacobowitz, D. M. and Palkovits, M., Topographic atlas of catecholamine and acetylcholinesterase-containing neurons in the rat brain. I. Forebrain (telencephalon, diencephalon), *J. Comp. Neurol.*, 157, 13, 1974.

Jaeger, C. B., Ruggiero, D. A., Albert, V. R., Park, D. H., Joh, T. H., and Reis, D. J., Aromatic L-amino acid decarboxylase in the rat brain: immunohistochemical localization in monoamine and non-monoamine neurons of the brain stem, *Neuroscience*, 11, 691, 1984.

Jennes, L., Beckman, W. C., Stumpf, W. E., and Grzanna, R., Anatomical relationships of serotoninergic and noradrenalinergic projections with the GnRH system in septum and hypothalamus, *Exp. Brain Res.*, 46, 331, 1982.

Kalra, S. P., Neural loci involved in naloxone-induced luteinizing hormone release: effects of a norepinephrine synthesis inhibitor, *Endocrinology*, 109, 1805, 1981.

Kalra, S. P. and Crowley, W. R., Epinephrine synthesis inhibitors block naloxone-induced LH release, *Endocrinology*, 111, 1403, 1982.

Kalra, S. P. and Kalra, P. S., Opioid-adrenergic-steroid connection in regulation of luteinizing hormone secretion in the rat, *Neuroendocrinology*, 38, 418, 1984.

Kalra, S. P. and Simpkins, J. W., Evidence for noradrenergic mediation of opioid effects on luteinizing hormone secretion, *Endocrinology*, 109, 776, 1981.

Kawano, H. and Daikoku, S., Functional topography of the rat hypothalamic dopamine neuron systems: retrograde tracing and immunohistochemical study, *J. Comp. Neurol.*, 265, 242, 1987.

Kawano, H. and Daikoku, S., Somatostatin-containing neuron systems in the rat hypothalamus: retrograde tracing and immunohistochemical studies, *J. Comp. Neurol.*, 271, 293, 1988.

Kent, O. L. and Sladek, J. R., Histochemical, pharmacological and microspectrofluorometric analysis of new sites of serotonin localization in the rat hypothalamus, *J. Comp. Neurol.*, 180, 221, 1978.

Khachaturian, H., Lewis, M. E., Tsou, K., and Watson, S. J., β-Endorphin, -MSH, ACTH and related peptides, in *Handbook of Chemical Neuroanatomy*, Vol. 4 (GABA and neuropeptides in the CNS), Björklund, A. and Hökfelt, T., Eds., Elsevier, Amsterdam, 1985, 216.

Kiss, J. and Halasz, B., Demonstration of serotoninergic axons terminating on luteinizing hormone-releasing hormone neurons in the preoptic area of the rat using a combination of immunocytochemistry and high resolution autoradiography, *Neuroscience*, 14, 69, 1985.

Kiss, J. Z. and Mezey, E., Tyrosine hydroxylase in magnocellular neurosecretory neurons: response to physiological manipulations, *Neuroendocrinology*, 43, 519, 1986.

Kizer, J. S., Palkovits, M., and Brownstein, M. J., The effect of bilateral lesions of the ventral noradrenergic bundle on endocrine-induced changes of tyrosine hydroxylase in the rat median eminence, *Endocrinology*, 98, 886, 1976a.

Kizer, J. S., Palkovits, M., and Brownstein, M. J., The projections of the A8, A9 and A10 dopaminergic cell bodies: evidence for a nigral-hypothalamic median eminence dopaminergic pathway, *Brain Res.*, 108, 363, 1976b.

Kobayashi, R. M., Palkovits, M., Kopin, I. J., and Jacobowitz, D. M., Biochemical mapping of noradrenergic nerves arising from the rat locus coeruleus, *Brain Res.*, 77, 269, 1974.

Krieg, R. J. and Sawyer, C. H., Effects of intraventricular catecholamines on luteinizing hormone release in ovariectomized, steroid-primed rats, *Endocrinology*, 99, 411, 1976.

Lechan, R. M., Nestler, J. L., and Jacobson, S., The tuberoinfundibular system of the rat as demonstrated by immunohistochemical localization of retrogradely transported wheat germ agglutinin (WGA) from the median eminence, *Brain Res.*, 245, 1, 1982.

Leibowitz, S. F., Impact of brain monoamines and neuropeptides on vasopressin release, in *Vasopressin: Cellular and Integrative Functions*, Cowley, A. W., Liard, J.-F., and Ausiello, D., Eds., Raven Press, New York, 1988, 379.

Leibowitz, S. F., Sladek, C., Spencer, L., and Tempel, D., Neuropeptide Y, epinephrine and norepinephrine in the paraventricular nucleus: stimulation of feeding and the release of corticosterone, vasopressin and glucose, *Brain Res. Bull.*, 21, 905, 1988.

Leibowitz, S. F., Diaz, S., and Tempel, D., Norepinephrine in the paraventricular nucleus stimulates corticosterone release, *Brain Res.*, 496, 219, 1989.

Li, Y. W., Halliday, G. M., Joh, T. H., Geffen, L. B., and Blessing, W. W., Tyrosine hydroxylase-containing neurons in the supraoptic and paraventricular nuclei of the adult human, *Brain Res.*, 461, 75, 1982.

Lightman, S. L. and Everitt, B. J., Eds., *Neuroendocrinology*, Blackwell Scientific, Oxford, 1986a.

Lightman, S. L. and Everitt, B. J., The neuroendocrinology of electrolyte and water balance, in *Neuroendocrinology*, Everitt, B. J. and Lightman, S. L., Eds., Blackwell Scientific, Oxford, 1986b, 197.

Lightman, S. L., Todd, K., and Everitt, B. J., Role for lateral tegmental noradrenergic neurons in the vasopressin response to hypertonic saline, *Neurosci. Lett.*, 42, 55, 1983.

Lightman, S. L., Todd, K., and Everitt, B. J., Ascending noradrenergic projections from the brainstem: evidence for a major role in the regulation of blood pressure and vasopressin secretion, *Exp. Brain Res.*, 55, 145, 1984.

Lindvall, O. and Björklund, A., Organization of catecholamine neurons in the rat central nervous system, in *Handbook of Psychopharmacology*, Vol. 9, Iversen, L. L., Iversen, S. D., and Snyder, S. H., Eds., Plenum Press, New York, 1978, 139.

Liposits, Zs., Phelix, C., and Paull, W. K., Electron microscopic analysis of tyrosine hydroxylase, dopamine-β-hydroxylase and phenylethanolamine-*N*-methyl transferase immunoreactive innervation of the hypothalamic paraventricular nucleus in the rat, *Histochemistry*, 84, 105, 1986a.

Liposits, Zs., Phelix, C., and Paull, W. K., Adrenergic innervation of corticotrophin releasing factor (CRF)-synthesizing neurons in the hypothalamic paraventricular nucleus of the rat, *Histochemistry*, 84, 201, 1986b.

Liposits, Zs., Paull, W. K., Wu, P., Jackson, I. M. D., and Lechan, R. M., Hypophysiotrophic thyrotrophin releasing hormone (TRH) synthesizing neurons: ultrastructure, adrenergic innervation and putative transmitter action, *Histochemistry*, 88, 1, 1987.

Luine, V. N. and Fischette, C. T., Inhibition of lordosis behaviour by intrahypothalamic implants of pargyline, *Neuroendocrinology*, 34, 237, 1982.

MacLeod, R. M. and Lehmeyer, J. E., Studies on the mechanism of dopamine-mediated inhibition of prolactin secretion, *Endocrinology*, 94, 1077, 1974.

Martensz, N. D., Goldstone, A. P., Stuart, E., and Everitt, B. J., Interactions between opioid peptides and adrenaline-containing neurons modulate luteinizing hormone secretion in male rats, *J. Neuroendocrinol.*, 2, 71, 1990.

McCann, S. M. and Ojeda, S. R., Synaptic transmitters involved in the release of hypothalamic releasing and inhibiting hormones, in *Reviews of Neuroscience*, Ehrenpreis, S. and Kopin, I. J., Eds., Raven Press, New York, 1976, 91.

McNeilly, A., Prolactin, in *Neuroendocrinology*, Lightman, S. L. and Everitt, B. J., Eds., Blackwell Scientific, Oxford, 1986, 537.

Meister, B. and Hulting, A. L., Influence of coexisting hypothalamic messengers on growth hormone secretion from rat anterior pituitary cells *in vitro*, *Neuroendocrinology*, 48, 516—526, 1987.

Meister, B. and Hökfelt, T., Peptide- and transmitter-containing neurons in the mediobasal hypothalamus and their relation to GABAergic systems: possible roles in control of prolactin and growth hormone secretion, *Synapse*, 6, 585, 1988.

Meister, B., Hökfelt, T., Vale, W., Sawchenko, P. E., Swanson, L. W., and Goldstein, M., Coexistence of tyrosine hydroxylase and growth hormone-releasing factor in a subpopulation of tuberoinfundibular neurons of the rat, *Neuroendocrinology*, 42, 237, 1986.

Meister, B., Hökfelt, T., Steinbusch, H. W. M., Skagerberg, G., Lindvall, O., Geffard, M., Joh, T. H., Cuello, A. C., and Goldstein, M., Do tyrosine hydroxylase-immunoreactive neurons in the ventrolateral arcuate nucleus produce dopamine by only D-DOPA? *J. Chem. Neuroanat.*, 1, 59, 1988a

Meister, B., Hökfelt, T., Tsuruo, Y., Hemmings, H., Owinet, C., Greengard, P., and Goldstein, M., DARPP-32, a dopamine and cyclic AMP-regulated phosphoprotein in tanycytes of the mediobasal hypothalamus: distribution and relation to dopamine and luteinizing hormone-releasing hormone neurons and other glial elements, *Neuroscience*, 27, 607—622, 1988b.

Meister, B., Ceccatelli, S., Hökfelt, T., Anden, N.-E., Anden, M., and Theodorsson, E., Neurotransmitters, neuropeptides and binding sites in the rat mediobasal hypothalamus: effects of monosodium glutamate (MSG) lesions, *Exp. Brain Res.*, 76, 343, 1989a.

Meister, B., Villar, M. J., Schalling, M., Ehrlich, M., Greengard, P., and Hökfelt, T., Demonstration of DARPP-32 in pituicytes of the neurohypophysis — decreased expression after administration of hyperosmotic stimuli, *Acta Physiol. Scand.*, 137, 461, 1989b.

Meister, B., Cortes, R., Villar, M. J., Schalling, M., and Hökfelt, T., Peptides and transmitter enzymes in hypothalamic magnocellular neurons after administration of hyperosmotic stimuli: comparison between messenger RNA and peptide/protein levels, *Cell Tiss. Res.*, 260, 279, 1990a.

Meister, B., Villar, M. J., Ceccatelli, S., and Hökfelt, T., Localization of chemical messengers in magnocellular neurons of the hypothalamic supraoptic and paraventricular nuclei: immunohistochemical study using experimental manipulations, *Neuroscience*, 37, 603, 1990b.

Melander, T., Hökfelt, T., Rökaeus, A., Cuello, A. C., Oertel, W. H., Verhofstad, A., and Goldstein, M., Coexistence of galanin-like immunoreactivity with catecholamines, 5-hydroxytryptamine, GABA and neuropeptides in the rat CNS, *J. Neurosci.*, 6, 3640, 1986.

Miller, M. A., Clifton, D. K., and Steiner, R. A., Noradrenergic and endogenous opioid pathways in the regulation of luteinizing hormone secretion in the male rat, *Endocrinology*, 117, 544, 1985.

Moore, R. T. and Bloom, F. E., Central catecholamine neuron systems: anatomy and physiology of the dopamine systems, *Annu. Rev. Neurosci.*, 1, 129, 1978.

Moore, R. T. and Bloom, F. E., Central catecholamine neuron systems: anatomy and physiology of the norepinephrine and epinephrine systems, *Annu. Rev. Neurosci.*, 2, 113, 1979.

Neill, J., Neuroendocrine regulation of prolactin secretion, in *Frontiers in Neuroendocrinology,* Vol. 6, Martini, L. and Ganong, W. F., Eds., Raven Press, New York, 1980, 129.

Nicholson, Greeley, G. G., Humm, J., Youngblood, W., and Kizer, J. S., Lack of effect of noradrenergic denervation of the hypothalamus and medial preoptic area on the feedback regulation of gonadotropin secretion and the estrous cycle of the rat, *Endocrinology*, 103, 559, 1978.

Okamura, H., Kitahama, K., Raynaud, B., Nagatsu, I., Borri-Voltatorni, C., and Weber, M., Aromatic L-amino acid decarboxylase (AADC)-immunoreactive cells in the tuberal region of the rat hypothalamus, *Biomed. Res.*, 9, 261, 1988.

Ouimet, C. C., Miller, P. E., Hemmings, H. C., Jr., Walaas, S. I., and Greengard, P., DARPP-32, a dopamine- and cyclic adenosine-3′:5′-monophosphate-regulated phosphoprotein enriched in dopamine-innervated brain regions. III. Immunocytochemical localization, *J. Neurosci.*, 4, 11, 1984.

Palkovits, M., Brownstein, M. J., Saavedra, J. M., and Axelrod, J., Norepinephrine and dopamine content of hypothalamic nuclei of rat, *Brain Res.*, 77, 137, 1974.

Palkovits, M., Fekete, M., Makara, G. B., and Herman, J. P., Total and partial hypothalamic deafferentations for topographical identification of catecholaminergic innervations of certain preoptic and hypothalamic nuclei, *Brain Res.*, 127, 127, 1977.

Parent, A., Descarries, L., and Beaudet, A., Organization of ascending serotonin systems in the adult rat brain. A radioautographic study after intraventricular administration of (^{3}H)5-hydroxytryptamine, *Neuroscience*, 6, 115, 1981.

Paxinos, G. and Watson, C., *The Rat Brain in Stereotaxic Coordinates.* Academic Press, Sydney, 1982.

Quabbe, H.-J., Growth hormone, in *Neuroendocrinology,* Lightman, S. L. and Everitt, B. J., Eds., Blackwell Scientific, Oxford, 1986, 409.

Racke, K., Holzbauer, M., Cooper, T. R., and Sharman, D. F., Dehydration increases the electrically evoked dopamine release from the neural and intermediate lobes of the rat hypophysis, *Neuroendocrinology*, 43, 6, 1986.

Ruggiero, D. A., Baker, H., Joh, T. H., and Reis, D. J., Distribution of catecholamine neurons in the hypothalamus and preoptic region of mouse, *J. Comp. Neurol.*, 1984.

Saavedra, J. M., Palkovits, M., Brownstein, M. J., and Axelrod, J., Serotonin distribution in the nuclei of the rat hypothalamus and preoptic region, *Brain Res.*, 77, 157, 1975.

Sawchenko, P. E. and Swanson, L. W., The organization of noradrenergic pathways from the brainstem to the paraventricular and supraoptic nuclei in the rat, *Brain Res. Rev.*, 4, 275, 1982.

Sawyer, C. H., Radford, H. M., Krieg, R. J., and Carrer, H. T., Control of pituitary-ovarian function by brain catecholamines and LH-releasing hormone, in *Neural Hormones and Reproduction,* Scott, D. E., Kozlowski, G. P., and Weindl, A., Eds., S. Karger, Basel, 1978, 263.

Selden, N. R. W., Cole, B. J., Everitt, B. J., and Robbins, T. J., Damage to ceruleo-cortical noradrenergic projections impairs locally cued but enhances spatially cued water maze acquisition, *Behav. Brain Res.,* 39, 29, 1990.

Selden, N. R. W., Everitt, B. J., and Robbins, T. W., Telencephalic but not diencephalic noradrenaline depletion enhances behavioural but not endocrine fear responses to contextual stimuli, *Behav. Brain Res.,* in press.

Shioda, S., Nakai, Y., Sato, A., Sunayama, S., and Shimoda, Y., Electron-microscopic cytochemistry of the catecholaminergic innervation of TRH neurons in the rat hypothalamus, *Cell Tiss. Res.,* 245, 247, 1986.

Simerly, R. B. and Swanson, L. W., The organization of neural inputs to the medial preoptic nucleus of the rat, *J. Comp. Neurol.,* 246, 312, 1986.

Simerly, R. B., Gorski, R. A., and Swanson, L. W., Neurotransmitter specificity of cells and fibres in the medial preoptic nucleus: an immunohistochemical study in the rat, *J. Comp. Neurol.,* 246, 363, 1986.

Spencer, S., Saper, C. B., Joh, T., Reis, D. J., Goldstein, M., and Raese, J. D., Distribution of catecholamine-containing neurons in the normal human hypothalamus, *Brain Res.,* 328, 73, 1985.

Steinbusch, H. W. M., Distribution of serotonin-immunoreactivity in the central nervous system of the rat — cell bodies and terminals, *Neuroscience,* 6, 557, 1981.

Steinbusch, H. W. M. and Nieuwenhuys, R., Localization of serotonin-like immunoreactivity in the central nervous system and pituitary of the rat, with special references to the innervation of the hypothalamus, *Adv. Exp. Med. Biol.,* 133, 1981.

Steinbusch, H. W. M., Verhofstad, A. A. J., Penke, B., Varga, J., and Joosten, H. W. J., Immunohistochemical characterization of mono-amine-containing neurons in the central nervous system by antibodies to serotonin and noradrenaline, *Acta Histochem., (Jena),* 1981.

Stoeckel, M. E., Tappaz, M., Hindelang, C., Seweryn, C., and Porte, A., Opposite effects of monosodium glutamate on the dopaminergic and GABAergic innervations of the median eminence and the intermediate lobe in the mouse, *Neurosci. Lett.,* 56, 249, 1985.

Swanson, L. W., The hypothalamus, in *Handbook of Chemical Neuroanatomy,* Vol. 5, (Part 1, Integrated systems of the CNS), Björklund, A., Hökfelt, T., and Swanson, L. W., Eds., 1987, 1.

Swanson, L. W. and Hartman, B. K., The central adrenergic system. An immunofluorescence study of the location of cell bodies and their efferent connections in the rat utilizing dopamine-β-hydroxylase as a marker, *J. Comp. Neurol.,* 163, 467, 1975.

Swanson, L. W. and Mogenson, C. J., Neural mechanisms for the functional coupling of autonomic, endocrine and somatomotor responses in adaptive behaviour, *Brain Res. Rev.,* 3, 1, 1981.

Swanson, L. W., Sawchenko, P. E., Berod, A., Hartman, B. K., Helle, K. E., and Van Orden, D. E., An immunohistochemical study of the organization of catecholaminergic cells and terminal fields in the paraventricular and supraoptic nuclei of the hypothalamus, *J. Comp. Neurol.,* 196, 271, 1981.

Swanson, L. W., Sawchenko, P. E., Rivier, J., and Vale, W. W., Organization of ovine corticotrophin-releasing factor immunoreactive cells and fibers in the rat brain: an immunohistochemical study, *Neuroendocrinology,* 36, 165, 1983.

Swanson, L. W., Sawchenko, P. E., and Lind, R. W., Regulation of multiple peptides in CRF parvocellular neurosecretory neurons: implications for the stress response, *Prog. Brain Res.,* 68, 169, 1986.

Treiman, M. and Greengard, P., D-1 and D-2 dopaminergic receptors regulate proteins phosphorylation in the rat neurohypophysis, *Neuroscience,* 15, 713—722, 1985.

Ungerstedt, U., Stereotaxic mapping of the monoamine pathways in the rat brain, *Acta. Physiol. Scand. (Suppl.),* 367, 1, 1971.

Van Den Pol, A. N. and Cassidy, J. R., The hypothalamic arcuate nucleus of rat — a quantitative Golgi analysis, *J. Comp. Neurol.,* 204, 65, 1982.

Van Den Pol, A. N., Herbst, R. S., and Powell, J. F., Tyrosine hydroxylase-immunoreactive neurons of the hypothalamus: a light and electron microscopic study, *Neuroscience*, 13, 1117, 1984.

Van Vugt, D. A., Aylsworth, C. A., Sylvester, P. W., Leung, F. C., and Meites, J., Evidence for hypothalamic noradrenergic involvement in naloxone-induced stimulation of luteinizing hormone release, *Neuroendocrinology*, 33, 261, 1981.

Vuillez, P., Carbajo, P. S., and Stoeckel, M. E., Colocalization of GABA and tyrosine hydroxylase immunoreactivities in the axons innervating and neurointermediate lobe of the rat pituitary: an ultrastructural immunogold study, *Neurosci. Lett.*, 79, 53, 1987.

Young, S. W., III, Warden, M., and Mezey, E., Tyrosine hydroxylase mRNA is increased by hyperosmotic stimuli in the paraventricular and supraoptic nuclei, *Neuroendocrinology*, 46, 349, 1987.

7

The Corticotropin-Releasing Factor System

PETER PETRUSZ AND ISTVÁN MERCHENTHALER
Department of Cell Biology and Anatomy
University of North Carolina
Chapel Hill, North Carolina
and
Functional Morphology Section
Laboratory of Molecular and Integrative Neuroscience
National Institute of Environmental Health Sciences
Research Triangle Park, North Carolina

I. Introduction

An essential and common feature of all living organisms is their ability to maintain a relatively stable internal structure and composition in the face of constant and often threatening changes in their external environment. This concept of adaptation was first recognized and expressed clearly by the French physiologist Claude Bernard more than a century ago. Studies aimed at clarifying the precise nature and components of the body's response to noxious or stressful stimuli have continued throughout this century and are still under way today.

Initially, almost all the emphasis was placed on the release of epinephrine (adrenalin) from the adrenal medulla. Medullary activity is increased tremendously in response to a variety of "emergencies" that may be either internal or external (e.g., hypoglycemia, injury, hemorrhage, extreme changes of temperature, attack, combat, etc.). This "fight or flight" reaction, as it became known mainly from Walter B. Cannon's work during the first three decades of this century, depends on a massive activation of the autonomic nervous system. The sympathetic division produces rapid and widespread reactions, while the responses of the parasympathetic division are slower and highly localized. Under these conditions, the animal shows typical signs of intense emotion and a readiness to fight: elevated heart rate, blood pressure and respiration, dilated pupils, sweating, increased pilomotor activity, increased blood sugar, decreased blood flow to the skin, increased blood flow to striated muscles, and decreased gastrointestinal activity.

Although the autonomic nervous system and the hormones of the adrenal medulla play a very important role in adaptation mechanisms under normal conditions, early experiments to prove their exclusive role failed because they did not take into account the role of the steroid hormones of the adrenal cortex, mainly the glucocorticoids. Attention shifted dramatically from studies of the adrenal medulla to those of the cortex in the mid-1930s, when Hans Selye first introduced the concept of the "general adaptation syndrome" or stress syndrome (Selye, 1936) that was based on the recognition of a specific and well-defined pathologic response to varied and nonspecific noxious stimuli. The central component of this response was the adrenal cortex.

It was clear by this time that the activation of the adrenal cortex could not be explained by sympathetic nervous outflow or by the actions of epinephrine alone, but depended on a peptide hormone of the anterior pituitary, adrenocorticotropic hormone (ACTH) or corticotropin (cf. Harris and George, 1969). The pituitary, in turn, appeared to be under the control of the hypothalamus, via humoral mechanisms first postulated by Geoffrey W. Harris (1948). The initial efforts to define these humoral mechanisms, i.e., to isolate the hypothetical hypothalamic "releasing factors" were driven to a great extent by the all-pervasive influence of Selye's work and the interest it generated in the hypothalamo-pituitary-adrenocortical (HPA) axis. Naturally, corticotropin-releasing factor (CRF) became the subject of the first studies designed specifically to demonstrate the presence of such substances in the hypothalamus. These studies (Saffran and Schally, 1955; Guillemin and Rosenberg, 1955) provided the first convincing evidence that the hypothalamus contained a chemical compound (or several compounds) with the ability to release ACTH from the pituitary both *in vitro* and *in vivo*. However, it required more than two decades of intensive research (which will be summarized briefly in the following section) to achieve the final purification and identification of a peptide that fulfilled the criteria of a major hypothalamic CRF (Spiess et al., 1981; Vale et al., 1981). This 41-residue peptide is produced by neurons in the hypothalamus, transported in their axons to the median eminence, released into portal capillaries, and functions as the major physiologic stimulator of ACTH release from the pituitary. This, in turn, results in the release of glucocorticoids from the adrenal cortex. Thus the key efferent (effector) components of the adrenocortical stress response are now known. As will be discussed later in this Chapter, much of the current work is directed toward the precise definition of the neural and humoral inputs received by hypothalamic CRF neurons, i.e., the afferent components of the response.

In addition, one of the most important outcomes of current studies with CRF-41 is the emerging recognition that this peptide may serve not only as a regulator of pituitary ACTH release, but also as a neurotransmitter or modulator. The neurotransmitter nature of CRF-41 is supported by several sets of observations (for a review, see Fisher, 1989): it is released from various brain regions, in a calcium-dependent manner, in response to depolarizing stimuli; it modifies the electrical discharge of neurons when applied to brain tissue both *in vivo* and *in vitro;* it binds to specific, high-affinity, adenylate cyclase-linked receptors present both in the pituitary and throughout the brain; finally, it has potent and distinct pharmacological actions when applied directly into brain tissue or injected into the cerebral ventricles. The most striking manifestation of the nonendocrine central effects of CRF-41 is the activation of the autonomic nervous system resulting, in turn, in the release of epinephrine and in all of the symptoms of the "fight or flight" reaction described earlier. Thus, it appears that at least one of the key elements in the central regulation of both adrenal cortical and medullary activity is a single neuropeptide, CRF-41.

This chapter will review the detailed anatomical and the essential physiological and pharmacological evidence that supports the role of CRF-41 as a mediator of the body's integrated endocrine and neural (autonomic) responses to stress. In addition, available evidence for the possible role of CRF-41 in certain pathological-clinical processes will also be reviewed briefly.

II. Early Studies on the Hypothalamic Control of ACTH Secretion

Although it was relatively easy to demonstrate ACTH-releasing activity in hypothalamic homogenates and in crude hypothalamic extracts, isolation of the "true" CRF proved to be extremely difficult. This was due partly to the extremely low concentrations of CRF in normal brain tissue (compounded by the relatively low sensitivity and resolution of the early purification and assay techniques) and partly to the fact that a large number of different substances extracted from the hypothalamus have been shown to possess ACTH-releasing activity (for reviews, see Vale et al., 1980; Yasuda et al., 1982). These include arginine-vasopressin (AVP), α-melanocyte stimulating hormone, norepinephrine, and fragments of proteins such as hemoglobin and myelin basic protein. The problem was further complicated by the findings that both extrahypothalamic brain tissue (cf. Saffran and Schally, 1955) and plasma or peripheral tissue extracts (cf. Lymangrove and Brodish, 1973) also contained ACTH-releasing activities. These results, although confusing, permitted at least two firm conclusions, (1) that there were multiple molecular species in the hypothalamus with ACTH-releasing activity, and (2) that AVP appeared to be distinct from, but to be a partial agonist of, the still uncharacterized CRF (cf. Vale et al., 1980).

Early studies (i.e., those before 1981) had to rely on indirect methods also in trying to determine the location of the neurons responsible for the hypothalamic control of ACTH secretion and thus (it was hoped) for the production of CRF. The experimental approaches applied to this problem included the following, alone or in combination: (1) interruption of the connections between the hypothalamus and the pituitary either by pituitary stalk section or by transplantation of pituitary tissue into hypophysectomized animals, (2) selective destruction of various hypothalamic areas or transection of neural pathways thought to project to the median eminence, (3) localized electrical stimulations of various hypothalamic areas, and (4) administration of various drugs, primarily central nervous system (CNS) depressants, steroid hormones, and neurotransmitters or their agonists. The (often conflicting) results of these studies have been reviewed in detail by Harris and George (1969), Ganong (1970), Yates and Maran (1974), and Saffran and Schally (1977). In summary, three major hypotheses emerged from the results of these indirect studies regarding the distribution of the postulated CRF neurons: they were believed to be located either in the medial-basal hypothalamus (Halász et al., 1967; Feldman et al., 1968; Greer and Rockie, 1968; Palka et al., 1969; Dunn and Critchlow, 1973; Csernus et al., 1975; Yasuda and Greer, 1976; Krieger et al., 1977), in the paraventricular nucleus (PVN) (Makara et al., 1981), or scattered "diffusely" throughout the hypothalamus (Brodish, 1963). Contrary to the seemingly overwhelming evidence for a medial-basal hypothalamic location of the postulated CRF neurons, Palkovits et al. (1976), Stark et al. (1978), and Makara et al. (1981) maintained that the source of CRF reaching the portal capillaries must be outside the boundaries of the medial-basal hypothalamus. This controversy became resolved only after 1981, when it became possible to localize CRF-producing neurons directly by immunocytochemistry (see Section III.B).

III. CRF-41

A.   Chemistry and Molecular Biology

The definitive isolation and characterization of a hypothalamic peptide that possessed all the characteristics expected of a physiologic CRF was finally achieved in 1981 by Vale and coworkers. As starting material, they used a fraction prepared from extracts of 490,000 ovine hypothalami. Other fractions that also contained some ACTH-releasing activity were not available for this work, since they had been used previously for the isolation of gonadotropin-releasing hormone (cf. Vale et al., 1981). The active moiety in the fractions studied turned out to be a 41-amino acid straight-chain peptide (ovine CRF-41) with a molecular weight of 4670. The synthetic peptide has the same ACTH-releasing potency as native oCRF-41 both *in vitro* and *in vivo* (Vale et al., 1981, Turkelson et al., 1981; Rivier et al., 1982). The full carboxy-terminal region of the peptide is required for biological activity, while some variability in the amino terminus is apparently tolerated without loss of potency (cf. Vale et al., 1981).

There are interesting structural homologies between CRF-41 and three other known peptide hormones (Figure 1): sauvagine, a 40-residue peptide first isolated from frog skin (Montecucchi et al., 1979), urotensin I, a 38-residue peptide found in the urophysis, a neurosecretory organ in fishes (Lederis et al., 1982), and angiotensinogen (renin substrate), the precursor protein of angiotensin (not shown in Figure 1).

The structure of oCRF-41 was confirmed by recombinant DNA technology, which also permitted the deduction of the amino acid sequence of the entire precursor, preproCRF-41 (Figure 2).

The precursor contains 190 amino acids and the sequence of CRF-41 is found near its C-terminal region, at positions 148 to 188. This sequence is preceded by a pair of basic amino acids (Arg-Arg) marking a cleavage site for trypsin-like processing enzymes. The C terminus of CRF-41 is followed by a Gly residue that is converted to a C-terminal amide — a posttranslational modification found in many other neuropeptides. The oCRF-41 sequence itself contains a pair of basic amino acid residues (Arg-Lys) at positions 35 and 36. There is some evidence that *in vivo* cleavage may occur at this site as well, to yield smaller, biologically inactive peptide fragments; it has been proposed that such cleavage may be glucocorticoid sensitive (cf. Smith et al., 1987). The physiological significance of these posttranslational modifications remains an open question.

Two additional dibasic sites (Arg-Arg at positions 116 and 117 and Lys-Arg at positions 127 and 128; see Figure 2) demarcate two additional peptide fragments that may be cleaved from preproCRF-41. It is not known at this time whether one or both of these fragments are indeed produced *in vivo*.

Characterization of CRF-41 from other species indicates that its structure is highly conserved: the human and rat peptides (cf. Rivier et al., 1983) are identical and differ only by seven amino acid residues from oCRF-41 (Figure 1) and by two residues from porcine CRF (Patthy et al., 1986; not shown). The highly conserved nature of CRF-41 is further supported by the results of immunocytochemical studies that, using antisera to oCRF-41, succeeded in detecting CRF-like peptides in the CNS of annelid worms (Remy et al., 1982), insects

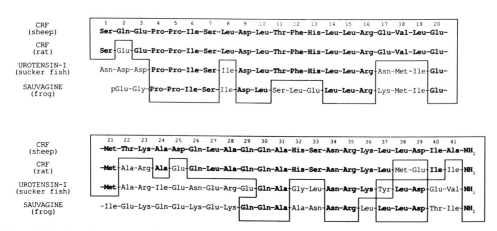

Figure 1. Amino acid sequences of sheep CRF-41, rat CRF-41 (identical with human), urotensin I (isolated from the sucker fish), and sauvagine (isolated from frog skin). The homologous residues, representing in each instance approximately half of the molecule, are indicated by the boxed area. [Based on data from Lederis et al. (1982), Montecucchi et al. (1979), Rivier et al. (1983), Spiess et al. (1981), and Vale et al. (1981).]

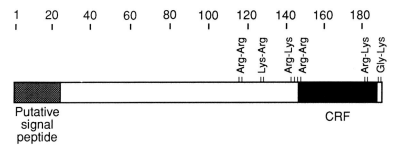

Figure 2. Schematic illustration of the amino acid sequence of human CRF-41 precursor derived by recombinant DNA techniques. The sequence coding for CRF-41 occurs at the C terminus of the prohormone. Actual and potential cleavage sites (adjacent pairs of basic amino acids) are shown. [Redrawn from the data of Shibahara et al. (1983).]

(Verhaert et al., 1984), fishes (Olivereau et al., 1984; Onstott and Elde, 1986; Yulis et al., 1986; Yulis and Lederis, 1987), amphibians (Fasolo et al., 1984; Verhaert et al., 1984; Olivereau et al., 1987), reptiles (Williamson and Eldred, 1989), and birds (Józsa et al., 1984; Yamada and Mikami, 1985; Bons et al., 1988).

The nucleotide sequences of the ovine (Furutani et al., 1983), rat (Jingami et al., 1985b), and human (Robinson et al., 1989) CRF-41 cDNA and the human (Shibahara et al., 1983) and rat (Thompson et al., 1987) CRF-41 genes have been determined. The human CRF-41 gene has been localized to chromosome 8 (Arbiser et al., 1988). It appears that the CRF-41 gene is also highly conserved through evolution. The gene sequences encoding human and rat CRF-41 show very high (94%) homology, and for the rest of the precursor the homology is still about 80%; in addition, both precursors contain highly conserved (94%) 5′-flanking DNA sequences assumed to represent regulatory elements affecting the expression of the CRF-41 gene (cf. Thompson et al., 1987). Not surprisingly, there is increasing evidence that expression of the CRF-41 gene is under multifactorial control: e.g., it is suppressed by glucocorticoids (Jingami et al., 1985a; Roche et al., 1988) and stimulated by cAMP (Seasholtz et al., 1988). *In situ* hybridization studies (see below) have confirmed and extended these fundamental observations on the regulation of CRF-41 gene expression.

B.   Distribution of CRF Neurons

Knowledge of the distribution of CRF-containing structures in the brain is derived mainly from immunocytochemical, immunoassay, and *in situ* hybridization experiments. With the characterization of the structure of CRF-41 from ovine (Spiess et al., 1981; Vale et al., 1981) and human and rat tissues (Rivier et al., 1983) and the availability of specific antibodies to localize (Merchenthaler et al., 1982; Olschowka et al., 1982; Swanson et at., 1983), measure (Fischman and Moldow, 1982; Vigh et al., 1982; Hashimoto et al., 1983), and neutralize *in vivo* (Rivier et al., 1982; Ono et al., 1985; Rivier and Vale, 1985) this peptide, the previously proposed heterogeneity of substances with corticotropin-releasing activity has been confirmed. However, several regions in the CNS that possess biological CRF activity are devoid of specific immunoreactivity, probably indicating the presence of ACTH secretagogues other than CRF-41. On the other hand, it also should be kept in mind that the antibodies raised against CRF-41 or against its fragments recognize only relatively short amino acid sequences and not necessarily the authentic CRF-41. Consequently, the demonstration of immunological but not biological CRF activity may result from detection of biologically inactive fragments of CRF-41 or structurally related but biologically irrelevant molecules. The terms "immunoreactive

CRF" (iCRF) or "CRF-immunoreactive" (CRFi) in this chapter refer to any and all tissue antigen(s) recognized by antisera raised against the ovine or human (=rat) CRF-41 peptides.

CRF-41 is expressed in many regions of the CNS. These can be divided into three major classes (Petrusz et al., 1985): (1) anatomic sites clearly involved in the control of ACTH release from the pituitary, (2) the cerebral cortex, and (3) subcortical areas associated with the regulation of autonomic functions. The distribution of CRFi perikarya as seen by immunocyto-chemistry is summarized in a series of drawings through the rostrocaudal extent of the rat brain and spinal cord (Figure 3).

In brain of intact animals, only a few faintly stained cells can be detected by immunocyto-chemistry. Following intracerebroventricular colchicine treatment, the CRF content of many perikarya in the CNS is elevated to detectable levels (Merchenthaler et al., 1982; Olschowka et al., 1982; Swanson et al., 1983). Colchicine treatment, however, since it blocks axoplasmic transport (Weisenberg et al., 1968), results in decreased CRF content in nerve fibers and terminals (Merchenthaler, 1984; Merchenthaler et al., 1982). Within the hypothalamus, entire CRF neurons (perikarya, fibers, and terminals) can be seen in animals in which the negative feedback effect of glucocorticoids and/or ACTH was interrupted by long-term adrenalectomy or hypophysectomy (Merchenthaler et al., 1983a; Paull and Gibbs, 1983; see Section IV.A). In the human brain, CRFi perikarya can be detected without previous manipulation (Figure 4; Mouri et al., 1984; Bresson et al., 1985).

Detection of mRNA content by *in situ* hybridization is another powerful tool to localize CRF-producing perikarya (Wolfson et al., 1985; Davis et al., 1986; Young and Zoeller, 1989; Young et al., 1986; Swanson and Simmons, 1989). This technique has the advantage that the detection of mRNA can be made in intact animals. The results of these studies on the location of CRF-producing perikarya are in good agreement with previous immunocytochemical observations.

1.   Hypophysiotropic CRF Neurons

Within the hypothalamus, the paraventricular nucleus (PVN) contains the most prominent group of CRF neurons (Figure 5 A to C). The majority of these cells is located throughout the parvocellular subdivisions of the PVN, with the largest number in the medial parvocellular part (Swanson et al., 1983; Figure 6).

CRF is also expressed in a small group of PVN neurons that project to the lower brain stem and the spinal cord (Sawchenko and Swanson, 1985; Swanson et al., 1986), as well as in a subset of oxytocin-containing neurons in the magnocellular subdivision of the PVN (Burlet et al., 1983; Sawchenko et al., 1984a; Kawano et al., 1988) that send their axons to the posterior lobe, which contains CRFi nerve processes and fibers (Bloom et al., 1982; Merchenthaler et al., 1983). Thus, CRF in the rat PVN appears to be expressed by at least three morphologically and functionally distinct cell types, although the largest group by far consists of parvocellular CRF neurons concentrated in the medial parvocellular subdivision (Figure 6). The total number of CRFi cells in the PVN is estimated to be around 2000 to 3000 in the rat brain, and 20% of these (about 400 cells) are located in the magnocellular subdivisions (Swanson et al., 1983).

2.   CRF Neurons in the Cerebral Cortex

The neocortex contains mostly bipolar, vertically oriented cell bodies (Figure 7B and C). The majority of these are located in the second and third layers, but occasionally perikarya are found in deeper layers as well. Cell bodies in the second and third layers are somewhat smaller than those in the deeper layers. Scattered cells in deeper layers might be classified as pyramidal cells, while those in the superficial layers might be classified as interneurons. Although all parts of the neocortex appear to contain CRF perikarya, these cells are much more frequent in the prefrontal, insular, and cingulate areas (Merchenthaler, 1984; Merchenthaler et al., 1982; Sakanaka et al., 1987a).

3.   CRF Neurons Involved in Autonomic Regulation
a.   Diencephalon

The second largest CRFi cell group within the diencephalon is located in the medial preoptic area (MPOA) (Figure 5D). The largest density of immunostained cell bodies is found in a dorsomedial cluster just ventral to the anterior commissure, a smaller number is found in the sexually dimorphic nucleus (Gorski et al., 1980), and others are scattered in the MPOA (Petrusz et al., 1985). Scattered CRFi cells are found in the dorsomedial nucleus (DMN), the arcuate nucleus, the posterior hypothalamus (Merchenthaler et al., 1982; Olschowka et al., 1982), the mammillary nuclei (Kovács et al., 1985), and the medially located thalamic nuclei (Figure 7A; Merchenthaler et al., 1982, 1984b; Sakanaka et al., 1987a; Foote and Cha, 1988). Interestingly, the supraoptic nucleus, which is a major locus of synthesis of vasopressin and oxytocin, contains only a few CRFi perikarya in the rat, but a more substantial number in other mammals (Lederis, 1987), including the human (Merchenthaler, unpublished observations). In marsupials (e.g., opossum), the supraoptic nucleus contains a dense plexus of CRFi nerve fibers around oxytocin- and vasopressin-producing perikarya, suggesting that CRF, through synaptic contacts, might influence the synthesis and/or release of these peptides (Merchenthaler, unpublished observations).

b.   Telencephalon

Dense accumulations of CRFi perikarya are present in the bed nucleus of the stria terminalis (Figure 7E), the central nucleus of the amygdala (Figure 7F), and the substantia innominata. Scattered cells are seen in the cortical, medial, and lateral nuclei of the amygdala, the medial septum, the diagonal band of Broca, and the olfactory bulb, and in different parts of the hippocampus, such as the indusium griseum, fasciola cinerea, septal half of the dentate gyrus, the CA3 and CA1 fields of Ammon's horn and the subiculum (Figure 7D; Merchenthaler, 1984; Merchenthaler et al., 1982; Olschowka et al., 1982; Cummings et al., 1983; Swanson et al., 1983).

c.   Brain Stem and Spinal Cord

Within the mesencephalon, perikarya with CRF immunoreactivity are present in the periaqueductal gray, medial to the Edinger-Westphal nucleus, the dorsal nucleus of the raphe, and the dorsal portion of the ventral tegmental nucleus. Scattered cells are seen in the colliculi, the deep mesencephalic nuclei, the interpeduncular nucleus, and the reticular formation.

In the pons, dense accumulations of CRFi perikarya are located in the ventral half of the locus coeruleus (Figure 8A), the dorsal and ventral portions of the parabrachial nucleus (Figure 8B and C), the medial vestibular nucleus, the paragigantocellular nucleus, and the periaqueductal gray.

No CRF-containing cell bodies are present in the cerebellum.

In the medulla, the majority of CRFi perikarya is present in the nucleus of the solitary tract and the dorsal vagal complex. Scattered cells are seen in the medullary reticular formation (Figure 8D), the spinal trigeminal nucleus, the external cuneate nucleus, and the inferior olive (Merchenthaler, 1984; Merchenthaler et al., 1982; Olschowka et al., 1982, Cummings et al., 1983; Swanson et al., 1983; Sakanaka et al., 1987a; Palkovits et al., 1987).

In the spinal cord CRFi perikarya are present in laminae V to VII, and X, and in the intermediolateral column at thoracic and lumbar levels (Figure 8G and H; Merchenthaler et al., 1983b; Sakanaka et al., 1987a). It has been proposed that iCRF neurons in the spinal cord are mainly sympathetic preganglionic neurons (Krukoff, 1986).

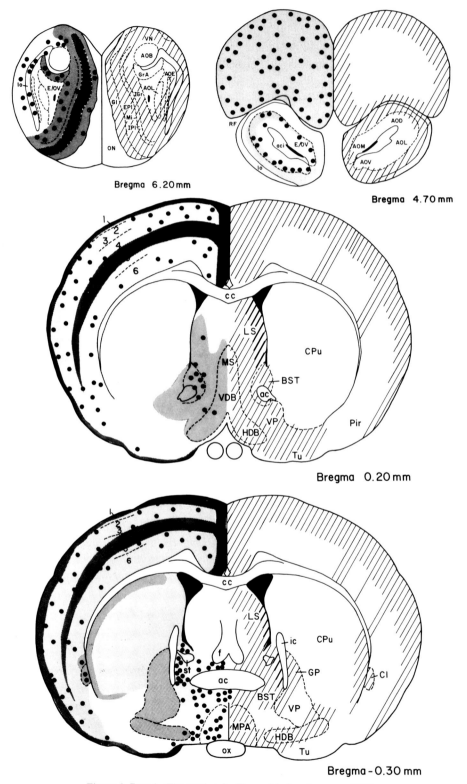

Bregma 6.20 mm

Bregma 4.70 mm

Bregma 0.20 mm

Bregma -0.30 mm

Figure 3, Part 1. (The caption for Figure 3 is found on page 142.)

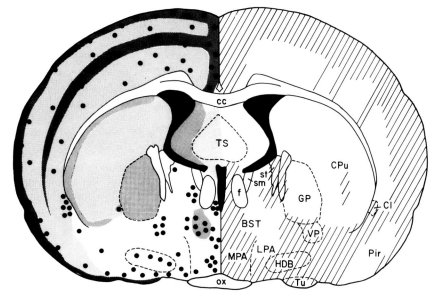

Bregma - 0.80 mm

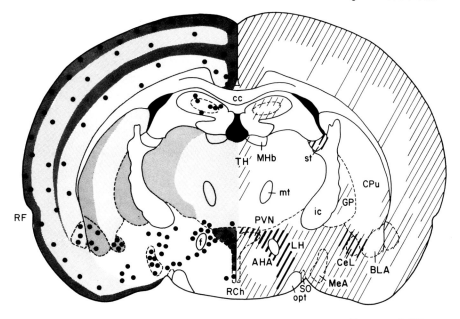

Bregma - 1.80 mm

Figure 3, Part 2.

4.   CRF-Containing Fibers and Terminals
a.   The Hypothalamo-Infundibular CRF System

In intact or colchicine-treated animals, due to the low levels of CRF, afferents to the median eminence cannot be detected by immunocytochemistry except at their termination around portal capillaries in the external zone of the median eminence itself. However, as discussed earlier, in adrenalectomized and/or hypophysectomized rats entire CRF neurons

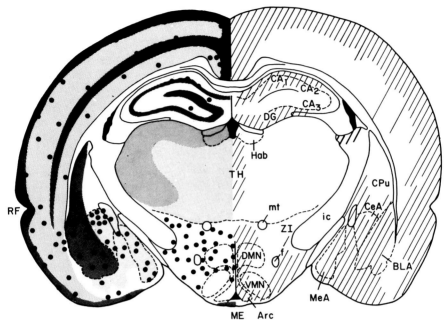

Bregma - 3.14 mm

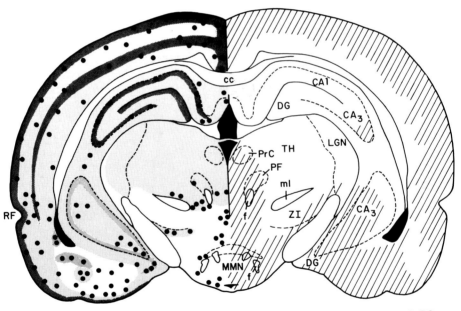

Bregma - 4.52 mm

Figure 3, Part 3.

(perikarya, processes, and terminals) can be labeled easily (Figures 5C and 9; Merchenthaler et al., 1983a).

The majority of CRFi fibers leave the PVN laterally, or lateroventrally, above or below the fornix, respectively, then form a curved, fanlike projection toward the optic chiasm in the hypothalamus. The vast majority of these fibers turn medially and enter the medial basal

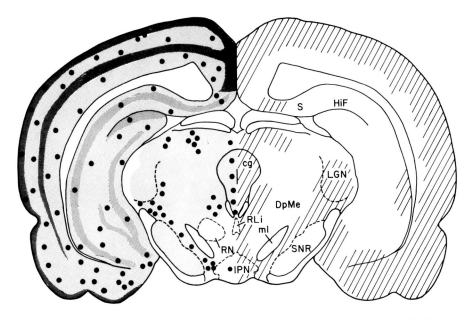

Bregma - 5.60 mm

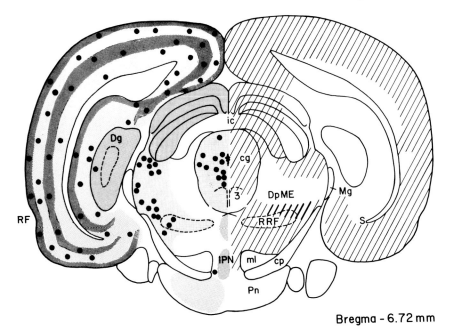

Bregma - 6.72 mm

Figure 3, Part 4.

hypothalamus through the lateral basal retrochiasmatic area (Palkovits, 1984). A small number of fibers from the periventricular subdivision of the PVN turns ventrally and reaches the medial basal hypothalamus at the midportion of the retrochiasmatic region (Merchenthaler et al., 1984a). Results of lesioning experiments in combination with CRF immunocytochemistry indicate that a smaller portion of CRFi fibers do not reach the medial basal hypothalamus through the basal retrochiasmatic area. These fibers from the PVN and the dorsomedial nuclei

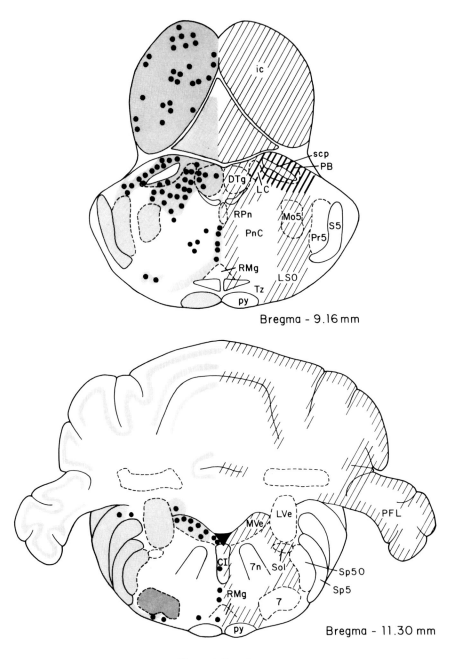

Figure 3, Part 5.

run caudally and then, similarly to the more anteriorly located fibers, reach the median eminence in a fan-like manner (Figure 10; Merchenthaler et al., 1984a). Here, even in intact animals, densely labeled nerve fibers and terminals are seen ending in pericapillary spaces, where they apparently release CRF into the portal circulation and thereby cause the release of ACTH from the pituitary.

These morphological data strongly indicate that the parvocellular part of the PVN is the major site of CRF neurons (hypophysiotropic CRF neurons) that send axon terminals to

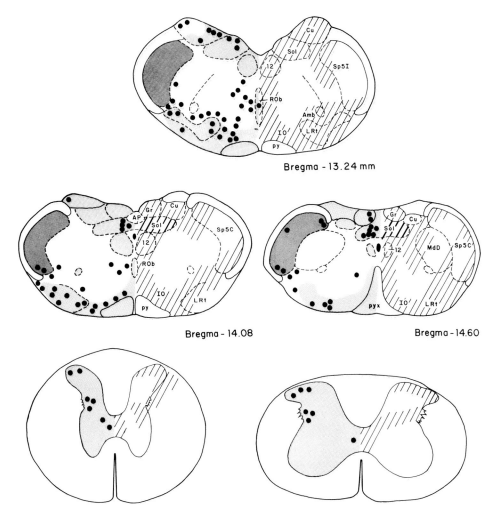

Bregma -13.24 mm

Bregma - 14.08

Bregma -14.60

Figure 3, Part 6.

capillaries of the median eminence. These are the neurons directly responsible for the regulation of the secretion of ACTH from the anterior pituitary. Surgical knife cuts around the medial basal hypothalamus (Antoni et al., 1983; Merchenthaler et al., 1984a), lesions in the PVN (Liposits et al., 1983; Bruhn et al., 1984), or retrograde labeling followed by CRF immunocytochemistry (Figure 11; Nimi et al., 1988; Kawano et al., 1988) have provided further support for the anatomical organization described above.

The hypothalamic location of iCRF neurons is highly conserved: the PVN is the major location of hypophysiotropic CRF neurons in all species studied (Lederis, 1987), including the human (Bresson et al., 1985; see Figure 4A).

b.   Extrahypothalamic CRF Fibers and Terminals

Except for a few well-defined fiber systems, i.e., the stria terminalis and the ventral amygdalofugal pathway, through which CRFi fibers interconnect the amygdala with the hypothalamus and the bed nucleus of the stria terminalis (Moga and Gray, 1985; Sakanaka et al., 1986), only a few CRFi fibers can be seen in the basal telencephalon. An interesting projection has been described by Crawley et al. (1985) from the dorsal-lateral tegmental

Figure 3 (seen on pages 138 to 143). Immunocytochemical mapping of CRF-41-containing neurons (solid circles) and fibers (cross-hatched areas) and CRF-41-binding sites (shaded areas) in the rat central nervous system. The distribution of CRF-immunoreactivity is based on the work of Merchenthaler et al. (1982), Swanson et al. (1983), and Sakanaka et al. (1987). The distribution of CRF receptors is based on the studies of Wynn et al. (1984), De Souza et al. (1985), De Souza and Kuhar (1986), and Aguilera et al. (1987). Abbreviations: Amb, ambiguus nucleus; ac, anterior commissure; aci, anterior commissure, intrabulbar part; AHA, area hypothalamica anterior; AOB, accessory olfactory bulb; AOE, anterior olfactory nucleus, external part; AOL, anterior olfactory nucleus, lateral part; AOM, anterior olfactory nucleus, medial part; AOP, anterior olfactory nucleus, posterior part; AP, area postrema; Arc, arcuate nucleus; BLA, basolateral amygdaloid nucleus; BST, bed nucleus of the stria terminalis; CA1-CA3: fields of Ammon's horn; cc, corpus callosum; CeA, central amygdaloid nucleus, anterior part; CeL, central amygdaloid nucleus, lateral part; cg, central gray; Cl, claustrum; cp, cerebral peduncle; CPu, caudate putamen (striatum); Dg, dentate gyrus; DMN, dorsomedial nucleus; DpME, deep mesencephalic nucleus; DTg, dorsal tegmental nucleus; EPI, external plexiform layer of the olfactory bulb; f, fornix; Gl, granular insular cortex; GP, globus pallidus; Gr, gracile fasciculus; GrA, granular cell layer of the accessory olfactory bulb; Hab, habenula; HDB, nucleus of the horizontal limb of the diagonal band; HiF, hippocampal fissure; ic, internal capsule; IGr, internal granular layer of the olfactory bulb; IPN, interpeduncular nucleus; IO, inferior olive; LC, locus coeruleus; LGN, lateral geniculate nucleus; LH, lateral hypothalamus; lo, lateral olfactory tract; LPA, lateral preoptic area; LRt, lateral reticular nucleus; LS, lateral septum; LSO, lateral superior olive; LVe, lateral vestibular nucleus; ME, median eminence; MeA, medial amygdaloid nucleus; MdD, medullary reticular nucleus; Mg, medial geniculate nucleus; Mi, mitral cell layer of the olfactory bulb; ml, medial lemniscus; MMN, medial mammillary nucleus; MO5, motor nucleus of the trigeminal nerve; MPA, medial preoptic area; MS, medial septum; mt, mammillothalamic tract; MVe, medial vestibular nucleus; ON, olfactory nerve layer; Opt, optic tract; ox, optic chiasm; PB, parabrachial nucleus; PF, parafascicular thalamic nucleus; PFL, paraflocculus Pir, piriform cortex; Pn, pontine nuclei; PnC, pontine reticular nucleus; PrC, precommissual nucleus; Pr5, principal sensory trigeminal nucleus; PVN, paraventricular nucleus; py, pyramidal tract; pyx, pyramidal decussation; RCh, retrochiasmatic area; RF, rhinal fissure; RLi, rostral linear nucleus of the raphe; RMg, raphe magnus nucleus; RN, red nucleus; ROb, raphe obscurus nucleus; RPn, raphe pontis nucleus; RRF, retrorubral field; S, subiculum; scp, superior cerebellar peduncle; sm, stria medullaris thalami; SNR, substantia nigra; SO, supraoptic nucleus; sol, solitary tract; S5, sensory root of the trigeminal nerve; Sp5C, spinal trigeminal nucleus, caudal part; Sp5I, spinal trigeminal nucleus, interpolar part; st, stria terminalis; TH, thalamus; Ts, tectospinal tract; Tu, olfactory tubercle; Tz, trapezoid body; VDB, nucleus of the vertical limb of the diagonal band; VMN, ventromedial nucleus; VN, vomeronasal nerve layer; VP, ventral pallium; ZI, zona incerta.

nucleus to several brain areas, including the medial frontal cortex, the septum, and the thalamus. The results suggest that CRF coexists with substance P and acetylcholine in some of these neurons and that it exerts an inhibiting modulation of the cholinergic response in the frontal cortex. Scattered CRFi fibers are present in the lateral septum and many of these seem to surround non-CRFi perikarya. Within the brain stem, the distribution of CRFi fibers is similar to that of CRFi perikarya. In addition, diffuse CRFi nerve fibers and terminals are present in the medial forebrain bundle, the reticular formation, the red nucleus, the pars reticulata of the substantia nigra, the superior cerebellar peduncle, the molecular layer of the cerebellar cortex (apparently in close association with the dendritic tree of Purkinje cells), the inferior olive and the spinal trigeminal nucleus (Merchenthaler et al., 1982; Olschowka et al., 1982, Swanson et al., 1983; Palkovits et al., 1987; Sakanaka et al., 1987a; Cha and Foote, 1988; Cummings et al., 1989). Recently, Palkovits et al. (1987) have demonstrated that CRFi fibers communicating with Purkinje cells are derived from the inferior olive, and exhibit the characteristics and termination pattern of climbing fibers. A well-characterized CRFi pathway exists between the parabrachial nucleus and the medial preoptic area (Lind and Swanson, 1984). CRFi neurons in the lateral hypothalamus and zona incerta send extensive projections to the inferior colliculus (Sakanaka et al., 1987b). Within the spinal cord, the majority of CRFi fibers forms an ascending system, probably terminating in the reticular formation, the vestibular complex, the central gray, and the thalamus (Merchenthaler et al., 1984b). Descending CRFi fibers in the spinal cord arise from CRF cell bodies in the PVN (Sawchenko and Swanson, 1985).

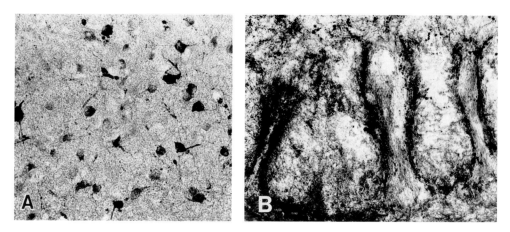

Figure 4. CRF in the human hypothalamus. CRFi perikarya in the PVN (A) and nerve terminals in the median eminence (B).

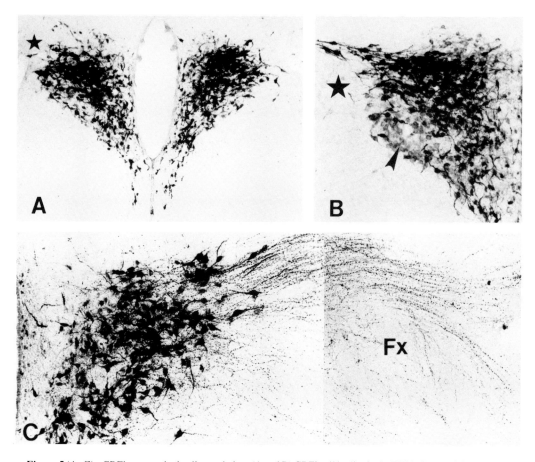

Figure 5 (A–C). CRFi neurons in the diencephalon. (A and B) CRFi cell bodies in the PVN of a colchicine-treated rat. The majority of immunoreactive perikarya is located in the dorsal medial parvocellular subdivisions of the PVN; however, the magnocellular subdivision (star) also contains faintly stained cell bodies (arrowhead). (C) The central part of the paraventriculoinfundibular CRF system as demonstrated in long-term adrenalectomized rat. The perikarya are concentrated in the medial parvocellular subdivision of the PVN. Their processes run either lateral or medial to the fornix (Fx), forming a curved fan of fibers at the level of the PVN.

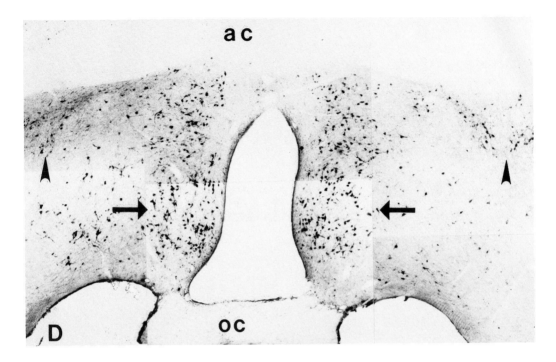

Figure 5 (continued). (D) CRFi perikarya in the anterior hypothalamus. The majority of cells is concentrated in the medial preoptic area (arrows) and in the bed nucleus of the stria terminalis below the anterior commissure (ac) (arrowheads). oc, Optic chiasm. (Silver-intensified frontal sections from Merchenthaler, I., Gallyas, F., and Liposits, Z., in *Techniques in Immunocytochemistry,* Vol. 4, Bullock, G. R. and Petrusz, P., Eds., Academic Press, New York, 1989, 217.)

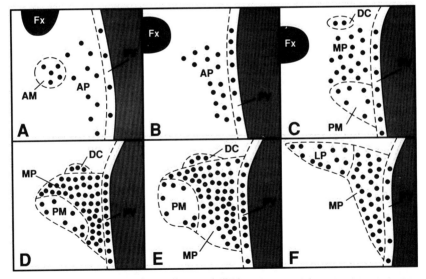

Figure 6. Schematic representation of the distribution of CRFi perikarya (solid circles) through the rostrocaudal extent of the PVN. The various subdivisions of the PVN are indicated by the following abbreviations: AM, anterior magnocellular; AP, anterior parvocellular; DC, dorsal cap; LP, lateral parvocellular; MP, medial parvocellular; PM, posterior magnocellular; PV, periventricular parvocellular; Fx, fornix. [Redrawn after the data of Sawnson et al. (1986) and Ceccatelli et al. (1989a).]

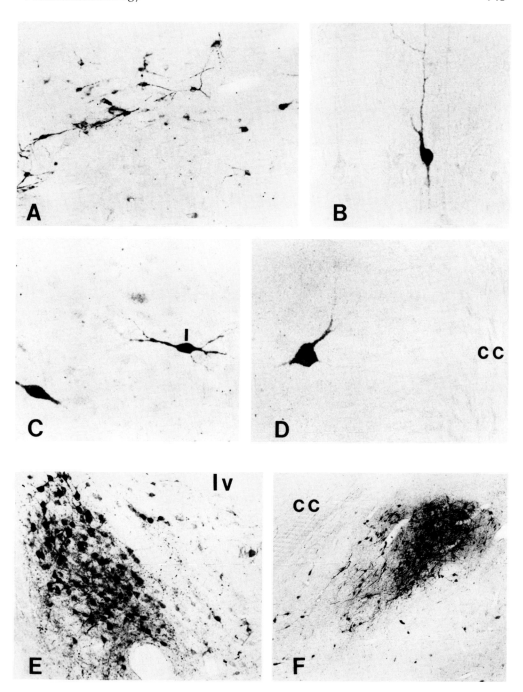

Figure 7. CRFi perikarya in the thalamus and the telencephalon. (A) The majority of immunoreactive cell bodies in the thalamus is located in the medial nuclei. CRFi perikarya (B) among unlabeled pyramidal cells in layer III and (C) in layers V and VI of the cortex. (D) CRFi perikaryon in the subiculum of the hippocampus, lateral to the corpus callosum (cc). (E) CRFi cell bodies in the bed nucleus of the stria terminalis and (F) the central nucleus of the amygdala. lv, Lateral ventricle.

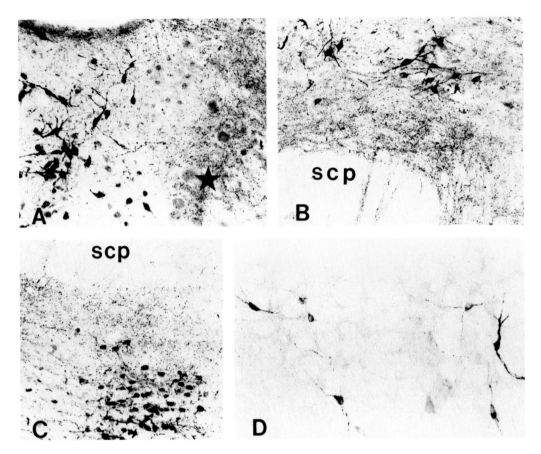

Figure 8. CRFi perikarya in the brain stem and the spinal cord. (A) Immunoreactive cells in the locus coeruleus, medial to the mesencephalic trigeminal nucleus (star). (B and C) CRFi cell bodies in the dorsal and ventral portions of the parabrachial nucleus, above and below the superior cerebellar peduncle (scp), respectively. (D) Scattered immunopositive cells in the medullary reticular formation. (E) CRFi fibers in the molecular layer (m) of the cerebellar cortex. g, Granular layer; w, white matter. Stars mark the cortical surface. Arrowheads point to unstained Purkinje cells. (F) Immunoreactive fibers in the dorsal horn of the spinal cord of a sheep. Most of these fibers are seen in the superficial layer of the dorsal horn, and in the intermediolateral column. (G) CRFi fibers around unstained cells in the intermediolateral column (sheep). (H) Immunopositive perikarya in the intermediolateral column (sheep). (A–F) Frontal sections; (G and H) Longitudinal vibratome sections.

5.   CRF in Body Fluids

The presence of CRF has been demonstrated in hypophysial portal blood in rats in concentrations of the order of $10^{-10} M$ (Gibbs and Vale, 1982; Plotsky and Vale, 1984); however, it has not been possible to detect CRF immunoreactivity reliably and consistently in the peripheral circulation in normal animals. Interestingly, immunoreactive CRF has been detected in human maternal plasma during the third trimester of pregnancy (Sasaki et al., 1984).

Similarly to other hypothalamic and pituitary hormones (Lenhard and Deftos, 1982), CRF is present in the cerebrospinal fluid (CSF) (Nemeroff et al., 1984; Hedner et al., 1989). The CSF may constitute a physiologic pathway for the dispersal of CRF to potential sites of action throughout the CNS. This hypothesis is consistent with the widespread distribution of CRF within the CNS described above, the wide range of pharmacological effects of CRF-41

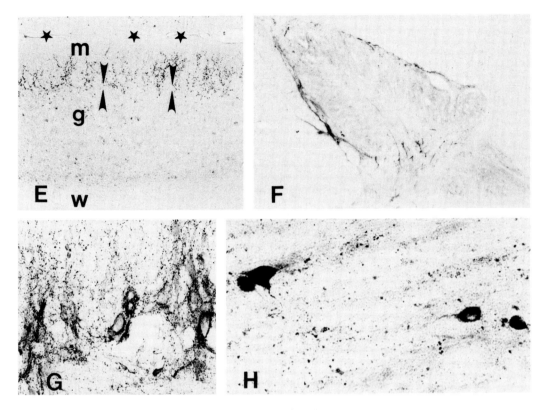

Figure 8 (continued).

injected into the CSF, and the broader integrative and behavioral functions of this peptide in the CNS (see Section IV.D.2).

CRF levels in the human CSF vary in a circadian rhythm paralleling that of pituitary-adrenal function. Furthermore, CSF levels of CRF may be lower in patients with Cushing's disease (Tomori et al., 1983) and normal or elevated in those with major depressive disorders (Nemeroff et al., 1984; cf. Section V).

C.   Colocalization of CRF with Other Neurotransmitters and Neuromodulators

As has been discussed above (see Section III.B.1), within the PVN the majority of CRFi perikarya are present in the medial parvocellular subdivision. This subdivision contains at least three distinct cell groups with entirely separate projections: one group of neurons projects to the median eminence, a second to the posterior lobe of the pituitary, and a third to the brainstem and spinal cord (Swanson and Kuypers, 1980). Each of these groups of cells appears to express a variety of neuroactive substances (Table 1). The hypophysiotropic or neuroendocrine CRF cells have been shown to express a large number of other peptides, including vasopressin (Tramu et al., 1983; Kiss et al., 1984; Sawchenko et al., 1984a), cholecystokinin (CCK; Mezey et al., 1986), angiotensin II, peptide histidine isoleucine (PHI; Hökfelt et al., 1983), vasoactive intestinal peptide (VIP; Hökfelt et al., 1987), enkephalin (Hisano et al., 1987; Hökfelt et al., 1987; Sakanaka et al., 1989), oxytocin (Dreyfuss et al., 1984; Sawchenko et al., 1984b), neurotensin (Sawchenko et al., 1984b), galanin (Ceccatelli et al., 1989a), and the classical

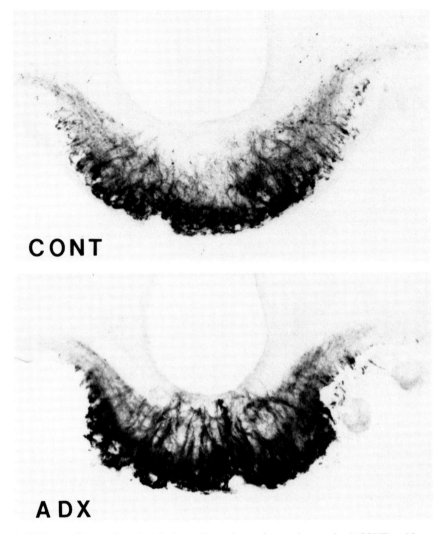

CONT

ADX

Figure 9. CRFi nerve fibers and terminals in the median eminence from an intact animal (CONT) and from a long-term adrenalectomized animal (ADX).

neurotransmitter γ-aminobutyric acid or GABA (Meister et al., 1988). There is evidence that some neurons may contain CRF plus two other peptides. For example, CCK and vasopressin (Mezey et al., 1986), enkephalin and vasopressin (Hisano et al., 1987), and enkephalin and VIP (Hökfelt et al., 1987) have been demonstrated in CRFi perikarya. However, it is important to note that only a relatively small population of the CRF neurons seems to express another peptide or neurotransmitter. Quantitative analysis reveals that about one third of the CRF neurons contains neurotensin, and about 20% enkephalin, whereas the other peptides (CCK, galanin, VIP/PHI), only occur in even smaller numbers of the CRF neurons. It is interesting that CRF neurons seem to represent a neuronal population separate from the thyrotropin-releasing hormone (TRH) neurons, which are also abundant in the PVN. This observation supports the concept that the major hypophysiotropic releasing and inhibiting hormones are found in distinct neuronal systems (cf. Swanson et al., 1987).

Many observations support the intriguing concept of chemical plasticity in CRF neurons,

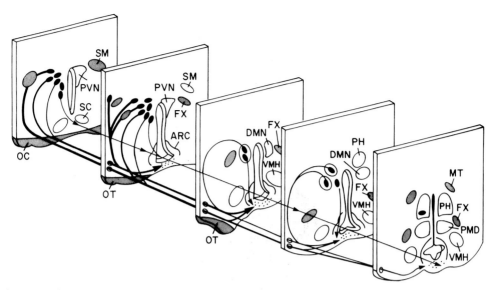

Figure 10. Schematic illustration of the hypothalamoinfundibular CRF system of the rat. The majority of the hypophysiotropic cells is located in the parvocellular subdivisions of the PVN. These neurons send their processes either lateral or medial to the fornix, forming a curved fan of fibers. At the level of the lateral basal retrochiasmatic area they turn medially and enter the medial basal hypothalamus and form axon terminals on capillaries of the portal circulatory system within the median eminence. In addition, scattered cells in the dorsal hypothalamic area and dorsomedial nucleus also send their processes to the median eminence. Abbreviations: ARC, arcuate nucleus; FX, fornix; DMN, dorsomedial nucleus; MT, mammillothalamic tract; OC, optic chiasm; OT, optic tract; PH, posterior hypothalamus; PMD, dorsal premammillary nucleus; SC, suprachiasmatic nucleus; SM, stria medullaris thalami; VMN, ventromedial nucleus.

i.e., that the extent of coexpression varies with regulatory influences. For example, adrenalectomy results in an increased immunostaining for vasopressin (Tramu et al., 1983, Kiss et al., 1984, Sawchenko et al., 1983), angiotensin (Lind et al., 1985a), CCK (Mezey et al., 1986), as well as CRF (Merchenthaler et al., 1983a) in many CRF neurons. In contrast, angiotensin and vasopressin immunostaining is decreased after adrenalectomy in magnocellular PVN neurons (cf. Swanson et al., 1986).

The physiological significance of colocalization of peptides and/or neurotransmitters and the mechanisms underlying the differential expression of the genes involved in their synthesis are not well understood. The colocalization of CRF and vasopressin in the PVN, however, is a topic of considerable interest, since the synergistic action of CRF and vasopressin on ACTH secretion is one of the few examples in which the physiological significance of colocalization appears established. As discussed above, the coexpression of CRF, vasopressin, and to some extent angiotensin II in perikarya of the PVN had been demonstrated only in adrenalectomized rats (Tramu et al., 1983; Kiss et al., 1984; Sawchenko et al., 1984). Recently, however, the colocalization of CRF-41 and vasopressin both in perikarya in the PVN and in nerve terminals of the median eminence has been reported even in intact animals. Approximately half of the CRFi axon terminals contain vasopressin or vasopressin-associated neurophysin, with both peptides packed into the same secretory vesicle (Whitnall et al., 1985, 1987). Following adrenalectomy, CRF and vasopressin levels within the PVN (Tramu et al., 1983; Kiss et al., 1984, Sawchenko et al., 1984) and mRNAs coding for both CRF-41 (Jingami et al., 1985; Young et al., 1986) and vasopressin (Davis et al., 1986) precursors are elevated. The increase in vasopressin mRNA was reported to occur only in CRFi neurons of the PVN (Wolfson et al., 1985). This finding has been further refined by recent electron microscopic immunocyto-

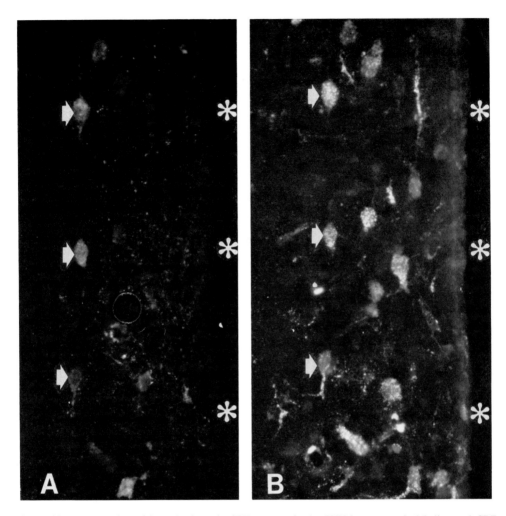

Figure 11. Demonstration of hypophysiotropic CRF neurons in the PVN by retrograde labeling and CRF immunostaining. The retrograde tracer Fluoro-Gold (FG) was injected intraperitoneally. Four days later the animals were given colchicine and sacrificed 1 day later. Thin paraffin sections were immunostained for CRF by the indirect immunofluorescence technique. CRF (A) and the retrograde tracer (B) were simultaneously examined in a fluorescent microscope. Arrows in (A) and (B) label FG-accumulating perikarya immunoreactive for CRF. The asterisks indicate the third ventricle.

chemical studies indicating the existence of two populations of CRFi neurons: one that coexpresses vasopressin extensively and one that is deficient in vasopressin. Following adrenalectomy, almost all of the CRFi neurons (Whitnall and Gainer, 1988) and nerve terminals become vasopressin immunopositive (Hisano et al., 1987; Whitnall et al., 1987). The two subpopulations of CRFi neurons show distinct anatomical distribution in the PVN. Following adrenalectomy, more than 90% of CRFi neurons in the PVN show intense vasopressin staining and these perikarya are highly concentrated in the midstrocaudal region of the PVN, while vasopressin-deficient CRFi neurons are predominant in the caudal part (Whitnall, 1988). According to Whitnall (1988), the caudal CRFi cell group is more sensitive for circulating levels of glucocorticoids. While in intact colchicine-treated animals vasopressin is present in the rostral CRF cell group, it is completely suppressed by normal levels of

Table 1

Neurotransmitters in Neuronal Perikarya of the
Paraventricular Nucleus[a]

Magnocellular	Magno- and parvocellular	Parvocellular
Oxytocin	CRF-41	TRH
Dynorphins	Vasopressin	Neurotensin
CGRP	CCK	Enkephalins
	Galanin	Somatostatin
	Angiotensin II	VIP
	NPY	PHI-27
		Substance P
		ANF
		FMRFamide
		GHRH
		Bradykinin
		Dopamine

[a]Abbreviations. ANF: atrial natriuretic peptide; CCK: cholecystokinin; CGRP: calcitonin gene-related peptide; GHRH: growth
hormone-releasing hormone; NPY: neuropeptide Y; PHI-27:
peptide histidine isoleucine amide; TRH: tyrotropin releasing
hormone; VIP: vasoactive intestinal peptide. For references see
Palkovits (1987).

glucocorticoids in the caudal group. Following adrenalectomy, almost all CRF neurons become immunopositive for vasopressin. These observations suggest that the two CRF cell groups are independently regulated by glucocorticoids (cf. Bondy et al., 1989).

The hypothesis of a functionally distinct subpopulation of CRF neurosecretory cells is further supported by the finding that the vasopressin-rich and vasopressin-deficient subsets of CRF neurons respond differently to acute stress (Whitnall, 1989). The vasopressin-rich population mediates rapid changes in ACTH secretion in response to homeostatic challenges. The vasopressin-deficient type of CRF neurons may serve other functions, such as maintaining a baseline level of ACTH secretion, responding to prolonged stress, or mediating the diurnal rhythm of ACTH output. In any case, the ratio of vasopressin to CRF in portal blood should rise during short-term stress, increasing the secretion of ACTH due to the potentiating effect of vasopressin on CRF-induced ACTH secretion (Gillies et al., 1982; Antoni, 1986; Bondy et al., 1989). Consistent with this hypothesis, changes of vasopressin in portal blood without comparable changes of CRF have been reported (Gibbs, 1985; Plotsky, 1985). In addition, recent evidence suggests that subpopulations of corticotropes in the anterior pituitary respond differently to CRF and vasopressin (Schwartz and Vale, 1988). Thus, differential activation of the vasopressin-rich and vasopressin-deficient CRF neuronal subpopulations may cause selective responses in populations of target cells with distinct functional properties (cf. Bondy et al., 1989).

The above results demonstrate that (1) the parvocellular CRF neuronal system is a probable source of portal vasopressin in normal as well as adrenalectomized animals; (2) in view of the packaging of both vasopressin and CRF in the same secretory vesicle, independent regulation of their release from a single axon terminal is extremely unlikely; but (3) the ratio of vasopressin and CRF in portal blood may be modulated by differential regulation of the two types of CRF neurons (vasopressin rich and vasopressin deficient). Existing data support the conclusion that the two populations of CRF cells are regulated differentially.

It is also important to consider the changes of CRF and vasopressin levels in the median eminence and the portal blood with respect to the length of time after adrenalectomy. About 24 hr after the removal of the adrenals, there is a marked depletion of both CRF-41 and vasopressin from fibers in the external zone of the median eminence (Zimmerman et al., 1977; Bugnon et al., 1984). A few days later, the CRF staining is similar to that seen in intact animals, and the staining for vasopressin becomes more prominent. After about a week, the levels of both vasopressin and CRF are elevated as shown by immunocytochemistry and radioimmuno-assay (Merchenthaler et al., 1983, Holmes et al., 1986). The release of CRF-41 from isolated median eminences decreased by 40% 4 days after adrenalectomy and increased 60% at 4 weeks, while the release of vasopressin rose by 150 and 500% at 4 days and 4 weeks after adrenalectomy, respectively. Thus, the ratio of vasopressin to CRF-41 released in the median eminence increased from approximately 2:1 in control animals to 9:1 in long-term adrenalectomized rats (Holmes et al., 1986). These results have important implications for the physiological significance of colocalization in general, as they suggest that the coexisting messengers in neurons may undergo long-term modulation by changes of the hormonal environment.

Any neuron that synthesizes and releases more than one chemical messenger has the potential to influence more than one type of receptor on single target cells or to influence multiple cell types. Both of these possibilities occur as target cells in the pituitary interact with neuropeptides released from CRF neurons (Hökfelt et al., 1983). Thus, CRF, vasopressin, angiotensin, and CCK all stimulate the release of ACTH, thyroid-stimulating hormone (TSH) (Lumpkin et al., 1987) and prolactin (Schramme and Denef, 1984). It is well known that stressful stimuli result in decreased luteinizing hormone (LH) and gonadal steroid levels (Rivier and Vale, 1984a). Besides other mechanisms, such as CRF innervation of luteinizing hormone-releasing hormone (LHRH) perikarya in the preoptic area (MacLusky et al., 1988), paracrine or synaptic mechanisms operating in the median eminence may be responsible for some of the actions of CRF. CRF may act at this level to inhibit the release of LHRH (Gambacciani et al., 1986). CRF may also exert its effects indirectly, e.g., by stimulating the release of β-endorphin, which, in turn, would inhibit the secretion of LHRH.

D.   CRF Receptors and Their Distribution

Consistent with the known actions of CRF, receptors for this peptide have been found in the anterior and intermediate lobes of the pituitary, in many regions of the CNS, and at several peripheral sites (cf. De Souza et al., 1985; De Souza and Kuhar, 1986; Aguilera et al., 1987).

1.   CRF Receptors in the Anterior Pituitary

In all species studied, autoradiographic analysis of the binding of radiolabeled CRF has indicated that binding sites are present in the anterior and intermediate lobes, but not in the neural lobe. In spite of differences in distribution among species, the binding properties (length of time to reach a steady state, optimal temperature, dissociation constant on the order of 10^{-9} M) of CRF receptors are similar in pituitary membranes from rat and primates (Millan et al., 1987). CRF receptors in the anterior pituitary are linked to changes in the G-regulatory component of the receptor, which is coupled to adenylate cyclase in the plasma membrane and finally cAMP production (Aguilera et al., 1986). The concentrations of CRF reported in portal blood (10^{-10} M; Plotsky and Vale, 1984; Gibbs, 1985) are in a suitable range for the affinity of CRF receptors of the pituitary (Aguilera et al., 1987). Following adrenalectomy, when ACTH levels and responsiveness to CRF are increased, pituitary CRF receptor concentration is reduced without changes in binding affinity (Wynn et al., 1985; Aguilera et al., 1987). The reduction of CRF receptor concentration after adrenalectomy is accompanied by a significant decrease in CRF-stimulated adenylate cyclase activity and cAMP production. These changes can be prevented by dexamethasone treatment.

It is well known that increased exposure of target cells to peptide hormones is accompanied by down regulation of the corresponding receptors (Catt et al., 1979). Thus, the elevated levels of CRF in portal blood following adrenalectomy (Holmes et al., 1986) might be responsible for the loss of CRF receptors. The mechanisms of this loss are not entirely clear. It may occur as a result of simple internalization of the existing receptors or reduced synthesis of newly produced receptor proteins (Aguilera et al., 1987). However, since prolonged infusion of CRF in intact rats has resulted in less pronounced decrease in pituitary CRF receptors than that seen after adrenalectomy, it is likely that other factors, probably vasopressin, are also involved in this process (Holmes et al., 1987). Furthermore, glucocorticoids inhibit ACTH release whether it is induced by receptor agonists such as CRF, vasopressin, angiotensin, and norepinephrine, or by postreceptor stimulants, such as 8-bromo-cyclic AMP and phorbol esters (Abou-Samra et al., 1986). Therefore, the inhibitory effect of glucocorticoids on ACTH release is explained only partially by down regulation of CRF receptors in the pituitary.

2.   CRF Receptors in the Central Nervous System

The distribution of CRF receptors in the CNS correlates well with the distribution of CRF-containing nerve terminals (see Figure 3 and Table 2). The binding properties of brain CRF receptor sites are identical to those seen in the pituitary. In contrast to the marked reduction in CRF receptors in the anterior pituitary, CRF receptor concentration in the brain and intermediate lobe of the pituitary are not affected by adrenalectomy (De Sousa and Kuhar, 1986, Wynn et al., 1985), stress, or glucocorticoid administration (Hauger et al., 1987). CRF receptors in the rat and monkey are located predominantly in two functionally distinct systems: the neocortex and the limbic system (Wynn et al., 1985, Millan et al., 1986; De Souza et al., 1985; De Souza and Kuhar, 1986). Both of these areas are known to contain CRFi perikarya and nerve terminals (Merchenthaler et al., 1982; Sakanaka et al., 1987a).

The following account of the distribution of CRF receptors is based on the data of Wynn et al. (1983, 1985), De Souza et al. (1985); De Souza and Kuhar (1986), and Aguilera et al. (1987).

High concentrations of CRF receptors are present throughout the cerebral cortex. A somewhat greater density of receptors is seen in the somatosensory, striate, and entorhinal cortex than in the motor and cigulate cortex. The highest concentration is found in layer IV, followed by layers I and III. In the pyriform cortex, a high density of binding is present in lamina I, with much lower densities in the remaining laminae.

The hippocampus contains a relatively low concentration of CRF receptors. Most of them are found in the subiculum, the molecular layer of the dentate gyrus, and the CA1 region.

Within the olfactory bulb, CRF-binding sites are highly localized to the external plexiform layer and the adjacent glomerular layer. The internal plexiform, mitral cell body, and internal granule layers contain only moderate levels of CRF receptors. A high density of binding sites is found in the external plexiform layer of the olfactory tubercle, and low density is found in the pyramidal and polymorphic layers as well as in the islands of Calleja.

In the corpus striatum, moderate levels of CRF receptors are present in the caudate-putamen, the globus pallidus, and the claustrum.

In the basal forebrain, low to moderate levels of CRF receptors are seen in the nucleus accumbens, the diagonal band of Broca, the medial and lateral septal nuclei, the triangular septal nucleus, and the bed nucleus of the stria terminalis. In the amygdala, more binding sites are found in the lateral than the medial and central nuclei.

Within the thalamus, higher concentration of receptors are present in the lateral than the medial nuclei.

In the hypothalamus, only the paraventricular nucleus, the external zone of the median eminence, and the mammillary peduncle contain CRF receptors.

Table 2

Distribution and Density of CRF Binding Sites in the Central Nervous System

Region	Density[a]	Region	Density
Cortex		Midbrain	
Layers I and IV	H	Inferior colliculus	M
Layers II, III, V, VI	M	Central gray	L
		Dorsal raphe	L
Olfactory bulb			
External plexiform layer	H	Pons-medulla	
Internal plexiform layer	L	Nuclei of cranial nerves III, IV, V, VII	H
Glomerular layer	L	Medial vestibular nucleus	M
Granular layer	L	Lateral vestibular nucleus	M
		Cuneate nucleus	M
Olfactory tubercle	M	Gracilis nucleus	M
		Lateral reticular nucleus	M
Hippocampus	L	Inferior olive	M
		Superior olive	M
Basal ganglia		Ventral tegmental nucleus	M
Caudate-putamen	M	Nucleus of cranial nerve XII	M
Globus pallidus	M	Parabrachial nuclei	M
Claustrum	M	Paragigantocellular nucleus	L
		Nucleus of solitary tract	L–M
Septum		Dorsal tegmental nucleus	L–M
Nucleus accumbens	M	Pyramids	L–M
Diagonal band of Broca	M	Locus coeruleus	L
Medial and lateral septum	L		
BNST	L	Cerebellum	H
Amygdala		Spinal cord	
Basolateral nucleus	M	Dorsal horn, Rexed	
Central, medial nuclei	L	laminae 1–4	L
		Dorsal horn, Rexed	
Thalamus	L	laminae 4–6	M–L
		Ventral horn	M–L
Habenula	L		
Hypothalamus			
Median eminence	H		
Paraventricular nucleus	H		
Medullary peduncle	H		
Other regions	O		

[a] L, low; M, medium; H, high; O, none detected.

In the midbrain, a moderate level of CRF receptors is present in the inferior colliculus. Somewhat lower levels can be observed in the trochlear nucleus, the interpeduncular nucleus, the periaqueductal gray, the dorsal raphe nucleus, and the superior colliculus. Only very low concentrations are seen in the substantia nigra.

In the pons, very high concentrations of CRF-binding sites are present in the facial, trigeminal, cochlear, and vestibular nulcei. High concentration is found in the medial vestibular nucleus and the lateral cervical nucleus. The spinal trigeminal nucleus, the nucleus of the hypoglossal nerve, the paragigantocellular, the parabrachial, dorsal, and ventral tegmental, and the pontine nuclei contain only a low density of binding sites.

In the medulla, the highest receptor densities are found in the cuneate and gracilis nuclei. Moderate densities are present in the inferior olive, the nucleus of the solitary tract, and throughout the pyramids.

In the cerebellum, CRF receptors are present in all layers, with somewhat greater concentrations in the granular layer and in the medial and interpositus nuclei.

In the spinal cord, moderate levels of receptors are present in the gray matter, with lower levels in the dorsal horn layers 1 and 4.

In general, the reported distribution of CRF receptors in most regions of the rat CNS appears to be quantitatively consistent with the distribution of CRFi nerve terminals. For example, the highest concentration of CRF receptors within the hypothalamus is present in the median eminence, where the greatest concentration of CRF nerve terminals is also found. The cerebral cortex, the diagonal band of Broca, the lateral septum, and several brain stem nuclei also belong to the areas with relatively good correspondence. However, there are some regions in the rat CNS in which the distributions of CRFi nerve terminals and CRF receptors do not correlate well. Some of these areas include the olfactory bulb, the amygdala, the cerebellum, and the spinal cord. The cerebellum provides a very striking example. In the rat (Merchenthaler, 1984; Merchenthaler et al., 1982; Cummings et al., 1983; Sakanaka et al., 1987a) only moderate densities of CRFi nerve fibers and terminals are present in the stratum moleculare. In contrast, the concentration of CRF-binding sites in the cerebellum is one of the highest within the CNS, and most of them are located in the stratum granulosum (De Souza et al., 1985).

The presence of a high concentration of CRF-binding sites in the median eminence is somewhat surprising, since the median eminence is not considered generally as a major "effector site" for CRF. The receptors present here may be presynaptic autoreceptors or receptors for axo-axonal communication, which may play a role in regulating the release of CRF and other neuropeptides into the portal vasculature (De Souza et al., 1985). They may also interact with ependymal tanycytes, which may function to transport CRF (and other compounds) from the third ventricle to the hypophysial portal vasculature (Zimmerman et al., 1977). However, it must be noted that neither CRF nor other neuropeptides have been identified in tanycytes by electron microscopic immunocytochemistry. Thus, the functional significance of CRF receptors in the median eminence remains unclear and should be the subject of further investigations.

IV. Regulation of CRF Neurons

A.   Feedback Regulation of CRF Neurons

Effective removal of glucocorticoid feedback by adrenalectomy or hypophysectomy markedly enhances the staining for CRF in the parvocellular subdivisions of the PVN (see Figure 5C; Antoni, 1986; Antoni et al., 1983; Burlet et al., 1983; Merchenthaler et al., 1983a, Paull and Gibbs, 1983). A slight increase in immunostaining within perikarya is also detected in the magnocellular subdivisions of the PVN, the central nucleus of the amygdala, the dorsal hypothalamic area, the dorsomedial nucleus, the BNST (Merchenthaler, 1984; Merchenthaler et al., 1983a; Paull and Gibbs, 1983; Swanson et al., 1987), and the spinal cord (Merchenthaler et al., 1983b), but not elsewhere in the CNS. Following adrenalectomy, the cells in the PVN ultrastructurally show hypertrophy of the rough endoplasmic reticulum, dilated cysternae in the Golgi complex, and an increased number and size of secretory granules (120 vs. 90 nm), indicative of increased protein synthesis and secretory activity (Liposits et al., 1985; Alonso et al., 1988). Interestingly (see Section III.C), in such animals about 70 to 90% of the CRFi perikarya in the PVN also express vasopressin (Tramu et al., 1983; Kiss et al., 1984, Sawchenko et al., 1984). Moreover, the two peptides are colocalized in single secretory granules not only

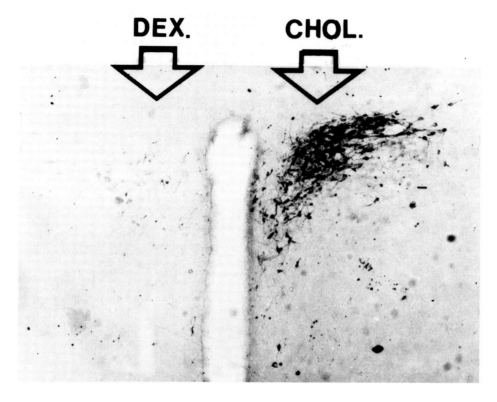

Figure 12. Effect of unilateral dexamethasone microimplant on CRF immunostaining in the PVN of an adrenalectomized rat. The implant was placed on the left side. Note the total disappearance of CRF-immunostaining from the PVN on the side of the implant. DEX: Dexamethasone-implanted side; C, control. (Reproduced with permission from Kovács, K., Kiss, J. Z., and Makara, G. B., *Neuroendocrinology*, 44, 229, 1986.

within perikarya but in terminals of the median eminence as well (Whitnall et al., 1985). This increase in the amount of immunoreactive peptide within the perikarya is accompanied by an increase in the amount of mRNA transcripts of both the CRF-41 and vasopressin genes (Wolfson et al., 1985; Davis et al., 1986; Young and Zoeller, 1989; Young et al., 1986). The signs of increased synthesis of CRF in the PVN and, to some extent, in some other brain regions following adrenalectomy or hypophysectomy are also detected in nerve processes within the hypothalamus (Figure 5C) and nerve terminals within the median eminence (Figure 9; Merchenthaler et al., 1983; Paull and Gibbs, 1983).

The increased CRF content observed in adrenalectomized and in hypophysectomized animals can be prevented or reversed by glucocorticoid or mineralocorticoid treatments (Paull and Gibbs, 1983; Itoi et al., 1987; Sawchenko, 1987a, 1987b) or implantation of glucocorticoids (e.g., dexamethasone) in the vicinity of the PVN (Figure 12; Kovács et al., 1986; Kovács and Mezey, 1987), suggesting that adrenal steroids act directly on neurons in the PVN to depress levels of CRF (cf. Sawchenko, 1988). Recent studies on the hypothalamic distribution of glucocorticoid receptor (see Figure 3) either by immunocytochemistry (Fuxe et al., 1985, 1987; Liposits et al., 1987b) or radioimmunoassay in microdissected areas (Reul and De Kloet, 1985) have confirmed that the parvocellular subdivisions of the PVN contain feedback-sensitive glucocorticoid receptors. With the aid of double-labeling immunocytochemistry it

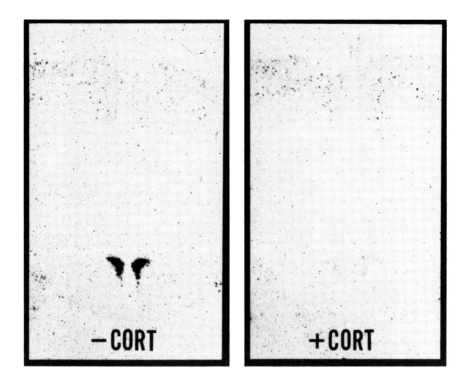

Figure 13. Photomicrographs of Cronex 4 film over frontal sections to show CRF mRNA hybridization over the PVN in an adrenalectomized rat (–CORT) and in another that had received 800-mg pellets of corticosterone 1 week before sacrifice (+CORT). Note the complete disappearance of CRF mRNA labeling induced by adrenalectomy in animals treated with corticosterone. (Reproduced with permission from Swanson, L. W. and Simmons, D. M., *J. Comp. Neurol.,* 285, 413, 1989.

has been shown that at least some CRF cells in the medial parvocellular cell group are also immunoreactive for the glucocorticoid receptor (Agnati et al., 1985).

Although it seems well established that glucocorticoids act directly on CRF neurons in the PVN, the mechanism of their action is not entirely clear. It appears certain that they act, at least in part, at the level of gene expression (Figures 13 to 15; Swanson and Simmons, 1989; Kovács and Mezey, 1987; Kovács et al., 1986; Wolfson et al., 1985; Young et al., 1986; Young and Zoeller, 1987. However, glucocorticoids may also influence posttranslational processing (cf. Smith et al., 1987), transport, or release of CRF-41 (Wolfson et al., 1985). Nevertheless, most of the results available to date suggest that glucocorticoids inhibit CRF production by acting primarily on CRF neurons in the PVN to suppress the expression of CRF and vasopressin genes, presumably via glucocorticoid receptors present in the appropriate neurons (Hollenberg et al., 1985).

B.   Neurnal Regulation of CRF Neurons

1.   Neural Afferents to the Paraventricular Nucleus

Exogenous and endogenous stressful stimuli are first encoded as neurochemical signals and are then processed in the CNS, leading to the activation of a widespread neuronal network involved in the stress response. Markers of metabolic activity (e.g., expression of the c-*fos*

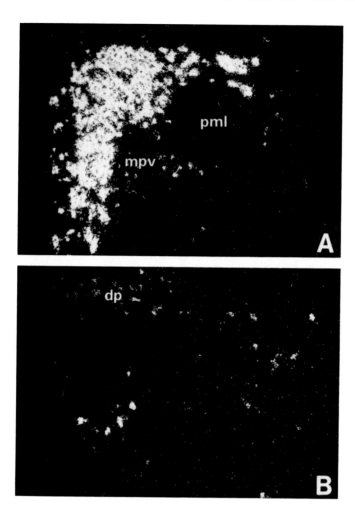

Figure 14. Photomicrographs of dipped autoradiographs to show CRF-41 mRNA hybridization over the PVN of an adrenalectomized animal (A) and an animal that had received 800-mg pellets of corticosterone for 1 week (B). Dark-field illumination of 20-μm thick frontal sections. Abbreviations: dp, dorsal parvicellular subdivision; mpv, medial parvocellular subdivision; pml, posterolateral magnocellular subdivision of the PVN. (Reproduced with permission from Swanson, L. W. and Simmons, D. M., *J. Comp. Neurol.*, 285, 413, 1989.)

oncogene protein) can be used to identify these neurons (Ceccatelli et al., 1989b). Subsequently, these signals are transported via multiple pathways to CRF neurons in the PVN, where they are transformed into a hypophysiotropic message. The hypophysiotropic message is of complex chemical nature, and may include CRF, vasopressin, oxytocin, angiotensin II, and several other compounds (cf. Figure 17). These compounds are secreted in a stimulus-specific fashion from nerve terminals of the median eminence into the hypophysial portal circulation, through which they reach ACTH cells in the anterior pituitary (see Figure 17).

Retrograde and anterograde tracing studies in combination with immunocytochemistry have been used to identify the source and the chemical nature of neuronal inputs to the medial parvocellular subdivision of the PVN. Since the hypophysiotropic CRF neurons constitute by far the largest population of neurons in this subdivision, inputs to this general area potentially represent afferents to CRF neurons. Some of these connections have already been substanti-

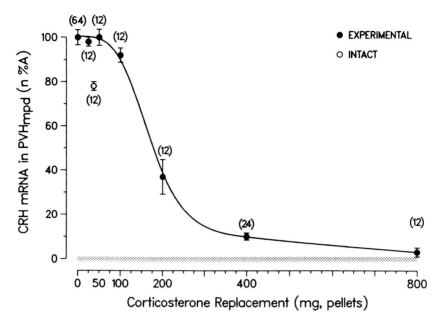

Figure 15. The relationship between CRF mRNA levels in the dorsal medial parvocellular subdivision of the PVN and replacement doses of corticosterone. Zero corticosterone corresponds to adrenalectomized animals, and all values were normalized to this maximum level (100%) of hybridization. For comparison, the hybridization levels in intact animals are shown. The SEM and number of measurements (parentheses) from Cronex 4 films are shown for each point. The mean (±SEM) blood levels of corticosterone for each group were as follow: adrenalectomized, undetectable; 25-mg pellets, 9 ± 3; 50-mg pellets, 63 ± 11; 100-mg pellets, 60 ± 10; 200-mg pellets, 109 ± 17; 400-mg pellets, 192 ± 18; 800-mg pellets, 244 ± 33; intact (decapitated), 19 ± 7. (Reproduced with permission from Swanson, L. W. and Simmons, D. M., *J. Comp. Neurol.,* 285, 413, 1989.)

ated by electron microscopic immunocytochemistry (see below); however, in many cases further ultrastructural and physiological studies will be required to demonstrate direct functional interactions.

a.   Afferents Containing Classical Neurotransmitters

At least six catecholaminergic cell groups in the brain stem project to the PVN (cf. Swanson et al., 1981; Sawchenko and Swanson, 1982; Tucker et al., 1987). The axons of the A2 noradrenergic cell group, which is located in the nucleus of the solitary tract, reach the PVN either directly or indirectly through the parabrachial nucleus (Norgren, 1978; Saper and Loewy, 1980). Some of these noradrenergic cells coexpress neuropeptide Y (NPY) (Sawchenko et al., 1985). The PVN also receives inputs from the A1 noradrenergic cell group in the ventrolateral medulla. Some of these neurons are also immunopositive for NPY (Sawchenko et al., 1985) and galanin (Levin et al., 1987). Adrenergic afferents arrive from three discrete cell groups in the rostral medulla. These include the C1 cell group in the rostral ventrolateral medulla, the C2 cell group in the rostral nucleus of the solitary tract, and the C3 cell group in the rostral dorsomedial medulla (Cunningham and Sawchenko, 1988; Swanson and Sawchenko, 1981). Some of the neurons in the C1 to C3 medullary cell groups also contain NPY (Sawchenko et al., 1985). Much less is known about the distribution of dopaminergic inputs, although immunofluorescence (Lindwall et al., 1984) and immunocytochemical (Buijs et al., 1984; Decavel et al., 1987) studies have described dopamine fibers and terminals in the

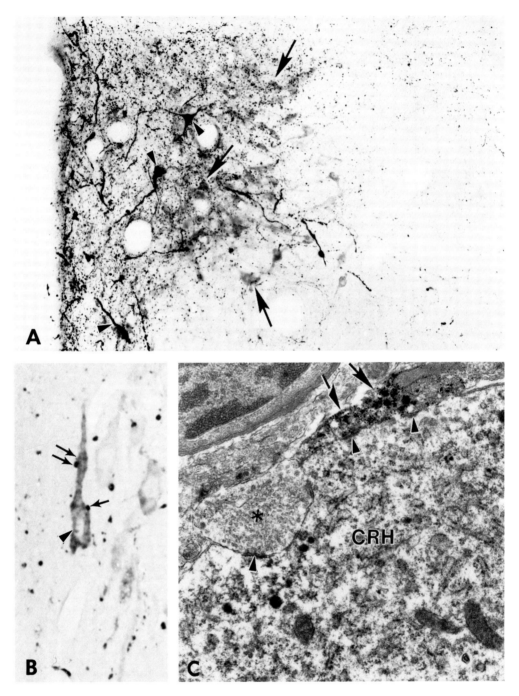

Figure 16. Simultaneous immunocytochemical detection of tyrosine hydroxylase (TH)-immunoreactive (THi) and CRFi neuronal structures in the PVN. (A) Whereas the entire parvicellular portion of the PVN is filled with brown diaminobenzidine (DAB)-labeled CRF cell bodies (arrows), THi neurons (arrowheads) and fibers are indicated by the black silver gold-intensified DAB end product (Merchenthaler et al., 1989). Note that the CRF-containing neurons are densely surrounded by THi fibers. Magnification: × 370. (B) THi fibers in close association with the dendrite (double arrows) and the soma (arrow) of a CRFi perikaryon (arrowhead) as demonstrated in a semithin section. Magnification: × 570. (C) CRFi perikaryon (CRH) forms synaptic specialization (arrowheads) with both THi (arrow) and chemically unidentified (*) axon terminals. Magnification: ×27,800. (Reproduced with permission from Liposits, Z., *Prog. Histochem. Cytochem.*, 2, No. 2, 1990.)

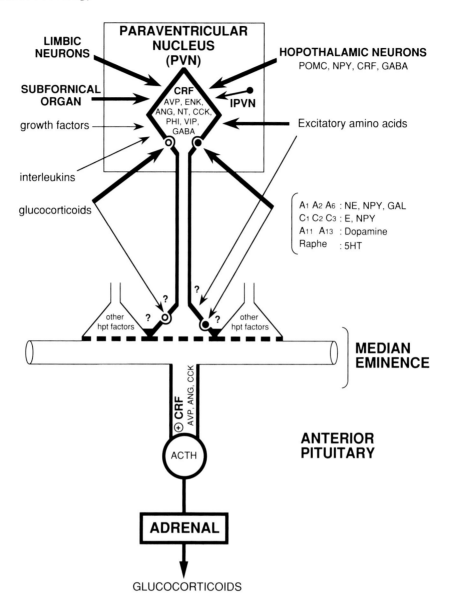

Figure 17. Schematic representation of the integrated neuroendocrine control of ACTH secretion. CRF cells receive neuronal afferents from the hypothalamus, limbic structures, the subfornical organ, the brainstem, and the PVN itself. Excitatory amino acids of unknown origin also affect the activity of CRF neurons. Humoral factors, such as glucocorticoids, interleukins, growth factors, and so on, directly influence the activity of CRF neurons. Some of these act through specific receptors on the perikarya or on nerve terminals. CRF neurons coexpress a variety of chemical messengers, including vasopressin (AVP), enkephalins (ENK), angiotensin II (ANG), neurotensin (NT), cholecystokinin (CCK), peptide histidine-isoleucine (PHI), vasoactive intestinal polypeptide (VIP), and γ-aminobutyric acid (GABA). CRF and the coexpressed substances are transported from the perikarya by axoplasmic transport to nerve terminals in the median eminence, where they are released into capillaries of the portal circulatory system. Through axoaxonic or other type of connections, these chemical messengers may interact within the median eminence. From the median eminence CRF and the coreleased substances are transported to the anterior pituitary via the portal circulatory system, where CRF stimulates the secretion of ACTH into the general circulation. In the adrenal cortex, ACTH stimulates the secretion of glucocorticoids, which, in turn, inhibit CRF production and ACTH secretion by acting through specific receptors present both in the brain and the pituitary. For further details see the text.

parvocellular part of the PVN. They probably originate from the arcuate nucleus (A12), the zona incerta (A13), and the periventricular area (A14).

Several studies have indicated that serotonin influences the function of the pituitary-adrenal axis; however, the site and nature of its action are controversial (see Section IV.D.1). Serotonergic neurons that project to the PVN are located in the dorsal raphe (B7 cell group), the median raphe (B8 cell group), and the medial lemniscus (B9 cell group).

The medullary catecholaminergic fibers ascend rather diffusely through the medullary tegmentum up to the level of the locus coeruleus. Here the afferents divide into two distinct components: the more prominent central tegmental tract and the less prominent ventral noradrenergic bundle (Ungerstedt, 1971; Sawchenko and Swanson, 1982). More rostrally, these components reunite and enter the medial forebrain bundle, through which they reach the PVN. The noradrenergic pathways, which are interconnected in a complex network and receive a diverse array of visceral and somatosensory inputs, are among the cadidates for mediating activation of the PVN (including its CRF neurons) in response to a number of visceral and somatic stimuli.

b.   Afferents Containing Neuropeptides

Among telencephalic areas, the BNST and the zona incerta have direct connections with the PVN. Through these connections the BNST may relay limbic informations from the amygdala and the hippocampus, while the zona incerta may transmit information concerning the regulation of fluid balance (Sawchenko and Swanson, 1983). Among hypothalamic regions, several areas have been shown to send afferents to the PVN. These include the preoptic periventricular nucleus, the medial and lateral preoptic areas, the suprachiasmatic nucleus, the anterior hypothalamic area, the ventromedial nucleus, the ventral premammillary nucleus, the supramammillary nuclei, the posterior hypothalamus, the lateral hypothalamus, and the arcuate nucleus (cf. Swanson et al., 1987; Watts et al., 1987). The role of the medial preoptic area might be of particular importance since it receives a massive angiotensin input from the subfornical organ (Lind and Swanson, 1984), which also sends angiotensin-containing fibers to the PVN (Sawchenko and Swanson, 1983; Lind et al., 1984, 1985b). Since the subfornical organ is sensitive to circulating levels of angiotensin, this circuitry might play an important role in fluid balance.

2.   Chemically Identified Synapses on CRF Neurons

By using double-labeling techniques at the electron microscopic level, axon terminals containing the following neurotransmitters and/or neuropeptides have been reported to be in direct contact with CRFi neurons: epinephrine and norepinephrine (Liposits et al., 1986a, b; Figure 16), dopamine (Liposits and Paull, 1989), serotonin (Liposits et al., 1987a), GABA (Olschowka, 1987), ACTH (Pilscher and Joseph, 1984; Liposits et al., 1985), CRF (Liposits et al., 1988; Silverman et al., 1989), NPY (Liposits et al., 1988), and vasopressin and oxytocin (Leranth et al., 1983; Liposits et al., 1985). For a detailed review of this subject, see Liposits (1990).

C.   Interactions Between CRF Neurons and the Immune System

In addition to neural and classical endocrine responses to stress, mammalian organisms have the important ability to respond, in a similar manner, to microbial infections, inflammatory processes, and immunological challenges. It has been learned in recent years that the acute phase of this response is mediated primarily by interleukin-1 (IL-1), a polypeptide cytokine produced by many cell types, especially monocytes (Dinarello, 1984). IL-1 activates T and B lymphocytes, promotes the production of other cytokines, and acts, in general, to integrate the broad and complex cellular reactions involved in the acute immune response (for reviews, see Harrison and Campbell, 1988; Bateman et al., 1989). There is now convincing evidence that IL-1 has another important function: it stimulates CRF gene expression in rat hypothalamus (Suda et al., 1990). It also stimulates CRF and ACTH release and thus, indirectly, increases glucocorticoid output (Besedowsky et al., 1986; Berkenbosch et al., 1987; Sapolsky et al., 1987; Uehara et al., 1987; Tsagarakis et al., 1989). One of the well-known effects of glucocorticoids is to suppress immune reactions, including the production of IL-1 (e.g., Snyder and Unanue, 1982; Staruch and Wood, 1985). Thus, IL-1 forms an important link between the neuroendocrine and immune systems, participating in their activation on the one hand and preventing their excessive reaction on the other (cf. Lumpkin, 1987). The CRF- and ACTH-releasing effects of IL-1 appear to explain the early controversy regarding the existence of a peripheral "tissue CRF" (cf. Brodish, 1979). The precise mechanisms by which IL-1 activates the HPA axis are not entirely clear. Circulating IL-1 is unlikely to cross the blood-brain barrier, although it can still be active at brain sites that normally lack the barrier, such as the median eminence or the organum vasculosum of the lamina terminalis (Katsuura et al., 1990). In addition, recent observations have demonstrated the presence of endogenous IL-1 in the hypothalamus (Breder et al., 1988; Lechan et al., 1990). High-affinity receptors for IL-1 have also been identified in the rat brain (Katsuura et al., 1988). The PVN seems to be particularly densely innervated by IL-1-immunoreactive nerve fibers — an observation that lends further support to the hypothesis that IL-1 may function as one of the central regulators of CRF production and release.

D.   Pharmacology of CRF Neurons

Two topics will be discussed in this section: (1) neurotransmitter regulation of CRF neurons and (2) the pharmacological effects of CRF-41 in the CNS.

1.   Neurotransmitter Regulation of CRF Neurons

Experiments addressing this subject and carried out prior to 1981 suffered from the same disadvantage as did the efforts to characterize the physiological CRF and define the hypothalamic mechanisms controlling ACTH secretion: the end point of the assays used, i.e., ACTH release either from pituitary cells *in vitro* or *in vivo*, was inherently unable to distinguish between the effects of true CRF and its endogenous or exogenous agonists such as vasopressin, angiotensin, epinephrine, or several drugs. Taken together, these early results suggested that acetylcholine, serotonin, angiotensin, and opioid peptides stimulated, whereas norepinephrine and GABA inhibited, the release of ACTH (cf. Gillies and Lowry, 1986; Jones and Gillham, 1988). More recent studies, which included the specific measurement and/or localization of CRF-41, have confirmed some, but not all, of these early conclusions (cf. Assenmacher et al., 1987).

Chemically identified synapses on paraventricular CRF neurons and the pathways through which these fibers may reach the PVN are described in Section III.B.2.

The role of catecholamines had been studied most extensively, even before direct innervation of CRF neurons by catecholaminergic fibers was demonstrated (Liposits et al., 1986a, b; Liposits and Paull, 1989). Upon release from nerve endings, catecholamines diffuse to interact with pre- and postsynaptic adrenergic receptors which have been classified into four subtypes (α_1, α_2, β_1, and β_2) according to their ligand specificities (Lands et al., 1967; Minneman et al., 1979; Wikberg, 1979). CRF neurons in the PVN express a mixed population of adrenergic receptors. Individual receptor subtypes appear to be differentially regulated by a variety of factors, such as the light-dark cycles, nutritional state, afferent neural input, glucocorticoid hormone levels, etc. The α_2-receptors are particularly sensitive to changes in the levels of glucocorticoids (Jhanwar-Uniyal et al., 1986). Removal of endogenous glucocorticoids is associated with a decline in hypothalamic α_2-receptor binding and this change is reversible by corticosterone replacement (Cummings and Seybold, 1988). In addition to their effects on the PVN, catecholamines appear to be capable of modulating CRF-41 release at the level of the median eminence as well as directly at the level of the pituitary (Spinedi et al., 1988). Although earlier studies emphasized the inhibitory nature of catecholamines on CRF release (e.g., see reviews by Ganong, 1980; Gillies and Lowry, 1986; Jones and Gillham, 1988), recent *in vivo* and *in vitro* experiments have established that catecholamines exert an overall facilitatory effect on CRF neurons (cf. Plotsky, 1987, 1989; however, see Al-Damluji et al., 1987).

Serotonin (5-HT), derived from ascending pathways that originate in the raphe nuclei and innervate a variety of forebrain structures (Steinbusch, 1981), plays an important, although incompletely understood, role in the regulation of the HPA axis. Immunocytochemical evidence indicates direct innervation of the PVN, including the neurons that produce CRF-41 (Sawchenko et al., 1983; Steinbusch, 1984; Liposits et al., 1987a), and biochemical-physiological studies support the conclusion that 5-HT at this level stimulates the release of CRF-41 into portal capillaries (Gibbs and Vale, 1983). However, other, indirect mechanisms may also be important. One of these is the dense 5-HT innervation of the suprachiasmatic nucleus (SCN). The SCN is responsible for the generation of circadian neuroendocrine rhythms and is known to project directly to the PVN. Disruption of the 5-HT innervation of the SCN suppresses the normal diurnal ACTH-corticosterone rhythm (cf. Ganong, 1980; Assenmacher et al., 1987). However, this effect may be mediated by noradrenergic mechanisms (Szafarczyk et al., 1985). Serotoninergic innervation of the hippocampus and the amygdala may also be important in the regulation of the HPA axis. A fairly good correlation exists between the concentrations of receptors for 5-HT and corticosterone in these regions (Biegon et al., 1982). There is some evidence that 5-HT at these sites may act as a modulator of the negative feedback control by glucocorticoids (Beaulieu et al., 1986).

Direct innervation of paraventricular CRF neurons by GABA-containing terminals has been demonstrated (Olschowka, 1987). The most likely source of these fibers is the population of scattered GABA-ergic neurons present in the hypothalamus (Ottersen and Storm-Mathisen, 1984). *In vivo* and *in vitro* studies agree that GABA exerts an overall tonic inhibition on CRF/ACTH release (cf. Assenmacher et al., 1987; Plotsky et al., 1987). The situation may be more complicated, however, since it is known that GABA is colocalized with CRF-41 in a small population of paraventricular neurons (Meister et al., 1988) and that CRF neurons in the PVN establish synaptic contacts with each other (Liposits et al., 1985). These observations underline the degree of complexity and "fine-tuning" of the mechanisms controlling the function of the HPA axis.

Although direct cholinergic input to paraventricular CRF cells has not been demonstrated, it seems clear that acetylcholine stimulates CRF release through a mixed population of nicotinic and muscarinic receptors under a variety of experimental conditions (Calegoro et al., 1988; Rivier and Plotsky, 1986; Plotsky et al., 1987). The neuroanatomical substrate of these effects is unknown.

Histamine, when injected into the cerebral ventricles, stimulates ACTH secretion and this effect can be blocked by H1-receptor antagonists. However, the effect of histamine may be indirect, mediated by α-adrenergic receptors (Bugajski and Gadek, 1984; cf. Assenmacher et al., 1987). Available immunocytochemical evidence, at least in the rat, appears to support the latter possibility, since the histaminergic innervation of the parvocellular regions of the PVN is quite limited (Steinbusch and Mulder, 1984).

Among the neuropeptides, vasopressin, angiotensin II, enkephalins, proopiomelanocortin-derived peptides (mainly β-endorphin), and NPY appear to be the most important in modulating CRF release from the PVN; their effects are stimulatory. However, synaptic contacts with CRF cells have not been demonstrated for all these peptides (see Section IV.B.2). The pathways from which peptidergic innervation of paraventricular CRF neurons may derive are largely unknown, except for the angiotensin II-containing pathway, which originates from the subfornical organ and is likely to be involved in the regulation of thirst and water intake (Lind et al., 1985a, b), the pathways carrying proopiomelanocortin-derived peptides, which originate from neurons in the medial basal hypothalamus, and those containing NPY, which arise from neurons in the arcuate nucleus and in the brain stem (cf. Palkovits, 1987).

2.   Central Pharmacological Effects of CRF-41

The pharmacological responses to injection of CRF-41 are characteristic of, and dependent on, the route of administration. Peripherally administered CRF-41 does not cross the blood-brain barrier; nevertheless, presumably acting through specific receptors located in peripheral tissues, it induces characteristic dose-dependent responses that are different from those elicited by central administration, i.e. by injection into the cerebral ventricles (i.c.v.) or directly into brain tissue. Only the central effects will be discussed in this section.

The primary effect of CRF-41, when injected into the cerebral ventricles at appropriate doses, is the release of ACTH from the pituitary. In addition to CRF-41, centrally administered oxytocin and epinephrine also elevate plasma ACTH levels, but their effect can be abolished by simultaneous administration of CRF-41-neutralizing antibodies (Rivier and Vale, 1985). CRF-41 has been shown to affect the secretion of pituitary hormones other than ACTH: it inhibits the secretion of luteinizing hormone (LH), but not of follicle-stimulating hormone (FSH) (Rivier and Vale, 1984a). This effect also seems to be indirect, since CRF-41 does not affect LH secretion from cultured pituitary cells (cf. Rivier and Vale, 1985). CRF-41 stimulates the secretion of somatostatin from neurons maintained in culture (Peterfreund and Vale, 1982); consistent with this observation, i.c.v. injection of CRF-41 results in a dramatic inhibition of spontaneous growth hormone (GH) release (Rivier and Vale, 1984b), probably by suppressing the pulsatile release of growth hormone-releasing factor (GRF) from the hypothalamus. CRF-41 may also play a role in the regulation of prolactin secretion from the pituitary, although the exact nature of this role is not yet clear (Rivier and Vale, 1985). Thus, CRF-41 can, directly or indirectly, influence the secretion of pituitary ACTH, LH, GH, and probably also prolactin. In this respect, CRF-41 follows the pattern seen previously with other hypothalamic releasing factors, i.e., it shows a certain degree of (initially unexpected, but physiologically probably significant) "nonspecificity" with regard to its effects on the pituitary.

Immediately after the discovery of CRF-41, immunocytochemical (Merchenthaler et al., 1982; Olschowka et al., 1982; Swanson et al., 1983) and radioimmunoassay (Fischman and Moldow, 1982; Palkovits et al., 1985) results emerged indicating that CRF-41, reminiscent of other hypophysiotropic peptides, is widely distributed in the CNS. These observations have led to the suspicion that this neuropeptide, like many others, may serve as a neurotransmitter or modulator in addition to its well-defined neuroendocrine role. Interestingly, the anatomical pattern of distribution of extrahypothalamic CRF-41 suggested a prominent involvement of this peptide in the central regulation of autonomic functions (cf. Swanson et al., 1983). The first experimental evidence to suggest this hypothesis was reported by Brown et al. (1982) who demonstrated that i.c.v. administration of CRF-41 in rats or dogs elicited a dose-dependent increase of plasma epinephrine, norepinephrine, glucagon, and glucose concentrations. These effects are not associated with elevated CRF-41 levels in the general circulation and are not prevented by hypophysectomy, indicating that they are mediated by central, and not peripheral, mechanisms. Indeed, neurons in the locus coeruleus have been shown to increase their firing rate in response to CRF-41 (Valentino et al., 1983). The increase in plasma catecholamine concentration after CRF-41 administration is associated with increased adrenal sympathetic nerve activity (Kurosawa et al., 1986). Furthermore, the stimulating effect of CRF-41 on sympathetic outflow can be prevented by ganglionic blocking agents such as chlorisondamine (Brown et al., 1982; Lenz, 1987). While the increase in plasma epinephrine concentration is abolished by adrenalectomy, the increase in norepinephrine can be abolished only by treatment with bretylium tosylate, an agent that prevents the release of norepinephrine from peripheral nerve terminals (cf. Lenz, 1987). Also, CRF-41 receptor antagonists, given i.c.v., prevent the CRF-induced catecholamine release (Brown et al., 1985). These results support the hypothesis that CRF-41, acting centrally as a neurotransmitter, may be a physiological mediator of the stress-induced activation of the sympathetic nervous system.

In addition, parasympathetic activity is also affected by central administration of CRF-41. In contrast to its stimulatory effect on sympathetic outflow, CRF-41 acts in the CNS to reduce parasympathetic activity. As a result, central administration of CRF-41 is followed by a remarkable combination of endocrine, metabolic, gastrointestinal, cardiovascular, and behavioral effects that mimic those seen after a variety of stressful stimuli.

The gastrointestinal effects of centrally administered CRF-41 include the inhibition of gastric acid secretion (Tache et al., 1983), gastric emptying, and gastrointestinal motility. These effects are apparently mediated by the PVN and its projections to the intermediolateral column of the spinal cord, since microinjections of CRF-41 into either of these sites reproduce the gastric responses seen after i.c.v. administration, while injections into other brain areas do not (Tache and Gunion, 1985). In dogs, but not in rats, the gastric effects of centrally administered CRF-41 are partially mediated by endogenous vasopressin and opioid peptides (Lenz et al., 1985; Druge et al., 1989).

CRF-41 and the related nonmammalian peptides urotensin I and sauvagine have dramatic effects on the cardiovascular system. These effects are also reminiscent of those seen in stress: increased mean arterial pressure, increased cardiac output (due to increased heart rate and stroke volume), and decreased peripheral vascular resistance — all favoring maximum tissue perfusion (Brown et al., 1982; Fisher et al., 1982, 1983; Scoggins et al., 1984). Pretreatment of the animals with ganglion blockers completely abolishes the CRF-induced hypertension and tachycardia, suggesting that these effects are also mediated by the autonomic nervous system (Fisher et al., 1982).

The observed behavioral effects of centrally administered CRF-41 include increased motor activity, decreased food and water intake, and decreased sexual activity (Brown et al., 1982; Sutton et al., 1982; Morley and Levine, 1982; Sirinathsinghji et al., 1983). These and other behavioral effects of CRF-41 can only partially be explained by the activation of the sympathetic nervous system (Britton and Indyk, 1989). The inhibition of ingestive behavior appears to depend on adrenomedullary activation (Gosnell et al., 1983), while the suppression of sexual activity is mediated by β-endorphin neurons projecting from the hypothalamus to the brain stem (Sirinathsinghji et al., 1983). Recently it has been proposed that the IL-1-induced inhibition of food intake may be mediated by CRF (Uehara et al., 1989). In dogs, i.c.v. administration of CRF-41 produces arousal, aggressive behavior, and increased vocalization (cf. Lenz, 1987); in rhesus monkeys, it results in huddling and lying down behavior (Kalin et al., 1983). Understandably, precise knowledge of the anatomical pathways and mechanisms mediating these complex and varied behaviors is still lacking.

E.   Pathology of CRF Neurons

1.   *Diseases of the Hypothalamo-Pituitary-Adrenal Axis*

Relatively little is known at present about the precise role of CRF neurons in diseases of the nervous system. Even in patent endocrine disturbances such as adrenal hypo- or hyperfunction, attempts to demonstrate a direct role of CRF have resulted in complex and often contradictory results (for a review, see Taylor and Fishman, 1988). Destruction of the hypothalamic CRF neuronal system, as expected, leads to secondary adrenal insufficiency with low circulating levels of CRF (Suda et al., 1985; Sasaki et al., 1987). In contrast, current evidence seems to indicate that most cases of adrenal hyperfunction (Cushing's disease) are not directly linked to increased hypothalamic CRF secretion but rather to ACTH-secreting pituitary adenomas (cf. Taylor and Fishman, 1988), even though CRF may play a role in the pathogenesis of these tumors (Orth et al., 1982). CRF definitely plays a key role in recently described forms of Cushing's syndrome due to ectopic CRF production by a variety of central and peripheral tumors (e.g., Carey et al., 1984; Asa et al., 1984). Another form of Cushing's syndrome, that caused by alcohol (Lamberts et al., 1979), may also be the result, at least in part, of hypersecretion of CRF (cf. Rivier et al., 1984).

2.   *Nonendocrine Diseases of the Nervous System*

It is well known that major depression and certain other psychiatric disorders, such as anorexia nervosa, bulimia, and obsessive-compulsive neurosis, are often associated with disturbances of the HPA axis, particularly with hypersecretion of cortisol. In view of the striking behavioral effects of CRF, it is not surprising that much work has been aimed at defining the possible role of CRF in psychiatric disorders, especially depression (Nemeroff et al., 1984; Gold et al., 1984). It stands to reason that the HPA abnormalities in such patients are likely to be mediated by the hypothalamic CRF system; however, neither specific anatomical nor functional data are available to date regarding the mechanisms responsible for this abnormality in patients with psychiatric disorders.

The CRF neuronal system has also been implicated in several degenerative neurological diseases. Bisette et al. (1985) reported reduced CRF concentrations in the striatum and cortex of patients with Alzheimer's disease (AD) and this has been confirmed by several other groups. Interestingly, the reduced cortical CRF concentrations are associated with a marked increase of CRF receptor binding activity — an effect explained by an increased number of receptors (De Souza et al., 1986). The involvement of CRF in AD is further supported by its decreased concentration in the cerebrospinal fluid (Mouradian et al., 1986) and by the demonstration of abnormalities in CRF-immunoreactive fibers in senile plaques in the amygdala from patients with AD (Powers et al., 1987). In rodents, the cerebral cortex contains a well-defined population of intrinsic CRF neurons (see Section III.B.3; Merchenthaler et al., 1982; Olschowka et al., 1982; Sakanaka et al., 1987a). Recently, an extensive population of CRF-41 immunoreactive neurons has been demonstrated in the monkey neocortex (Lewis et al., 1989); however, we are not aware of similar data regarding the human brain. Kelley and Kowall (1989) reported that CRF-41-immunoreactive neurons in the hippocampal formation, hypothalamus, and cerebellum of AD brains showed only minor differences from normal age-matched controls. Unfortunately, observations of the neocortex were not included in this report. Our knowledge of CRF-containing cortical afferents is also fragmentary. There is some evidence that these afferents, in addition to containing CRF and/or other neuropeptides, are cholinergic (e.g., Crawley et al., 1985). The possible relationship between brain cholinergic systems and cortical CRF receptors was explored by De Souza and Battaglia (1986), who demonstrated that chronic treatment with atropine, a muscarinic cholinergic receptor antagonist, resulted in a significant and selective increase of CRF receptor concentration in the frontoparietal cortex of rats.

Decreased CRF content in the cerebral cortex was also demonstrated in cases of Parkinson's disease associated with dementia and in patients with progressive supranuclear palsy (cf. De Souza et al., 1987). As in AD, it is not known whether these changes indicate primary involvement of CRF neurons or are secondary to the degenerative changes affecting other neuronal systems. Similarly, the anatomical distribution of the affected CRF neurons in all these neurodegenerative diseases remains to be determined.

In summary, although relatively little is known about the involvement of CRF-containing neurons in various disease processes, a significant number of data indicate that CRF may be involved in the pathogenesis or pathophysiology of several forms of endocrine, psychiatric and neurologic disorders. In addition, it can be expected that CRF and its agonists and antagonists will find increasing utility both as diagnostic tools and therapeutic agents.

V. Integrated Neuroendocrine Control of the Stress Response

A well-coordinated, generalized, and effective response to noxious stimuli is of fundamental survival value for mammalian organisms. Therefore, it is not surprising that in the CNS a distinct and widespread neuronal system, chemically defined by the common ability of its neurons to synthesize, store and release CRF-41, is dedicated to this task. As we have seen, these neurons and their axons occur or extend into practically every major part of the CNS. In spite of the large number and complex distribution of CRF neurons, functionally they can be divided quite clearly into three groups: (1) the large cluster of neurons in the PVN, projecting to the median eminence (ME), directly responsible for the regulation of ACTH production and release from the anterior pituitary; thus, these neurons represent the final common pathway in the activation of the HPA axis; (2) a large number of neurons scattered in the basal forebrain, limbic structures, brain stem, and spinal cord, responsible for the activation and coordination of autonomic, metabolic, emotional, and behavioral responses to stress; (3) finally, neurons in the cerebral cortex, which have been regarded as a separate group; their function is largely unknown, but it may be assumed that they play an important role in the organization and coordination of cortical responses associated with the stress reaction.

Because of the great variety of stimuli to which the organism must respond by activation the HPA axis, an unusually high number of afferents converge on hypothalamic CRF neurons. It is well known that, even in absence of stressful stimuli, there is an important diurnal rhythm of corticosteroid secretion, driven by input from the suprachiasmatic nuclei. Pain and trauma are perceived through the primary sensory systems and the impulses travel to the PVN via spinothalamic and bulbothalamic pathways and the reticular formation. Osmotic stimuli reach the PVN through an identified pathway from the subfornical organ. Emotional stresses are conveyed via the limbic system, with some components probably emanating from the cortex. There is an inhibitory input from the tractus solitarius via baroreceptors. Perhaps the most important physiological regulatory mechanism is humoral: the negative feedback by glucocorticoids, mediated through glucocorticoid receptors present in both the hypothalamus and the pituitary (see Section IV.A). There is some evidence that the responsiveness of CRF neurons to glucocorticoid feedback is not restricted to the PVN but extends (albeit to a lesser extent) to distant brain regions as well (Merchenthaler et al., 1983a; see Section IV.A). Additional peripheral humoral factors, such as IL-1 and perhaps others, may exert a stimulatory effect on CRF neurons. These and other relationships are schematically represented in Figure 17. The neural input on paraventricular CRF neurons is exerted via synaptic contacts from the large number of pathways reaching this area from other brain regions, as summarized in Section IV.B.1. Chemically defined synapses on CRF neurons include those containing CRF-41 itself, opioid peptides, NPY, galanin, norepinephrine, epinephrine, dopamine, serotonin, GABA, excitatory amino acids, and certain growth factors.

The CRF-producing neurons in the PVN display perhaps the greatest chemical complexity of all neurons in the mammalian CNS (see Figure 17). They have been shown to contain, in addition to CRF, a large number of other neuropeptides and transmitters, including vasopressin, opioid peptides, angiotensin, neurotensin, CCK, VIP, and GABA. Thus, activation of these neurons leads not only to CRF release in the ME and subsequent ACTH release from the anterior pituitary, but to the release of several other chemical modulators in the ME, where they can interact with neighboring terminals and can enter portal capillaries as well. Consequently, the secretion of several pituitary hormones other than ACTH (e.g., gonadotropins, TSH, prolactin) is also affected. Last but not least, some of the substances coexpressed by CRF neurons (most notably vasopressin) modulate directly the action of CRF on corticotropes (see Figure 17).

An additional level of complexity is introduced by collateral projections from axons of paraventricular CRF neurons and other neurons in surrounding hypothalamic areas (cf. Swanson et al., 1987). These can exert further modulating effects on the pituitary ACTH response.

The functional roles of the three major CRF neuronal systems (as described above) are now reasonably well understood, even though many of the fine details remain to be clarified. The role of the hypothalamoinfundibular system as the major activator of the HPA axis is self-evident. The extrahypothalamic CRF systems are responsible for the activation of the autonomic nervous system and the adrenal medulla and the coordination of the behavioral and emotional responses to stress. The distribution of CRF receptors and CRF-containing nerve terminals in the central nervous system and the pituitary is consistent with these concepts.

In summary, recent results identify the CRF-41 neuronal system as a widespread and complex system that appears to be dedicated, perhaps uniquely among chemically defined neurons, to a single task: the regulation and coordination of the body's endocrine, autonomic, metabolic, behavioral, and emotional responses to stressful stimuli. In addition, an increasing number of data indicates that the entire CRF system, but especially its limbic and cortical components, may be involved in the pathophysiology of several endocrine, neurological, and psychiatric disorders.

VI. Acknowledgments

Work in the authors' laboratories was supported in part by USPHS Grant No. NS 14904 and by joint grants from the National Science Foundation and the Hungarian Academy of Sciences (INT-8602688). The authors are grateful to Drs. Krisztina Kovács, Zsolt Liposits, and Larry W. Swanson for their generous permission to include their previously published illustrations in this chapter.

References

Abou-Samra, A. B., Catt, K. J., Aguilera, G., Involvement of protein kinase C in the regulation of adrenocorticotropin release from rat anterior pituitary cells, *Endocrinology*, 118, 212, 1986.

Agnati, L. F., Fuxe, K., Yu, Z. Y., Harfstrand, A., Okret, S., Wickstrom, A. C., Goldstein, M., Zoli, M., Vale, W., Gustafsson, J. A., Morphometrical analysis of the distribution of corticotropin releasing factor, glucocorticoid receptor and phenylethanolamine-*N*-methyltransferase immunoreactive structures in the paraventricular hypothalamic nucleus of the rat, *Neurosci. Lett.*, 54, 147, 1985.

Aguilera, G., Wynn, P. V., Harwood, J. P., Hauger, R. L., Millan, M. A., Grewe, C., Catt, K. J., Receptor mediated action of corticotropin releasing factor in pituitary gland and nervous system, *Neuroendocrinology*, 43, 79, 1986.

Aguilera, G., Millan, M. A., Hauger, R. L., Catt, K. J., Corticotropin-releasing factor receptors: Distribution and regulation in brain, pituitary, and peripheral tissues, *Ann. N.Y. Acad. Sci.*, 512, 48, 1987.

Al-Damluji, S., Perry, L., Tomlin, S., Bouloux, P., Grossman, A., Rees, L. H., and Besser, G. M., Alpha-adrenergic stimulation of corticotropin secretion by a specific central mechanism in man, *Neuroendocrinology*, 45, 68, 1987.

Alonso, G., Siaud, P., and Assenmacher, I., Immunocytochemical ultrastructural study of hypothalamic neurons containing corticotropin releasing-factor in normal and adrenalectomized rats, *Neuroendocrinology*, 24, 553, 1988.

Antoni, F. A., Hypothalamic control of adrenocorticotropin secretion: advances since the discovery of 41-residue corticotropin-releasing factor, *Endocrinol. Rev.*, 7, 351, 1986.

Antoni, F. A., Palkovits, M., Makara, G. B., Linton, E. A., Lowrey, P. J., Kiss, J. Z., Immunoreactive corticotropin releasing hormone (CRF) in the hypothalamo-infundibular tract, *Neuroendocrinology*, 36, 415, 1983.

Arbiser, J. L., Morton, C. C., Burns, C. A. P., Majzoub, J. A., Human corticotropin releasing hormone gene is located on the long arm of chromosome 8, *Cytogenet. Cell Genet.*, 47, 113, 1988.

Asa, S. L., Kovacs, K., Tindall, G. T., Barrow, D. L., Horvath, E., and Vecsei, P., Cushing's disease associated with an intrasellar gangliocytoma producing corticotrophin-releasing factor, *Ann. Intern. Med.*, 101, 789, 1984.

Assenmacher, I., Szafarczyk, A., Alonso, G., Ixart, G., Barbanel, G., Physiology of neural pathways affecting CRH secretion, *Ann. N.Y. Acad. Sci.*, 512, 149, 1987.

Bateman, A., Singh, A., Kral, T., and Solomon, S., The immune-hypothalamic-pituitary-adrenal axis, *Endocrinol, Rev.*, 10, 92, 1989.

Beaulieu, S., DiPaolo, T., and Barden, N. Control of ACTH secretion by the central nucleus of the amygdala: implication of the serotoninergic system and its relevance to the glucocorticoid delayed negative feedback mechanism, *Neuroendocrinology*, 44, 247, 1986.

Berkenbosch, F., Van Oers, J., Del Rey, A., Tilders, F., and Besedowsky, H., Corticotropin releasing factor-producing neurons in the rat activated by interleukin-1, *Science*, 238, 524, 1987.

Besedowsky, H., Del Rey, A., Sorkin, E., and Dinarello, C. A., Immunoregulatory feedback between interleukin-1 and glucocorticoid hormones, *Science*, 233, 652, 1986.

Biegon, A., Rainbow, T. C., and McEwen, B. S., Quantitative autoradiography of serotonin receptors in the rat brain, *Brain Res.*, 242, 197, 1982.

Bisette, D., Reynolds, G. P., Kilts, C. D., Widerlov, E., and Nemeroff, C. B., Corticotropin-releasing factor-like immunoreactivity in senile dementia of the Alzheimer type. Reduced cortical and striatal concentrations, *JAMA*, 254, 3067, 1985.

Bloom, F. E., Battenberg, L. F., Rivier, J., Vale, A., Corticotropin releasing factor (CRF): immunoreactive neurons and fibers in rat hypothalamus, *Regul. Pept.*, 4, 43, 1982.

Bondy, C. A., Whitnall, M. H., Brady, L. S., and Gainer, H., Coexisting peptides in hypothalamic neuroendocrine systems: some functional implications, *Cell Mol. Neurobiol.*, 9, 427, 1989.

Bons, N., Bouille, C., Tonon, M. C., and Guillaume, V., Topographical distribution of CRF immunoreactivity in the pigeon brain, *Peptides*, 9, 697, 1988.

Breder, C. D., Dinarello, C. A., and Saper, C. B., Interleukin-1 immunoreactive innervation of the human hypothalamus, *Science*, 240, 321, 1988.

Bresson, J. L., Clavequin, M. V., Fellmann, D., and Bugnon, C., Anatomical and ontogenetic studies of the human paraventriculo-infundibular corticoliberin system, *Neuroscience*, 14, 1077, 1985.

Britton, D. R. and Indyk, E., Effects of ganglionic blocking agents on behavioral responses to centrally administered CRF, *Brain Res.*, 478, 205, 1989.

Brodish, A., Diffuse hypothalamic system for the regulation of ACTH secretion, *Endocrinology*, 73, 727, 1963.

Brodish, A., Control of ACTH secretion by corticotropin releasing factor(s), *Vitam. Horm.*, 37, 111, 1979.

Brown, M. R., Fisher, L. A., Rivier, J., Spiess, J., Rivier, C., and Vale, W., Corticotropin releasing factor: Effect on the sympathetic nervous system and metabolism, *Endocrinology*, 111, 928, 1982.

Brown, M. R., Fisher, L. A., Webb, V., Vale, W. W., and Rivier, J. J., Corticotropin-releasing factor: a physiologic regulator of adrenal epinephrine secretion, *Brain Res.*, 328, 355, 1985.

Bruhn, T. O., Plotsky, P. M., and Vale, W. W., Effect of paraventricular lesion on corticotropin-releasing factor (CRF)-like immunoreactivity in the stalk-median eminence: studies on the adreno-corticotropin response to ether stress and exogenous CRF, *Endocrinology*, 114, 57, 1984.

Bugajski, J. and Gadek, A., The effect of adrenergic and cholinergic antagonists on central histaminergic stimulation of pituitary-adrenocortical response under stress in rats, *Neuroendocrinology*, 38, 447, 1984.

Bugnon, C., Fellman, D., Gouget, A., Bresson, J., Clavequin, M. C., Hadjiyiassemis, M., and Cardot, J., Corticoliberin neurons: cytophysiology, phylogeny and ontogeny, *J. Steroid Biochem.*, 20, 183, 1984.

Buijs, R., Geffard, M., Pool, C., and Hoorneman, E. D., The dopaminergic innervation of the supraoptic and paraventricular nucleus. A light and electron microscopical study, *Brain Res.*, 323, 65, 1984.

Burlet, A., Tonon, M. C., Tankosic, P., Coy, D., and Vaudry, H., Comparative immunocytochemical localization of corticotropin-releasing factor (CRF-41) and neurohypophyseal peptides in the brain of Brattleboro and Long-Evans rats, *Neuroendocrinology*, 367, 64, 1983.

Calegoro, A. E., Golucci, W., Bernardini, R., Sauotis, C., Gold, P., and Chrousos, G., Effect of cholinergic agonists and antagonists on rat hypothalamic corticotropin releasing factor secretion *in vitro*, *Neuroendocrinology*, 47, 303, 1988.

Carey, R. M., Varma, S. K., Drake, C. R., Jr., Thorner, M. O., Kovacs, K., Rivier, J., and Vale, W., Ectopic secretion of corticotropin-releasing factor as a cause of Cushing's syndrome: a clinical, morphologic, and biochemical study, *N. Engl. J. Med.*, 311, 13, 1984.

Catt, K. J., Harwood, J. P., Aguilera, G., and Dufau, M. L., Hormonal regulation of peptide receptors and target cell responses, *Nature (London)*, 280, 109, 1979.

Ceccatelli, S., Eriksson, M., and Hökfelt, T., Distribution and existence of corticotropin-releasing factor-, neurotensin-, enkephalin-, cholecystokinin-, galanin- and vasoactive intestinal polypepitide/peptide histidine isoleucine-like peptides in the parvocellular part of the paraventricular nucleus, *Neuroendocrinology*, 49, 309, 1989a.

Ceccatelli, S., Villar, M. J., Goldstein, M., and Hökfelt, T., Expression of c-Fos immunoreactivity in transmitter-characterized neurons after stress, *Proc. Natl. Acad. Sci. U.S.A.*, 86, 9569, 1989b .

Cha, C. I. and Foote, S. L., Corticotropin-releasing factor in olivocerebellar climbing-fiber system of monkey (*Saimiri sciures* and *Macaca fascicularis*): parasagittal and regional organization visualized by immunohistochemistry, *J. Neurosci.*, 8, 4121, 1988.

Crawley, J. N., Olschowka, J. A., Diz, D. I., and Jacobowitz, D. M., Behavioral investigation of the coexistence of substance P, corticotropin releasing factor, and acetylcholinesterase in lateral dorsal tegmental neurons projecting to the medial frontal cortex of the rat, *Peptides*, 6, 891, 1985.

Csernus, V., Lengvari, I., and Halász, B., Further studies on ACTH secretion from pituitary grafts in the hypophysiotrophic area, *Neuroendocrinology*, 17, 18, 1975.

Cummings, S. and Seybold, V., Relationship of alpha-1- and alpha-2-adrenergic-binding sites to regions of the paraventricular nucleus of the hypothalamus containing corticotropin-releasing factor and vasopressin neurons, *Neuroendocrinology*, 47, 523, 1988.

Cummings, S., Elde, R., Ells, J., and Lindall, A., Corticotropin-releasing factor immunoreactivity is widely distributed in the central nervous system of the rat: an immunocytochemical study, *J. Neurosci.*, 3, 1355, 1983.

Cummings, S. L., Young, W. S., Bishop, G. A., De Souza, E. B., and King, J. S., Distribution of corticotropin releasing factor in the cerebellum and precerebellar nuclei of the opossum: a study utilizing immunohistochemistry, in situ hybridization histochemistry, and receptor autoradiography, *J. Comp. Neurol.*, 280, 501, 1989.

Cunningham, E. T. and Sawchenko, P. E., Anatomical specificity of noradrenergic inputs to the paraventricular and supraoptic nuclei of the rat hypothalamus, *J. Comp. Neurol.*, 274, 60, 1988.

Davis, L. G., Arentzen, R., Reid, J. M., Manning, R. W., Wolfson, B., Lawrence, K. L., and Baldino, F. Glucocorticoid sensitivity of vasopressin mRNA levels in the paraventricular nucleus of the rat, *Proc. Natl. Acad. Sci. U.S.A.*, 83, 1145, 1986.

Decavel, C., Geffard, M., and Calas, A., Comparative study of dopamine- and noradrenaline-immunoreactive terminals in the paraventricular and supraoptic nuclei of the rat, *Neurosci. Lett.*, 77, 149, 1987.

De Souza, E. B. and Battaglia, G., Increased corticotropin-releasing factor receptors in rat cerebral cortex following chronic atropine treatment, *Brain Res.*, 397, 401, 1986.

De Souza, E. B. and Kuhar, M. J., Corticotropin-releasing factor receptors in the pituitary gland and central nervous system, *Methods Enzymol.*, 124, 560, 1986.

De Souza, E. B., Insel, T. R., Perrin, M. P., Rivier, J., Vale, W. W., and Kuhar, M. J., Corticotropin-releasing factor receptors are widely distributed within the rat central nervous system: an autoradiographic study, *J. Neurosci.*, 5, 3189, 1985.

De Souza, E. B., Whitehouse, P. J., Kuhar, M. J., Price, D. L., and Vale, W. W., Reciprocal changes in corticotropin-releasing factor (CRF)-like immunoreactivity and CRF receptors in cerebral cortex of Alzheimer's disease, *Nature (London)*, 319, 593, 1986.

De Souza, E. B., Whitehouse, P. J., Price, D. L., and Vale, W. W., Abnormalities in corticotropin-releasing hormone (CRH) in Alzheimer's disease and other human disorders, *Ann. N.Y. Acad. Sci.*, 512, 237, 1987.

Dinarello, C. A., Interleukin-1 and the pathogenesis of the acute-phase response, *N. Engl. J. Med.*, 311, 1413, 1984.

Dreyfuss, F., Burlet, A., Tonon, M. C., and Vaudry, H., Comparative immune electron microscopic localization of corticotropin releasing factor (CRF-LI) and oxytocin in the rat median eminence, *Neuroendocrinology*, 39, 84, 1984.

Druge, G., Raedler, A., Greten, H., and Lenz, H. J., Pathways mediating CRF-induced inhibition of gastric acid secretion in rats, *Am. J. Physiol.*, 256 (Pt 1), G214, 1989.

Dunn, J. and Critchlow, V., Pituitary-adrenal function following ablation of the medial basal hypothalamus, *Proc. Soc. Exp. Biol. Med.*, 142, 749, 1973.

Fasolo, A., Andreone, C., and Vandesande, F. Immunohistochemical localization of corticotropin-releasing factor (CRF)-like immunoreactivity in the hypothalamus of the newt, *Triturus cristatus*, *Neurosci. Lett.*, 49, 135, 1984.

Feldman, S., Conforti, N., Chowers, I., and Davidson, J. M., Differential effects of hypothalamic deafferentation on responses to different stresses, *Israel J. Med. Sci.*, 4, 908, 1968.

Fischman, A. J. and Moldow, R. L., Extrahypothalamic distribution of CRF-like immunoreactivity in the rat brain, *Peptides*, 1, 149, 1982.

Fisher, L. A., Corticotropin-releasing factor: endocrine and autonomic integration of responses to stress, *Trends Pharmacol. Sci.*, 10, 189, 1989.

Fisher, L. A., Rivier, J., Rivier, C., Spiess, J., Vale, W. W., and Brown, M. R., Corticotropin-releasing factor (CRF): Central effect on mean arterial pressure and heart rate in rats, *Endocrinology*, 110, 2222, 1982.

Fisher, L. A., Jessen, G., and Brown, M. R., Corticotropin-releasing factor (CRF): mechanism to elevate mean arterial pressure and heart rate, *Regul. Pept.*, 5, 153, 1983.

Foote, S. L. and Cha, C. I., Distribution of corticotropin-releasing factor-like immunoreactivity in brain stem of two monkey species (*Saimiri sciureus* and *Macaca fascicularis*): an immunhistochemical study, *J. Comp. Neurol.*, 276, 239, 1988.

Furutani, Y., Morimoto, Y., Shibahara, S., Noda, M., Takahashi, H., Hirose, T., Asai, M., Inayama, S., Hayashida, H., Miyata, T., and Numa, S., Cloning and sequence analysis of cDNA for ovine corticotropin-releasing factor precursor, *Nature (London)*, 301, 537, 1983.

Fuxe, K., Wikstrom, A. C., Okret, S., Agnati, L. F., Hafstrand, A., Yu, Z. Y., Granholm, L., Zdi, M., Vale, W., and Gustafsson, J. A., Mapping of glucocorticoid receptor immunoreactive neurons in the rat tel- and diencephalon using monoclonal antiobody against rat liver glucocorticoid receptor, *Endocrinology*, 117, 1803, 1985.

Fuxe, K., Cintra, A., Harfstrand, A., Agnati, L. F., Kalia, M., Zoli, M., Wikstrom, A. C., Okret, S., Aronsson, M., and Gustafsson, J. A., Central glucocorticoid receptor immunoreactive neurons: new insights into the endocrine regulation of the brain, *Ann. N.Y. Acad. Sci.,* 512, 362, 1987.

Gambacciani, M., Yem, S. S. C., and Rasmussen, D. D., GnRH release from the medial basal hypothalamus: *in vitro* inhibition by corticotropin-releasing factor, *Neuroendocrinology*, 43, 533, 1986.

Ganong, W. F., Control of adrenocorticotropin and melanocyte-stimulating hormone secretion, in *The Hypothalamus,* Martini, L., Motta, M., and Fraschini, F., Eds., Academic Press, New York, 1970, 313.

Ganong, W. F., Neurotransmitters and pituitary function: regulation of ACTH secretion, *Fed. Proc.,* 39, 2923, 1980.

Gibbs, D., Measurement of hypothalamic corticotropin-releasing factors in hypophyseal portal blood, *Fed. Proc.,* 44, 203, 1985.

Gibbs, D. M. and Vale, W., Presence of corticotropin-releasing factor-like immunoreactivity in hypophyseal portal blood, *Endocrinology*, 111, 1418, 1982.

Gibbs, D. M. and Vale, W., Effect of serotonin reuptake inhibitor fluoxetine on corticotropin-releasing factor and vasopressin secretion into hypophyseal portal blood, *Brain Res.,* 280, 176, 1983.

Gillies, G. E. and Lowry, P. J., Adrenal function, in *Neuroendocrinology*, Lightman, S. L. and Everitt, B. J., Eds., Blackwell Scientific, Oxford, 1986 360.

Gillies, G. E., Linton, E. A, and Lowrey, P. J., Corticotropin releasing activity of the new CRF is potentiated several times by vasopressin, *Nature (London),* 299, 355, 1982.

Gold, P. W., Chrousos, G., Kellner, C., Post, R., Roy, A., Augerinos, P., Schulte, H., Oldfield, E., and Loriaux, D. L., Psychiatric implications of basic and clinical studies with corticotropin-releasing factor, *Am. J. Psychiatr.,* 141, 619, 1983.

Gorski, R. A., Harlan, R. E., Jacobson, C. D., Shryne, J. E., and Southam, A. M., Evidence for the existence of a sexually dimorphic nucleus in the preoptic area of the rat, *J. Comp. Neurol.,* 193, 529, 1980.

Gosnell, B. A., Morley, J. E., and Levine, A. S., Adrenal modulation of the inhibitory effect of corticotropin releasing factor on feeding, *Peptides*, 4, 807, 1983.

Greer, M. A. and Rockie, C., Inhibition by pentobarbital of ether-enduced ACTH secretion in the rat, *Endocrinology*, 103, 528, 1968.

Guillemin, R. and Rosenberg, B., Humoral hypothalamic control of the anterior pituitary: a study with combined tissue cultures, *Endocrinology*, 57, 599, 1955.

Halász, B., Slusher, M., and Gorski, R. A., Adrenocorticotrophic hormone secretion in rats after partial or total deafferentation of the medial basal hypothalamus, *Neuroendocrinology*, 2, 43, 1967.

Harris, G. W., Neural control of the pituitary gland, *Physiol. Rev.,* 28, 139, 1948.

Harris, G. W. and George, R., Neurohumoral control of the adenohypophysis and the regulation of the secretion of TSH, ACTH and growth hormone, in *The Hypothalamus,* Haymaker, W., Anderson, E., Nauta, W. J. H., Eds., Charles C Thomas, Springfield, IL, 1969, 326.

Harrison, L. C. and Campbell, I. L., Cytokines: an expanding network of immuno-inflammatory hormones, *Mol. Endocrinol.,* 2, 1151, 1988.

Hashimoto, K., Murakami, K., Ohno, N., Kageyama, J., Aoki, Y., Takahara, J., and Ota, Z., A specific radioimmunoassay for corticotropin releasing factor (CRF) using synthetic ovine CRF, *Life Sci.,* 32, 1001, 1983.

Hauger, R. L., Millan, M. A., Catt, K. J., Aguilera, G., Differential regulation of brain and pituitary corticotropin releasing factor receptors by corticosterone, *Endocrinology*, 120, 1527, 1987.

Hedner, J., Hedner, T., Lundell, K. H., Bissette, G., O'Connor, L., and Nemeroff, C. B., Cerebrospinal fluid concentrations of neurotensin and corticotropin releasing factor in pediatric patients, *Biol. Neonate,* 55, 260, 1989.

Hisano, S., Tsuruo, Y., Katoh, S., Daikoku, S., Yanaihara, N., and Shibasaki, T., Intragranular colocalization of arginine vasopressin and methionin-enkephalin-octapeptide in CRF-axons in the rat median eminence, *Cell Tissue Res.,* 249, 497, 1987.

Hökfelt, T., Fahrenkrug, J., Tatemoto, K., Mutt, V., Werner, S., Hultings, A. L., Terenius, L., Chang, K. J., The PHI (PHI-27)/corticotropin-releasing factor/enkephalin immunoreactive hypothalamic neuron: Possible morphological basis for integrated control of prolactin, corticotropin, and growth hormone secretion, *Proc. Natl. Acad. Sci. U.S.A.*, 80, 895, 1983.

Hökfelt, T., Johansson, O., and Goldstein, M., Central catecholamine neurons as revealed by immunocytochemistry with special reference to adrenal neurons, in *Handbook of Chemical Neuroanatomy*, Vol. 2, Björklund, A. and Hökfelt, T., Eds., Amsterdam, Elsevier, 1984, 157.

Hökfelt, T., Tsuruo, Y., Meister, B., Melander, T., Schalling, M., and Everitt, B., Localization of neuroactive substances in the hypothalamus with special reference to coexistence of messenger molecules, *Adv. Exp. Med. Biol.*, 219, 21, 1987.

Hollenberg, S. M., Weinberger, C., Ong, E. S., Cerelli, G., Oro, A., Lebo, R., Thompson, E. B., Rosenfeld, M. G., and Evans, R. M., Primary structure and expression of a functional human glucocorticoid receptor cDNA, *Nature (London)*, 318, 635, 1985.

Holmes, M. C., Antoni, F. A., Catt, K. J., and Aguilera, G., Predominant release of vasopressin vs. corticotropin releasing factor from the isolated median eminence after adrenalectomy, *Neuroendocrinology*, 43, 245, 1986.

Holmes, M. C., Catt, K. J., and Aguilera, G., Involvement of vasopressin in the down-regulation of pituitary corticotropin releasing factor receptors after adrenalectomy, *Endocrinology*, 121, 2093, 1987.

Itoi, K., Moiri, T., Takahashi, K., Murakami, O., Imai, Y., Sasaki, S., Yoshinaga, K., and Sorono, N., Suppression by glucocorticoids of the immunoreactivity of corticotropin releasing factor and vasopressin in the paraventricular nucleus of the rat hypothalamus, *Neurosci. Lett.*, 73, 231, 1987.

Jhanwar-Uniyal, M., Roland, C., and Leibowitz, S., Diurnal rhythm of alpha 2-noradrenergic receptors in the paraventricular nucleus and other brain areas: relation to circulating corticosterone and feeding behavior, *Life Sci.*, 38, 473, 1986.

Jingami, H., Matsukura, S., Numa, S., and Imura, H., Effects of adrenalectomy and dexamethasone administration on the level of prepro-corticotropin-releasing factor messenger ribonucleic acid (mRNA) in the hypothalamus and adrenocorticotropin/beta-lipotropin precursor mRNA in the pituitary in rats, *Endocrinology*, 117, 1314, 1985a.

Jingami, H., Mizuno, N., Takahashi, H., Shibahara, S., Furutani, Y., Imura, H., and Numa, S., Cloning and sequence analysis of cDNA for rat corticotropin-releasing factor precursor, *FEBS Lett.*, 191, 63, 1985b.

Jones, M. T. and Gillham, B., Factors involved in the regulation of adrenocorticotropic hormone/beta-lipotropic hormone, *Physiol. Rev.*, 68, 743, 1988.

Jozsa, R., Vigh, S., Schally, A. V., and Mess, B., Localisation of corticotropin-releasing factor-containing neurons in the brain of the domestic fowl. An immunohistochemical study, *Cell Tissue Res.*, 236, 245, 1984.

Kalin, N. H., Shelton, S. E., Kraemer, G. W., and McKinney, W. T., Corticotropin-releasing factor administered intraventricularly to rhesus monkeys, *Peptides*, 4, 217, 1983.

Katsuura, G., Gottschall, P. E., Arimura, A., Identification of a high affinity receptor for interleukin-1-beta in rat brain, *Biochem. Biophys. Res. Commun.*, 156, 1, 1988.

Katsuura, G., Arimura, A., Koves, K., and Gottschall, P. E., Involvement of organum vasculosum of lamina terminalis and preoptic area in interleukin-1 beta-induced ACTH release, *Am. J. Physiol.*, in press.

Kawano, H., Daikoku, S., and Shibasaki, T., CRF-containing neuron systems in the rat hypothalamus: retrograde tracing and immunhistochemical studies, *J. Comp. Neurol.*, 272, 260, 1988.

Kelley, M. and Kowall, N., Corticotropin-releasing factor neurons persist throughout the brain in Alzheimer's disease, *Brain Res.*, 501, 392, 1989.

Kiss, J. Z., Mezey, E., Skirboll, L., Corticotropin-releasing factor-immunoreactive neurons of the paraventricular nucleus become vasopressin positive after adrenalectomy, *Proc. Natl. Acad. Sci. U.S.A.*, 81, 1854, 1984.

Kovács, K. and Mezey, E., Dexamethasone inhibits corticotropin-releasing factor gene expression in the rat paraventricular nucleus, *Neuroendocrinology*, 46, 365, 1987.

Kovács, K., Kiss, J. Z., and Makara, G. B., Glucocorticoid implants around the hypothalamic paraventricular nucleus prevent the increase of corticotropin-releasing factor and arginine vasopressin immunostaining induced by adrenalectomy, *Neuroendocrinology*, 44, 229, 1986.

Kovacs, M., Lengvari, I., Liposits, Z., Vigh, S., Schally, A. V., and Flerko, B., Corticotropin-releasing factor (CRF)-immunoreactive neurons in the mammillary body of the rat, *Cell Tissue Res.*, 240, 455, 1985.

Krieger, D. T., Liotta, A., and Brownstein, M. J., Corticotropin-releasing factor distribution in normal and Brattleboro rat brain, and effect of deafferentation, hypophysectomy and steroid treatment in normal animals, *Endocrinology*, 100, 227, 1977.

Krukoff, T. L., Segmental distribution of corticotropin-releasing factor and vasoactive intestinal polypeptide-like immunoreactivities in presumptive sympathetic preganglionic neurons in the cat, *Brain Res.*, 382, 153, 1986.

Kurosawa, M., Sato, A., Swenson, R. S., and Takahashi, Y., Sympatho-adrenal medullary functions in response to intracerebroventricularly injected corticotropin-releasing factor, *Brain Res.*, 367, 250, 1986.

Lamberts, S. W. J., Klijn, J. G. M., de Jong, F. H., and Birkenhager, J. C., Hormone secretion in alcohol-induced pseudo-Cushing's syndrome: differential diagnosis with Cushing's disease, *JAMA*, 242, 1640, 1979.

Lands, A., Arnold, A., McAnliff, J. P., Luduena, F., and Brown, T., Differentiation of receptor systems activated by sympathomimetic amines, *Nature (London)*, 214, 597, 1967.

Lechan, R. M., Toni, R., Clark, B. D., Cannon, J. G., Shaw, A. R., Dinarello, C. A., and Reichlin, S., Immunoreactive interleukin-1 localization in the rat forebrain, *Brain Res.*, 514, 135, 1990.

Lederis, K., Non-mammalian corticotropin release-stimulating peptides, *Ann. N.Y. Acad. Sci.*, 512, 129, 1987.

Lederis, K., Letter, A., McMaster, D., Moore, G., and Schlesinger, D., Complete amino acid sequence of urotensin I, a hypotensive and corticotropin-releasing neuropeptide from *Catostomus*, *Science*, 218, 162, 1982.

Lenhard, L., Deftos, L. J., Adenohypophyseal hormones in the CSF, *Neuroendocrinology*, 34, 303, 1982.

Lenz, H. J., Extrapituitary effects of corticotropin-releasing factor, *Horm. Metab. Res. Suppl.*, 16, 17, 1987 .

Lenz, H. J., Hester, S. E., and Brown, M. R., Corticotropin-releasing factor. Mechanisms to inhibit gastric acid secretion in conscious dogs, *J. Clin. Invest.*, 75, 889, 1985.

Leranth, C., Antoni, F. A., and Palkovits, M., Ultrastructural demonstration of ovine CRF-like immunoreactivity (oCRF-LI) in the rat hypothalamus: processes of magnocellular neurons establish membrane specializations with parvocellular neurons containing oCRF-LI, *Regul. Pept.*, 6, 179, 1983.

Levin, M. C., Sawchenko, P. E., Howe, P. R. C., Bloom, S. R., and Polak, J. M., The organization of galanin-immunoreactive inputs to the paraventricular nucleus of the hypothalamus with special reference to their relationship to catecholaminergic afferents, *J. Comp. Neurol.*, 261, 562, 1987.

Lewis, D. A., Foote, S. L., and Cha, C. I., Corticotropin-releasing factor immunoreactivity in monkey neocortex: an immunohistochemical analysis, *J. Comp. Neurol.*, 290, 599, 1989.

Lind, R. W. and Swanson, L. W., Evidence for corticotropin-releasing factor and Leu-enkephalin in the neural projection from the lateral parabrachial nucleus to the median preoptic nucleus: a retorgrade transport, immunhistochemical double labeling study in the rat, *Brain Res.*, 321, 217, 1984.

Lind, R. W., Swanson, L. W., and Ganten, D., Angiotensin II immunoreactive pathways in the central nervous system of the rat: evidence for the projections from the subfornical organ to the paraventricular nucleus of the hypothalamus, *Clin. Exp. Hypertension,* A6, 1915, 1984.

Lind, R. W., Swanson, L. W., Bruhn, T. O., and Ganten, D., The distribution of angiotensin II-immunoreactive cells and fibers in the paraventriculo-hypophyseal system of the rat, *Brain Res.*, 338, 81, 1985a.

Lind, R. W., Swanson, L. W., and Sawchenko, P. E., Anatomical evidence that neural circuits related to the subfornical organ contain angiotensin II, *Brain Res. Bull.*, 15, 79, 1985b.

Lindwall, O., Björklund, A., and Skakerberg, G. Seletive histochemical demonstration of dopamine terminal system in rat di- and telencephalon: new evidence for dopaminergic innervation by hypothalamic neurosecretory nuclei, *Brain Res.*, 306, 19, 1984.

Liposits, Z., Ultrastructural immunocytochemistry of the hypothalamic corticotropin releasing hormone synthesizing system, *Prog. Histochem. Cytochem.*, 2, No. 2, Gustav Fisher Verlag, Stuttgart, 21 (No. 2), 1, 1990.

Liposits, Z. and Paull, W. K., Ultrastructural alterations of the paraventriculo-infundibular neuronal system in long-term adrenalectomized rats, *Peptides*, 6, 1021, 1985.

Liposits, Z. and Paull, W. K., Association of dopaminergic fibers with corticotropin releasing hormone (CRH)-synthesizing neurons in the paraventricular nucleus of the rat hypothalamus, *Histochemistry*, 93, 119, 1989.

Liposits, Z., Lengvari, I., Vigh, S., Schally, A. V., and Flerko, B., Immunohistological detection of degenerating CRF-immunoreactive nerve fibers in the median eminence after lesion of paraventricular nucleus of the rat. A light and electron microscopic study, *Peptides*, 4, 941, 1983.

Liposits, Z., Paull, W. K., Setalo, G., Vigh, S., Evidence for local corticotropin releasing factor (CRF)-immunoreactive neuronal circuits in the paraventricular nucleus of the rat hypothalamus. An electron microscopic immunohistochemical analysis, *Histochemistry*, 83, 5, 1985.

Liposits, Z., Phelix, C., and Paull, W. K., Adrenergic innervation of corticotropin releasing factor (CRF)-synthesizing neurons in the hypothlamic paraventricular nucleus of the rat, *Histochemistry*, 84, 201, 1986a.

Liposits, Z., Sherman, D., Phelix, C., and Paull, W. K., A combined light and electron microscopic immunocytochemical method for the simultaneous localization of multiple tissue antigens, *Histochemistry*, 85, 95, 1986b.

Liposits, Z., Phelix, C., and Paull, W. K., Synaptic intercation of serotoninergic axons and corticotropin releasing factor (CRF) synthesizing neurons in the hypothalamic paraventricular nucleus of the rat, *Histochemistry*, 86, 541, 1987a.

Liposits, Z., Uht, R. M., Harrison, R. W., Gibbs, F. P., Paull, W. K., and Bohn, M. C., Ultrastructural localization of glucocorticoid receptor (GR) in hypothalamic paraventricular neurons synthesizing corticotropin-releasing factor (CRF), *Histochemistry*, 87, 407, 1987b.

Liposits, Z., Sievers, L., and Paull, W. K., Neuropeptide-Y and ACTH-immunoreactive innervation of corticotropin releasing factor (CRF)-synthesizing neurons in the hypothalamus of the rat, *Histochemistry*, 88, 227, 1988.

Lumpkin, M. D., The regulation of ACTH secretion by IL-1, *Science*, 238, 452, 1987.

Lumpkin, M. D., Samson, W. K., and McCann, S. M., Arginin vasopressin as a thyrotropin releasing hormone, *Science*, 235, 1070, 1987.

Lymangrove, J. R. and Brodish, A., Tissue CRF: an extra-hypothalamic corticotropin releasing factor (CRF) in the peripheral blood of stressed rats, *Neuroendocrinology*, 12, 225, 1973.

MacLusky, N. J., Naftolin, F., and Leranth, C., Immunocytochemical evidence for direct synaptic connections between corticotropin-releasing factor (CRF) and gonadotropin-releasing hormone (GnRH)-containing neurons in the preoptic area of the rat, *Brain Res*, 439, 391, 1988.

Makara, G. B., Stark, E., Karteszi, M., Palkovits, M., and Rappay, G., Effect of paraventricular lesions on stimulated ACTH release and CRF in stalk-median eminence of the rat, *Am. J. Physiol.*, 240, E441, 1981.

Meister, B., Hökfelt, T., Geffard, M., and Oertel, W., Glutamic acid decarboxylase- and gamma-aminobutyric acid-like immunoreactivities in corticotropin-releasing factor-containing parvocellular neurons of the hypothalamic paraventricular nucleus, *Neuroendocrinology*, 48, 516, 1988.

Merchenthaler, I., Corticotropin-releasing factor (CRF)-like immunoreactivity in the rat central nervous system. Extrahypothalamic distribution, *Peptides*, 5 (Suppl. 1), 53, 1984.

Merchenthaler, I., Vigh, S., Petrusz, P., and Schally, A. V., Immunocytochemical localization of corticotropin-releasing factor (CRF) in the rat brain, *Am. J. Anat.*, 165, 385, 1982.

Merchenthaler, I., Vigh, S., Petrusz, P., and Schally, A. V., The paraventriculo-infundibular corticotropin-releasing factor (CRF) pathways as revealed by immunocytochemistry in long-term hypophysectomized or adrenalectomized rats, *Regul. Pept.*, 5, 295, 1983a.

Merchenthaler, I., Hynes, M. A., Vigh, S., Schally, A. V., and Petrusz, P., Immunocytochemical localization of corticotropin releasing factor (CRF) in the spinal cord, *Brain Res.,* 275, 373, 1983b.

Merchenthaler, I., Hynes, M. A., Vigh, S., Schally, A. V., and Petrusz, P., Corticotropin-releasing factor (CRF): origin and course of afferent pathways to the median eminence (ME) of the rat hypothalamus, *Neuroendocrinology*, 39, 296, 1984a.

Merchenthaler, I., Vigh, S., Schally, A. V., Stumpf, W. E., and Arimura, A., Immunocytochemical localization of corticotropin-releasing factor (CRF)-like immunoreactivity in the thalamus of the rat, *Brain Res.,* 323, 119, 1984b.

Merchenthaler, I., Gallyas, F., and Liposits, Z., Silver intensification in immunocytochemistry, in *Techniques in Immunocytochemistry,* Vol 4, Bullock, G. R. and Petrusz, P., Eds., Academic Press, New York, 1989, 217.

Mezey, E., Reisine, T. D., Skirboll, L., Beinfeld, M., and Kiss, J. Z., Role of cholecystokinin in corticotropin release: coexistence with vasopressin and corticotropin-releasing factor in cells of the rat hypothalamic paraventricular nucleus, *Proc. Natl. Acad. Sci. U.S.A.,* 83, 3510, 1986.

Millan, M. A., Jacobowitz, D. M., Hauger, R. L., Catt, K. J., and Aguilera, G., Distribution of corticotropin-releasing factor receptors in the primate brain, *Proc. Natl. Acad. Sci. U.S.A.,* 83, 1921, 1986.

Millan, M. A., Abou-Samra, A. B., Wynn, P. C., Catt, K. J., and Aguilera, G., Receptors and action of corticotropin-releasing factor in the primate pituitary gland, *J. Clin. Endocrinol. Metab.,* 64, 1036, 1987.

Minneman, K., Hegstrand, L., and Molinoff, P., The pharmacological specificity of beta-1 and beta-2 adrenergic receptors in rat heart and lung *in vitro, Mol. Pharmacol.,* 16, 21, 1979.

Moga, M. M. and Gray, T. S., Evidence for corticotropin-releasing factor, neurotensin, ans somatostatin in the neural pathway from the central nucleus of the amygdala to the parabrachial nucleus, *J. Comp. Neurol.,* 241, 275, 1985.

Montecucchi, P. C., Henschen, A., and Erspamer, V., Structure of sauvagine, a vasoactive peptide from the skin of a frog, *Hoppe-Seyler's Z. Physiol. Chem.,* 360, 1178, 1979.

Morley, J. E. and Levine, A. S., Corticotropin releasing factor, grooming and ingestive behavior, *Life Sci.,* 31, 1459, 1982.

Mouradian, M. M., Farah, J. M., Mohr, E., Fabbrini, G., O'Donohue, T. L., and Chase, T. N., Spinal fluid CRF reduction in Alzheimer's disease, *Neuropeptides*, 8, 393, 1986.

Mouri, T., Suda, T., Sasano, N., Andoh, N., Takei, Y., Takashe, M., Sasaki, A., Murakami, O., and Yoshinaga, K., Immunocytochemical identification of CRF in the human hypothalamus, *J. Exp. Med.,* 142, 423, 1984.

Nemeroff, C. B., Widerlov, E., Bissette, G., Walleus, H., Karlson, I., Eklund, K., Kilts, C. D., Loosen, P. T., and Vale, W., Elevated concentrations of CSF corticotropin-releasing factor-like immunoreactivity in depressed patients, *Science*, 226, 1342, 1984.

Nimi, M., Takahara, J., Hashimoto, K., and Kawanishi, K., Immunohistochemical identification of corticotropin releasing factor-containing neurons projecting to the stalk-median eminence of the rat, *Peptides*, 9, 589, 1988.

Norgren, R., Projections from the nucleus of the solitary tract in the rat, *Neuroscience*, 3, 207, 1978.

Olivereau, M., Ollevier, F., Vandesande, F., and Verdonck, W., Immunocytochemical identification of CRF-like and SRIF-like peptides in the brain and the pituitary of cyprinid fish, *Cell Tissue Res.,* 237, 379, 1984.

Olivereau, M., Vandesande, F., Boucique, E., Ollevier, F., and Olivereau, J. M., Immunocytochemical localization and spatial relation to the adenohypophysis of a somatostatin-like and a corticotropin-releasing factor-like peptide in the brain of four amphibian species, *Cell Tissue Res.,* 247, 317, 1987.

Olschowka, J. A., GABA-ergic innervation of corticotropin releasing factor neurons in the rat paraventricular nucleus: an electron microscopic immunocytochemical study, *Soc. Neurosci. Abstr.,* 13, 1656, 1987.

Olschowka, J. A., O'Donohue, T. L., Mueller, G. P., and Jacobowitz, D. M., The distribution of corticotropin-releasing factor-like immunoreactive neurons in rat brain, *Peptides*, 3, 995, 1982.

Ono, N., Samson, W. K., McDonald, J. K., Lumpkin, M. D., Berdan de Castro, J., and McCann, S. M., Effect of intravenous and intraventricular injection of antisera directed against corticotropin releasing factor on the secretion of anterior pituitary hormones, *Proc. Natl. Acad. Sci. U.S.A.*, 82, 7787, 1985.

Onstott, D. and Elde, R., Immunohistochemical localization of urotensin I/corticotropin-releasing factor, urotensin II, and serotonin immunoreactivities in the caudal spinal cord of nonteleost fishes, *J. Comp. Neurol.*, 249, 205, 1986.

Orth, D. N., DeBold, C. R., DeCherney, G. S., Jackson, R. V., Alexander, A. N., Rivier, J., Rivier, C., Spiess, J., and Vale, W., Pituitary microadenomas causing Cushing's disease respond to corticotropin-releasing factor, *J. Clin. Endocrinol. Metab.*, 55, 1017, 1982.

Ottersen, O. P. and Storm-Mathisen, J., Neurons containing or accumulating transmitter amino acids, in *Handbook of Chemical Neuroanatomy*, Vol. 3 (Part II, Classical trasmitters and transmitter receptors in the CNS), Björklund, A., Hökfelt, T., and Kuhar, M. J., Eds., Elsevier, Amsterdam, 1984, 141.

Palka, Y., Coyer, D., and Critchlow, V., Effects of isolation of medial basal hypothalamus on pituitary-adrenal and pituitary-ovarian functions, *Neuroendocrinology*, 5, 333, 1969.

Palkovits, M., Neuropeptides in the hypothalamo-hypophyseal system: lateral retrochiasmatic area as a common gate for neuronal fibers towards the median eminence, *Peptides*, 5 (Suppl. 1), 35, 1984.

Palkovits, M., Anatomy of neural pathways affecting CRH secretion, *Ann. N.Y. Acad. Sci.*, 512, 139, 1987.

Palkovits, M., Makara, G. B., and Stark, E., Hypothalamic region and pathways responsible for adrenocortical response to surgical stress in the rat, *Neuroendocrinology*, 21, 280, 1976.

Palkovits, M., Browstein, M. J., and Vale, W., Distribution of corticotropin-releasing factor in rat brain, Fed. Proc., 44, 215, 1985.

Palkovits, M., Leranth, C., Gorcs, T., and Young, W. S., Corticotropin-releasing factor in the olivocerebellar tract of the rat: demonstration by light- and electron microscopic immunohisto-chemistry and *in situ* hybridization histochemistry, *Proc. Natl. Acad. Sci. U.S.A.*, 84, 3911, 1987.

Patthy, M., Horvath, J., Mason-Garcia, M., Szoke, B., Schlesinger, D. H., and Schally, A. V., Isolation and amino acid sequence of corticotropin-releasing factor from pig hypothalami, *Proc. Natl. Acad. Sci. U.S.A.*, 82, 8762, 1986.

Paull, W. K. and Gibbs, F. B., The corticotropin releasing factor (CRF) neurosecretory system in intact, adrenalectomized and adrenalectomized-dexamethasone treated rats, *Histochemistry*, 78, 303, 1983.

Peterfreund, R. A. and Vale, W. W., Ovine corticotropin-releasing factor stimulates somatostatin-secretion from cultured brain cells, *Endocrinology*, 112, 1275, 1982.

Petrusz, P., Merchenthaler, I., Maderdrut, J. L., and Heitz, P. U., Central and peripheral distribution of corticotropin-releasing factor, *Fed. Proc.*, 44, 229, 1985.

Pilscher, W. E. and Joseph, S. A., Co-localization of CRF-ir oerikarya and ACTH-ir fibers in rat brain, *Brain Res.*, 299, 91, 1984.

Plotsky, P., Hypophyseotropic regulation of adenohypophyseal adrenocorticotropin secretion, *Fed. Proc.*, 44, 207, 1985.

Plotsky, P., Facilitation of immunoreactive corticotropin-releasing factor secretion into the hypophysial-portal circulation after activation of catecholmaninergic pathways or central norepinephrine injection, *Endocrinology*, 121, 924, 1987.

Plotsky, P., Catecholaminergic modulation of corticotropin releasing factor and adrenocorticotropin secretion, *Endocrinol. Rev.*, 10, 437, 1989.

Plotsky, P. and Vale, W., Hemorrhage-induced secretion of corticotropin-releasing factor-like immu-noreactivity into the rat hypophysial portal circulation and its inhibition by glucocorticoids, *Endocrinology*, 114, 164, 1984.

Plotsky, P., Otto, S., and Sutton, S., Neurotransmitter modulation of corticotropin-releasing factor secretion into the hypophyseal portal circulation, *Life Sci.*, 41, 1311, 1987.

Powers, R. E., Walker, L. C., De Souza, E. B., Vale, W. W., Struble, R. G., Whitehouse, P. J., and Price, D. L., Immunohistochemical study of neurons containing corticotropin-releasing factor in Alzheimer's disease, *Synapse*, 1, 405, 1987.

Remy, C., Tramu, G., and Dubois, M. P., Immunohistochemical demonstration of a CRF-like material in the central nervous system of the annelid *Dendrobaena, Cell Tissue Res.*, 227, 569, 1982.

Reul, J. M. H. M. and De Kloet, E. R., Two receptor systems for corticosterone in rat brain: microdistribution and differential occupation, *Endocrinology*, 117, 2505, 1985.

Rivier, C. L. and Plotsky, P. M., Mediation by corticotropin-releasing factor (CRF) of adenohypophyseal hormone secretion, *Annu. Rev. Physiol.*, 48, 475, 1986.

Rivier, C. and Vale, W, Influence of corticotropin-releasing factor on reproductive functions in the rat, *Endocrinology*, 114, 914, 1984a.

Rivier, C. and Vale, W., Corticotropin-releasing factor (CRF) acts centrally to inhibit growth hormone secretion in the rat, *Endocrinology*, 114, 2409, 1984b.

Rivier, C. and Vale, W., Effects of corticotropin-releasing factor, neurohypophyseal peptides, and catecholmanines on pituitary function, *Fed. Proc.*, 44, 189, 1985.

Rivier, C., Brownstein, M., Spiess, J., Rivier, J., and Vale, W., In vivo corticotropin releasing factor induced secretion of adrenocorticotropin, beta-endorphin and corticosterone, *Endocrinology*, 110, 272, 1982.

Rivier, C., Rivier, J., and Vale, W., Inhibition of adrenocorticotropin secretion in the rat by immunoneutralization of corticotropin-releasing factor (CRF), *Science*, 218, 377, 1982.

Rivier, J., Spiess, J., and Vale, W., Characterization of rat hypothalamic corticotropin-releasing factor, *Proc. Natl. Acad. Sci. U.S.A.*, 80, 4851, 1983.

Rivier, C., Bruhn, T., and Vale, W., Effect of ethanol on the hypothalamic-pituitary-adrenal axis in the rat: role of corticotropin-releasing factor (CRF), *J. Pharmacol. Exp. Ther.*, 229, 127, 1984.

Robinson, B. G., D'Angio, L. A., Jr., Pasieka, K. B., and Majzoub, J. A., Preprocorticotropin releasing homrone: cDNA sequence and in vitro processing, *Mol. Cell Endocrinol.*, 61, 175, 1989.

Roche, P. J., Crawford, R. J., Fernley, R. T., Tregear, G. W., and Coghlan, J. P., Nucleotide sequence of the gene coding for ovine corticotropin-releasing factor and regulation of its mRNA levels by glucocorticoids, *Gene*, 71, 421, 1988.

Saffran, M. and Schally, A. V., The release of corticotropin by anterior pituitary tissues *in vitro, Can. J. Physiol.*, 33, 408, 1955.

Saffran, M. and Schally, A. V., The status of the corticotrophin recleasing factor (CRF), *Neuroendocrinology*, 24, 359, 1977.

Sakanaka, M., Shibasaki, T., and Lederis, K., Distribution and efferent projections of corticotropin-releasing factor-like immunoreactivity in the rat amygdaloid complex, *Brain Res.*, 382, 213, 1986.

Sakanaka, M., Shibasaki, T., Lederis, K., Corticotropin releasing factor-like immunoreactivity in the rat as revealed by a modified cobalt-glucose oxidase-diaminobenzidine method, *J. Comp. Neurol.*, 260, 256, 1987a.

Sakanaka, M., Shibasaki, T., Lederis, K., Corticotropin-releasing factor-containing afferents of the inferior colliculus of the rat brain, *Brain Res.*, 414, 68, 1987b.

Sakanaka, M., Magari, S., Shibasaki, T., and Inoue, N., Co-localization of corticotropin-releasing factor- and enekephalin-like immunoreactivities in nerve cells of the rat hypothalamus and adjacent areas, *Brain Res.*, 487, 357, 1989.

Saper, C. B. and Loewy, A. D., Efferent connections of the parabrachial nucleus in the rat, *Brain Res.*, 197, 291, 1980.

Sapolsky, R., Rivier, C., Yamamoto, G., Plotsky, P., and Vale, W., Interleukin-1 stimulates the secretion of hypothalamic corticotropin-releasing factor, *Science*, 238, 522, 1987.

Sasaki, A., Liotta, A. S., Luckey, M. M., Suda, T., and Krieger, D., Immunoreactive corticotropin releasing factor is present in human maternal plasma during the third trimester of pregnancy, *J. Clin. Endocrinol. Metab.*, 59, 812, 1984.

Sasaki, A., Sato, S., Murakami, O., Go, M., Inoue, M., Shimizu, Y., Hanew, K., Andoh, N., Sato, I., Sasano, N., and Yoshinaga, K., Immunoreactive corticotropin-releasing hormone present in human plasma may be derived from both hypothalamic and extrahypothalamic sources, *J. Clin. Endocrinol. Metab.*, 65, 176, 1987.

Sawchenko, P. E., Evidence for local site of action for glucocorticoids in inhibiting CRF and vasopressin in the paraventricular nucleus, *Brain Res.*, 403, 303, 1987a.

Sawchenko, P. E., Adrenalectomy-induced enhancement of CRF and vasopressin immunoreactivity in parvocellular neurosecretory neurons: autonomic, peptide, and steroid specificity, *J. Neurosci.*, 7, 1093, 1987b.

Sawchenko, P. E., Evidence for differential regulation of corticotropin-releasing factor and vasopressin immunoreactivities in parvocellular neurosecretory and autonomic-related projections of the paraventricular nucleus, *Brain Res.*, 437, 253, 1987c.

Sawchenko, P. E., Effect of catecholamine-depleting medullary knife cuts on corticotropin-releasing factor and vasopressin immunoreactivity in the hypothalamus of normal and steroid-manipulated rats, *Neuroendocrinology*, 48, 459, 1988.

Sawchenko, P. E. and Swanson, L. W., Immunohistochemical identification of neurons in the paraventricular nucleus of the hypothalamus that project to the medulla or to the spinal cord in the rat, *J. Comp. Neurol.*, 205, 260, 1982.

Sawchenko, P. E. and Swanson, L. W., The organization of forebrain afferents to the paraventricular and supraopric nuclei of the rat, *J. Comp. Neurol.*, 218, 121, 1983.

Sawchenko, P. E. and Swanson, L. W., Localization, co-localization, and plasticity of corticotropin-releasing factor immunoreactivity in rat brain, *Fed. Proc.*, 44, 221, 1985

Sawchenko, P. E., Swanson, L. W., Steinbusch, H. W. M., and Verhofstad, A. A. J., The distribution and cells of origin of serotonergic inputs to the paraventricular and supraoptic nuclei of the rat, *Brain Res.*, 277, 355, 1983.

Sawchenko, P. E., Swanson, L. W., and Vale, W., Co-expression of corticotropin-releasing factor and vasopressin immunoreactivity in parvocellular neurosecretory neurons of the adrenalectomized rat, *Proc. Natl. Acad. Sci. U.S.A.*, 81, 1883, 1984a.

Sawchenko, P. E., Swanson, L. W., and Vale, W., Corticotropin-releasing factor: co-expression within distinct subsets of oxytocin-, vasopressin-, and neurotensin-immunoreactive neurons in the hypothalamus of the male rat, *J. Neurosci.*, 4, 1118, 1984b.

Sawchenko, P. E., Swanson, L. W., Grzanna, R., Howe, P. R. C., Bloom, S. R., Polak, J. M., Colocalization of neuropeptide Y immunoreactivity in brain stem catecholaminergic neurons that project to the paraventricular and supraoptic nuclei in the rat, *J. Comp. Neurol.*, 241, 138, 1985.

Schramme, C. and Denef, C., Stimulation of spontaneous and dopamine-inhibited prolactin release from anterior pituitary reaggregate cell cultures by angiotensin peptides, *Life Sci.*, 34, 1651, 1984.

Schwartz, J. and Vale, W., Dissociation of the adrenocorticotropin secretory responses to corticotropin-releasing factor (CRF) and vasopressin or oxytocin by using a specific cytotoxic analog of CRF, *Endocrinology*, 122, 1695, 1988.

Scoggins, B. A., Coghlan, J. P., Denton, D. A., Fei, D. W., Nelson, M. A., Treager, G. W., Tresham, J., and Wang, Z. M., Intracerebroventricular infusion of corticotropin-releasing factor (CRF) and ACTH raise blood pressure in sheep, *Clin. Exp. Pharmacol. Physiol.*, 11, 65, 1984.

Seasholtz, A. F., Thompson, R. C., and Douglass, J. O., Identification of a cyclic adenosine monophosphate-responsive element in the rat corticotropin-releasing hormone gene, *Mol. Endocrinol.*, 12, 1311, 1988.

Selye, H., A syndrome produced by diverse nocuous agents, *Nature (London)*, 138, 32, 1936.

Shibahara, S., Morimoto, Y., Furutani, Y., Notake, M., Takahashi, H., Shimizu, S., Horikawa, S., and Numa, S., Isolation and sequence analysis of the human corticotropin-releasing factor precursor gene, *EMBO J.*, 2, 775, 1983.

Silverman, A. J., Hou-Yu, A., and Chen, W. P., Corticotropin-releasing factor synapses within the paraventricular nucleus of the hypothalamus, *Neuroendocrinology*, 49, 291, 1989.

Sirinathsinghji, D. J. S., Rees, L. H., Rivier, J., Vale, W., Corticotropin releasing factor is a potent inhibitor of sexual receptivity in the female rat, *Nature (London)*, 305, 232, 1983.

Smith, I. A., Engler, D., Fullerton, M. J., Pham, T., Wallace, C., Morgan, F. J., Clarke, I. J., and Funder, J. W., Posttranslational processing of corticotropin-releasing factor in the ovine tuberoinfundibular system and pituitary, *Ann. N.Y. Acad. Sci.*, 512, 24, 1987.

Snyder, D. S. and Unanue, E. R., Corticosteroids inhibit murine macrophage Ia expression and interleukin-1 production, *J. Immunol.*, 129, 1803, 1982.

Spiess, J., Rivier, J., Rivier, C., and Vale, W. W., Primary structure of corticotropin-releasing factor from ovine hypothalamus, *Proc. Natl. Acad. Sci. U.S.A.*, 78, 6517, 1981.

Spinedi, E., Johnston, C., Chisari, A., Negro-Vilar, A., Role of central epinephrine in the regulation of corticotropin-releasing factor and adrenocorticotropin secretion, *Endocrinology*, 122, p. 1977, 1988.

Stark, E., Makara, G. B., Palkovits, M., Karteszi, M., Mihaly, K., Basal levels of pituitary corticotropin and plasma corticosterone after complete or frontal cuts around the medial basal hypothalamus, *Endocrinol. Exp.*, 12, 209, 1978.

Staruch, M. J. and Wood, D. D., Reduction of serum interleukin 1 like activity after treatment with dexamethasone, *J. Leukocyte Biol.*, 37, 193, 1985.

Steinbusch, H. W. M., Distribution of serotonin-immunoreactivity in the central nervous system of the rat-cell bodies and terminals, *Neuroscience*, 6, 557, 1981.

Steinbusch, H. W. M., Serotonin-immunoreactive neurons and their projections in the CNS, in *Handbook of Chemical Neuroanatomy*, Vol. 3 (Classical trasmitters and transmitter receptors in the CNS), Björklund, A., Hökfelt, T., and Kuhar, M. J., Eds., Elsevier, Amsterdam, 1984, 68.

Steinbusch, H. W. M. and Mulder, A. H., Immunohistochemical localization of histamine in neurons and mast cells in the rat brain, in *Handbook of Chemical Neuroanatomy*, Vol. 3 (Classical transmitters and transmitter receptors in the CNS, Björklund, A., Hökfelt, T., and Kuhar, M. J., Eds., Elsevier, Amsterdam, 1984, 126.

Suda, T., Tomori, N., Yajima, F., Sumimoto, T., Nakajimi, Y., Ushiyama, T., Dumura, H., and Shizume, K., Immunoreactive corticotropin-releasing factor in human plasma, *J. Clin. Invest.*, 76, 2026, 1985.

Suda, T., Tozawa, F., Ushiyama, T., Sumitomo, T., Yamada, M., Demura, H., Interleukin-1 stimulates corticotropin-releasing factor gene expression in rat hypothalamus, *Endocrinology*, 126, 1223, 1990.

Sutton, R. E., Koob, G. F., LeMoal, M., Rivier, J., and Vale, W., Corticotropin releasing factor produces behavioral activation in rats, *Nature (London)*, 297, 331, 1982.

Swanson, L. W. and Kuypers, G. G. J. M., The paraventricular nucleus of the hypothalamus: cytoarchitectonic subdivisions and organization of projections to the pituitary, dorsal vagal complex, and spinal cord as demonstrated by retrograde fluorescence double-labeling methods, *J. Comp. Neurol.*, 194, 555, 1980.

Swanson, L .W. and Simmons, D. M., Diffenrential steroid hormone and neural influences on peptide mRNA levels in CRH cells of the paraventricular nucleus: a hybridization histochemical study in the rat, *J. Comp. Neurol.*, 285, 413, 1989.

Swanson, L. W., Sawchenko, P. E., Berod, A., Hartman, B. K., Helle, K. B., and Van Orden, D. E., An immunohistochemical study of the organization of catecholaminergic cells and terminal fields in the paraventricular and supraoptic nuclei of the hypothalamus, *J. Comp. Neurol.*, 196, 271, 1981.

Swanson, L. W., Sawchenko, P. E., Rivier, J., and Vale, W., Organization of ovine corticotropin-releasing factor immunoreactive cells and fibers in the rat brain: an immunohistochemical study, *Neuroendocrinology*, 36, 165, 1983.

Swanson, L. W., Sawchenko, P. E., and Lind, R. W., Regulation of multiple peptides in CRF parvocellular neurosecretory neurons: Implications for the stress response, *Prog. Brain Res.*, 68, 169, 1986.

Swanson, L. W., Sawchenko, P. E., Lind, R. W., and Rho, J. H., The CRH motoneuron: differential peptide regulation in neurons with possible synaptic, paracrine, and endocrine outputs, *Ann. N.Y. Acad. Sci.*, 512, 12, 1987.

Szafarczyk, A., Alonso, G., Ixart, G., Malaval, F., and Assenmacher, I., Diurnal-stimulated and stress-induced ACTH release is mediated by ventral noradrenergic bundle, *Am. J. Physiol.*, 249, E219, 1985.

Tache, Y. and Gunion, M., Corticotropin-releasing factor: central action to influence gastric secretion, *Fed. Proc.*, 44, 255, 1985.

Tache, Y., Goto, Y., Gunion, M. W., Vale, W. W., Rivier, J., and Brown, M., Inhibition of gastric acid secretion in rats by intracerebral injection of corticotropin-releasing factor, *Science*, 222, 935, 1983.

Taylor, A. L. and Fishman, L. M., Corticotropin-releasing hormone, *N. Engl. J. Med.*, 319, 213, 1988.

Thompson, R. T., Seasholtz, A. F., Douglass, J. O., Herbert, E., The rat corticotropin-releasing hormone gene, *Ann. N.Y. Acad. Sci.*, 512, 1, 1987.

Tomori, N., Suda, T., Tozawa, F., Demura, H., Shizume, K., and Mouri, T., Immunoreactive corticotropin releasing factor concentrations in cerebrospinal fluid from patients with hypothalamic-pituitary-adrenal disorders, *J. Clin. Endocrinol. Metab.*, 57:1305, 1983.

Tramu, G., Croix, C., and Pillez, A., Ability of CRF immunoreactive neurons of the paraventricular nucleus to produce a vasopressin-like material, *Neuroendocrinology*, 37, 467, 1983.

Tsagarakis, S., Gillies, G., Rees, L. H., Besser, M., and Grossmann, A., Interleukin-1 directly stimulates the release of corticotropin releasing factor from rat hypothalamus, *Neuroendocrinology*, 49:98, 1989.

Tucker, D. C., Saper, C. B., Ruggiero, D. A., and Reis, D. J., Organization of central noradrenergic pathways. I. Relationship of ventral medullary projections to the hypothalamus and spinal cord, *J. Comp. Neurol.*, 259, 591, 1987.

Turkelson, C. M., Arimura, A., Culler, M. D., Fishback, J. B., Groot, K., Kanda, M., Luciano, M., Thomas, C. R., Chang, D., Chang, J. K., and Shimizu, M., In vivo and in vitro release of ACTH by synthetic CRF, *Peptides*, 2, 425, 1981.

Uehara, A., Gottschall, P. E., Dahl, R. R., and Arimura, A., Interleukin 1 stimulates ACTH release by an indirect action which requires endogenous corticotropin-releasing factor, *Endocrinology*, 121, 1580, 1987.

Uehara, A., Sekiya, C., Takasugi, Y., Namiki, M., and Arimura, A., Anorexia induced by interleukin 1: involvement of corticotropin releasing factor, *Am. J. Physiol.*, 257, R613, 1989.

Ungerstedt, W., Stereotaxic mapping of the monoamine pathways in the rat brain, *Acta Physiol. Scand. (Suppl.)*, 367, 1, 1971.

Vale, W., Rivier, C., and Brown, M., Physiology and pharmacology of hypothalamic regulatory peptides, in *Handbook of the Hypothalamus*, Vol. 2 (Physiology of the hypothalamus), Morgane, P. J. and Panksepp, J., Eds., Marcel Dekker, New York, 1980,165.

Vale, W., Spiess, J., Rivier, C., and Rivier, J., Characterization of a 41-residue ovine hypothalamic peptide that stimulates secretion of corticotropin and beta-endorphin, *Science*, 213, 1394, 1981.

Valentino, R. J., Foote, S. L., and Aston-Jones, G., Corticotropin-releasing factor activates noradrenergic neurons of the locus ceruleus, *Brain Res.*, 270, 363, 1983.

Verhaert, P., Marivoet, S., Vandesande, F., and De Loof, A., Localization of CRF immunoreactivity in the central nervous system of three vertebrate and one insect species, *Cell Tissue Res.*, 238, 49, 1984.

Vigh, S., Merchenthaler, I., Torres-Aleman, I., Sueiras-Diaz, J., Coy, D. H., Carter, W. H., Petrusz, P., Schally, A. V., Corticotropin releasing factor (CRF): immunocytochemical localization and radioimmunoassay (RIA), *Life Sci.*, 31, 2441, 1982.

Watts, A. G., Sawnson, L. W., and Sanchez-Watts, G., Efferent projections of the suprachiasmatic nucleus. I. Studies using anterograde transport of *Phaseolus vulgaris* leucoagglutinin in the rat, *J. Comp. Neurol.*, 258, 204, 1987.

Weisenberg, R. C., Borisy, G. G., and Taylor, E. W., The colchicine-binding protein of mammalian brain and its relation to microtubules, *Biochemistry*, 7, 4466, 1968.

Whitnall, M. H., Distributions of pro-vasopressin expressing and pro-vasopressin-deficient CRH neurons in the paraventricular hypothalamic nucleus of colchicine-treated adrenalectomized rats, *J. Comp. Neurol.*, 275, 3, 1988.

Whitnall, M. H., Stress selectively activates the vasopressin-containing subset of corticotropin-releasing hormone neurons, *Neuroendocrinology*, 50, 702, 1989.

Whitnall, M. H. and Gainer, H., Major pro-vasopressin expressing and pro-vasopressin deficient CRH neurons in the paraventricular hypothalamic nucleus of colchicine-treated normal and adrenalectomized rats, *J. Comp. Neurol.*, 275, 13, 1988a.

Whitnall, M. H. and Gainer, H., Major pro-vasopressin-expressing and pro-vasopressin deficient subpopulation of corticotropin- releasing factor neurons in normal rats, *Neuroendocrinology*, 47, 176, 1988b.

Whitnall, M. H., Mezey, E., and Gainer, H., Co-localization of corticotropin-releasing factor and vasopressin in median eminence neurosecretory vesicles, *Nature (London)*, 317, 248, 1985.

Whitnall, M. H., Key, S., and Gainer, H., Vasopressin-containing and vasopressin deficient subpopulation of corticotropin-releasing factor axons are differentially affected by adrenalectomy, *Endocrinology*, 120, 2180, 1987a.

Whitnall, M. H., Smyth, D., Gainer, H., Vasopressin coexists in half of the corticotropin-releasing factor axons present in the external zone of the median eminence, *Neuroendocrinology*, 45, 420, 1987b.

Wikberg, J., The pharmacological classification of adrenergic alpha 1 and alpha 2 receptors and their mechanisms of action, *Acta Physiol. Scand. Suppl.*, 468, 1, 1979.

Williamson, D. E. and Eldred, W. D., Amacrine and ganglion cells with corticotropin-releasing factor-like immunoreactivity in the turtle retina, *J. Comp. Neurol.*, 280, 424, 1989.

Wolfson, B., Manning, R. W., Davis, L. G., and Arentzen, R., Co-localization of corticotropin releasing factor and vasopressin mRNA in neurons after adrenalectomy, *Nature (London)*, 315, 59, 1985.

Wynn, P. C, Aguilera, G., Morell, J., and Catt, K. J., Properties and regulation of high-affinity pituitary receptors for corticotropin-releasing factor, *Biochem. Biophys. Res. Commun.*, 110, 602, 1983.

Wynn, P. C., Harwood, J. P., Catt, K. J., and Aguilera, G., Regulation of corticotropin-releasing factor receptors in the rat pituitary gland: effect of adrenalectomy on CRF receptors and corticotroph responses, *Endocrinology*, 116, 1653, 1985.

Yamada, S. and Mikami, S., Immunohistochemical localization of corticotropin-releasing factor (CRF)-containing neurons in the hypothalamus of the Japanese quail, *Coturnix coturnix, Cell Tissue Res.*, 239, 299, 1985.

Yasuda, N., Greer, M. A., Rat hypothalamic corticotropin-releasing factor (CRF) content remains constant despite marked acute or chronic changes in ACTH secretion, *Neuroendocrinology*, 22, 48, 1976.

Yasuda, N. and Greer, M. A., and Aizawa, T., Corticotropin-releasing factor, *Endocrinol. Rev.*, 3, 123, 1982.

Yates, F. E. and Maran, J. W., Stimulation and inhibition of adrenocorticotropin release, in *Handbook of Physiology* (Section 7, Endocrinology, Vol. IV, The pituitary gland and its neuroendocrine control), Knobil, E. and Sawyer, W. H., Eds., American Physiological Society, Bethesda, MA, 1974, 367.

Young, S. W. and Zoeller, R. T. L., Neuroendocrine gene expression in the hypothalamus: *in situ* hybridization histochemical studies, *Cell Mol. Endocrinol.*, 7, 353, 1987.

Young, S. W., Mezey, E., and Siegel, R. E., Quantitative *in situ* hybridization histochemistry reveals increased levels of corticotropin releasing factor mRNA after adrenalectomy in rats, *Neurosci. Lett.*, 70, 198, 1986.

Yulis, C. R. and Lederis, K., Co-localization of the immunoreactivities of corticotropin-releasing factor and arginine vasotocin in the brain and pituitary system of the teleost *Catostomus commersoni, Cell Tissue Res.*, 247, 267, 1987.

Yulis, C. R., Lederis, K., Wong, K. L., and Fisher, A. W., Localization of urotensin I- and corticotropin-releasing factor-like immunoreactivity in the central nervous system of *Catostomus commersoni, Peptides*, 7, 79, 1986.

Zimmerman, E. A., Stillman, M. A., Recht, L. D., Antunes, J. L., Carmel, P. W., and Goldsmith, P. C., Vasopressin and corticotropin-releasing factor: an axonal pathway to portal capillaries in the zona externa of the median eminence containing vasopressin and its interaction with adrenal corticoids, *Ann. N.Y. Acad. Sci.*, 297, 405, 1977.

8

Gonadotropin Releasing Hormone (GnRH)

GLORIA E. HOFFMAN AND WEN-SEN LEE
Department of Physiology
University of Pittsburgh
Pittsburgh, Pennsylvania

and

SUSAN WRAY
Laboratory of Neurochemistry
National Institute for Neurologic Disease and Stroke
National Institutes of Health
Bethesda, Maryland

The release of luteinizing hormone (LH) and follicle-stimulating hormone (FSH) from the pituitary, essential for gonadal function, is under the control of neuroendocrine cells residing in the forebrain and relies on the correct expression of a single gene that encodes the precursor protein for the decapeptide gonadotropin-releasing hormone, (GnRH, also known as LH/FSH-RH or LHRH). The purification and characterization of GnRH in 1971, and subsequent generation of specific antibodies against the peptide, provided the tools for determining the organization and function of this important releasing hormone. Yet despite the availability of antibodies and workable strategies, the lack of a precise site in the brain where GnRH neurons are concentrated, as well as the difficulties encountered in measuring GnRH in the pituitary portal blood, made investigation of the physiology of the GnRH system extremely difficult and controversy regarding the role of GnRH in the regulation of the reproductive cycle resulted. Only recently, with the isolation of the gene for GnRH, acquisition of new evidence on the origin of the GnRH system, and application of new strategies for examining GnRH activity, have some of these controversies been resolved.

I. Function of GnRH

GnRH release by the hypothalamus is required for LH release and, in most instances, for FSH release as well. The actions of GnRH are exerted via abundant nerve terminals located within the median eminence of the hypothalamus that release their product into the hypophysial portal circulation. The concept that the brain regulated gonadotropin secretion from the pituitary via neurohumoral substances discharged from the hypothalamus into the hypophysial portal vasculature was formulated by Harris in 1947. Hypophysectomy caused reproductive dysfunction in the female rat, and these functions were restored when the excised gland was transplanted back to its original site or into the median eminence, but not to other places, such as the temporal lobe of the brain. The first evidence of LH-releasing activity in hypothalamic extracts was presented by McCann et al. (1960) and later confirmed by Campbell et al. (1961) and Nikitovitch-Winer (1962). Intrapituitary infusions of median eminence extracts effectively caused ovulation in the rabbit and in the pentobarbital-blocked rat; intravenous infusion of the same extract was effective in causing ovulation only if introduced in greater amounts. Control extracts (such as extracts of cerebral cortex, corpus callosum, caudate nucleus, and hypothalamus from which the median eminence had been removed) were inactive.

In 1971, the chemical composition of the hypothalamic neurohumoral substance responsible for evoking LH release was elucidated (Amos et al., 1971; Schally et al., 1971) and subsequent assays confirmed that GnRH is released from portal blood in concordance with changes in plasma LH (Sarkar et al., 1976). The 10-amino acid peptide has the following structure: pGlu-His-Trp-Ser-Tyr-Gly-Leu-Arg-Pro-Gly-NH$_2$. GnRH is now recognized as the primary hypothalamic neural factor responsible for controlling LH release from the pituitary gonadotrophs. The peptide also releases FSH along with LH, but other factors may have FSH-releasing capabilities in addition to GnRH. GnRH can stimulate LH secretion from the anterior pituitary *in vitro* and *in vivo* . The immunoneutralization of the blood-borne GnRH suppresses the secretion of LH and blocks the preovulatory LH surge and ovulation (Fraser and Baker, 1978). Furthermore, the reproductive deficiency of the adult hypogonadal mutant mouse (*hpg*), which cannot produce active GnRH due to a truncation of the GnRH gene (Mason et al., 1986a), is overcome at least in part by the implantation of normal fetal or neonatal septal-preoptic tissue containing GnRH neurons into the third ventricle (Gibson et al., 1984a, b; Krieger and Gibson, 1984). In addition, the reproductive capacity of the *hpg* mouse is completely restored by gene therapy, in which the wild-type mouse GnRH gene is introduced into the mutant mouse germ line (Mason et al., 1986b). These results indicate that in mammals, reproductive functions are heavily (if not solely) dependent on the GnRH gene and its products.

A.   Pulsatile Secretion of LH

In all animals, LH secretion is pulsatile, and the pattern of LH secretion is dictated by a pulse generator consisting of the GnRH neurons or systems driving the GnRH cells. The importance of pulsatile presentation of GnRH is well illustrated by comparing LH release in animals bearing hypothalamic lesions that receive identical amounts of GnRH by constant vs. pulsatile replacement (Figure 1). LH secretion is strongly stimulated by pulsatile administration of GnRH; in the absence of pulsatile release, LH secretion is markedly attenuated (Belchetz et al., 1978). In females of many species, the pattern of pulsatility of LH varies with the reproductive cycle. In the female rat, for example, LH concentrations in serum reach a maximum on the afternoon of proestrus, then decline to basal levels during estrus and diestrus (Gay and Midgley, 1969). The pattern of basal LH secretion during diestrus-1, diestrus-2, and during proestrus before the LH surge is pulsatile, while during estrus, LH pulses are undetectable (Fox and Smith, 1985; Higuchi and Kawakami, 1982). LH interpulse intervals are similar during diestrus-1, diestrus-2, and proestrus before the LH surge, with average values of 50 min. In contrast, the amplitude of LH pulses varies throughout the estrus cycle. A low level of LH secretion essential for follicle growth and maturation characterizes the diestrus period. The pattern of LH release changes abruptly on the afternoon of proestrus (Fox and Smith, 1985). The onset of the proestrus LH surge is typified by an abrupt and sharp increase of plasma LH levels. The proestrus LH surge peaks within 3 hr, with concentrations reaching approximately 100 times basal levels. The fall in LH levels occurs rapidly over the first 3 hr after the peak but then slows considerably, so that basal concentrations are not reached until the early morning of estrus. LH secretion during the transition to surge LH release is still pulsatile. However, LH secretion during the rising phase of the LH surge appears to occur smoothly and in a nonpulsatile fashion.

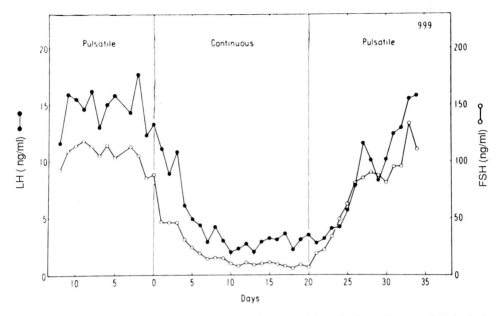

Figure 1. Comparison of plasma LH (filled circles) and FSH (open circles) after intermittent (1 μg/min for 6 min, once per hour) vs. continuous (1 μg/min) GnRH infusion in an ovariectomized rhesus monkey with a radio-frequency lesion in the hypothalamus; gonadotropin secretion was markedly suppressed by continuous infusion, but was reestablished by the intermittent mode of GnRH stimulation. The vertical lines beneath the LH data points on days 10 and 13 of continuous infusion indicate values below the sensitivity of the radioimmunoassay. (From Belchetz, P. E., Plant, T. M., Nakai, Y., Keogh, E. J., and Knobil, E., *Science*, 202, 631, 1978.)

B.   Role of GnRH in LH Secretion: Passive or Active?

While the notion that GnRH is required for LH release is well accepted, great controversy has surrounded the issue of whether GnRH *actively* regulates the ovulatory LH surge. Rhesus monkeys bearing a hypothalamic lesion that abolished endogenous GnRH production show ovulatory menstrual cycles after unvarying, pulsatile GnRH replacement (Knobil et al., 1980). This finding suggested that GnRH plays a permissive role in the menstrual cycle and that the preovulatory surge of LH in rhesus monkeys is dependent on estrogen-induced increases in the pituitary responses to GnRH. Yet the weight of more recent evidence suggests an alternate hypothesis. An increase in GnRH content has been reported in samples from hypophysial portal blood or in push-pull perfusates from the median eminence during the LH surge in the rat (Levine and Ramirez, 1982; Sarkar et al., 1976), rabbit (Kaynard et al., 1990; Tsou et al., 1977), monkey (Levine et al., 1985; Neill et al., 1977), and sheep (Clarke and Cummins, 1982; Schillo et al., 1985). Changing GnRH levels were temporally correlated with the preovulatory LH surges (Sarkar et al., 1976), as is shown in Figure 2.

Gonadal estrogens dictate the changes in GnRH secretion. In rats, ovariectomy on the morning of diestrus significantly reduces the concentration of GnRH in hypophysial portal blood on the afternoon of expected proestrus, while the subcutaneous injection of estradiol benzoate immediately after ovariectomy restored the GnRH concentration in the hypophysial blood to that seen on the afternoon of proestrus in intact female rats (Fink et al., 1978; Sarkar and Fink, 1979). These results suggested that increased GnRH secretion accompanies the estradiol-induced LH surge. The fact that estradiol changes can support an LH surge does not preclude the presence of a GnRH surge. Thus, in species like primates, the pituitary-driven LH surge may have evolved as a "fail safe" mechanism that operates along with a GnRH surge to ensure successful induction of ovulation.

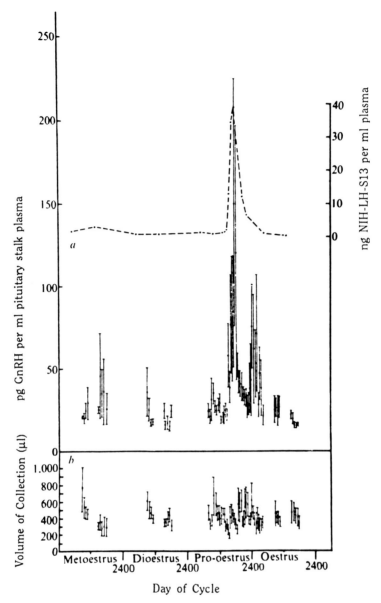

Figure 2. Pattern of plasma LH concentration (dotted line), GnRH concentration (a), and sample volume (b) during the estrous cycle. Note that a clear surge of GnRH accompanies the LH surge on the afternoon of proestrus. (From Sarkar, D. M., Chiappa, S. A., and Fink, G., *Nature (London)*, 264, 461, 1976.)

Studies in ewes illustrate that both GnRH surges and hypothalamic independent steroid-induced changes in LH secretion can coexist. Using an experimental model similar to that described above for the monkey, Clarke and Cummins (1984) induced surge-like LH secretion in the sheep with injections of estrogen. The GnRH-clamped steroid-induced response was smaller than the normal surge, suggesting that enhanced sensitivity of the gonadotroph to GnRH cannot completely account for the normal LH surge in the sheep. More recently, advances in technology have permitted monitoring of portal blood in ambulatory ewes at the same time peripheral plasma was collected (Moenter et al., 1990). With this approach, a clear surge of GnRH accompanied the LH surge induced by estrogen treatment (Figure 3). More-

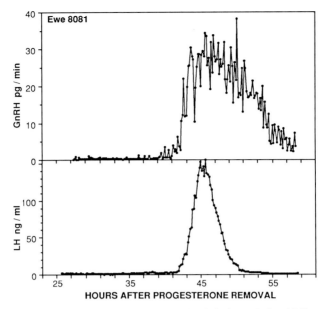

Figure 3. Patterns of GnRH (portal blood) and LH (jugular blood) during an induced LH surge in a ewe. (From Moenter, S. M., Caraty, A., and Karsch, F. J., *Endocrinology,* 127, 1375, 1990.)

over, at times other than the preovulatory surge, LH pulses were driven by GnRH bursts. These data confirm the notion that GnRH plays an active role in LH secretion and demonstrate that while gonadal steroids can support an LH surge without changes in GnRH secretion, a GnRH preovulatory surge still occurs. How GnRH surges are regulated is now under active investigation. As will be discussed below, the diffuse nature of GnRH neurons is one factor that has hampered investigation of the activity of individual GnRH neurons.

II. The GnRH Gene

The GnRH gene expressed in neural tissue has four exons. The first contains the 5′-untranslated region. Exon 2 codes for the signal peptide, the GnRH decapeptide, the enzymatic amidation site, the precursor processing site, and the N-terminal 11 amino acids of the gonadotropin-releasing hormone associate peptide (GAP). Exon 3 codes for the next 32 GAP residues and exon 4 contains the coding region for the last 13 amino acids of GAP, the termination codon, and the entire 3′-untranslated region of the mRNA (Adelman et al., 1986; Seeburg and Adelman, 1984). The large GAP protein, found within all GnRH-containing structures in the brain, is released along with GnRH, but its function remains unknown.

III. Neuroanatomy of the GnRH System

An understanding of the neuroanatomical localization of GnRH and its circuitry is fundamental to understanding the physiological regulation of GnRH activity. Mapping the GnRH system using immunocytochemical techniques proved difficult compared to other peptide systems. Controversies over the localization of GnRH arose because (1) the organization of GnRH systems in vertebrates varies; (2) unlike other neuroendocrine systems such as the magnocellular vasopressin and oxytocin neurons or the CRH neuroendocrine system, the

GnRH system is not confined to discrete classical anatomical nuclei, (3) the total number of GnRH neurons is small; and (4) GnRH within neurons is labile owing to the ease with which the peptide is extracted during routine histological preparation.

A.   GnRH Cell Location

The initial descriptions of GnRH cell location were confusing and there was resistance to relinquishing the expectation that GnRH neurons should reside in defined cytoarchitectonic boundaries. As techniques for localizing GnRH improved, the controversies resolved. With both immunocytochemistry of LHRH (reviewed by Barry et al., 1984) or portions of its precursor (Ronnekleiv et al., 1989) a consistent pattern of GnRH neuron location in the rat has emerged. The location of GnRH cells in the rat (Ronnekleiv et al., 1989; Seeburg et al., 1987; Zoeller et al., 1988), mouse (Mason et al., 1986b), and primate (Standish et al., 1987) has been confirmed with *in situ* hybridization techniques localizing the mRNA for GnRH. In the rat, GnRH cells form a diffuse Y-shaped network with the single stem of the 'Y' arching through the midline septum and diagonal band of Broca into the medial aspect of the olfactory bulbs along the nervus terminalis, and the two other limbs stretching caudally and ventrolaterally into the anterior hypothalamus (Figure 4). The GnRH perikarya are most heavily concentrated in the vicinity of the organum vasculosum of the lamina terminalis (OVLT) (Wray and Hoffman, 1986a) and the GnRH-positive fibers are most dense in the median eminence and the OVLT (Barry et al., 1984). The projections of the GnRH cells to the median eminence are diverse (Figure 5), with four prominent tracts to the median eminence in the rat: one that arises in the preoptic area and which follows the ventral surface of the brain between the optic nerves and then courses beneath the optic chiasm to enter the median eminence from the ventral surface (Figure 6), a second tract that courses along the floor of the third ventricle to the rostral median eminence, a third tract from the preoptic area and rostral septum that courses along the lateral walls of the third ventricle and then fans out through the arcuate nucleus to the median eminence, and a fourth tract that arises from the more lateral and caudal GnRH cells and which courses along with the medial forebrain bundle to the median eminence. The lateral tract is most prominent in the rat. However, when lesions are made that sever the ventricular and lateral paths, reproductive function can be maintained by the subchiasmatic tract (Hoffman and Gibbs, 1982).

In other species, the perikaryal staining patterns were less controversial (Barry et al., 1984), but comparisons between species were equally confusing (Table 1). In cat, sheep, pig, and hamster, like the murine rodents (shown for the rat in Figure 7), the GnRH neurons are concentrated within the forebrain in or near the preoptic area, with only a few cells extending into the hypothalamus. In the guinea pig, the pattern generally was similar to the other rodents, but a greater number of GnRH neurons were found within the arcuate nucleus. Location of GnRH neurons in primates and humans revealed a large number of GnRH cells located in the ventrolateral hypothalamus near the median eminence as well as in the preoptic area (Figure 8); scattered GnRH neurons in the anterior hypothalamus bridge these populations. Similarly, in dog and rabbit, the GnRH neurons are evenly spread throughout the preoptic area and hypothalamus. In bats and ferrets (shown for the ferret in Figure 9), GnRH neurons are concentrated in the medial basal hypothalamus and extend into the pituitary stalk; only a few cells are found within the preoptic area. In contrast, in the South American opossum, GnRH neurons are clustered in a ganglion-like structure at the rostral-most tip of the forebrain. In nonmammalian vertebrates similar diversity is noted. In many of the species discussed above, "stray" GnRH neurons can be found in any location where GnRH axons project, including the cerebral cortex, amygdala, midbrain central gray, and hippocampus (Hoffman, 1983). While it appeared initially that species differences in GnRH cell location might make generalization from one species to another impossible, there are two unifying principles of GnRH cell distribution: GnRH neurons avoid defined nuclear clusters and the cells lay interspersed between cytoarchitectonically defined nuclei rather than within them (Figure 10); GnRH neurons are certain to lie within a continuum extending from the olfactory bulbs, at varying distances through the midline septum to the ventral hypothalamus (Figure 11).

B.   GnRH Development

Since GnRH neurons in the forebrain spanned neuronal areas normally arising from different sites on the neuroepithelium, it had been assumed that the GnRH system had multiple embryonic origins (Krey and Silverman, 1983). Curiously, throughout the vertebrate class, GnRH neurons were found outside the central nervous system as well as within it. Immunopositive GnRH neurons resided in olfactory areas, specifically within the nervus terminalis, in a number of postnatal animals (Jennes, 1987; Muske and Moore, 1987; Schwanzel- Fukuda and Silverman, 1980; Silverman et al., 1982). The nervus terminalis is a structure that originates, along with the vomeronasal complex, from the olfactory placode and migrates centrally to contact the developing forebrain (Bojsen-Moller, 1975; Brown, 1987; Oelschlager et al., 1987). From this contact point, along the ventral surface of the telencephalon, the nervus terminalis continues into the brain along the ventromedial surface of the olfactory bulbs to septal and preoptic areas (Bojsen-Moller, 1975; Brown, 1987; Garcia et al., 1987; Oelschlager et al., 1987). These same forebrain areas contain GnRH neurons. Comparison of the topography of the nervus terminalis and GnRH neurons in a variety of adult amphibians led Muske and Moore (1987) to speculate that forebrain GnRH neurons do not develop from the ventricular epithelium, but arise with the nervus terminalis from the olfactory placode.

Recently, a number of independent studies have reevaluated the prenatal development of the GnRH system in the mouse (Schwanzel-Fukuda and Pfaff, 1989; Wray, 1989; Wray et al., 1989a, b), rhesus monkey (Ronnekliev and Resko, 1990), and chicken (Norgren and Lehman, 1990), using immunocytochemistry. Each study indicated that GnRH neurons are first found in the vicinity of the olfactory placode and then the GnRH cells appear to migrate through the nasal septum into the forebrain. One example is illustrated in Figure 12. *In situ* hybridization histochemical techniques offered further understanding of the origin of GnRH neurons. In the mouse, the numbers of cells expressing GnRH mRNA 1 day after the GnRH neurons left the mitotic cycle equalled that seen in adults; yet 90% of the cells were located within the nasal regions. Over the next 4 days, the number of cells expressing GnRH decreased in nasal regions and concomitantly increased in forebrain areas, with no change in the total cell number (Wray, 1989; Wray et al., 1989c). Moreover, birth-dating studies of GnRH neurons using combined autoradiography of [³H] thymidine and immunocytochemistry showed that (1) within hours after [³H] thymidine labeling, labeled GnRH neurons were only found next to the olfactory pit, not the ventricles of the forebrain (Schwanzel-Fukuda and Pfaff, 1989), and (2) GnRH neurons arose as a single population, leaving the mitotic cycle shortly after differentiation of the olfactory placode at a time just prior to GnRH mRNA expression in cells of the olfactory pit (Wray, 1989; Wray et al., 1989c). These studies strengthen the evidence for a nasal origin of all GnRH cells, including those found in the central nervous system, and demonstrate a migratory path of GnRH neurons through nasal and then forebrain areas to establish the adult-like GnRH distribution.

Species differences in GnRH position within the brain appear to result from greater (bat, ferret, human, monkey, dog, rabbit, guinea pig) or lesser (opossum, birds, fish, reptiles, amphibians, rodents, cat) penetration along the olfactory-forebrain-hypothalamic continuum

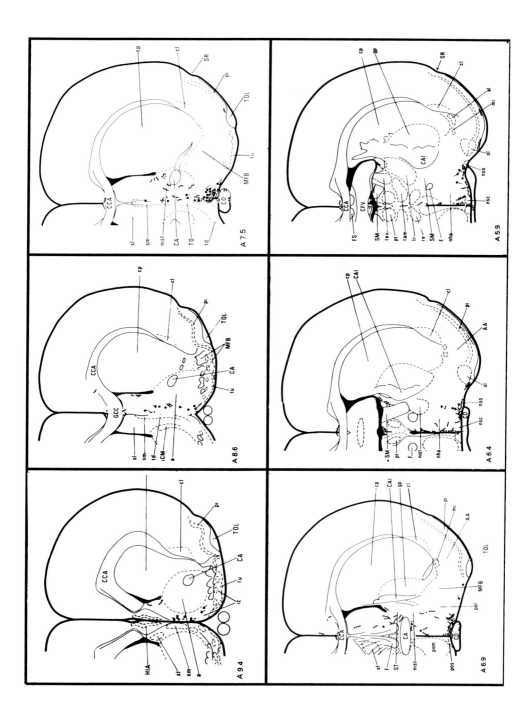

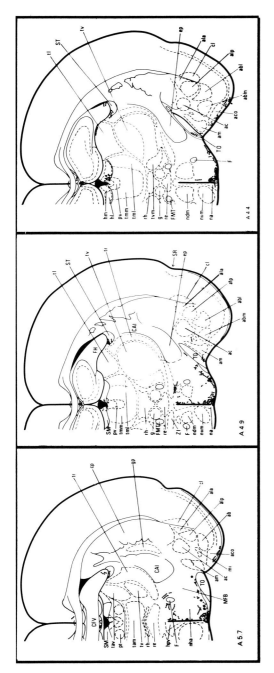

Figure 4. The organization of the GnRH system in the rat, illustrated in a series of coronal sections throughout the rostral forebrain and hypothalamus. (Modified from Barry et al., 1984.)

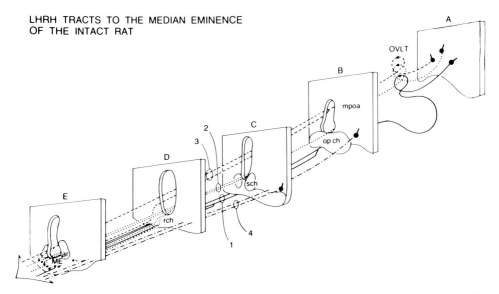

Figure 5. Illustration of the course that GnRH axons take to the median eminence. (From Hoffman, G. and Gibbs, F., *Neuroscience*, 7, p. 1979, 1982.)

(Figure 11) to the median eminence. Moreover, this unusual developmental pattern explains another of the odd characteristics of GnRH neurons: like olfactory epithelial cells that remain in the nasal cavities, GnRH neurons have cilia (Jennes et al., 1985; Kozlowski et al., 1980). From a functional perspective, the association of the GnRH neurons with the nasal epithelium may represent a vestige of the pheromonal control of reproductive function. Evidence that a link between olfactory function and GnRH activity in humans was thought to be provided by Kallmann's disorder, a syndrome characterized by hypogonadism and anosmia. In a familial subclass of the syndrome, premature closure or thickening of the cribiform plate locks out both the migrating GnRH neurons and the axons of the olfactory nerves (Schwanzel-Fukuda et al., 1989). It is likely that other forms of the syndrome result from similar processes.

C.   GnRH Morphology and Synchrony

In the rat, GnRH neurons are small (approximately 10 to 12 μm in diameter) and relatively few in number (approximately 1200; Wray and Hoffman, 1986b). In primates the numbers are somewhat increased (approximately 5000) but the GnRH population remains small in comparison to other neuroendocrine systems. In rat, GnRH neurons are categorized as smooth or spiny according to their contour (Jennes et al., 1985; Kozlowski et al., 1980; Krisch, 1980; Liposits et al., 1984; Wray and Hoffman, 1986b). The two subtypes are illustrated in Figure 13. At the time of birth, most GnRH neurons are smooth (Wray and Hoffman, 1986b). However, during postnatal life there is a shift from smooth to spiny that plateaus at the time of puberty. Removal of the GnRH neurons from the brain and placement in culture arrests the shift from smooth to spiny (Wray et al., 1988), suggesting that extrinsic connections or hormonal factors are necessary for the maturational process. One study suggested that spiny cells receive a more dense innervation than smooth cells (Jennes et al., 1985). However, Witkin and Demasio (1990) later demonstrated that there was no difference in the incidence of synapses or in the density of synaptic input in smooth and spiny GnRH neurons. Spiny GnRH neurons did possess significantly greater numbers of Golgi complexes and mitochondria, suggesting that the two subtypes have different metabolic states. A survey of GnRH cell morphology across

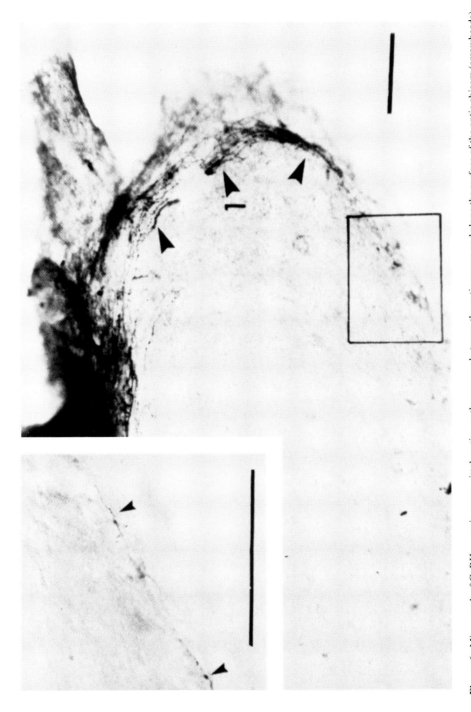

Figure 6. Micrograph of GnRH axons in parasagittal section as they course between the optic nerves and along the surface of the optic chiasm (arrowheads). The inset shows a GnRH axon coursing underneath the optic chiasm. Bar: 100 μm. (From Hoffman, G. and Gibbs, F., *Neuroscience*, 7, p. 1979, 1982.)

Table 1
Diversity of Distribution of GnRH Neurons in Mammals

	Septum	Preoptic area	Anterior Hypothalamus	Medial Hypothalamus	Premammilary body
Rodents					
Mouse	++	++++	++	+/−	−
Hamster	+++	++++	+	−	−
Rat	++	++++	++	+/−	−
Guinea pig	+	+++	++	+	−
Lagomorphs					
Rabbit	++	+++	+	+	+
Chiroptera					
Bats	−/+	−/+	+	++++	−
Carnivores					
Ferrets	−/+	+	+	++++	−
Dogs	+	++	++	++	+
Cats	+	+++	++	−	−
Ungulates					
Sheep	++	++++	+	−	−
Pigs	++	++++	+	−	−
Marsupials					
South American opossum	+++	−	−	−	−
Primates					
Rhesus monkey	++	++++	++	+++	+
Baboon	++	++++	++	+++	+

different species reveals that spines do not accompany GnRH neurons in all species, as is shown for the ferret in Figure 14, casting doubt on the applicability of spines as a marker of cell activity. To date, the significance of this interesting characteristic still remains a mystery.

Apart from spines, the morphology of GnRH neurons is varied and intriguing and may underlie the ability of GnRH neurons to synchronously burst. For example, GnRH neurons receive GnRH synapses (Leranth et al., 1985b; Pelletier, 1987; Witkin and Silverman, 1985; Wray and Gainer, 1987); examples of this interaction at the light and electron microscopic level are shown in Figures 15 and 16. The synaptic connections between GnRH neurons may explain the synchronization of GnRH signals responsible for the induction of the LH surge. In addition, GnRH neurons may interact through dendrodendritic communication. In primates, for example, dendritic processes from one GnRH neuron appear to contact neighboring GnRH cells (Marshall and Goldsmith, 1980; Hoffman, unpublished), as shown in Figure 17.

Another striking feature of GnRH neurons is their relationship with the vasculature. GnRH neurons, or their dendrites, lie closely apposed to small blood vessels (Figure 18) (Hoffman, 1983). Ultrastructural examination of this relationship reveals GnRH perikarya or dendrites lying immediately outside the basement membrane of the capillaries (Figure 19). This anatomical relationship may facilitate the delivery of blood-borne factors, such as gonadal steroids, capable of crossing the blood-brain barrier to influence GnRH function.

D.   Neuroendocrine Nature of Most GnRH Neurons

The broad spatial distribution of GnRH neurons and their unique morphology beg the

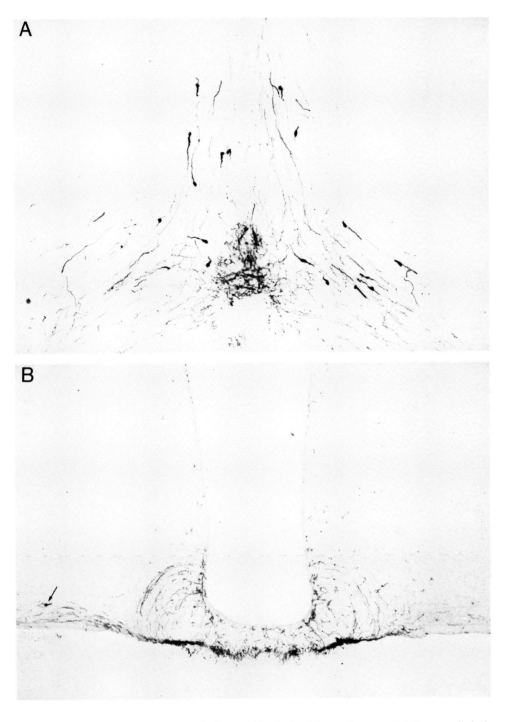

Figure 7. Concentration of GnRH neurons in the rostral forebrain of the rat. Numerous GnRH neurons lie in the region of the organum vasculosum of the lamina terminalis (A), while only an occasional GnRH neuron (arrow) is found in the medial basal hypothalamus (B).

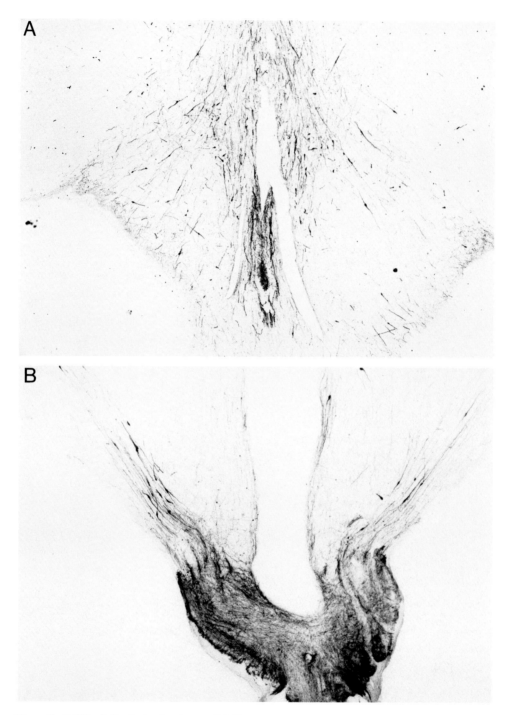

Figure 8. GnRH cell distribution in primates. GnRH neurons are numerous both within the preoptic area (A) and basal hypothalamus (B).

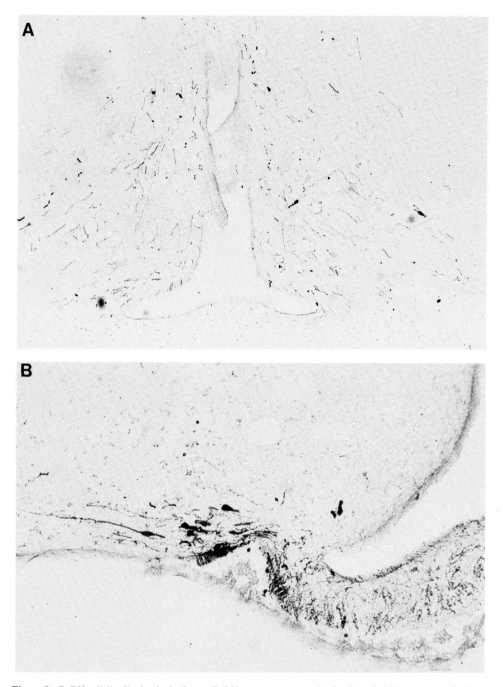

Figure 9. GnRH cell distribution in the ferret. GnRH neurons are sparsely distributed within the rostral forebrain, including the preoptic area (A); rather, most GnRH neurons are found within the region immediately surrounding the median eminence (B).

Gloria E. Hoffman, Wen-Sen Lee, and Susan Wray

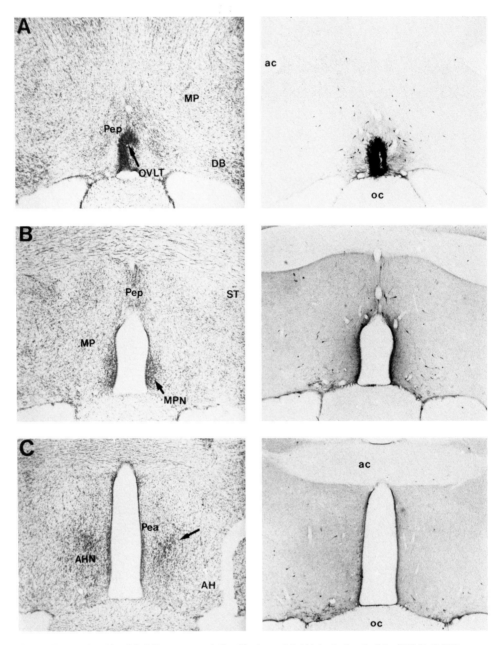

Figure 10. Relationship of GnRH neurons to defined brain nuclei. (A) At the level of the OVLT, GnRH neurons appear to ignore cytoarchitectonic boundaries of the medial preoptic nucleus (MPN), preoptic periventricular nucleus (Pe), and other nuclei. Rather, the cells are scattered about as if the boundaries were absent. (B) At a more caudal area, the GnRH neurons lie between the medial preoptic area (MPO) and lateral preoptic area (LPO), as well as along the midline above the anterior commissure. (C) At the level of the sexual dimorphic nucleus (arrow) GnRH neurons are now located along the border between the medial and lateral preoptic nuclei. (Micrograph provided by courtesy of Dr. Stanley Wiegand.)

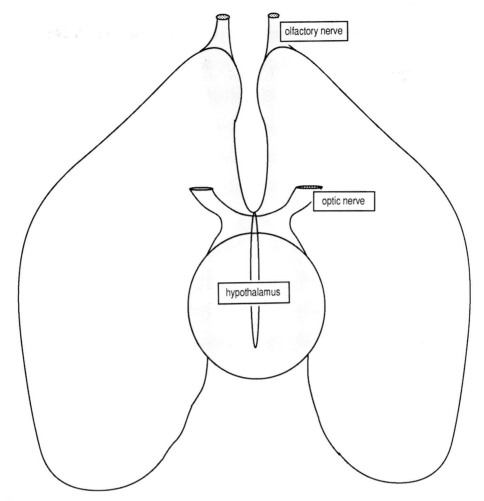

Figure 11. Diagrammatic view of the brain seen from its ventral surface. The shaded area, which extends from the olfactory nerves, through the olfactory bulbs, rostral forebrain, preoptic area, and hypothalamus, marks the possible areas where GnRH neurons generally lie.

question of whether GnRH neurons throughout the GnRH cell field participate in the regulation of LH secretion, or whether discrete subpopulations have different roles. Long before the GnRH neurons were identified, Halasz and Gorski (1967) proposed that two populations of gonadotrophin-releasing hormone neurons existed: one in the medial basal hypothalamus that was responsible for tonic release of LH, and another in the preoptic area that affected the phasic release of LH during the surge. While GnRH neurons are not present in significant numbers in the rodent medial basal hypothalamus, there is reason to suspect that there are functionally distinct populations of GnRH neurons that project to the median eminence. Virtually all GnRH neurons project to circumventricular organs of the brain that lack a blood-brain barrier (Witkin, 1990), with approximately 70% projecting to the median eminence (Merchanthaler et al., 1989). The neurons that project to the median eminence are scattered throughout the entire GnRH cell field. King et al. (1987) have examined changes in GnRH staining following

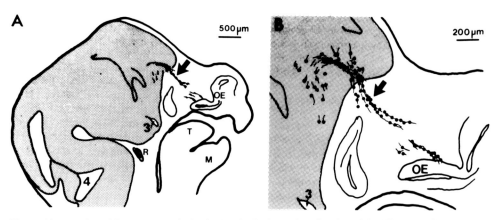

Figure 12. Location of GnRH neurons in the fetal rat brain shows the migration of GnRH neurons from the nasal placode into the forebrain. (From Wray, S., Neiburgs, A., and Elkabes, S., *Dev. Brain Res.*, 46, 309, 1989a.)

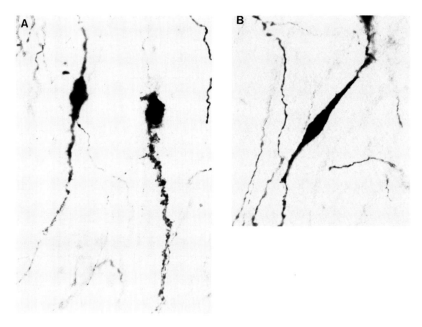

Figure 13. GnRH neurons are of two morphologic types in the rat: (a) spiny and (b) smooth.

castration using GnRH antisera that recognize different epitopes on the GnRH molecule. Select populations of GnRH neurons differ in their intensity of staining during times of increased LH secretion. Furthermore, these same subpopulations of GnRH neurons appear to have altered levels of mRNA for GnRH as revealed with *in situ* hybridization (Wray et al., 1989b; Zoeller et al., 1988). While these data suggest that activity in a subpopulation of GnRH neurons is changing, direct evidence that the synthetic activity is linked to neuronal activity is lacking.

E.   Activation of GnRH Neurons During an GnRH Surge: Which Cells?

Until recently, the difficulty in addressing the issue of changing activity within GnRH

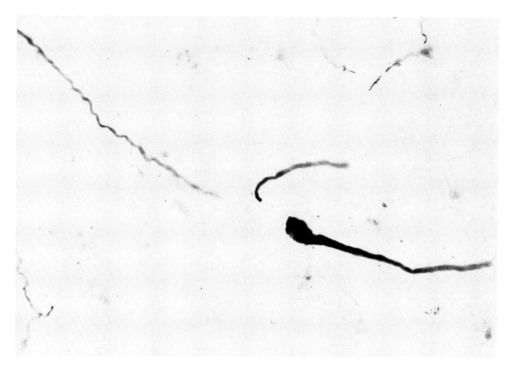

Figure 14. GnRH neurons appear to lack spines in the ferret.

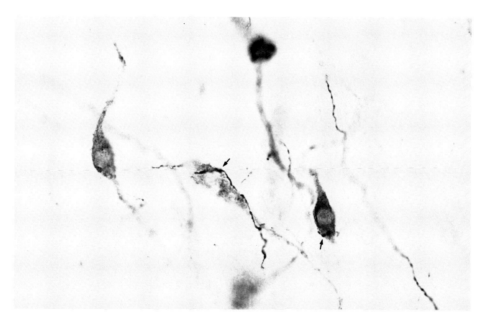

Figure 15. GnRH neurons are contacted by axons from nearby GnRH neurons (arrow).

neurons was largely due to the absence of experimental techniques for measuring responses of individual GnRH neurons. For such small and diffusely scattered GnRH neurons, electrical measurements are not practical. Alternative approaches, using such as 2-[^{3}H]deoxyglucose, lacked the cellular resolution required for identification of GnRH cells within the midst of

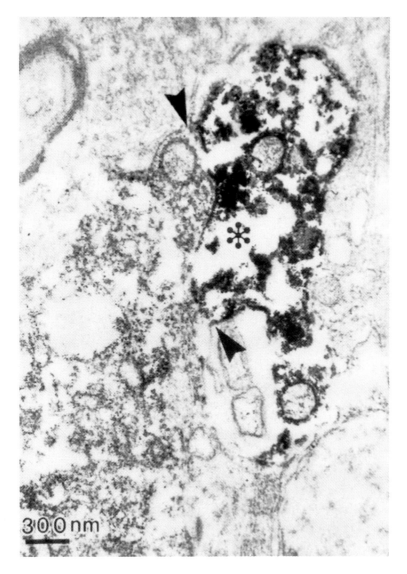

Figure 16. A GnRH neuron receives a synapse from a GnRH terminal. (From Wray, S. and Gainer, H., *Neuroendocrinology*, 45, 413, 1987.)

other neurons. Recently a marker has become available that allows stimulated neurons to be identified and distinguished from neurons that are not activated (Sagar et al., 1988). The marker is the protooncogene product c-Fos. GnRH neurons normally do not express c-Fos. However c-Fos expression is induced within 45 min following electrochemical stimulation and during induced or spontaneous LH surges (Hoffman et al., 1990; Lee et al., 1990a, b). An analysis of the location of stimulated GnRH neurons expressing c-Fos during the peak of an LH surge identifies a subpopulation of GnRH neurons in the vicinity of the organum vasculosum of the lamina terminalis (OVLT) below the anterior commissure, extending into the preoptic area and anterior hypothalamus, which actively participates in the LH surge (Figure 20). Interestingly, the GnRH neurons located above the anterior commissure and rostral to the

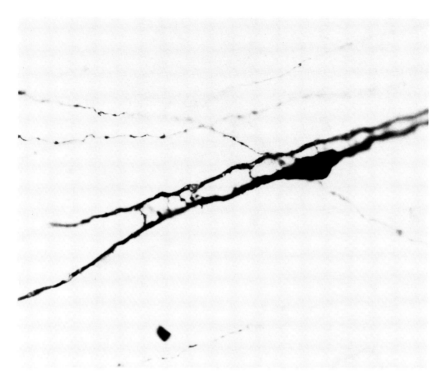

Figure 17. Two neighboring GnRH neurons in the monkey hypothalamus appear to share numerous bridge-like processes.

OVLT remain "quiet" during an LH surge. The activated GnRH population may have been targeted by selective innervation of GnRH neurons. GnRH neurons contacted by catecholamine or neurotensin axons (Hoffman, 1985) are distributed in a pattern similar to that observed for *fos* expression in GnRH neurons during a surge.

F.   Afferents to the GnRH Neurons

One of the first reports of GnRH ultrastructure suggested that GnRH neurons are not innervated. Following more rigorous examination, GnRH neurons are innervated (Figure 21), although sparsely compared to neighboring neurons (Lehman, 1988; Witkin and Silverman, 1985). Yet a vast literature (Kalra, 1986, for review) supports the notion that specialized afferents stimulate or inhibit the release of GnRH. Light microscopic examination of GnRH and other transmitter systems suggested that catecholamines (Hoffman, 1985; Hoffman et al., 1982; Jennes et al., 1982, 1983; Lehman et al., 1988), serotonin (Jennes et al., 1982), substance P (Hoffman, 1985), neurotensin (Hoffman, 1985), opioid peptides (Hoffman et al., 1988), corticotropin-releasing hormone (CRH) (MacLusky et al., 1988), and γ-aminobutyric acid (GABA) (Jennes et al., 1983) provide direct regulation of GnRH neurons. Electron microscopy has verified synaptic relations between the GnRH neurons and ACTH/endorphin (Leranth et al., 1988), catecholamines (Kuljis and Advis, 1989; Leranth et al., 1989), corticotropin-releasing factor (CRF) (MacLusky et al., 1988), GABA (Leranth et al., 1985a), 5-hydroxytryptamine (5-HT) (Kiss and Halasz, 1985), neuropeptide Y (Norgren and Lehman, 1989), and substance P (Tsuruo et al., 1990) terminals. An example of a synaptic contact of an NPY terminal on a GnRH neuron is shown in Figure 22. From a physiological standpoint our understanding of the

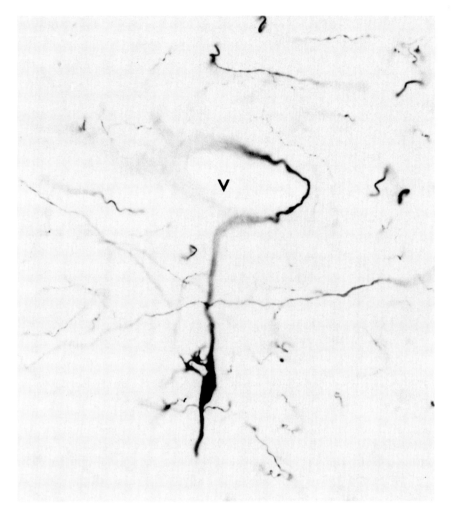

Figure 18. GnRH processes are found in close apposition to small blood vessels. This cell, from a rhesus monkey, has a dendritic process that appears to wrap around a small blood vessel.

control of GnRH release is still growing. Yet through the scores of reports demonstrating pharmacologic effects of agonists and antagonists on these systems, a more focused picture of GnRH regulation is emerging with the catecholamines, excitatory amino acids, and opioid peptides as key regulators of GnRH release.

1. Catecholamines

Abundant evidence indicates that catecholamines may be involved in triggering the proestrous surges of LH and GnRH. Sawyer and associates first demonstrated that administration of norepinephrine into the third ventricle of estrous rabbits increased LH secretion and resulted in ovulation (Sawyer, 1952; Sawyer et al., 1975) whereas injection of an α-adrenergic antagonist, dibenamine, inhibited ovulation (Sawyer et al., 1947). These observations led to the hypothesis that norepinephrine-containing neurons play a stimulatory role in the release of LH.

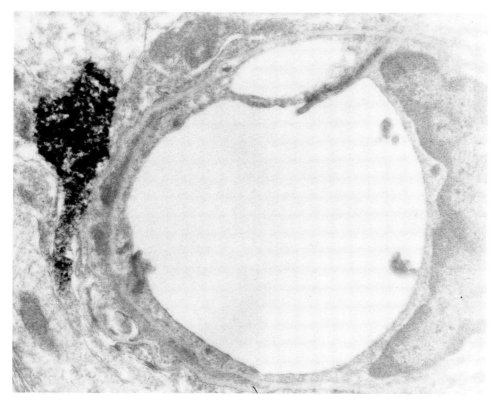

Figure 19. Electron micrograph of a GnRH neuron process lying adjacent to the basement membrane of a small capillary.

a.   Norepinephrine

A role for norepinephrine in the induction of the proestrous LH surge was further supported by several findings. (1) Hypothalamic norepinephrine content (Stefano and Donoso, 1967), synthesis (Zschaeck and Wurtman, 1973), and turnover (Donoso and Moyano, 1970) are increased prior to the LH surge in adult cyclic rats or in prepubertal females treated with serum gonadotropin from a pregnant mare (Agnati et al., 1977; Lofstrom, 1977; Negro-Vilar et al., 1977). (2) Intraventricular injection of norepinephrine stimulated ovulation in animals showing constant vaginal cornification after anterior hypothalamic lesions, continuous illumination, or neonatal administration of androgen (Tima and Flerko, 1974, 1975). (3) Intrahypothalamic infusions of norepinephrine into the median eminence of pentobarbital-blocked, iproniazid-treated rats induced ovulation (Craven and McDonald, 1971). (4) Administration of DBH (dopamine β-hydroxylase) inhibitors prior to the critical period blocked the preovulatory LH surge (Drouva and Gallo, 1976; Kalra and McCann, 1974). (5) The proestrous LH surge can be reduced or eliminated by blocking this afternoon rise of norepinephrine turnover (Akabori and Barraclough, 1986; Rance and Barraclough, 1981), by the administration of an α_1-adrenergic antagonist such as phenoxybenzamine (Weick, 1978) or by destruction of the ventral norepinephrine pathway (Martinovic and McCann, 1977).

b.   Epinephrine

The role of epinephrine in the regulation of LH and GnRH secretion is similar to norepinephrine. Single intraventricular injections of epinephrine stimulated LH secretion in

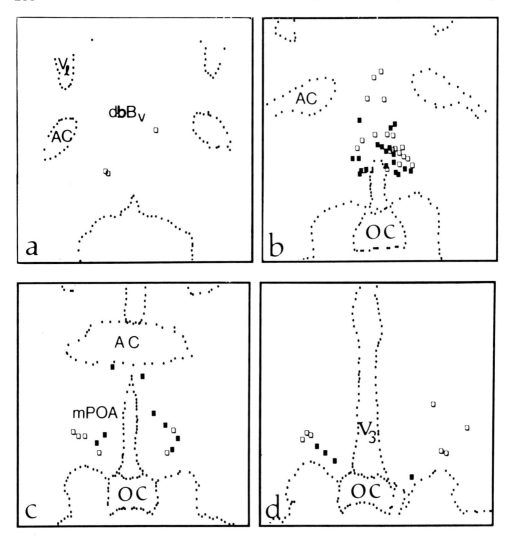

Figure 20. Pattern of c-Fos expression within GnRH neurons during the afternoon of proestrus at the time of the LH surge. The distribution is shown within four levels of the GnRH cell field selected at 300-μm intervals. The level of the vertical limb of the diagonal band of Broca (dbBv) in the rostral forebrain (a); the level of the OVLT where LHRH neurons are most abundant (b); the level of the crossing of the anterior commissure (AC) and the medial preoptic area (mPOA) (c); and the juncture of the caudal pole of the preoptic area and anterior hypothalamus (d). Filled squares, GnRH neurons containing c-Fos immunoreactivity; open squares, GnRH neurons devoid of c-Fos immunoreactivity. Note that the activated GnRH neurons lie near the OVLT or caudal to it and lie below the anterior commissure. (From Lee, W.-S., Smith, M. S., and Hoffman, G. E., *Proc. Natl. Acad. Sci. U.S.A.*, 1990b.)

ovariectomized estrogen/progesterone-primed rats (Vijayan and McCann, 1978). Intraventricular administration of epinephrine was effective in overriding the blockade of ovulation by pentobarbital in the rat (Rubenstein and Sawyer, 1970). Some of the lesion studies cited above also could be interpreted as evidence for an effect of epinephrine since the noradrenergic and adrenergic axons travel together as they ascend to the hypothalamus and preoptic area. The presence of immunoreactivity for the enzyme that converts norepinephrine to epinephrine in the preoptic area recently in apposition to GnRH neurons (Casteneyra-Perdomo et al., 1988), offers more direct evidence that epinephrine-secreting neurons may regulate GnRH secretion.

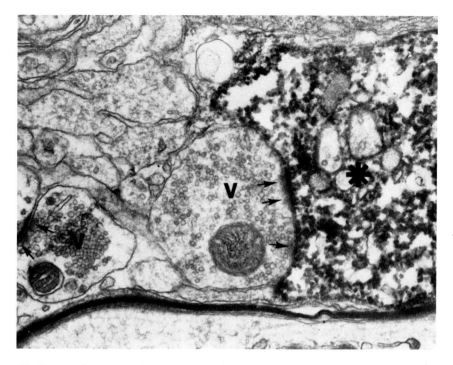

Figure 21. Synapse of a nerve terminal (arrows) on an immunoreactive GnRH neuron (asterisk). (From Lehman, M. N., *J. Comp. Neurol.*, 273, 447, 1988.)

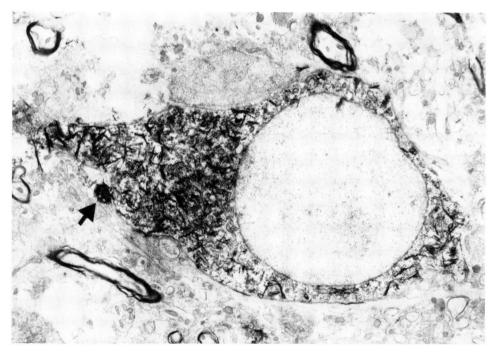

Figure 22. NPY terminal synapses on an immunoreactive GnRH neuron (arrow). (From Norgren, R. B. and Lehman, M. N., *Neurosci. Abstr.*, 16, 649, 1990.)

c.   Dopamine

In contrast to the roles of central norepinephrine and epinephrine systems, the role of dopaminergic system in the regulation of LH and GnRH release still remains a matter of dispute. Dopamine has been postulated to have both stimulatory and inhibitory actions in the regulation of LH secretion. Intraventricular administration of dopamine stimulates LH secretion in the ovariectomized estrogen/progesterone-primed rat (Vijayan and McCann, 1978), and dopamine also stimulates GnRH release from the mediobasal hypothalamus and median eminence *in vitro* (Negro-Vilar et al., 1979; Rotszstein et al., 1976), suggesting a GnRH-stimulating function of the dopaminergic system. However, there is considerable evidence that the central dopaminergic systems inhibit GnRH and LH release. Intraperitoneal administration of dopamine receptor agonists, such as ET 495 or apomorphine, reduces LH concentrations in intact or ovariectomized rats (Drouva and Gallo, 1977; Mueller et al., 1976). In castrated rats, blockade of dopamine receptors either has no effect on LH concentrations (Drouva and Gallo, 1976; Drouva and Gallo, 1977) or causes a further elevation (Gnodde and Schuiling, 1976). Moreover, several dopamine receptor agonists inhibit the LH surge induced in immature females by pregnant mare serum, but some dopamine receptor blockers, such as chlorpromazine, had the same effect (Agnati et al., 1977). Anatomic evidence indicates that catecholamine terminals on GnRH neurons persist after lesioning the noradrenergic and adrenergic axons ascending from the brainstem (Leranth et al., 1989). By virtue of the fact that the only remaining catecholamine systems are dopaminergic, these results support a direct dopaminergic input to GnRH neurons. Alternatively, these data may reflect a slow degeneration of noradrenergic axons following deafferentation. Clearly more direct evidence is needed to resolve this issue. With the new knowledge that neuropeptide Y is released along with the catecholamines, the entire issue of how these transmitters act is being reevaluated.

2.   Excitatory Amino Acids

Recently, the excitatory amino acids have been implicated in regulation of the preovulatory surges of LH and GnRH. Peripheral administration of L-glutamate or *N*-methyl-D-aspartic acid (NMDA) induces acute elevations of plasma LH levels in prepubertal and adult rats (Arslan et al., 1989; Ondo et al., 1976; Price et al., 1976). On the other hand, intraventricular administration of glutamate receptor antagonists such as 2-amino-7-phosphoheptanoic acid (AP-7) at 1300-hr blocks the estradiol-induced LH surge (Lopez et al., 1990). Since excitatory amino acids do not have a direct LH-releasing action on the pituitary (Schainker and Cicero, 1980), and the effects of NMDA can be blocked by the administration of a GnRH antagonist (Cicero et al., 1988), the action of excitatory amino acids on LH secretion seems to be exerted by modulating the secretion of GnRH from hypothalamus. *In vitro* studies confirm the direct stimulatory effect of excitatory amino acids on GnRH release. In male adult rats, excitatory amino acids such as L-glutamate, kainate, NMDA, and quisqualate stimulate GnRH release from nerve terminals in the arcuate nucleus-median eminence (Bourguignon et al., 1989; Donoso et al., 1990). Although it seems clear that excitatory amino acids can increase GnRH activity and trigger LH surges, the pathways by which these substances affect GnRH neurons have not been resolved. Difficulties in localizing excitatory amino acids in nerve terminals have left open the question of where these agents exert their actions.

3.   Opioid Peptides

A critical role in the timing of GnRH activity is played by opioid peptides. The natural proestrous stimulation of GnRH neurons is timed and predictable. The "critical period" for activation of GnRH neurons takes place 8 to 10 hr after the onset of daylight, during the afternoon of proestrus. Intravenous administration of the opioid antagonist naloxone will advance the LH surge on proestrus to as early as 1100 hr (Allen and Kalra, 1986; Allen et al., 1988). The advanced LH surge resembles the natural one in respect to its magnitude and duration. Steroids influence both opioid peptide synthesis and receptor number in the hypothalamus (Allen et al., 1988). Whether opioid influences are exerted directly on the GnRH neurons as is implied by synapses containing β-endorphin on GnRH neurons (Chen et al., 1988a, b; Leranth et al., 1988) and apposition of methionine enkephalin axons on GnRH neurons (Hoffman et al., 1988), or indirectly through effects on catecholamine systems (Kalra and Simpkins, 1981), is not yet resolved.

Acknowledgments

The authors would like to express their appreciation to Mr. Thomas Waters for expert photographic assistance. This research was supported by NIH Grant HD 13254 and NSF Grant BNS 8919953.

References

Adelman, J. P., Mason, A. J., and Seeburg, P. H., Isolation of the gene and hypothalamic cDNA for the common precursor of gonadotropin-releasing hormone and prolactin release inhibiting factor in human and rat, *Proc. Natl. Acad. Sci. U.S.A.*, 83, 179, 1986.

Agnati, L., Fuxe, K., Logstrom, A., and Hökfelt, T., Dopaminergic drugs and ovulation: studies on the PMS induced ovulation and changes in median eminence DA and NE turnover in immature female rats, *Adv. Biochem. Psychopharmacol.*, 16, 159, 1977.

Akabori, A. and Barraclough, C. A., Effects of morphine on luteinizing hormone secretion and catecholamine turnover in the hypothalamus of estrogen-treated rats, *Brain Res.*, 362, 221, 1986.

Allen, L. G. and Kalra, S.P., Evidence that a decrease in opioid tone may evoke preovulatory luteinizing hormone release in the rat, *Endocrinology*, 118, 2375, 1986.

Allen, L. G., Hahn, E., Caton, D., and Kalra, S. P., Evidence that a decrease in opioid tone on preestrus changes the episodic pattern of luteinizing hormone (LH) secretion: implications in the preovulatory LH hypersecretion, *Endocrinology*, 122, 1004, 1988.

Amos, M., Burgus, R., Blackwell, R., Vale, W., Fellows, R., and Guillemin, R., Purification, amino acid composition and N-terminis of the hypothalamic luteinizing hormone releasing factor (LRF) of bovine origin, *Biochem. Biophys. Res. Commun.*, 44, 205, 1971.

Arslan, M., Pohl, C. R., and Plant, T. M., DL-2-Amino-5-phosphopentanoic acid, a specific *N*-methyl-D-aspartic acid receptor antagonist suppresses pulsatile LH release in the rat, *Neuroendocrinology*, 47, 465, 1989.

Barry, J., Hoffman, G., and Wray, S., LHRH systems, in *Handbook of Chemical Neuroanatomy*, Bkörklund, A. and Hökfelt, T., Eds., Elsevier/North Holland, Amsterdam, 1984, 166.

Belchetz, P. E., Plant, T. M., Nakai, Y., Keogh, E. J., and Knobil, E., Hypophysial responses to continuous and intermittent delivery of hypothalamic gonadotropin-releasing hormone, *Science*, 202, 631, 1978.

Bojsen-Moller, F., Demonstration of terminalis olfactory, trigeminal, and perivascular nerves in the rat nasal septum, *J. Comp. Neurol.*, 159, 245, 1975.

Bourguignon, J. P., Gerard, A., and Francimont, P., Direct activation of gonadotropin-releasing hormone secretion through different receptors to neuroexcitatory amino acids, *Neuroendocrinology*, 49, 402, 1989.

Brown, J. W., The nervus terminalis in insectivorous bat embryos and notes on its presence during human ontogeny, in *The Terminal Nerve (Nervus Terminalis) Structure, Function and Evolution*, Dempski, L. and Schwanzel-Fukuda, M., Eds., N.Y. Academy of Sciences, New York, 1987, 184.

Campbell, H. J., Fever, G., Garcia , J., and Harris, G. W., The infusion of brain extracts into the anterior pituitary gland and the secretion of gonadotropic hormone, *J. Physiol. (London)*, 157, 30, 1961.

Casteneyra-Perdomo, A., Bennett, M., and Coen, C. W., Medullary projections to the luteinizing hormone releasing hormone formation of the rat: studies involving retrograde tracing and immuno-histochemistry for neuropeptide Y and phenylethanolamine *N*-methyltransferase, *Soc. Neurosci. Abstr.*, 14, No. 471.6, 1988.

Chen, W.-P., Witkin, J. W., and Silverman, A.-J., Beta endorphin and gonadotropin releasing hormone synaptic input to gonadotropin releasing hormone neurosecretory cells in the male rat, *J. Comp. Neurol.*, 286, 85, 1988a.

Chen, W.-P., Witkin, J. W., and Silverman, A.-J., Gonadotropin releasing hormone (GnRH) neurons are directly innervated by catecholamine terminals, *Synapse*, 3, 288, 1988b.

Cicero, T. J., Meyer, E. R., and Bell, R. D., Characterization and possible opioid modulation of *N*-methyl-D-aspartic acid induced increases in serum luteinizing hormone levels in the developing male rat, *Life Sci.*, 42, 1725, 1988.

Clarke, I. J. and Cummins, J. T., The temporal relationship between gonadotropin releasing hormone (GnRH) and luteinizing hormone (LH) secretion in ovariectomized ewe, *Endocrinology*, 111, 1737, 1982.

Clarke, I. J. and Cummins, J. T., Direct pituitary effects of estrogen and progesterone on gonadotropin secretion in the ovariectomized ewe, *Neuroendocrinology*, 39, 267, 1984.

Craven, R. P. and McDonald, P. G., The effect of intrahypothalamic infusions of dopamine and noradrenaline on ovulation in the adult rat, *Life Sci.*, 10, 1409, 1971.

Donoso, A. O. and Moyano, M. B., Adrenergic activity in hypothalamus and ovulation, *Proc. Soc. Exp. Biol. Med.*, 135, 633, 1970.

Donoso, A. O., Lopez , F. J., and Negro-Vilar, A., Glutamate receptors of the non-*N*-methyl-D-aspartic acid type mediate the increase in luteinizing hormone-releasing hormone release by excitatory amino acids in vitro, *Endocrinology*, 126, 414, 1990.

Drouva, S. V. and Gallo, R. V., Catecholamine involvement in episodic luteinizing hormone release in adult ovariectomized rats, *Endocrinology*, 99, 651, 1976.

Drouva, S. V. and Gallo, R. V., Further evidence for inhibition of episodic luteinizing hormone release in ovariectomized rats by stimulation of dopamine receptors, *Endocrinology*, 100, 792, 1977.

Fink, G., Sarkar , D. K., and Chiappa, S. A., Gonadotrophin releasing hormone surge during prooestrus: role of steroid hormones, *J. Endocrinol.*, 75, 46p, 1978.

Fox, S. R. and Smith, M. S., Changes in the pulsatile pattern of luteinizing hormone secretion during the rat estrous cycle, *Endocrinology*, 116, 1485, 1985.

Fraser, H. and Baker, T., Changes in the ovaries of rats after immunization against luteinizing hormone releasing hormone, *J. Endocrinol.*, 77, 85, 1978.

Garcia, M. S., Schwanzel-Fukuda, M., Morrell, J. I., and Pfaff, D. W., Immunocytochemical studies of the location of luteinizing hormone releasing hormone neurons in the nervus terminalis of the mouse, in *The Terminal Nerve (Nervus Terminalis) Structure, Function and Evolution,* Dempski, L. and Schwanzel-Fukuda, M., Eds., N.Y. Academy of Sciences, New York, 1987, 465.

Gay, V. L. and Midgley, A. R. J., Response of the adult rat to orchidectomy and ovariectomy as determined by radioimmunoassay, *Endocrinology*, 84, 1359, 1969.

Gibson, M. J., Krieger, D. T., Charlton, H., Zimmerman, E. A., Silverman, A.-J., and Perlow, M. J., Mating and pregnancy can occur in genetically hypogonadal mice with preoptic area brain grafts, *Science*, 225, 949, 1984a.

Gibson, M. J., Perlow, M. J., Charlton, H. M., Zimmerman, E. A., Davies, T. F., and Krieger, D. T., Preoptic area brain grafts in hypogonadal (hpg) female mice abolish effects of congenital hypotha-lamic gonadotropin releasing hormone (GnRH) deficiency, *Endocrinology*, 114, 1938, 1984b.

Gnodde, H. P. and Schuiling, G. A., Involvement of catecholaminergic and cholinergic mechanisms in the pulsatile release of LH in the long-term ovariectomized rat, *Neuroendocrinology*, 20, 212, 1976.

Halasz, B. and Gorski, R. A., Gonadotropin hormone secretion in female rats after partial or total interruption of neural afferents to the medial basal hypothalamus, *Endocrinology*, 80, 608, 1967.

Higuchi, T. and Kawakami, M., Changes in the characteristics of pulsatile luteinizing hormone secretion during the oestrous cycle and after ovariectomy and estrogen treatment in female rats, *J. Endocrinol.*, 94, 177, 1982.

Hoffman, G. E., LHRH neurons and their projections, in *Structure and Function of Peptidergic and Aminergic Neurons*, Sano, Y., Ibata, Y., and Zimmerman, E. A., Eds., Japan Scientific Societies Press, Tokyo, 1983, 183.

Hoffman, G. E., Organization of LHRH cells: differential apposition of neurotensin, substance P and catecholamine axons, *Peptides*, 6, 439, 1985.

Hoffman, G. and Gibbs, F., Deafferentiation spares a subchiasmatic LHRH projection to the median eminence, *Neuroscience*, 7, 1979, 1982.

Hoffman, G. E., Wray, S., and Goldstein, M., Interrelationship of catecholamines and LHRH: a light microscope study, *Brain Res. Bull.*, 9, 417, 1982.

Hoffman, G. E., Fitzsimmons, M. D., and Watson, R. E., Jr., Relationship of endogenous opioid peptide axons to GnRH neurons in the rat, in *Opioid Peptides in Reproduction*, Eds., Oxford University Press, London, 1988.

Hoffman, G., Lee, W.-S., Attardi, B., Yann, V., and Fitzsimmons, M., LHRH neurons express c-*fos* after steroid activation, *Endocrinology*, 1990.

Jennes, L., The nervus terminalis in the mouse: light and electron microscopic immunocytochemical studies, in *The Terminal Nerve (Nervus Terminalis) Structure, Function and Evolution*, Demski, L. and Schwanzel-Fukuda, M., Eds., N.Y. Academy of Sciences, New York, 1987, 165.

Jennes, L., Beckman, W. C., Stumpf, W. E., and Grzanna, R., Anatomical relationships of serotoninergic and noradrenalinergic projections with the GnRH system in septum and hypothalamus, *Exp. Brain Res.*, 46, 331, 1982.

Jennes, L., Stumpf, W. E., and Tapaz, M. L., Anatomical relationships of dopaminergic and GABAergic systems with the GnRH systems in the septohypothalamic area, *Exp. Brain Res.*, 50, 91, 1983.

Jennes, L., Stumpf, W. E., and Sheedy, M. E., Ultrastructural characterization of gonadotropin-releasing hormone (GnRH)-producing neurons, *J. Comp. Neurol.*, 232, 543, 1985.

Kalra, S. P., Neural circuitry involved in the control of LHRH secretion: a model for preovulatory LH release, *Front. Neuroendocrinol.*, 9, 31 1986.

Kalra, S. P. and McCann, S. M., Effects of drugs modifying catecholamine synthesis on plasma LH and ovulation in the rat, *Neuroendocrinology*, 15, 79,1974.

Kalra, S. P. and Simpkins, J. W., Evidence for noradrenergic mediation of opioid effects on luteinizing hormone secretion, *Endocrinology*, 109, 776, 1981.

Kaynard, A. H., Pau, F. K.-Y., Hess, D. L., and Spies, H. G., Gonadotropin-releasing hormone and norepinephrine release from the rabbit mediobasal and anterior hypothalamus during the mating-induced luteinizing hormone surge, *Endocrinology*, 127, 1176, 1990.

King, J. C., Kugel, G., Zahnister, D., Wooledge, K., Damassa, D. A., and Alexsavich, B., Changes in populations of LHRH immunopositive cell bodies following gonadectomy, *Peptides*, 8, 721, 1987.

Kiss, J. and Halasz, B., Demonstration of serotoninergic axons terminating on luteinizing hormone releasing hormone neurons in the preoptic area of the rat using a combination of immunocytochemistry and high resolution autoradiography, *Neuroscience*, 14, 69, 1985

Knobil, E., Plant, T. M., Wildt, L., Belchetz, P. E., and Marshall, G., Control of the rhesus monkey menstrual cycle: permissive role of hypothalamic gonadotropin releasing hormone, *Science*, 207, 1371, 1980.

Kozlowski, G., Chu, L., Hostetter, G., and Kerdelhue, B., Cellular characteristics of immunolabeled luteinizing hormone-releasing hormone (LHRH) neurons, *Peptides*, 1 (Suppl. 1), 37, 1980.

Krey, L. C. and Silverman, A. J., Luteinizing hormone releasing hormone, in *Brain Peptides*, Krieger, D. T., Brownstein, M. J., and Martin, J., Eds., John Wiley & Sons, New York, 1983, 687.

Krieger, D. and Gibson, M., Correction of genetic gonadotropic hormone-releasing hormone deficiency by preoptic area transplants, in *Neural Transplants, Development and Function*, 1984, 187.

Krisch, B., Two types of luliberin-immunoreactive perikarya in the preoptic area of the rat, *Cell Tissue Res.*, 212, 443, 1980.

Kuljis, R. O. and Advis, J. P., Immunocytochemical and physiological evidence of a synapse between dopamine and luteinizing hormone releasing hormone-containing neurons in the ewe median eminence, *Endocrinology*, 124, 1579, 1989.

Lee, W.-S., Smith, M. S., and Hoffman, G. E., Progesterone enhances the surge of luteinizing hormone by increasing the activation of luteinizing hormone-releasing hormone neurons, *Endocrinology*, 127, 2604, 1990a.

Lee, W.-S., Smith, M. S., and Hoffman, G. E., Luteinizing hormone releasing hormone (LHRH) neurons express c-Fos during the proestrous LH surge, *Proc. Natl. Acad. Sci. U.S.A.*, 1990b.

Lehman, M. N., Ultrastructure and synaptic organization of luteinizing hormone-releasing hormone (LHRH) neurons in the anestrous ewe, *J. Comp. Neurol.*, 273, 447, 1988.

Lehman, M. N., Karsch, F. J., and Silverman, A.-J., Potential sites of interaction between catecholamines and LHRH in the sheep brain, *Brain Res. Bull.*, 20, 49, 1988.

Leranth, C., MacLusky, N. J., Sakamoto, H., Shanabrough, M., and Naftolin, F., Glutamic acid decarboxylase-containing axons synapse on LHRH neurons in the rat medial preoptic area, *Neuroendocrinology*, 40, 536, 1985a.

Leranth, C., Seguraum, L. M. G., Palkovits, M., MacLusky, N. J., Shanabrough, M., and Naftolin, F., The LH-RH containing neuronal network in the preoptic area of the rat: demonstration of LH-RH containing nerve terminals in synaptic contact with LHRH neurons, *Brain Res.*, 345, 332, 1985b.

Leranth, C., MacLusky, N. J., Shanabrough, M., and Naftolin, F., Immunohistochemical evidence for synaptic connections between pro-opiomelanocortin-immunoreactive axons and LH-RH neurons in the preoptic area, *Brain Res.*, 449, 167, 1988.

Leranth, C., MacLusky, N. J., Shanabrough, M., and Naftolin, F., Catecholaminergic innervation of LHRH and GAD immunopositive neurons in the rat medial preoptic area: an electron microscopic double immunostaining and degeneration study, *Neuroendocrinology*, 48, 581, 1988.

Levine, J. E. and Ramirez, V. D., Luteinizing hormone-releasing hormone release during the rat estrous cycle and after ovariectomy, as estimated with push-pull cannulae, *Endocrinology*, 111, 1439, 1982.

Levine, J. E., Norman, R. L., Gleissman, P. M., Oyama, T. T., Bangsberg, D. R., and Speis, H. G., In vivo gonadotropin-releasing hormone release and serum luteinizing hormone measurements in ovariectomized estrogen-treated rhesus monkeys, *Endocrinology*, 111, 1449, 1985.

Liposits, Z., Setalo, G., and Flerko, B., Application of the silver-gold intensified 3,3′-diaminobenzidine chromogen to the light and electron microscopic detection of the luteinizing hormone-releasing hormone system of the rat brain, *Neuroscience*, 13, 513, 1984.

Lofstrom, A., Catecholamine turnover alterations in discrete area of the median eminence of the 4- and 5-day cyclic rats, *Brain Res.*, 120, 113, 1977.

Lopez, F. J., Donoso, A. O., and Negro-Vilar, A., Endogenous excitatory amino acid neurotransmission regulates the estradiol-induced LH surge in ovariectomized rats, *Endocrinology*, 126, 1771, 1990.

MacLusky, N., Naftolin, F., and Leranth, C., Immunocytochemical evidence for direct synaptic connections between corticortropin releasing factor (CRF) and gonadotropin releasing hormone (GnRH)-containing neurons in the preoptic area of the rat, *Brain Res.*, 439, 391, 1988.

Marshall, P. E. and Goldsmith, P. C., Neuroregulatory and neuroendocrine GnRH pathways in the hypothalamus and forebrain of the baboon, *Brain Res.*, 193, 353, 1980.

Martinovic, J. V. and McCann, S. M., Effects of lesions in the ventral noradrenergic tract produced by microinjections of 6-hydroxydopamine on gonadotropin release in the rat, *Endocrinology*, 100, 1206, 1977.

Mason, A. J., Hayflick, J. S., Zoeller, R. T., Young, W. S., III, Phillips, H. S., Nikolics, K., and Seeburg, P. H., A deletion truncating the gonadotropin-releasing hormone gene is responsible for hypogonadism in the hpg mouse, *Science*, 234, 1366, 1986a.

Mason, A. J., Pitts, S. L., Nikolics, K., Szonyi, E., Wilcox, J. N., Seeburg, P. H., and Stewart, T. A., The hypogonadal mouse: reproductive functions restored by gene therapy, *Science*, 234, 1372, 1986b.

McCann, S. M., Taleisnik, S., and Friedman, H. M., LH releasing activity in hypothalamic extracts, *Proc. Soc. Exp. Biol. Med.*, 82, 432, 1960.

Merchanthaler, I., Setalo, G., Gorcs, T., Petrusz, P., and Flerko, B., Combined retrograde tracing and immunocytochemical identification of luteinizing hormone-releasing hormone- and somatostatin-containing neurons projecting to the median eminence of the rat, *Endocrinology*, 125, 2812, 1989.

Moenter, S. M., Caraty, A., and Karsch, F. J., The estradiol-induced surge of gonadotropin-releasing hormone in the ewe, *Endocrinology*, 127, 1375, 1990.

Mueller, G. P., Simpkins, J., Meites, J., and Moore, K. E., Differential effects of dopamine agonists and haloperidol on release of prolactin, thyroid-stimulating hormone, growth hormone and luteinizing hormone in rats, *Neuroendocrinology*, 20, 121, 1976.

Muske, L. E. and Moore, F. L., Luteinizing hormone releasing hormone immunoreactive neurons in the amphibian brain are distributed along the course of the nervus terminalis, in *The Terminal Nerve (Nervus Terminalis) Structure, Function and Evolution,* Demsky, L. and Schwanzel-Fukuda, M., Eds., N.Y. Academy of Sciences, New York, 1987, 433.

Negro-Vilar, A., Chiocchio, S. R., and Tramezzani, J. H., Changes in catecholamine content of the median eminence precede the proestrous surges of luteinizing hormone and prolactin, *J. Endocrinol.*, 75, 339, 1977.

Negro-Vilar, A., Ojeda, S. R., and McCann, S. M., Catecholaminergic modulation of luteinizing hormone-releasing hormone release by median eminence terminals in vitro, *Endocrinology*, 104, 1749, 1979.

Neill, J. D., Patton, J. M., Dailey, R. A., Tsou, R. C., and Tindall, G. T., Luteinizing hormone releasing hormone (LHRH) in pituitary stalk blood of rhesus monkeys: relationship to level of LH release, *Endocrinology*, 101, 430, 1977.

Nikitovitch-Winer, M. B., Induction of ovulation in rats by direct intrapituitary infusion of median eminence extracts, *Endocrinology*, 70, 350, 1962.

Norgren, R. B. and Lehman, M. N., Migration of LHRH neurons from the olfactory placode to the brain in the chick, *Soc. Neurosci. Abstr.,* 16, 649, 1990.

Norgren, R. B., Jr. and Norgren, M. N., A double-label pre-embedding immunoperoxidase technique for electron microscopy using diaminobenzidine and tetramethylbenzidine as markers, *J. Histochem. Cytochem.,* 37, 1283, 1989.

Oelschlager, H. A., Buhl, E. H., and Dann, J. F., Development of the nervus terminalis in mammals including toothed whales and humans, in *The Terminal Nerve (Nervus Terminalis) Structure, Function and Evolution,* Dempski, L. and Schwanzel-Fukuda, M., Eds., N.Y. Academy of Sciences, New York, 1987, 447.

Ondo, J. G., Pass, K. A., and Baldwin, R., The effects of neuronally active acids on pituitary gonadotroph secretion, *Neuroendocrinology*, 21, 79, 1976.

Pelletier, G., Demonstration of contacts between neurons staining for LHRH in the preoptic area of the rat brain, *Neuroendocrinology*, 46, 457, 1987.

Price, M. T., Olney, J. W., and Cicero, T. J., Acute elevations of serum luteinizing hormone induced by kainic acid, *N*-methyl aspartic acid and homocysteic acid, *Neuroendocrinology*, 26, 352, 1976.

Rance, N. and Barraclough, C. A., Effects of phenobarbital on hypothalamic LHRH and catecholamine turnover in proestrous rats, Proc. Soc. Exp. Biol. Med., 166, 425, 1981.

Ronnekleiv, O. K. and Resko, J. A., Ontogeny of gonadotropin-releasing hormone-containing neurons in early fetal development in rhesus monkeys, *Endocrinology*, 126, 498, 1990.

Ronnekleiv, O. K., Naylor, B. R., Bond, C. T., and Adelman, J. P., Combined immunohistochemistry for gonadotropin-releasing hormone (GnRH) and pro-GnRH, and *in situ* hybridization for GnRH messenger ribonucleic acid in rat brain, *Mol. Endocrinol.,* 3, 363, 1989.

Rotszstein, W. H., Charli, J. L., Pattou, E., Epelbaum, J., and Kordon, C., In vitro release of luteinizing hormone-releasing hormone (LHRH) from rat mediobasal hypothalamus: effects of calcium, potassium and dopamine, *Endocrinology*, 99, 1663, 1976.

Rubenstein, W. H. and Sawyer, C. H., Role of catecholamines in stimulating the release of pituitary ovulating hormone(s) in rats, *Endocrinology*, 86, 988, 1970.

Sagar, S. M., Sharp, F. R., and Curran, T., Expression of c-fos protein in brain: metabolic mapping at the cellular level, *Science*, 240, 1328, 1988.

Sarkar, D. K. and Fink, G., Effects of gonadal steroids on output of luteinizing hormone releasing factor into hypophysial portal blood in the female rat, *J. Endocrinol.*, 80, 1979.

Sarkar, D. M., Chiappa, S. A., and Fink, G., Gonadotropin-releasing hormone surge in proestrous rats, *Nature (London)*, 264, 461, 1976.

Sawyer, C. H., Stimulation of ovulation in the rabbit by the intraventricular injection of epinephrine or norepinephrine, *Anatom. Rec.*, 112, 385, 1952.

Sawyer, C. H., Markee, J. E., and Hollingshead, W. H., Inhibition of ovulation in the rabbit by the adrenergic blocking agent dibenamine, *Endocrinology*, 41, 395, 1947.

Sawyer, C. H., Hilliard, J., Kanematsu, S., Scaramuzzi, R., and Blake, C. A., Effects of intraventricular infusions of norepinephrine and dopamine on LH release and ovulation in the rabbit, *Neuroendocrinology*, 15, 328, 1975.

Schainker, B. and Cicero, T. J., Acute central stimulation of luteinizing hormone by parenterally administered N-methyl-D,L-aspartic acid in the male rat, *Brain Res.*, 184, 425, 1980.

Schally, A. V., Arimura, A., Baba, Y., Nair, R., Matsuo, J., Redding, T. W., Debeljuk, L., and White, W. F., Isolation and properties of the FSH- and LH-releasing hormone, *Biochem. Biophys. Res. Commun.*, 43, 393, 1971.

Schillo, K. K., Leshin, L. S., Kuehl, D., and Jackson, G. L., Simultaneous measurement of luteinizing hormone-releasing hormone and luteinizing hormone during estradiol-induced luteinizing hormone surges in the ovariectomized ewe, *Biol. Reprod.*, 33, 644, 1985.

Schwanzel-Fukuda, M. and Pfaff, D., Origin of luteinizing hormone-releasing hormone neurons, *Nature (London)*, 338, 161, 1989.

Schwanzel-Fukuda, M. and Silverman, A. J., The nervus terminalis of the guinea pig: a new luteinizing hormone releasing hormone (LHRH) neuronal system, *J. Comp. Neurol.*, 191, 213, 1980.

Schwanzel-Fukuda, M., Bick, D., and Pfaff, D. W., Luteinizing hormone releasing hormone (LHRH)-expressing cells do not migrate normally in an inherited hypogonadal (Kallmann) syndrome, *Mol. Brain Res.*, 6, 311, 1989.

Seeburg, P. H. and Adelman, J. P., Chacterization of cDNA for precursor of human luteinizing hormone releasing hormone, *Nature (London)*, 338, 666, 1984.

Seeburg, P. H., Mason, A. J., Stewart, T. A., and Nikolics, K., The mammalian GnRH gene and its pivotal role in reproduction, *Recent Prog. Horm. Res.*, 43, 69, 1987.

Silverman, A. J., Paden, C. M., and Witkin, J. W., The luteinizing hormone releasing hormone (LHRH) systems in the rat brain, *Neuroendocrinology*, 35, 429, 1982.

Standish, L. J., Adams, L. A., Vician, L., Clifton, D. K., and Steiner, R. A., Neuroanatomical localization of cells containing gonadotropin-releasing hormone messenger ribonucleic acid in the primate brain by *in situ* hybridization histochemistry, *Mol. Endocrinol.*, 1, 371, 1987.

Stefano, F. J. E. and Donoso, A. O., Norepinephrine levels ion the rat hypothalamus during the estrous cycle, *Endocrinology*, 81, 1405, 1967.

Tima, L. and Flerko, B., Ovulation induced by norepinephrine in rats made anovulatory by various experimental procedures, *Neuroendocrinology*, 15, 346, 1974.

Tima, L. and Flerko, B., Ovulation induced by intraventricular infusion of norepinephrine in rats made anovulatory by neonatal administration of various doses of testosterone, *Endocrinology*, 101, 218, 1975.

Tsou, R. C., Dailey, R. A., McLanahan, C. S., Parent, A. D., Tindall, G. T., and Neill, J. D., Luteinizing hormone releasing hormone (LHRH) levels in pituitary stalk plasma during the preovulatory gonadotropin surge of rabbits, *Endocrinology*, 101, 534, 1977.

Tsuruo, Y., Kawano, H., Hisano, S., Kagotani, Y., Daikoku, S., Zhang, T., and Yanaihara, N., Synaptic regulation of LHRH-containing neurons by substance P in rats, *Neurosci. Lett.*, 110, 261, 1990.

Vijayan, E. and McCann, S. M., Reevaluation of the role of catecholamines in control of gonadotropin and prolactin release, *Neuroendocrinology*, 25, 150, 1978.

Weick, R. F., Acute effects of adrenergic receptor blocking drugs and neuroleptic agents on pulsatile discharges of luteinizing hormone in the ovariectomized rat, *Neuroendocrinology*, 26, 108, 1978.

Witkin, J. W., Access of LHRH neurons to the vasculature in the rat, *Neuroscience*, 37, 501, 1990.

Witkin, J. W. and Demasio, K. A., Ultrastructural differences between smooth and thorny GnRH neurons, *Neuroscience*, 34, 777, 1990.

Witkin, J. W. and Silverman, A.-J., Synaptology of LHRH neurons in the rat preoptic area, *Peptides*, 6, 263, 1985.

Wray, S., Evidence that cells of the gonadotropin releasing hormone system are derived from progenitor cells in the olfactory placode, in *Control of the Onset of Puberty III*, Delemarre-van de Waal, H. A., et al., Eds., Elsevier, New York, 1989, 23.

Wray, S. and Gainer, H., Effect of neonatal gonadectomy on the postnatal development of LHRH cell subtypes in male and female rats, *Neuroendocrinology*, 45, 413, 1987.

Wray, S. and Hoffman, G. E., A developmental study of the quantitative distribution of LHRH neurons in postnatal male and female rats, *J. Comp. Neurol.*, 252, 522, 1986a.

Wray, S. and Hoffman, G. E., Postnatal morphological changes in rat LHRH neurons correlated with sexual maturation, *Neuroendocrinology*, 43, 93, 1986b.

Wray, S., Gahwiler, B. H., and Gainer, H., Slice cultures of LHRH neurons in the presence and absence of brainstem and pituitary, *Peptides*, 9, 1151, 1988.

Wray, S., Neiburgs, A., and Elkabes, S., Spatiotemporal cell expression of luteinizing hormone-releasing hormone in the prenatal mouse: evidence for an embryonic origin in the olfactory placode, *Dev. Brain Res.*, 46, 309, 1989a.

Wray, S., Zoeller, R. T., and Gainer, H., Differential effects of estrogen on luteinizing hormone-releasing hormone gene expression in slice explant cultures prepared from specific rat forebrain regions, *Mol. Endocrinol.*, 3, 1197, 1989b.

Wray, S., Grant, P., and Gainer, H., Evidence that cells expressing luteinizing hormone-releasing hormone mRNA in the mouse are derived from progenitor cells in the olfactory placode, *Proc. Natl. Acad. Sci. U.S.A.*, 86, 8132, 1989c.

Zoeller, R. T., Seeburgh, P. H., and Young, W. S., III, *In situ* hybridization histochemistry for messenger ribonucleic acid (mRNA) encoding gonadotropin releasing hormone (GnRH): effect of estrogen on cellular levels of GnRH mRNA in female rat brain, *Endocrinology*, 122, 2570, 1988.

Zschaeck, L. L. and Wurtman, R. J., Brain H3-catechol synthesis and the vaginal estrous cycle, Neuroendocrinology, 11, 144, 1973.

9

The Somatostatin and Growth Hormone-Releasing Factor Systems

BJÖRN MEISTER AND TOMAS HÖKFELT
Department of Histology and Neurobiology
Karolinska Institute
Stockholm, Sweden

I. Introduction

The hypothalamic control of growth hormone (GH) secretion from the anterior pituitary (Figure 1) primarily involves two hormones, one inhibitory peptide, somatostatin, and one stimulatory, growth hormone-releasing factor (GRF). These two peptides are synthesized within separate sets of hypothalamic neurons and are, after axonal transport, released from nerve endings in the median eminence to reach the anterior pituitary via the portal vascular plexus according to the classical concept of Harris (1955).

The first evidence for a neural control of GH secretion came from physiological studies employing bilateral lesions of the ventromedial nucleus of the hypothalamus that resulted in impaired growth (Reichlin, 1960). Some years later it was shown that crude or partially purified hypothalamic extracts possessed GH-releasing activity (Deuben and Meites, 1964; Knobil et al., 1968; Krulich et al., 1968; Wilber et al., 1971; Sandman et al., 1972) as well as GH release-inhibiting activity (Krulich et al., 1968, 1972; Dhariwal et al., 1969). With the introduction of radioimmunoassay it could later also be demonstrated that electrolytic lesions placed in the ventromedial and arcuate nuclei decreased pituitary and plasma GH levels (Frohman and Bernardis, 1968), whereas electrical stimulation in the same area increased plasma GH (Frohman et al., 1969; Martin, 1972). In 1971, while searching for the GH-releasing factor, Guillemin and colleagues isolated from ovine hypothalamus a factor that dramatically inhibited the secretion of GH from dispersed anterior pituitary cells (Vale et al., 1972). The substance was subsequently characterized as a tetradecapeptide and termed somatostatin (somatotropin-release inhibiting hormone, SRIF, or growth hormone release-inhibiting hormone) (Brazeau et al., 1973). Schally and colleagues later showed that an identical compound was present in porcine hypothalamic and intestinal extracts (Schally et al., 1976). When using the name somatostatin one should consider the fact that somatostatin has been found to inhibit, for example, the secretion of thyroid-stimulating hormone (TSH) (Vale et al., 1975) and that the peptide is found in many areas and tissues outside the hypothalamus, where it predominantly exerts direct inhibitory effects (see Vale et al., 1975; Luft et al., 1978; Reichlin, 1983, 1985; Harmar et al., 1986).

From the isolation of somatostatin it took another decade until GRF was chemically characterized. Because GRF is present in only very small quantities in the hypothalamus, as compared to the other hypophysiotropic hormones, efforts to determine its structure were hampered for many years. However, in 1982, the groups of Guillemin and Vale revealed the

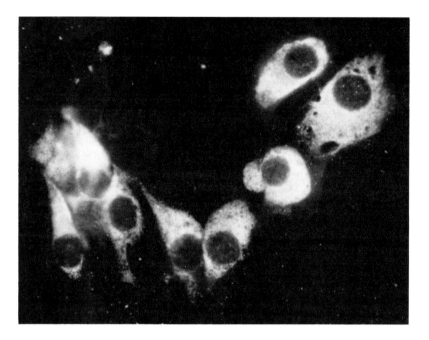

Figure 1. Growth hormone-producing rat anterior pituitary cells. The somatotrophs have been cultured and stained with an antiserum to human growth hormone.

structure of human peptides with GH-releasing activity (Guillemin et al., 1982; Rivier et al., 1982). Unlike the isolation of the previous hypothalamic hormones, which were extracted from hypothalamic tissue, GRF was first purified from two rare human pancreatic tumors that secreted GRF and caused acromegaly. The isolation and characterization of hypothalamic GRFs from other species have subsequently been reported (see Ling et al., 1985). Somatocrinin has been proposed as another name for GRF (Brazeau et al., 1982a). GRF/somatocrinin has, compared to somatostatin, been found to occur in restricted areas of the brain and only sparsely outside the nervous system.

In this chapter we will focus on the anatomical localization of the somatostatin- and GRF-containing neuronal systems in the brain. The GRF neurons have been shown to contain a number of other neuroactive compounds (see Meister and Hökfelt, 1988), one of which is galanin, a peptide of particular interest with regard to the regulation of GH secretion. This peptide will also be briefly considered.

II. Somatostatin

A.   Biochemistry

In their original work Guillemin and co-workers found both a linear and cyclic form of somatostatin isolated from ovine hypothalamus, and subsequent studies showed that the structure of the peptide exhibited considerable similarity between different species. In mammals, one gene located on chromosome 3 is responsible for transcription of somatostatin mRNA, which in both rats and humans encodes a polypeptide of 116 amino acids (preprosomatostatin) (Figure 2) (Shen et al., 1982; Goodman et al., 1983; Shen and Rutter, 1984). Prosomatostatin contains 92 amino acids and is formed after cleavage and removal of a

24-amino acid signal peptide (Figure 2) (Noe et al., 1987). As prosomatostatin passes from the endoplasmic reticulum to the Golgi apparatus to be packaged into secretory vesicles, a number of proteolytic cleavages take place to yield seven different peptides (Benoit et al., 1982). Four of these peptides contain the somatostatin sequence either as a tetradecapeptide (somatostatin-14, M_r 1638, amino acids 15 to 28) (Figure 3), an octacosapeptide (somatostatin-28, M_r 3149) (Figure 3), an M_r 6000 to 7500 form, or as the intact prosomatostatin molecule itself. The remaining peptides contain at the C-terminal end the first 12 amino acids of somatostatin-28 (Benoit et al., 1982).

Somatostatin-14 and -28 appear to have qualitatively similar biological actions, although the 28-amino acid form has higher affinity for receptors in the anterior pituitary, while the 14-amino acid peptide binds with higher affinity to receptors in the hypothalamus and cerebral cortex (Srikant and Patel, 1981). Somatostatin-28 has also a longer half-life time in plasma as compared to somatostatin-14 (Polonsky et al., 1982), accounting for the more prolonged action of somatostatin-28 in inhibiting GH release. Somatostatin-14 is in most tissues the predominantly biologically active end product of the biosynthetic pathway. In the nervous system, somatostatin-14 represents 65 to 80% of the total immunoreactivity and may play the dominant role in neurotransmission. The somatostatin-containing neurons in the anterior hypothalamic periventricular nucleus projecting to the median eminence, however, synthesize somatostatin-14 and -28 in almost equal amounts. Somatostatin-secreting cells in the intestinal tract predominantly secrete somatostatin-28, whereas the somatostatin cells in the pancreas mainly secrete somatostatin-14 (see Harmar et al., 1986). Synthetic somatostatin analogues are now available for clinical use in the treatment of diseases such as acromegaly, gastric ulcer, and endocrine tumors in the gut and pancreas (see Harmar et al., 1986).

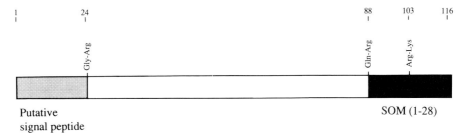

Figure 2. Structure of the human and rat preprosomatostatin-116 molecule. The putative signal peptide extends from amino acids 1 to 24 and is indicated by the gray area. Somatostatin (SOM)-28 extends from amino acid 88 and SOM-14 extends from amino acid 103. Amino acid sequences where proteolytic cleavages take place are indicated. Comparison of rat and human preprosomatostatin has revealed a high degree of homology, with only four amino acid substitutions. [Drawn after data from Shen et al. (1982) and Goodman et al. (1983)]

Somatostatin-14

```
      S────────────────────────────────S
      |                                 |
Ala-Gly-Cys-Lys-Asn-Phe-Phe-Trp-Lys-Thr-Phe-Thr-Ser-Cys
```

Somatostatin-28

```
Ser-Ala-Asn-Ser-Asn-Pro-Ala-Met-Ala-Pro-Arg-Glu-Arg-Lys-
      S────────────────────────────────S
      |                                 |
Ala-Gly-Cys-Lys-Asn-Phe-Phe-Trp-Lys-Thr-Phe-Thr-Ser-Cys
```

Figure 3. Amino acid sequences of somatostatin-28 (SOM$_{1-28}$) and SOM-14 (SOM$_{15-28}$).

B.   Localization of Somatostatin

After the characterization of somatostatin, antibodies to the peptide were raised and used in radioimmunological and immunohistochemical studies. High amounts of somatostatin-like immunoreactivity (LI) could, as expected, be demonstrated in the external layer of the median eminence (Dubois et al., 1974; Hökfelt et al., 1974; Brownstein et al., 1975; Elde and Parsons, 1974), i.e., the area where the hypothalamic hormones are released into the portal blood vessels for transport to the anterior pituitary.

It rapidly became apparent that somatostatin is not restricted to the hypothalamus, but has a widespread distribution in different species, both in the central and peripheral nervous system as well as in several types of endocrine cells (Hökfelt et al., 1975; Brownstein et al., 1975; Parsons et al., 1976). This extensive occurrence of somatostatin in various systems makes it reasonable to classify somatostatin as a neurohormone in the control of GH secretion, a neurotransmitter/neuromodulator in the central and peripheral nervous system, and as a hormone when released from endocrine cells in the gastrointestinal tract (see Vale et al., 1975; Luft et al., 1978; Reichlin, 1983; Harmar et al., 1986).

The present chapter will only briefly summarize the major somatostatin-containing systems. For more extensive descriptions of the anatomical localization of somatostatin in the brain the reader is referred to some immunohistochemical studies (see Bennett-Clarke et al., 1980; Finley et al., 1981; Johansson et al., 1984; Vincent et al., 1985). More recently, the distribution of somatostatin mRNA has been shown with *in situ* hybridization (Fitzpatrick-McElligott et al., 1988; Naus et al., 1988).

1.   Hypothalamic Systems

The hypothalamus contains by far the highest concentration of somatostatin in the brain, being found in cell bodies and nerve endings and has also been shown to be present in synaptic vesicles (Epelbaum et al., 1977; Berelowitz et al., 1978). Somatostatin occurs in several cell groups, as schematically depicted in Figure 6, and in many fiber systems in the hypothalamus of the rat. In some of these groups it is present in high concentrations and in a form recognizable to many antisera, and can therefore be visualized without pretreatment with the axonal transport inhibitor colchicine. This is true for somatostatin-containing cell bodies in the anterior periventricular nucleus, where the cells closely surround the entire third ventricle, extending from the posterior half of the suprachiasmatic region to the retrochiasmatic area (Figure 4). These small and fusiform cell bodies in the anterior periventricular region send axons laterally, forming an arch, turning ventrally, approaching the ventral surface of the brain, and then converging toward and into the external layer of the median eminence on the ipsilateral side (Figure 9). The periventricular cells send axons that terminate in the median eminence (Figure 8C), where the somatostatin-immunoreactive (IR) fibers are seen in dense aggregations around portal vessels in the external layer (Figure 8C). It has been calculated that about one third of all nerve endings in the external layer may contain somatostatin (Foster and Johansson, 1985). A similarly dense aggregation of somatostatin-IR varicosities is seen in the monkey median eminence (Figure 5). The somatostatin-containing fibers in the median eminence arise almost exclusively from the anterior periventricular cell group, as has been shown with a variety of different techniques, including deafferentations/lesions (Brownstein et al., 1977; Critchlow et al., 1978; Patel et al., 1979; Crowley and Terry, 1980; Kawano et al., 1982; Makara et al., 1983) and retrograde tracing (Ishikawa et al., 1987; Kawano and Daikoku, 1988; Merchenthaler et al., 1989). Lesioning of the somatostatin-containing pathway from the anterior periventricular nucleus to the median eminence leads to depletion of somatostatin in the median eminence and to increased serum levels of GH (Critchlow et al., 1978, 1981).

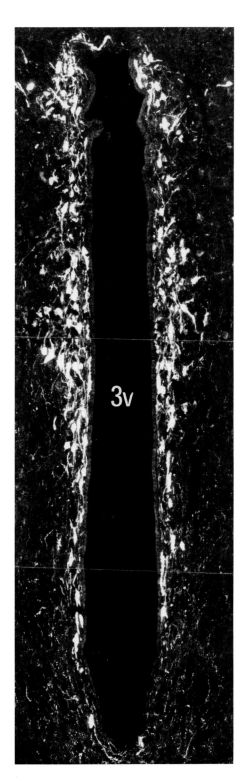

Figure 4. Somatostatin-containing neurons in the anterior periventricular hypothalamic nucleus. The cells densely surround the entire third ventricle (3v). The periventricular somatostatin neurons have been shown to project to the external zone of the median eminence.

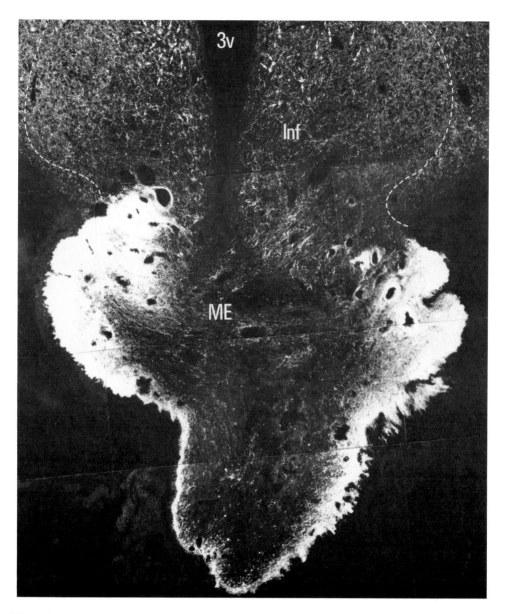

Figure 5. Somatostatin-immunoreactive neurons in the mediobasal hypothalamus of the monkey (Macaca fascicularis.). A dense plexus of somatostatin fibers is distributed in the external layer of the median eminence (ME), closely surrounding portal vessels. Somatostatin fibers are also seen in the infundibular nucleus (Inf; outlined with broken line). In the dorsal part of the infundibular nucleus, several somatostatin-containing cell bodies are found, see arrows).

Conversely, electrical stimulation of the anterior periventricular area causes increased levels of somatostatin in the portal blood and inhibition of GH secretion (Chihara et al., 1979). Thus, the periventricular cell group with its projections is directly responsible for the negative control of GH secretion. This is further illustrated in Figure 7, where periventricular hypothalamic somatostatin-containing neurons are shown to contain the retrograde tracer Fast Blue, which has presumably been taken up by nerve endings in the median eminence. Somatostatin-

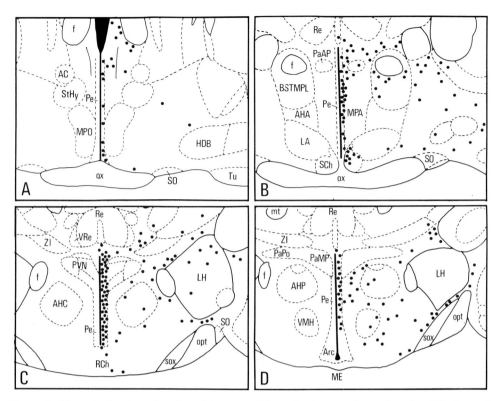

Figure 6. Schematic drawings of the hypothalamus at different levels, according to the atlas of Paxinos and Watson (1986), illustrate the distribution of somatostatin-containing cell bodies (dots). Abbreviations: AHP, anterior hypothalamic area, posterior; Arc, arcuate nucleus; DA, dorsal hypothalamic area; DM, dorsomedial hypothalamic nucleus; DMC, dorsomedial hypothalamic nucleus, compact; DMD, dorsomedial hypothalamic nucleus, diffuse; Do, dorsal hypothalamic nucleus; f, fornix; InfS, infundibular stem; LH, lateral hypothalamic area; ME, median eminence; mt, mammillothalamic tract; MTu, medial tuberal nucleus; opt, optic tract; PaMP, paraventricular hypothalamic nucleus, medial parvocellular part; PaPo, paraventricular hypothalamic nucleus, posterior part; Pe, periventricular hypothalamic nucleus; PMV, premammillary nucleus, ventral; Re, reuniens thalamic nucleus; sox, supraoptic decussation; SOR, supraoptic nucleus, retrochiasmatic; SPF, subparafascicular thalamic nucleus; Subl, subincertal nucleus; TMC, tuberal magnocellular nucleus; VMH, ventromedial hypothalamic nucleus; VMHC, ventromedial hypothalamic nucleus, central; VMHDM, ventromedial hypothalamic nucleus, dorsomedial; VMHVL, ventromedial hypothalamic nucleus, ventrolateral; ZI, zona incerta; VRe, ventral reuniens nucleus; 3V, third ventricle. (A) Bregma, -2.12 mm; (B) -2.30 mm; (C) -2.56 mm; (D) -2.80 mm; (E) -3.14 mm; (F) -3.30 mm; (G) -3.60 mm; (H) -3.80 mm.

containing cell bodies in the arcuate nucleus, however, do not accumulate the tracer Fast Blue after intravenous infusion (Meister et al., 1987a), indicating that they do not project to the median eminence.

Small somatostatin-IR cell bodies are also seen in the dorsal posterior aspect of the arcuate nucleus, the ventrolateral part of the ventromedial nucleus, and also in the suprachiasmatic nucleus, as well as being more diffusely distributed in other hypothalamic areas (Figure 6). The somatostatin-IR cell bodies in the arcuate nucleus do not seem to contribute to the fiber system in the median eminence, since neonatal administration of monosodium glutamate (MSG), a drug causing specific lesions in the arcuate nucleus (Olney, 1969), does not change the number of somatostatin fibers, in spite of a nearly total elimination of the cell bodies within the nucleus (Figure 8) (Kawano et al., 1982; Romagnano et al., 1982; Meister et al., 1989). This further suggests that somatostatin neurons in the arcuate nucleus do not project to the median eminence.

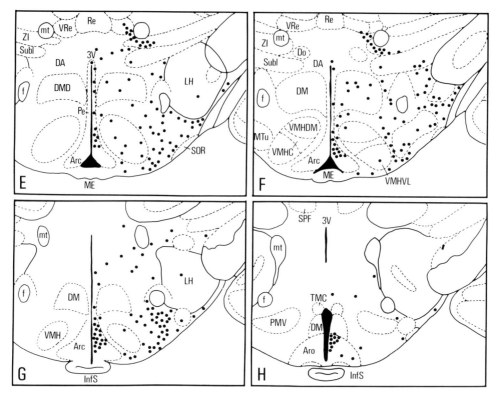

Figure 6. (continued).

Apart from the very dense aggregations of somatostatin-IR fibers in the median eminence, a dense plexus of somatostatin-IR fibers is located in the organum vasculosum of the lamina terminalis, an area that, just like the median eminence, contains nerve terminals located outside the blood-brain-barrier. Within the arcuate nucleus and in parts of the ventromedial nucleus, as well as in the suprachiasmatic nucleus, high concentrations of somatostatin-positive fibers are found. Remaining hypothalamic areas contain low-density or single somatostatin-IR fibers. The majority of the somatostatin fibers in the arcuate nucleus are most likely local (Willoughby et al., 1989), originating from somatostatin-containing cell bodies in the dorsal part of the arcuate nucleus, since MSG-treatment eliminates both somatostatin-IR cell bodies and fibers within the nucleus (Figure 8) (Kawano et al., 1982; Meister et al., 1989).

The ontogeny of at least some hypothalamic somatostatin cell groups is prenatal, and somatostatin-containing neurons in the anterior periventricular nucleus have been seen as early as on embryonic day 17 (Shiosaka et al., 1982; Daikoku et al., 1983).

In situ hybridization (Arentzen et al., 1985; Uhl and Sasek, 1986; Fitzpatrick-McElligott et al., 1988) and Northern blot analysis (Werner et al., 1988) have been used to demonstrate somatostatin mRNA in the anterior periventricular nucleus. The amount of somatostatin mRNA has been found to be higher in male rats than in proestrous females and to decrease 2 to 3 weeks after ovariectomy or orchidectomy (Werner et al., 1988; Baldino et al., 1988; Chowen-Breed et al., 1989). These effects can be reversed by treating gonadectomized female and male rats with estradiol or testosterone, respectively (Baldino et al., 1988; Chowen-Breed et al., 1989), indicating that the synthesis of somatostatin in the anterior periventricular nucleus is under the strong influence of gonadal steroids.

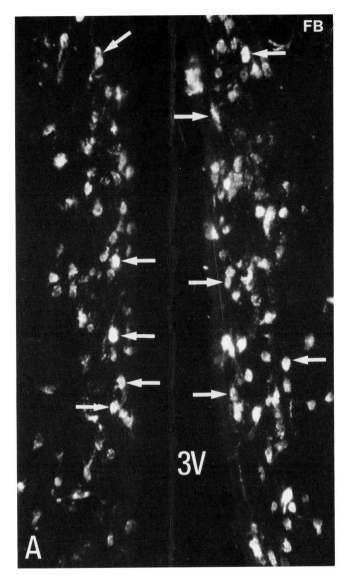

Figure 7. Fluorescence (A) and immunofluorescence (B) photomicrographs of sections of the anterior periventricular nucleus after intravenous injection of the retrograde tracer Fast Blue (FB) and subsequent incubation with somatostatin (SOM) antiserum. The tracer (FB) is taken up by nerve terminals in the median eminence and is retrogradely transported to the cell bodies in the anterior periventricular nucleus. Arrows point to cells containing FB fluorescence and that are somatostatin immunoreactive. 3V, Third ventricle.

2.   Other Forebrain Systems

Somatostatin-containing neurons have a wide distribution outside the hypothalamus (Figure 10). For instance, many somatostatin neurons are found in the amygdala, hippocampus, and striatum, and are thought to function as interneurons in these areas. All parts of the cortex contain somatostatin-IR cell bodies, mainly in layers II, III, and VI (Parnavelas and McDonald, 1983). The cells are mainly multipolar, but also bipolar and bitufted forms of nonpyramidal neurons contain somatostatin-LI (Parnavelas and McDonald, 1983; see Parnavelas

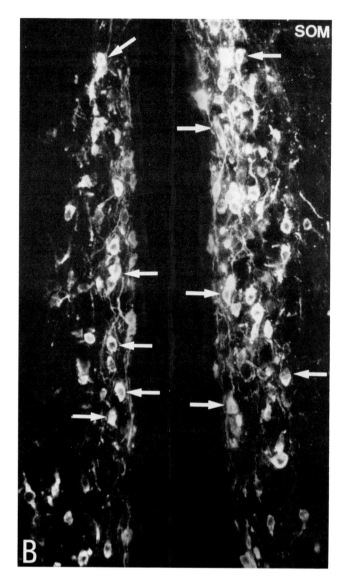

Figure 7. (continued).

et al., 1989). In the cerebellum, some Purkinje cells and Golgi cells in the granular layer are somatostatin-IR. Some amacrine cells in the retina also contain somatostatin-LI (see Brecha, 1983).

Several immunohistochemical studies have shown that somatostatin-LI appears only transiently in certain brain areas during development (Shiosaka et al., 1981a,b, 1982; Takatsuki et al., 1982; Laemle et al., 1982). For example, during embryogenesis of the cerebellum a large proportion of neurons exhibit somatostatin-LI that then subsequently disappears, with only regionally restricted Purkinje cells and Golgi cells retaining the peptide (Inagaki et al., 1982; Villar et al., 1989). This has also been confirmed with *in situ* hybridization (Inagaki et al., 1989).

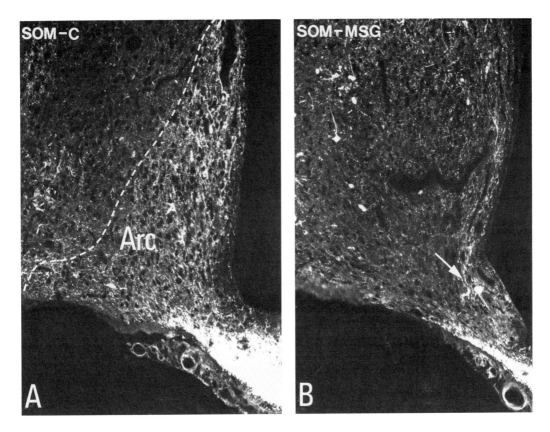

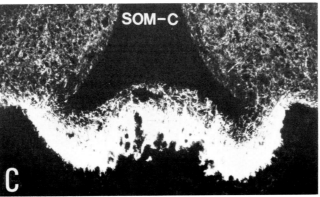

Figure 8. Immunofluorescence photomicrographs of sections of the arcuate nucleus (Arc; outlined with broken line) of control (C) (A,C) and rats treated neonatally with the neurotoxin monosodium glutamate (MSG) (B,D). The neurotoxin induces specific lesions in the Arc, resulting in a disappearance of somatostatin (SOM)-immunoreactive (IR) cell bodies. Note the elimination of SOM-IR fibers within the Arc and the remaining SOM-IR cell bodies (arrow in B) in the ventromedial part of the nucleus. In the median eminence, no change in density of SOM-IR fibers is seen.

3. Lower Brain Stem, Spinal Cord, and Sensory Systems

Somatostatin neurons are frequently found also in the lower brainstem, for example in the solitary tract nucleus and spinal trigeminal nucleus, in the gray matter around the ventricles and aqueduct, as well as in the reticular formation and in the cochlear complex. In the spinal cord, the substantia gelatinosa of the dorsal horn contains a dense plexus of somatostatin-IR

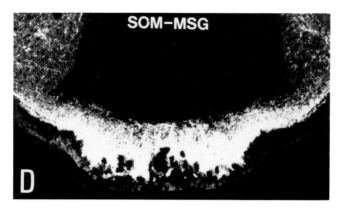

Figure 8. (continued).

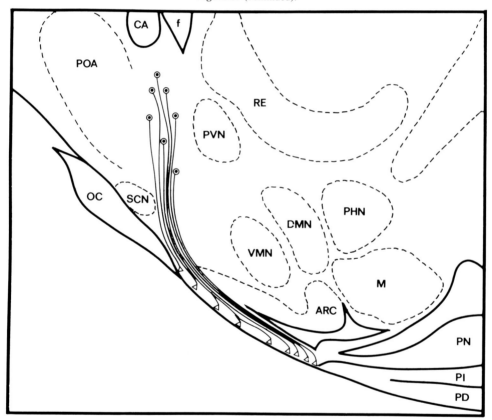

Figure 9. Schematic drawing (sagittal view) of the rat brain illustrating the location of somatostatin-containing neurons in the anterior hypothalamic periventricular nucleus projecting to the external layer of the median eminence. Abbreviations: ARC, arcuate nucleus; CA, anterior commissure; DMN, dorsomedial nucleus; f, fornix; M, mammillary nucleus; OC, optic chiasm; PHN, posterior hypothalamic nucleus; PD, pars distalis hypophysis; PI, pars intermedia hypophysis; PN, pars nervosa hypophysis; POA, preoptic area; SCN, suprachiasmatic nucleus; PVN, paraventricular nucleus; RE, reuniens nucleus of thalamus.

fibers (Figure 11A), which mainly originates from small cells in the superficial layers of the dorsal horn but to some extent also in dorsal root ganglion cells (Figure 11B) (see Hunt, 1983). Somatostatin cells are also present in smaller numbers in other parts of the spinal gray matter.

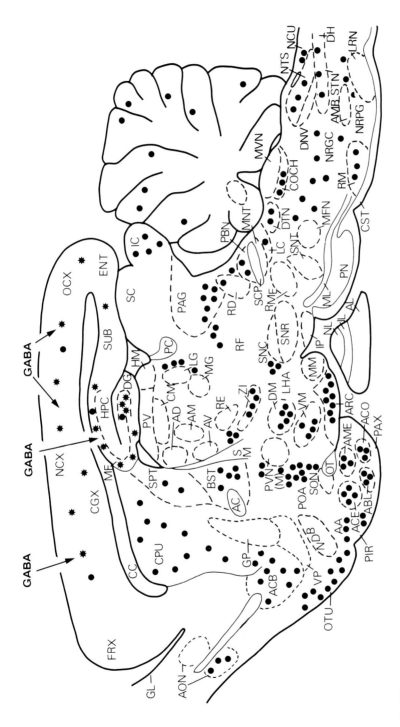

Figure 10. Schematic drawing illustrating the distribution of major somatostatin-containing cell groups (dots) in the rat brain (sagittal view). Some somatostatin cell groups also containing GABA are indicated by filled star. Abbreviations: AA, anterior amygdala; ABL, basolateral nucleus of amygdala; ACB, nucleus accumbens; ACE, central nucleus of amygdala; ACO, cortical nucleus of accumbens; AME, medial nucleus of accumbens; AON, anterior olfactory nucleus; ARC, arcuate nucleus; BST, bed nucleus of stria terminalis; CGX, cingulate cortex; COCH, cochlear nucleus; CPU, caudate-putamen; DG, dentate gyrus; DM, dorsomedial nucleus of hypothalamus; DTN, dorsal tegmental nucleus; ENT, entorhinal cortex; FRX, frontal cortex; HPC, hippocampus; IC, inferior colliculus; LC, nucleus locus coeruleus; LHA, lateral hypothalamic area; MF, mossy fibers of hippocampus; NCU, nucleus cuneatus; NCX, neocortex; NRGC, nucleus reticularis gigantocellularis; NRPG, nucleus reticularis paragigantocellularis; NTS, nucleus tractus solitarii; OCX, occipital cortex; OTU, olfactory tubercle; PAG, periaqueductal gray; PBN, parabrachial nucleus; POA, preoptic area; RF, reticular formation; SNT, spinal nucleus of trigeminal; nerve; SUC, subiculum; ZI, zona incerta.

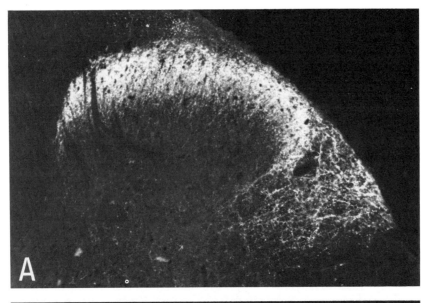

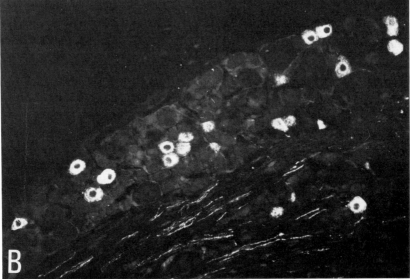

Figure 11. Somatostatin immunoreactivity in the dorsal horn of the rat spinal cord (A), rat dorsal root ganglion (B), and guinea pig inferior mesenteric sympathetic ganglion (C).

4.   Binding Sites/Receptors in the CNS

The distribution of somatostatin-binding sites in the brain has been studied in rats and humans with autoradiographic techniques, showing a high degree of correspondence with the distribution of somatostatin-LI (Tran et al., 1984, 1985; Reubi and Maurer, 1985; Reubi et al., 1986). A high density of somatostatin-binding sites has been found in cortex, hippocampus, and striatum. Low numbers of binding sites are seen in the cerebellum and brainstem, where also few somatostatin-containing fibers are found.

5.   Peripheral Nervous System

The gut is densely innervated by somatostatin-containing nerves located both in the

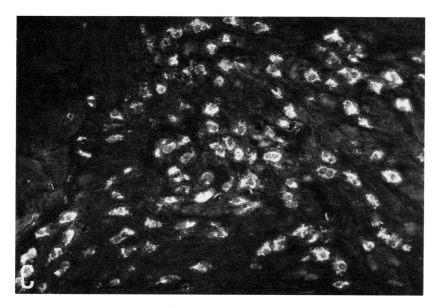

Figure 11. (continued).

submucous and myenteric plexus, with their cell bodies mainly in the intestinal wall but with some originating in prevertebral ganglia (Figure 12) (see Furness and Costa, 1987). The intestinal systems have also been studied in the human gut. Both in the small and large intestine many somatostatin-IR fibers are found, and they are especially abundant in the duodenum (Keast et al., 1984).

Cell bodies in sympathetic autonomic ganglia, such as the superior cervical ganglia and especially the prevertebral celiac, superior, and inferior mesenteric ganglia, contain somatostatin-LI (Figure 11C) (Hökfelt et al., 1977; see Schultzberg and Lindh, 1988).

6. Endocrine Cells

Shortly after the immunohistochemical identification of somatostatin in the hypothalamus, it was shown that somatostatin also was present in a number of endocrine cell types (Luft et al., 1974; Arimura et al., 1975; Dubois, 1975; Hökfelt et al., 1975; Orci et al., 1975). Thus, somatostatin is located in the endocrine cells of the pancreas (Figure 12D), where they constitute the D cells within the Langerhans cell islets, and thus stain intensely with silver, and are distinct from the ones containing insulin (B cells), glucagon (A cells), or pancreatic polypeptide (PP) (F cells). In the rat, somatostatin, glucagon, and PP cells are distributed in the periphery of the islets (Figure 12D), whereas insulin is seen in the central core. However, in the human pancreas, the somatostatin-containing D cells are scattered throughout the islets. Somatostatin inhibits insulin as well as glucagon secretion, and the release of somatostatin is stimulated by glucose (see Gerich, 1980; Miller, 1981; Sorenson and Elde, 1983).

Apart from being present in nerves throughout the gastrointestinal tract, somatostatin is also present in epithelial endocrine cells (D cells) (Figure 12) (see Sundler and Håkansson, 1988). These cells are most abundant in the antral region of the stomach and decrease in distal direction to the lower colon, where they are found deep in the crypts of the epithelium and possess processes that have contact with the lumen of the digestive tract. They appear to be sensitive to concentrations of hydrogen ions and certain nutrients. Apart from having local paracrine effects within interstitial space of the gut, the somatostatin-containing endocrine cells secrete their contents into the intestinal venous blood to enter the portal circulation

Figure 12. Somatostatin-immunoreactive cells and nerve fibers in the stomach (A), small intestine (B and C), large intestine (E), and pancreas (D). (A) In the stomach, the somatostatin-immunoreactivity is located in endocine epithelial cells with small processes extending into the lumen (see inset in A). (B and C) Somatostatin-containing nerve fibers are distributed in the lamina propria starting from the small intestine (see B and C) and decrease in number toward the large intestine (see E). Few endocrine-like cells are also seen in the small and large intestine (see inset in E). (D) Endocrine cells in the Langerhans islets of the pancreas contain somatostatin immunoreactivity. These cells are found in the peripheral part of the islands and are referred to as D cells. The central part of the cell islet contains the insulin-producing cells.

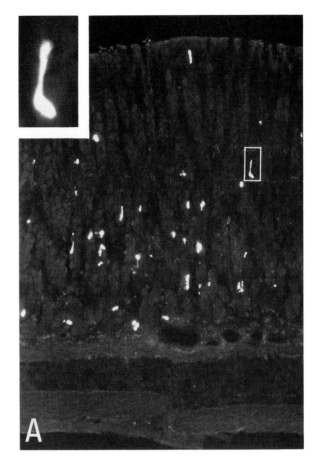

(Pradayrol, 1988); there is also an intralumenal secretion (Uvnäs-Wallensten, 1980). Somatostatin has been shown to have an inhibitory effect on most exocrine secretions in the gut (see Gerich, 1980; Miller, 1981).

Somatostatin is also present in some of the calcitonin-producing (C cells) interstitial parafollicular cells of the thyroid (see Hökfelt et al., 1975), where it has been found to inhibit the secretion of calcitonin, most likely via autocrine mechanisms, i.e., diffusion of somatostatin to the interstitial space and binding to the somatostatin-binding site at the cell membranes (Gordin et al., 1978). Both somatostatin-14 and -28 have been demonstrated in rat pituitary gland by radioimmunoassay and immunohistochemistry (Mesguich et al., 1988), and preprosomatostatin mRNA has also been detected in normal and tumorous anterior pituitary tissue in humans (Pagesy et al., 1989).

7. Afferents

Descending inputs from the telencephalon, ascending inputs from the brainstem, and inputs from the diencephalon constitute afferent pathways to the anterior periventricular zone (see Zaborsky, 1982; Swanson, 1987). Specific, chemically identified afferents making synaptic contact with the somatostatin cells in the anterior periventricular nucleus are, however, relatively unknown. Fibers originating in the lower brainstem carry the catecholamines noradrenaline and adrenaline. Noradrenergic fibers arising in the locus coeruleus innervate the anterior periventricular nucleus (Jones and Moore, 1977), and serotoninergic fibers originating in the dorsal raphe nucleus reach both the anterior periventricular nucleus and the arcuate

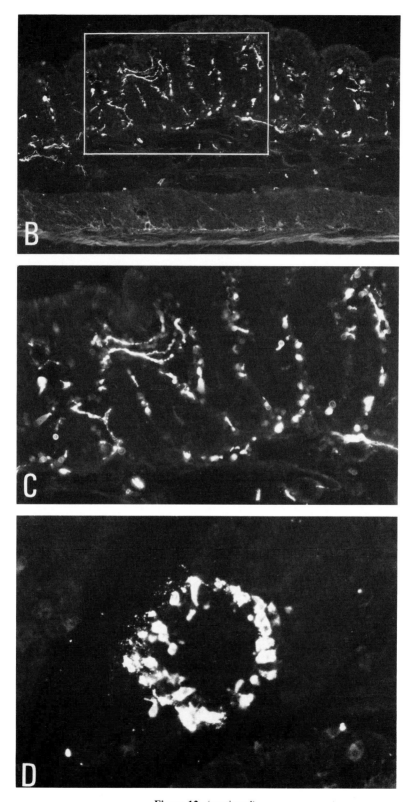

Figure 12. (continued).

Figure 12. (continued).

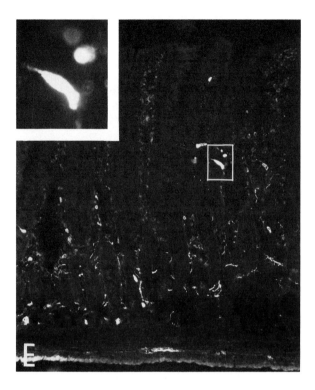

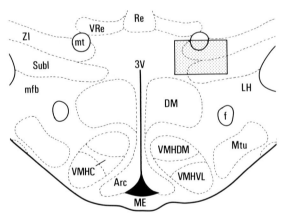

Figure 13. Somatostatin (SOM)-containing neurons located in the hypothalamic zona incerta (the A13 cell group) cocontaining the dopamine-synthesizing enzymes tyrosine hydroxylase (TH) and aromatic L-amino acid decarboxylase (AADC). The cell bodies are located just beneath the mammillothalamic tract (mt) (see schematic drawing). Arrows point at cells containing somatostatin, TH, and AADC immunoreactivity. 3V, Third ventricle, Arc, arcuate nucleus; DM, dorsomedial hypothalamic nucleus; f, fornix; LH, lateral hypothalamic area; ME, median eminence; mfb, medial forebrain bundle; mt, mammillothalamic tract; Mtu, medial tuberal nucleus; Re, reuniens thalamic nucleus; Subl, subincertal nucleus; VMHC, ventromedial hypothalamic nucleus, central; VMHVL, ventromedial hypothalamic nucleus, lateral; VMHDM, ventromedial hypothalamic nucleus, dorsomedial; VRe, ventral reuniens nucleus; ZI, zona incerta. (From Meister et al., 1987b, with permission.)

nucleus (see Swanson, 1987; see also Zaborsky, 1982). The cells in the anterior periventricular nucleus are densely surrounded by glutamic acid decarboxylase (GAD)- and γ-aminobutyric acid (GABA)-containing fiber networks (Mugnaini and Oertel, 1985; Meister and Hökfelt,

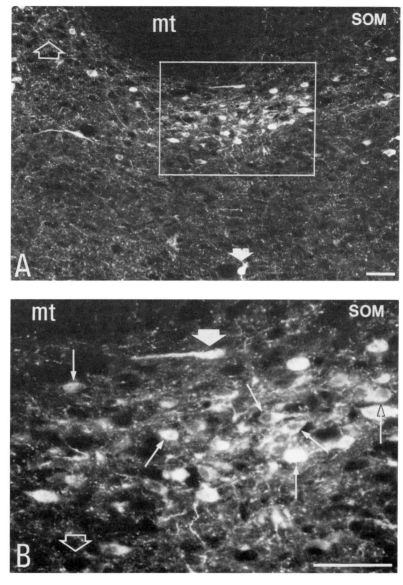

Figure 13. (continued).

1988; Sakaue et al., 1988). Of special interest is that a dense GRF-IR nerve plexus has been shown in the periventricular region, and ultrastructural studies have demonstrated that GRF-IR nerve endings directly contact somatostatin-IR cell bodies in the anterior periventricular nucleus (Horváth et al., 1989a). GRF neurons may therefore participate in the control of somatostatin release into the portal vessels.

8. Colocalization with Other Neuroactive Substances

A considerable amount of evidence has been presented to support the fact that both neurons and endocrine cells synthesize, store, and secrete more than one messenger molecule (see Hökfelt et al., 1986). The somatostatin and GRF systems are not excluded from this principle and both peptides have been observed together with classical transmitters as well as

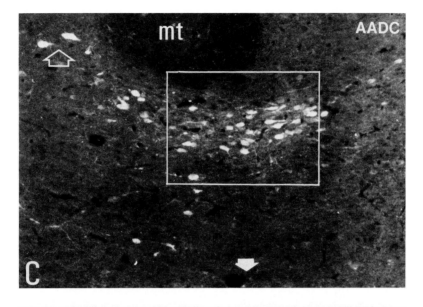

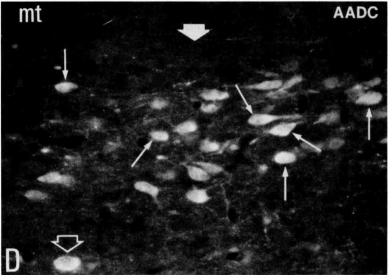

Figure 13. (continued).

other peptides. Although somatostatin colocalizes with several other bioactive compounds in the central and peripheral nervous system, the somatostatin-containing neurons in the periventricular nucleus projecting to the median eminence and being involved in GH control, as well as the somatostatin-containing cell bodies in the arcuate nucleus, have so far not been recognized to contain any other classical transmitter or any other peptide (see Everitt et al., 1986). However, in one hypothalamic cell group, the so-called A13 cell group in the zona incerta, somatostatin is seen together with dopamine in its caudal extension (Figure 13) (Meister et al., 1987b). This cell group most likely has intrahypothalamic projections (see Björklund and Lindvall, 1984). In the cortex and hippocampus, somatostatin is found together with neuropeptide Y (NPY) and GABA (Figure 14) (see Jones and Hendry, 1986).

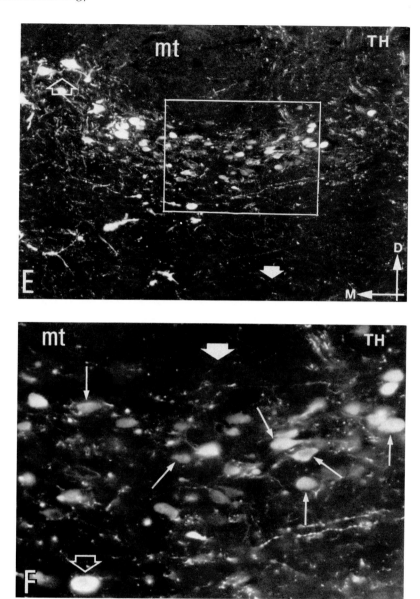

Figure 13. (continued).

III. GRF

A.   Biochemistry

Peptides with 44, 40, and 37 amino acids with GH-releasing activity were isolated from two different human pancreatic islet tumors that caused acromegaly (Guillemin et al., 1982; Rivier et al., 1982; Esch et al., 1983b). The GRF characterized by Vale and collaborators (Rivier et al., 1982) contained 40 amino acids with a free carboxy terminus, whereas the GRF characterized by Guillemin and colleagues (Guillemin et al., 1982) contained 44 amino acids

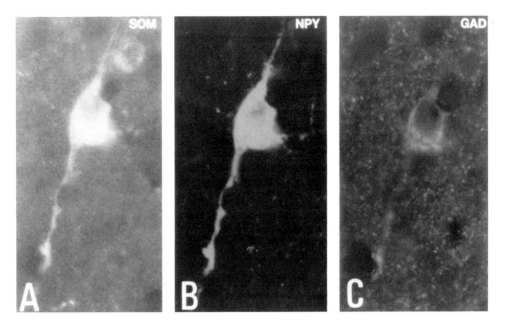

Figure 14. Three-color immunofluorescence histochemistry of the same section of the parietal cortex stained with antisera to somatostatin (SOM) (A), neuropeptide Y (NPY) (B), and glutamic acid decarboxylase (GAD) (C). One cell appears to contain all three immunoreactivities.

having an amidated carboxy terminus (Figure 15). In addition to these two peptides, Guillemin et al. (1982) extracted a nonamidated GRF with 37 amino acids. Interestingly, both $GRF_{1-44}NH_2$ and $GRF_{1-40}OH$ are encountered in the human hypothalamus (Böhlen et al., 1983a; Spiess et al., 1983; Ling et al., 1984), exhibit similar activity on GH release (see Frohman and Jansson, 1986), and are identical to the human pancreatic forms. In primary cultures of dispersed rat anterior pituitary cells, GRF stimulates dose dependently the secretion of GH (Guillemin et al., 1982; Brazeau et al., 1982a; Bilezikjian and Vale, 1983; Vale et al., 1983), but has no effect on the serum levels of follicle-stimulating hormone (FSH), luteinizing hormone (LH), TSH, or prolactin (Brazeau et al., 1982a). GRF has been shown to be a potent stimulator of the secretion of GH *in vivo* in all species of vertebrates studied so far (Wehrenberg et al., 1982a). The full biological activity of GRF is present in N-terminal fragments as short as 29 amino acids (Ling et al., 1984). Removal of further C-terminal amino acids from the peptide will result in a dramatic loss of the GH-releasing property (Rivier et al., 1982). Specific GRF antagonists have been synthesized with potent inhibitory effect on GH secretion and somatic growth (Mulroney et al., 1989; Lumpkin and McDonald, 1989; Lumpkin et al., 1989).

In 1983, Spiess et al. reported the isolation and characterization of rat hypothalamic (rh) GRF from acid extracts of 80,000 rat hypothalami. Rat hypothalamic GRF_{1-43} is a nonamidated peptide (Figure 15) that shows homology only in about two thirds of all amino acids with human pancreas (hp)GRF_{1-44} (Figure 16) (Spiess et al., 1983), and is three to six times more potent in stimulating the release of GH from rat somatotrophs than all other GRFs (Baird et al., 1986). The marked difference between human and rat GRF has led to confusion in the literature with regard to the cellular localization of GRF in rat brain (see below). GRFs have also been isolated from several other species, including bovine (Esch et al., 1983a), ovine (Brazeau et al., 1984), porcine (Böhlen et al., 1983b), and caprine (Brazeau et al., 1984) hypothalamus, and they all exhibit a high degree of homology with human GRF. In contrast, the newly characterized mouse GRF only shows about two thirds homology with both human and rat GRF (Frohman et al., 1989).

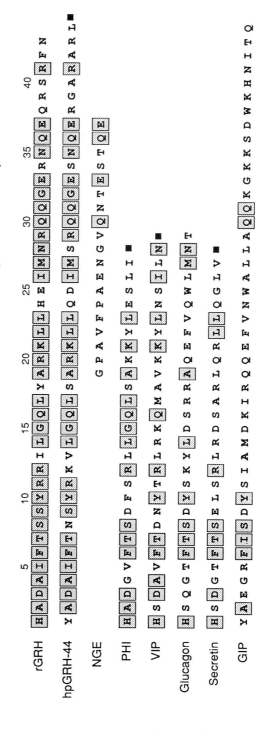

Growth hormone-releasing factor (Human)

Tyr-Ala-Asp-Ala-Ile-Phe-Thr-Asn-Ser-Tyr-Arg-Lys-Val-Leu-Gly-Gln-Leu-Ser-
Ala-Arg-Lys-Leu-Gln-Asp-Ile-Met-Ser-Arg-Gln-Gln-Gly-Glu-Ser-Asn-Gln-
Glu-Arg-Gly-Alal-Arg-Ala-Arg-Leu-NH₂

Growth hormone-releasing factor (Rat)

His-Ala-Asp-Ala-Ile-Phe-Thr-Ser-Ser-Tyr-Arg-Arg-Ile-Leu-Gly-Gln-Leu-Tyr-
Ala-Arg-Lys-Leu-Leu-His-Glu-Ile-Met-Asn-Arg-Gln-Gln-Gly-Glu-Arg-Asn-Gln-
Glu-Gln-Arg-Ser-Arg-Phe-Asn

Figure 15. Amino acid sequence of human and rat growth hormone-releasing factor (GRF.. Two forms of GRF are encountered in the human hypothalamus, a nonamidated peptide with 40 amino acid residues and an amidated peptide with 44 amino acid residues. Note the marked difference between human and rat GRF.

Sequence Comparison of rGRH with Other Members of the Glucagon-Secretin Family and NGE

Figure 16. Amino acid sequences of GRFs and other members of the glucagon-secretin peptide family, including peptide histidine-isoleucine (PHI), vasoactive intestinal polypeptide (VIP), glucagon, secretin, and gastric inhibitory peptide (GIP). Homologous sequences are indicated by shaded boxes and squares point at C-terminal amidation sites. NGE is a putative neuropeptide encoded by the salmon melanin-concentrating hormone (MCH) precursor. Five of eight amino acid residues at the C-terminal end of NGE exhibit identity with hpGRF30-37. Cross-reactivity of antisera to hpGRF with NGE is most likely the cause of artifactual staining of cells in the lateral hypothalamic area and zona incerta obtained with hpGRF antisera in the rat hypothalamus (see text). (Kindly provided by Dr. P. E. Sawchenko.)

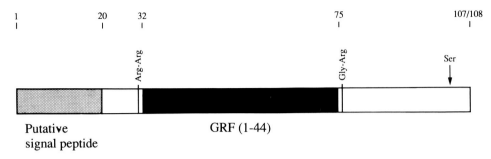

Figure 17. Structure of the human prepro-GRF-107 and -108 molecule. The prepro-GRF-108 molecule differs from prepro-GRF-107 by the insertion of a serine (Ser) residue in the carboxy-terminal portion of the precursor. The sequence of hpGRF₁-₄₄ extends from amino acid residues 32 to 75 (the black area). The putative signal peptide is indicated by the gray area. Amino acid residues where proteolytic cleavages take place are indicated. (Drawn from data of Gubler et al., 1983.)

Structurally, GRF belongs to the glucagon-secretin peptide family (Mutt, 1988), which includes glucagon, secretin, vasoactive intestinal polypeptide (VIP), peptide histidine-isoleucine (PHI), and gastric inhibitory peptide (GIP) (Guillemin et al., 1982; Rivier et al., 1982; Miller, 1984) (see Figure16). However, of all these peptides, only GRF has a significant direct effect on GH secretion from the somatotrophs.

The cDNAs encoding human (Gubler et al., 1983; Mayo et al., 1983) and rat (Mayo et al., 1985a) GRF have been cloned and characterized. Two GRF precursors of 13,000 Da with lengths of 107 and 108 amino acid residues have been identified, and they are identical except for a serine residue at the C-terminal end of the molecule (Figure 17). The entire human GRF gene has been structurally characterized and been found to be located on chromosome 20 (Mayo et al., 1985b).

B.   Localization of GRF

Physiological studies employing lesions or electrical stimulation within the hypothalamus previously indicated that the location of the GRF-containing neurons would be in the region of the ventromedial and arcuate nuclei (Reichlin, 1960; Frohman and Bernardis, 1968; Frohman et al., 1969; Martin, 1972). These observations have been confirmed by immunohistochemical detection of GRF-immunoreactive perikarya using immunohistochemistry.

In contrast to the broad distribution of neurons carrying the other hypothalamic hormones, GRF-like immunoreactivity is found, in all species investigated, in a very limited number of neurons within the brain, almost exclusively in the mediobasal hypothalamus (see Sawchenko et al., 1985; for review see Sawchenko and Swanson, 1990). Almost invariably it is necessary to use the mitosis inhibitor colchicine in order to arrest axonal transport and increase the levels of peptides in the cell soma to visualize GRF-IR perikarya in the rat brain. A detailed account of the distribution and localization of rhGRF-IR cell bodies and fibers in the rat hypothalamus has been presented by Sawchenko et al. (1985) (see Sawchenko and Swanson, 1990).

The principal GRF-containing cell group is found along the rostrocaudal extension of the arcuate nucleus, predominantly in the ventrolateral part of the nucleus (Figures 18-21). Around 1400 GRF-IR neurons have been counted in the arcuate nucleus on each side of the rat brain (Sawchenko et al., 1985), and the cell bodies are in general fusiform or ovoid (Beauvillain et al., 1987). The second major cell group extends from the lateral part of the arcuate nucleus, continuing dorsolaterally to surround and encapsulate the ventromedial nucleus (Figures 18, 20, and 21). This group continues to the anterior periventricular nucleus, the ventral part of the

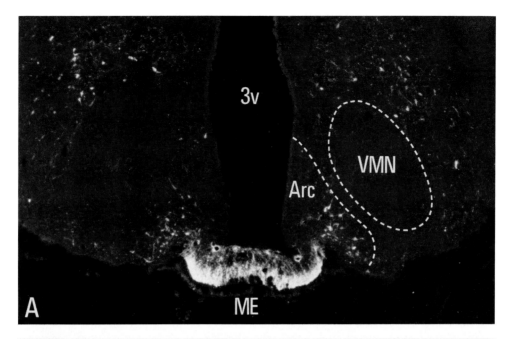

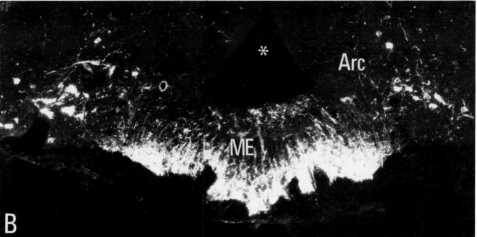

Figure 18. Growth hormone-releasing factor (GRF)-containing neurons in the mediobasal hypothalamus of the rat. GRF-immunoreactive cell bodies are located in the ventrolateral part of the arcuate nucleus (Arc) (B) and encapsulate the ventromedial nucleus (VMN) (A). A very dense plexus of GRF-immunoreactive fibers is distributed in the external zone of the median eminence (ME). 3v, *: third ventricle.

parvocellular portion of the paraventricular nucleus, and the dorsomedial nucleus (Figure 20) (Sawchenko et al., 1985; Bruhn et al., 1987). The latter cells in the paraventricular and dorsomedial nuclei have been particularly difficult to visualize, and the use of more sensitive immunohistochemical techniques have been of special importance here. Apart from the above-mentioned locations, no evidence for the existence of GRF-IR cell bodies in any other part of the central nervous system has been reported.

Immediately after the characterization of hpGRF, antisera were produced against the human pancreatic peptides. The use of some antisera to *human* GRF in immunohistochemical

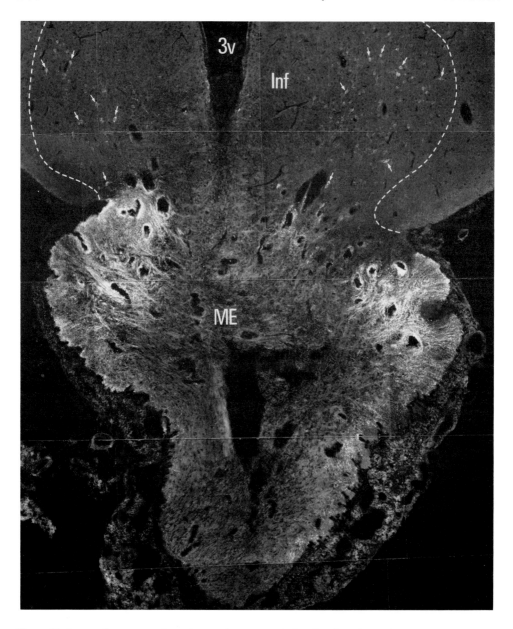

Figure 19. Immunofluorescence photomicrographs (montages) of sections from the monkey (Macaca fascicularis) mediobasal hypothalamus showing the infundibular nucleus (Inf; outlined with broken lines) and median eminence (ME) after incubation with monoclonal antibodies to human GRF$_{1-44}$. Dense aggregations of GRF-immunoreactive (IR) fibers surrounding portal vessels are observed in the external layer of the median eminence. Note the presence of several GRF-IR cell bodies (small arrows) in the infundibular nucleus (Inf). The GRF-IR cell bodies are located in the ventrolateral part of the infundibular nucleus. 3v, Third ventricle.

experiments in *rat* has led to some confusion in the literature. Initial studies on the localization of GRF in both rat (Bloch et al., 1983a; Jacobowitz et al., 1983; Tramu et al., 1983) and primate brain (Bloch et al., 1983b; Lechan et al., 1984) revealed hpGRF-IR cell bodies in the arcuate nucleus (infundibular nucleus in the primate brain) with a dense plexus of immunoreactive fibers in the median eminence. However, in the *rat*, cell bodies were in addition detected in the

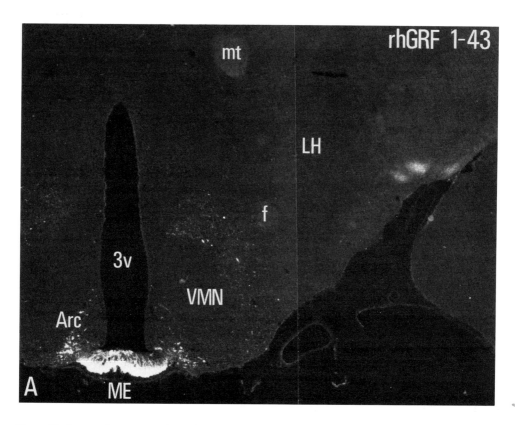

Figure 20. Immunofluorescence photomicrographs of two adjacent sections of the rat hypothalamus incubated with antisera to rat hypothalamic (rh) GRF$_{1-43}$ (A) and human pancreatic (hp) GRF$_{1-37}$ (B). The rhGRF$_{1-43}$ antiserum labels cell bodies in the arcuate nucleus (Arc) and surround the ventromedial nucleus (VMN) and fibers in the external part of the median eminence (ME), whereas the hpGRF$_{1-37}$ antiserum in addition labels cells in the lateral hypothalamic area (LH). f, Fornix; mt, mammillothalamic tract; 3v, third ventricle.

lateral hypothalamic area and zona incerta (Figure 20) (Jacobowitz et al., 1983; Merchenthaler et al., 1984a). When later rhGRF was characterized and antisera were generated against this peptide, it was shown that rhGRF-IR cell bodies were exclusively located in the mediobasal hypothalamus (Figure 20) (Sawchenko et al., 1985; Merchenthaler et al., 1984b, 1986; Daikoku et al., 1986; VandePol et al., 1986). The reason for this discrepancy may be explained by some later observations made by Fellmann et al. (1985), who reported that an antiserum against hpGRF$_{1-37}$, but not an antiserum to rat GRF, stained a cell group in the lateral hypothalamus and zona incerta (Figure 20). Their hpGRF antiserum recognized a part of the GRF molecule corresponding to amino acids 29 to 37 of the human GRF. It was later demonstrated that the hpGRF$_{1-37}$-IR cells in the lateral hypothalamic area and zona incerta also stained positively for melanocyte-stimulating hormone (MSH), salmon melanin-concentrating hormone (MCH), and rat corticotropin-releasing factor (CRF) (Fellmann et al., 1986, 1987). Recently, the MCH precursor was cloned and it has become apparent that eight amino acid residues in the MCH prohormone, referred to as the putative neuropeptide NGE, shares five identical amino acids with hpGRF$_{30-37}$ (Figure 16) (Breton et al., 1989; Fellmann et al., 1989; Nahon et al., 1989). Absorption of the hpGRF$_{1-37}$ antiserum with NGE eliminates the staining in the lateral hypothalamic area (see Sawchenko and Swanson, 1990). Thus, the initial immunohistochemical studies in the rat using antisera to hpGRF in all probability detected the

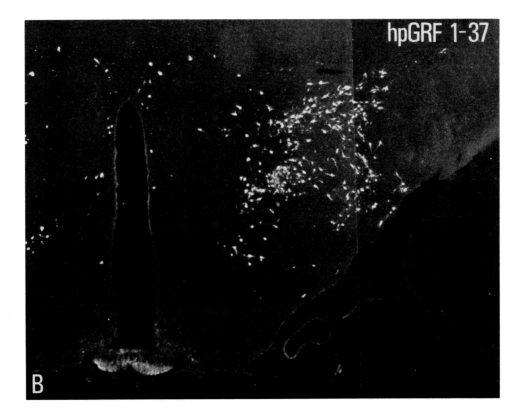

Figure 20. (continued).

prohormone to MCH, giving rise to a 'false' positive cell group in the lateral hypothalamic area and zona incerta not containing genuine rat GRF.

The localization of rhGRF-IR perikarya in the hypothalamus has recently been confirmed by *in situ* hybridization histochemistry (see Sawchenko and Swanson, 1990), showing that GRF is synthesized exclusively in the mediobasal hypothalamus. No GRF mRNA has been detected in the lateral hypothalamus, further supporting that the initial immunohistochemical studies with antisera to human GRF detected antigens other than the one(s) they were originally produced against.

Ontogenetic studies have shown that, in the rat arcuate nucleus and median eminence, GRF-IR neurons can be detected as early as on gestational day 18 (Daikoku et al., 1985; Ishikawa et al., 1986; Jansson et al., 1987). In agreement, GH secretion from the anterior pituitary (Baird et al., 1984) and GH in the circulation (Wilson and Frohman, 1974) are detected on embryonic day 18. The GRF neurons encapsulating the ventromedial nucleus, however, seem to express detectable levels of GRF just after birth (Daikoku et al., 1985; Ishikawa et al., 1986). In the human fetus, GRF-IR cell bodies and fibers are found as early as the 18th week of gestation (Bresson et al., 1984). It has been observed that the GRF-LI in the median eminence decreases with increasing age (Fuxe et al., 1988; Morimoto et al., 1988), and the GH responses to GRF are greater in newborn rats as compared to older individuals both *in vivo* (Cella et al., 1985) and *in vitro* (Szabo and Cuttler, 1986), in agreement with studies in humans (see Thorner et al., 1987).

Evidence has accumulated indicating that GRF-LI also is present in several peripheral

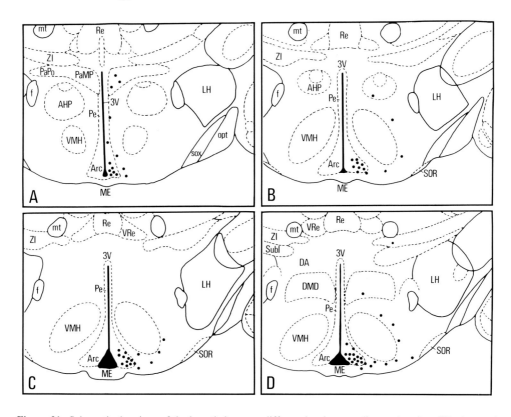

Figure 21. Schematic drawings of the hypothalamus at different levels, according to the atlas of Paxinos and Watson (1986), illustrate the distribution of GRF-containing cell bodies (dots). Abbreviations: AHP, anterior hypothalamic area, posterior; Arc, arcuate nucleus; DA, dorsal hypothalamic area; DM, dorsomedial hypothalamic nucleus; DMC, dorsomedial hypothalamic nucleus, compact; DMD, dorsomedial hypothalamic nucleus, diffuse; Do, dorsal hypothalamic nucleus; f, fornix; InfS, infundibular stem; LH, lateral hypothalamic area; ME, median eminence; mt, mammillothalamic tract; MTu, medial tuberal nucleus; opt, optic tract; PaMP, paraventricular hypothalamic nucleus, medial parvocellular part; PaPo, paraventricular hypothalamic nucleus, posterior part; Pe, periventricular hypothalamic nucleus; PMV, premamillary nucleus, ventral; Re, reuniens thalamic nucleus; sox, supraoptic decussation; SOR, supraoptic nucleus, retrochiasmatic; SPF, subparafascicular thalamic nucleus; Subl, subincertal nucleus; TMC, tuberal magnocellular nucleus; VMH, ventromedial hypothalamic nucleus; VMHC, ventromedial hypothalamic nucleus, central; VMHDM, ventromedial hypothalamic nucleus, dorsomedial; VMHVL, ventromedial hypothalamic nucleus, ventrolateral; ZI, zona incerta; VRe, ventral reuniens nucleus; 3V, third ventricle. (A) Bregma, −2.12 mm; (B) −2.30 mm; (C) −2.56 mm; (D) −2.80 mm; (E) −3.14 mm; (F) −3.30 mm; (G) −3.60 mm; (H) −3.80 mm.

tissues, including sensory ganglia (Jósza et al., 1987), testis (Berry and Pescovitz, 1988), duodenum (Bruhn et al., 1985), stomach (Bosman et al., 1984), placenta (Baird et al., 1985; Meigan et al., 1988), anterior pituitary (Morel et al., 1984), and normal pancreas (Bosman et al., 1984).

1. Projections

Neurons in the arcuate nucleus belong to the so-called tuberoinfundibular system, known to possess projections to the median eminence (Szentagothai et al., 1972; Wiegand and Price, 1980; Lechan et al., 1982), and it was early shown that the GRF-containing cell bodies in the arcuate nucleus give rise to the dense GRF-IR fiber plexus in the median eminence (Figure 17) (Bloch et al., 1984). This conclusion was based on experiments in rats with the neurotoxin MSG, which is known to cause selective lesions in the arcuate nucleus, especially in its ventral

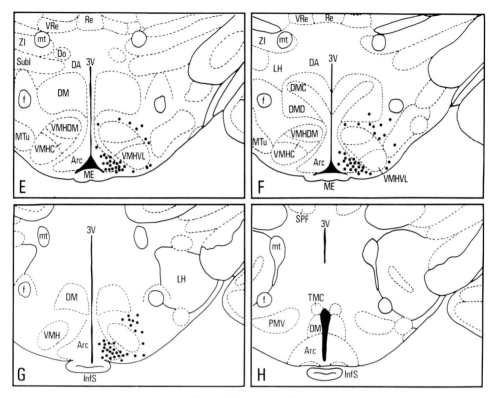

Figure 21. (continued).

part (Figure 22) (see Meister et al., 1989). After MSG treatment during the neonatal period all GRF-IR cell bodies in the arcuate nucleus are eliminated, combined with a marked reduction in the number of GRF-IR fibers in the median eminence (Figure 22) (Bloch et al., 1984; Daikoku et al., 1986; Meister et al., 1989). Destruction of the hypothalamic GRF neurons by MSG causes stunted growth and a decrease in plasma and pituitary GH (W. J. Millard et al., 1982). In spite of the complete elimination of the GRF-IR cell bodies in the arcuate nucleus, a few remaining fibers are still encountered in the median eminence after this treatment. The remaining fibers may originate in the parvocellular part of the paraventricular nucleus, which is relatively insensitive to the toxic effects of MSG (see Meister et al., 1989). GRF-containing neurons projecting to the median eminence are located in the ventrolateral division of the arcuate nucleus, as shown by administering retrograde tracers either into the median eminence (Niimi et al., 1989, 1990) or intravenously (Figure 23) (Meister et al., 1987a). The GRF-IR cell bodies encapsulating the ventromedial nucleus do not appear to send projections to the median eminence (Wiegand and Price, 1980; Lechan et al., 1982; Daikoku et al., 1986).

Besides the tuberoinfundibular projection, two major GRF-IR fiber systems may be distinguished (Sawchenko et al., 1985). The first fiber system is ascending and goes dorsally to the anterior periventricular nucleus, the ventral parts of the dorsomedial nucleus, and the parvocellular paraventricular nucleus. The second fiber system is both ascending and descending. The ascending part goes via the ventromedial margin of the hypothalamus to the preoptic region, whereas the descending part travels dorsally from the dorsomedial nucleus through the lateral hypothalamic area to the medial nucleus of the amygdala. Terminal fields derived from the descending pathway are also found in the posterior periventricular and ventral premammillary nuclei as well as the tuberomammillary and supramammillary nuclei. In the tuberoinfundibular system, ultrastructural studies have shown that GRF is localized in secretory granules (diam-

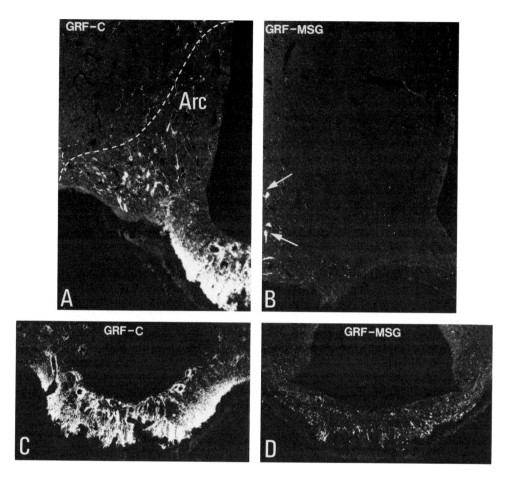

Figure 22. Immunofluorescence photomicrographs of sections of the arcuate nucleus (Arc; outlined with broken line) of control (A,C) and rats treated neonatally with the neurotoxin monosodium glutamate (MSG) (B,D). The neurotoxin induces specific lesions in the Arc, resulting in a total disappearance of growth hormone-releasing factor (GRF)-immunoreactive (IR) cell bodies. Some remaining GRF-IR cell bodies (arrows in D) are seen lateral to the remaining part of the Arc. In the median eminence there is an almost complete disappearance of GRF-IR fibers after MSG treatment. Remaining GRF-IR fibers in the median eminence may arise from the parvocellular part of the paraventricular nucleus.

eter 100 to 200 nm) that are transported to the median eminence (Ibata et al., 1986; Beauvillain et al., 1987; Daikoku et al., 1988).

2.   Afferents

Little is known with regard to specific afferents synapsing on GRF neurons. However, it is well established that the arcuate nucleus receives a variety of inputs from aminergic cell groups in the brainstem, from several nuclei in the hypothalamus, and from limbic structures (see Swanson, 1987). Most of the noradrenergic and adrenergic input to the arcuate nucleus, anterior periventricular nucleus, and median eminence derives from cell groups in the lower brainstem and from the locus coeruleus (see Zaborsky, 1982). The GRF-IR neurons in the arcuate nucleus have small numbers of somatostatin-containing synapses on their cell somata and dendrites (Ibata et al., 1986; Daikoku et al., 1988; Liposits et al., 1988; Horváth et al., 1989a). Somatostatin-binding sites have also been demonstrated in the arcuate nucleus (Uhl et

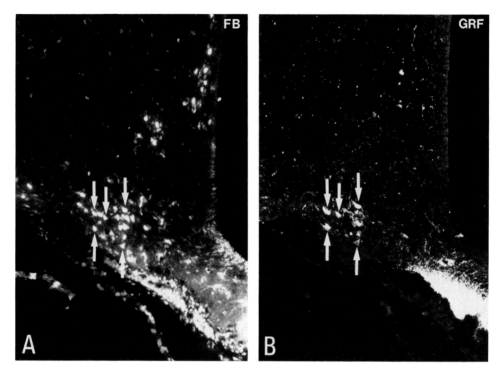

Figure 23. Fluorescence (A) and immunofluorescence (B) photomicrographs of sections of the arcuate nucleus after intravenous injection of the retrograde tracer Fast Blue (FB) and subsequent incubation with GRF antiserum. The tracer (FB) is taken up by nerve terminals in the median eminence and is retrogradely transported to the cell bodies in the anterior periventricular nucleus. Arrows point to cells containing FB fluorescence and GRF immunoreactivity.

al., 1985; Epelbaum et al., 1989). This has raised the exciting possibility that periventricular somatostatin neurons in the anterior hypothalamus, in addition to secreting somatostatin into portal vessels, may exert an inhibitory tone on GH secretion via an inhibitory influence on GRF neurons. However, the origin of the somatostatin-containing terminals in the arcuate nucleus is not fully clarified and both cells in the anterior periventricular nucleus and local somatostatin-IR cell bodies within the arcuate nucleus are possible sources. In fact, recent findings by Willoughby et al. (1989) suggest that at least most somatostatin synapses have a local origin (see also Meister et al., 1989).

In addition to the GRF-containing cell bodies in the arcuate nucleus, there exists a local network of GRF-IR fibers and varicosities in the nucleus (Horváth and Palkovits, 1988). By electron microscopy, it has been demonstrated that the GRF-IR nerve terminals are in synaptic contact with GRF-IR dendrites and perikarya (Horváth and Palkovits, 1988). It has been suggested that these neuronal circuits may allow GRF neurons to operate synchronously, alternatively providing morphological evidence for the existence of ultrashort feedback mechanisms for regulating GRF release (Horváth and Palkovits, 1988), i.e., a mechanism through which GRF may inhibit its own synthesis/secretion.

3.   Colocalization with Other Neuroactive Substances

The GRF-containing neurons in the ventrolateral part of the arcuate nucleus have been shown to be surprisingly rich in other neuroactive substances. One of the first compounds to be demonstrated in the GRF-containing cells of the arcuate nucleus was the catecholamine-synthesizing enzyme tyrosine hydroxylase (TH) (Meister et al., 1985, 1986; Okamura et al., 1985; Daikoku et al., 1986). Since TH-IR neurons in the arcuate nucleus lack dopamine β-hydroxylase, it has generally been assumed that they are dopaminergic (see Everitt et al., 1986; Meister et al., 1986, 1988). It has, however, to date not been possible to demonstrate dopa decarboxylase (the dopamine-synthesizing enzyme) in the ventrolateral GRF-IR cells, raising the possibility that they may produce only L-dopa (Meister et al., 1988). Recently, TH has also been demonstrated within the GRF neurons in the parvocellular part of the paraventricular nucleus (Horváth et al., 1989b). The GRF-IR cell bodies have in addition been found to contain glutamic acid decarboxylase (GAD; the GABA-synthesizing enzyme) (Meister and Hökfelt, 1988), choline acetyltransferase (ChAT; the acetylcholine-synthesizing enzyme) (Meister and Hökfelt, 1988), and the neuropeptides neurotensin (Sawchenko et al., 1985; Everitt et al., 1986; Meister and Hökfelt, 1988) and galanin (Everitt et al., 1986; Meister and Hökfelt, 1988; Niimi et al., 1990; Meister et al., 1990) (see Figures 24, 25, and 27). The coexistence of GRF with these compounds in cell bodies of the arcuate nucleus has also been partly confirmed in nerve fibers and terminals of the median eminence (Figure 26) (Meister and Hökfelt, 1988; Meister et al., 1990), pointing to a corelease of these substances into the pericapillary space in the external layer of the median eminence. In general, the GRF- and NPY-IR neurons constitute two separate cell populations, located in the ventrolateral and ventromedial part of the arcuate nucleus, respectively (see Everitt et al., 1986). However, Ciofi et al. (1987, 1988, 1990) have reported that a subset of GRF neurons also contain NPY-LI. Finally, the presence of the glucocorticoid receptor in GRF neurons of the arcuate nucleus has been reported, supporting the view that glucocorticoids influence GH secretion via GRF (Cintra et al., 1987).

In view of the complete coexistence of GRF and galanin as well as some interesting findings on a role of galanin in control of GH secretion, we will briefly discuss the peptide galanin in the following section.

IV. Galanin

A 29-amino acid peptide with an N-terminal *glycine* and a C-terminal *alanine* residue, and hence termed galanin, was isolated in 1983 from porcine small intestine (Tatemoto et al., 1983). The mRNAs encoding the precursor proteins for porcine (Rökaeus and Brownstein, 1986), bovine (Rökaeus and Carlquist, 1988), and rat (Vrontakis et al., 1987; Kaplan et al., 1988a) have been characterized. Preprogalanin consists of 123 (pig, cow) and 124 (rat) amino acids, and the precursor protein contains four distinct regions, the putative signal peptide, a pregalanin message peptide (PGMP), galanin, and a 59- (pig, cow) or 60 (rat)-amino acid galanin message-associated peptide (GMAP) (see Rökaeus, 1987). Galanin-LI is widely distributed in the central and peripheral nervous system, with particularly high concentrations in the hypothalamus, as shown with radioimmunoassay (Skofitsch and Jacobowitz, 1985a; see Rökaeus, 1987 for review). Immunohistochemical analyses have shown a dense network of galanin-containing fibers in the external layer of the median eminence and cell bodies in several hypothalamic nuclei, including the supraoptic, paraventricular (parvocellular and magnocellular part), and arcuate nuclei (Melander et al., 1986; Skofitsch and Jacobowitz, 1985b). Specific binding sites for galanin have also been found in the median eminence (Skofitsch et al., 1986; Melander et al., 1987, 1988; Nordström et al., 1987), indicating a role for galanin at this site in the control of anterior pituitary function. Galanin has in particular been shown to be of importance for the regulation of GH secretion, but has other functions as well (see Rökaeus, 1987).

Within the arcuate nucleus, galanin is mainly located in the ventrolateral part and, in fact,

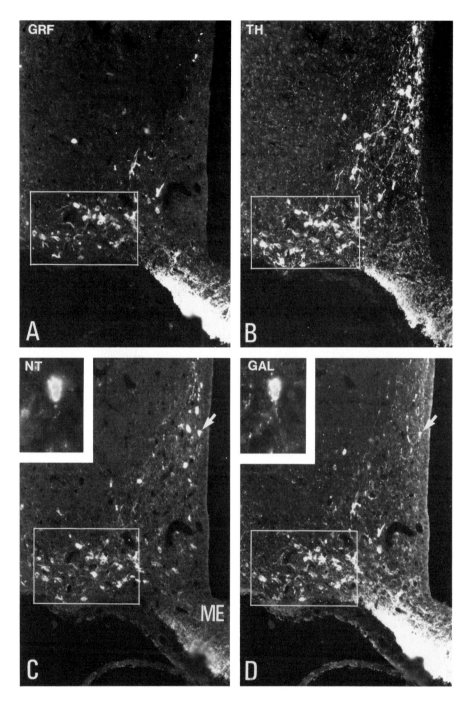

Figure 24. Immunofluorescence photomicrographs of the same section of the arcuate nucleus of the rat stained with antiserum to growth hormone-releasing factor (GRF) (A), tyrosine hydroxylase (TH) (B), neurotensin (NT) (C), and galanin, (GAL) (D). Two following double-staining procedures have been used. GRF-containing cell bodies are exclusively located in the ventrolateral part of the arcuate nucleus, whereas TH, and to a minor extent also NT and GAL, are found in both the ventrolateral and dorsomedial part of the nucleus. Note that virtually all cells in the ventrolateral part (see rectangles) contain all four compounds. Insets in (C) and (D) show a cell in the dorsomedial part of the arcuate nucleus that contains both NT and GAL (arrow). ME, Median eminence.

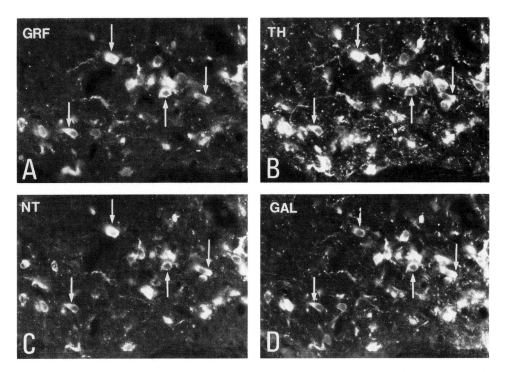

Figure 25. Higher magnifications of Figure 24A through D as indicated by rectangles. Arrows point to cells containing all four immunoreactivities.

to a large extent colocalizes with GRF (Everitt et al., 1986; Meister and Hökfelt, 1988; Meister et al., 1990; see above). Galanin mRNA has also been demonstrated in the ventrolateral arcuate neurons (Figure 28) (Meister et al., unpublished). The galanin-containing nerve fibers in the median eminence arise primarily from the arcuate nucleus, and to a minor extent from the parvocellular part of the paraventricular nucleus (Meister et al., 1989; Niimi et al., 1990). The development of galanin-IR neurons in the CNS has been studied with both immunohistochemistry and radioimmunoassay (Sizer et al., 1990), indicating that the ontogeny of galanin is entirely postnatal. The first apparent galanin-IR fibers in the median eminence are detected with immunohistochemistry on postnatal day 2, and radioimmunoassayable galanin is seen on day 3 (Sizer et al., 1990).

Galanin has been demonstrated to increase serum levels of GH when given intraventricularly (Ottlecz et al., 1985, 1988; Melander et al., 1987; Murakami et al., 1987a, 1989) or intravenously (Cella et al., 1988; Ottlecz et al., 1988; Murakami et al., 1989). A less prominent, but significant, increase in prolactin secretion by galanin has also been observed after intraventricular administration (Koshiyama et al., 1987; Melander et al., 1987; Ottlecz et al., 1988). Galanin also markedly increases plasma GH in humans after intravenous administration (Bauer et al., 1986; Davis et al., 1987; Loche et al., 1989). Passive immunoneutralization of galanin causes reduced plasma GH values (Ottlecz et al., 1988), reduced GH pulse amplitude and an increase in pulse frequency with a loss of the normal 3-hr periodicity, whereas the pulsatile secretion of prolactin is unaffected (Maiter et al., 1990). These results indicate that galanin is a physiological regulator of spontaneous pulsatile GH secretion. A mechanism by which galanin induces GH release may be via GRF, since it has been shown that galanin *in vitro* increases the release of GRF-LI from rat hypothalamic fragments (Murakami et al., 1989). It is in this context of special interest to consider that galanin colocalizes with GRF in

Figure 26. Immunofluorescence photomicrographs of a section of the rat median eminence after double-staining with antisera to the GABA-synthesizing enzyme glutamic acid decarboxylase (GAD) (A) and GRF (B). In the external layer, many nerve fiber varicosities exhibiting both GAD and GRF immunoreactivity are seen (see arrows), whereas the internal layer of the median eminence contains a GAD-positive/GRF-negative fiber plexus (large open arrows).

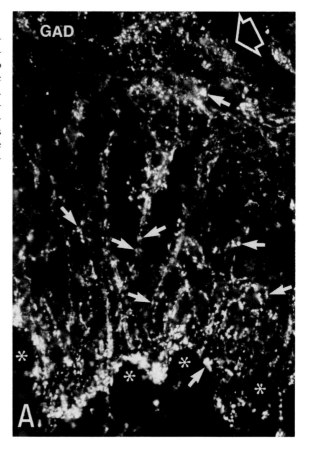

neurons of the arcuate nucleus both in rat and monkey (Everitt et al., 1986; Meister and Hökfelt, 1988; Meister et al., 1990; Niimi et al., 1990). Galanin also inhibits the release of dopamine from fragments of the mediobasal hypothalamus, an effect that may mediate the galanin-induced secretion of prolactin *in vivo* (Nordström et al., 1987). Little or no effect of galanin on basal or GRF-stimulated GH release from the anterior pituitary cells is seen *in vitro* (Ottlecz et al., 1985; Meister and Hulting, 1987; Gabriel et al., 1988), and lack of galanin-binding sites in the anterior pituitary has been observed (Gaymann and Falke, 1990). Galanin is also produced endogenously within the anterior pituitary, and the synthesis of galanin is increased after estrogen induction (Kaplan et al., 1988b; Vrontakis et al., 1987, 1989; Hulting et al., 1989; Gabriel et al., 1990). The levels of galanin-LI and galanin mRNA in the anterior pituitary are four- to five-fold higher in female than in male rats (Gabriel et al., 1989).

V. Secretory Patterns of Somatostatin and GRF

Growth hormone is secreted episodically in all species investigated (see Robinson and Clark, 1987), and exhibits a sexually dimorphic secretory pattern (Jansson et al., 1986). In male rats, the secretory bursts of GH appear at 3- to 3.5-hr intervals, and between these periods of secretion the GH is virtually undetectable (Tannenbaum and Martin, 1976). Female rats have a lower GH pulse amplitude but higher basal levels during the periods between the secretory pulses, resulting in more continuous exposure to GH than is seen in male rats. The

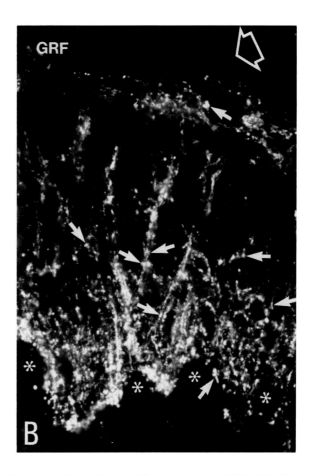

Figure 26. (continued).

mean plasma GH levels are similar in male and female rats (Jansson et al., 1986). This fact plays a major role in sexually dimorphic patterns of growth and metabolism. The episodic GH surges are entrained to the light-dark cycle via the retinohypothalamic tract and the suprachiasmatic nucleus. Lesions of the suprachiasmatic nucleus cause loss of entrainment but not loss of episodic secretion (Willoughby and Martin, 1978). In humans, the majority of the GH is secreted during the night, but smaller pulses may also occur during the day. It was shown early that selective lesioning of the arcuate/ventromedial nuclei will diminish or abolish episodic GH release (Frohman and Bernardis, 1968; Reichlin, 1974). Although the episodic nature of GH secretion has been confirmed in several studies, the mechanism underlying the generation of this ultradian rhythm remains unknown. Results from physiological experiments show that the secretion of somatostatin decreases in synchrony with the peaks of GH, whereas GRF secretion coincides with the GH pulses (see Figure 29) (Tannenbaum and Ling, 1984; Plotsky and Vale, 1985). Somatostatin is responsible for the GH pulse frequency, since a GH pulse occurs only if the somatostatin tone is withdrawn (Tannenbaum, 1988). Immunoneutralization of circulating GRF abolishes the episodic GH secretion, without affecting baseline GH values (Wehrenberg et al., 1982b,c). Episodic GH release is still observed in rats, whose endogenous somatostatin has been neutralized by passive immunization with anti-somatostatin serum (see Martin et al., 1978a,b). Somatostatin exerts an inhibitory effect on GH trough levels, since treatment with somatostatin antiserum raises the interpeak trough values (Ferland et al., 1976; Terry and Martin, 1981; Tannenbaum and Ling, 1984). Taken together, these findings suggest that both hypothalamic GRF and somatostatin are secreted in an episodic fashion to induce the

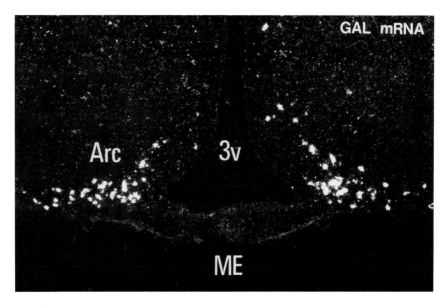

Figure 27. Galanin (GAL) mRNA-containing cell bodies in the arcuate nucleus (Arc) (dark-field photomicrograph of emulsion-dipped section). Cells containing GAL mRNA are mainly found in the ventrolateral part of the arcuate nucleus, similar to the distribution of GRF-containing neurons. ME, Median eminence; 3v, third ventricle.

periodic surges of GH in the male rat. The secretory patterns of GRF and somatostatin in relation to the episodic GH secretion are illustrated in Figure 29.

VI. Feedback Regulation

The regulation of GH secretion is under strong feedback regulation, involving short, long, and presumably ultrashort loops. Negative feedback effects of GH were first demonstrated by Krulich and McCann (1966), who showed that pituitary GH content was reduced in rats treated with bovine GH. Exogenous GH treatment suppresses endogenous GH secretion as a result of short-loop negative feedback (Katz et al., 1969; Voogt et al., 1971). Excess of GH leads to increased hypothalamic somatostatin content and secretion (Patel, 1979; Berelowitz et al., 1981b; Chihara et al., 1981). Recently, it has also been shown that hypophysectomy decreases the content of preprosomatostatin mRNA in cell bodies of the anterior periventricular nucleus, and that this effect can be reversed by GH administration (Rogers et al., 1988). In contrast, hypothalamic levels of GRF mRNA are increased after hypophysectomy, while the levels of GRF are decreased, and both these effects are partially reversed by GH replacement therapy (Chomczynski et al., 1988). This suggests that GH may operate to suppress GRF synthesis and release (Clark et al., 1988). GH thus exerts short-loop negative feedback by stimulating somatostatin gene expression/secretion and inhibiting GRF gene expression/secretion.

Intraventricularly injected GRF in high doses (0.2 or 2 µg) results in a dose-dependent elevation of plasma GH, indicating that the GRF is transported from the hypothalamus to the anterior pituitary (Arimura and Culler, 1985). Intriguingly, intraventricular administration of a low dose (0.02 µg) of GRF results in a suppression of GH release, suggesting that hypothalamic GRF regulates its own secretion via an ultrashort feedback mechanism. These findings are supported by morphological studies showning that GRF-IR terminals are in contact with GRF-IR cell bodies (Horváth and Palkovits, 1988). Alternatively, intraventricularly adminis-

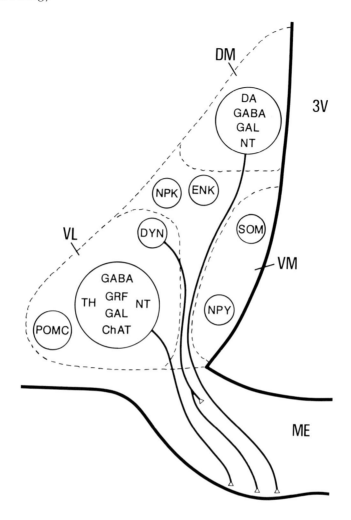

Figure 28. Schematic drawing illustrating the distribution of various neuroactive compounds in different parts of the rat arcuate nucleus and afferents to the median eminence (ME). The arcuate nucleus may be divided into the dorsomedial (DM), ventrolateral (VL), and ventromedial (VM) parts. ChAT, Choline acetyltransferase; DA, dopamine; DYN, dynorphin; ENK, enkephalin; GABA, γ-aminobutyric acid; GAL, galanin; GRF, growth hormone-releasing factor; NPK, neuropeptide K; NPY, neuropeptide Y; NT, neurotensin; POMC, proopiomelanocortin; SOM, somatostatin; TH, tyrosine hydroxylase; 3V, Third ventricle.

tered GRF suppresses GH secretion by increasing somatostatin release. There also exists anatomical support for an interaction between somatostatin and GRF, suggesting that both peptides may regulate each other's activity via specific pathways. A GRF-IR terminal network around somatostatin neurons in the anterior periventricular nucleus and GRF-IR terminals have been identified and at the ultrastructural level it is seen that GRF-IR neurons contact somatostatin neurons (Horváth et al., 1989a). Intraventricularly administered GRF causes a decrease in serum GH (Katakami et al., 1986), an effect that can be blocked by administration of antibodies to somatostatin, further indicating that GRF may stimulate the secretion of somatostatin. A stimulation of somatostatin release by GRF has also been demonstrated *in vitro* with fragments of the median eminence (Aguila and McCann, 1985). Conversely, a dense somatostatin-IR fiber plexus is located in the arcuate nucleus, closely surrounding and terminating on GRF-IR cell bodies (Liposits et al., 1988). In agreement, somatostatin-binding sites

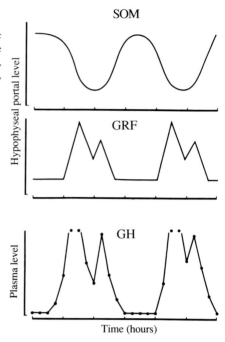

Figure 29. Schematic drawing illustrating postulated episodic secretion of (A) somatostatin (SOM) and (B) GRF into the hypophysial portal blood, with net result on GH secretion (C), as observed in plasma. (Modified after Tannenbaum and Ling, 1984, with permission.)

have also been demonstrated in the arcuate nucleus (Epelbaum et al., 1989). Moreover, intraventricular administration of somatostatin antiserum has in one study been reported to enhance GRF release during GH troughs in male rats, suggesting that somatostatin inhibits GRF release during the normal GH pulse cycle (Plotsky and Vale, 1985).

There is evidence that certain peripheral factors can exert an inhibitory long-loop feedback on GH release. Insulin-like growth factors (IGFs) and somatomedins are synonyms for the same class of peptides, which is under influence of GH (Hall and Sara, 1983; Nissley and Rechler, 1984; Van Wyk, 1984; Froesch et al., 1985). IGFs are found in high concentrations in plasma and are mainly produced in the liver, and the production of IGF-I is stimulated by GH (see Nissley and Rechler, 1984). High numbers of IGF-I receptors are present in the growth plate chondrocytes and most of the growth promoting effects on cartilage of GH are believed to be mediated through IGF-I (Van Wyk, 1984; Isaksson et al., 1987). Twenty-four hours after a single injection of GH there is a significant elevation of serum IGF-I (see Molitch, 1988). There exists a feedback regulation between GH and IGF-I and -II. Intraventricularly injected IGF-I abolishes spontaneous surges of GH (Abe et al., 1983; Tannenbaum et al., 1983). IGF-I is a potent stimulator of hypothalamic somatostatin secretion *in vitro* (Berelowitz et al., 1981) and inhibits both basal and GRF-stimulated secretion of GH *in vitro* (Berelowitz et al., 1981; Brazeau et al., 1982b; Goodyer et al., 1984; Ceda et al., 1985, 1987). Of special interest is that high concentrations of IGF-I binding sites have been demonstrated in the median eminence (Bohannon et al., 1986). IGF-I-mediated negative feedback operates via short-term suppression at the hypothalamic level via stimulation of somatostatin and inhibition of GRF secretion and long-term suppression mediated directly at the pituitary level.

VII. Neurotransmitter Control of Secretion

The release of GRF and somatostatin is controlled by complex neural regulatory mechanisms, and alterations in CNS activities such as sleep, stress, and exercise are often accompanied by changes in GH secretion, and there is a considerable amount of evidence indicating that several neurotransmitters influence the secretion of GH via indirect and direct effects (see Arimura and Fishback, 1981; Arimura and Culler, 1985).

Catecholamines such as dopamine and noradrenaline have a role in the control of GH secretion. The role of dopamine in control of GH secretion is, however, equivocal, since dopamine has effects both at the hypothalamic and pituitary level. *In vivo*, dopamine agonists such as apomorphine and bromocriptine cause an increase in GH (Lal et al., 1975a; Camanni et al., 1975; Bansal et al., 1981), as do infusions of dopamine (Leblanc et al., 1976; Camanni et al., 1977; Bansal et al., 1981; see Molitch, 1988). Dopamine does not cross the blood-brain barrier and can, therefore, affect GH secretion directly at the pituitary or through the median eminence, which is located outside the blood-brain barrier. In agreement with a central stimulatory role of dopamine are findings showing that dopamine stimulates somatostatin release from rat hypothalamus *in vitro* as well as in anesthetized rats (Wakabayashi et al., 1977; Negro-Vilar et al., 1978; Chihara et al., 1979). *In vitro*, dopamine and dopamine agonists inhibit GH release from pituitary cell cultures (see, e.g., Tallo and Malarkey, 1981; Marcovitz et al., 1982). This suggests that systemic dopamine stimulates GH release via the median eminence, and that the central stimulatory effect overrides the inhibitory effect exerted at the pituitary level.

Both the anterior periventricular nucleus and the arcuate nucleus receive a rich supply of noradrenergic/adrenergic afferents from the lower brainstem that can influence somatostatin and GRF secretion. Microinjections of noradrenaline into the ventromedial nucleus of monkeys result in GH release (Toivola and Gale, 1972), and α-adrenergic blockade with phentolamine in humans results in a blunting of the GH response to hypoglycemia, arginine, and surgical stress (Blackard and Heidingsfelder, 1968; Vigas et al., 1977; see Molitch, 1988). The α_2-receptor agonist clonidine induces release of GH (Durand et al., 1977) and this effect can be completely abolished by pretreatment with rabbit anti-rat GRF, indicating that the GH-releasing action of central α_2-adrenergic stimulation is mediated by endogenous GRF release (Miki et al., 1984). Episodic GH secretion is completely inhibited by α-adrenergic blockade induced by yohimbine, whereas GH trough values are unaffected. Furthermore, episodic GH secretion is inhibited by phenoxybenzamine (an α-adrenergic antagonist), FLA-63 (an inhibitor of dopamine β-hydroxylase), or α-methyl-*p*-tyrosine (an inhibitor of tyrosine hydroxylase) (see Martin et al., 1978b; Arimura and Culler, 1985). α-Adrenergic stimulation suppresses somatostatin secretion, thereby facilitating GH release (Torres et al., 1982; Chihara et al., 1984). β-Adrenergic blockade using propranolol results in an enhancement of the GH response to hypoglycemia (Vigas et al., 1977). Subsequent studies have shown that α-adrenergic mechanisms appear to have a general facilitatory influence on the regulation of GH secretion, where the stimulatory effect is mediated by α_2 receptors, whereas the inhibitory effect is exerted via α_1 and β_2 receptors (Lal et al., 1975b; Krulich et al., 1982; see Molitch, 1988).

Evidence exists indicating that serotonin may also be involved in the regulation of GH release (Imura et al., 1973). Administration of the serotonin precursors L-tryptophan and 5-hydroxytryptophan causes GH release in humans, and this effect can be blocked by the serotonin blocker cyproheptadine (Nakai et al., 1974; Woolf and Lee, 1977). *p*-Chlorophenylalanine, a tryptophan hydroxylase inhibitor, suppresses episodic GH secretion (Martin et al., 1978a). The inhibitory effect of metergoline, another serotonin receptor blocker, on GH secretion is reversed by anti-somatostatin serum (Arnold and Fernstrom, 1980), suggesting that the facilitatory influence of serotonin on GH secretion operates by decreasing hypothalamic somatostatin secretion.

The neurotransmitter acetylcholine has, in most studies stimulated GH release. Blockade of muscarinic cholinergic receptors results in a decrease in GH in response to various stimuli (Mendelsohn et al., 1978; Delitala et al., 1982, 1983). Recently, it has been shown that atropine is able to block the GH response to GRF in humans (Casanueva et al., 1986). *In vitro*, acetylcholine inhibits somatostatin release from fragments of the rat hypothalamus (Richardson et al., 1980; see Molitch, 1988).

Dual effects of GABA on GH secretion have been observed depending on route of administration. Increased GH release has been reported after intraventricular injection of GABA (Abe et al., 1977; Takahara et al., 1980), an effect that can be abolished by intraventricularly injected GRF antiserum (Murakami et al., 1985). Conversely, the GABA antagonists picrotoxin and bicuculline inhibit spontaneous GH pulses (Martin et al., 1978a; Katakami et al., 1981). However, after systemic administration of muscimol, a GABA agonist, or after pharmacological elevation of brain GABA levels, a decrease in GH release is seen, and increased GH release is observed after GABA receptor blockade or when brain GABA levels are lowered (Cocchi et al., 1981; Fiók et al., 1984). An inhibitory effect of systemically injected muscimol on GH secretion is also seen after hypothalamic anterolateral deafferentation, which removes the input of somatostatin-containing nerves, suggesting that GABA exerts an inhibitory effect on the GRF neuron (Fiók et al., 1984). The dual effects of GABA on GH secretion may be explained by the possibility that intraventricular GABA mainly affects cell bodies located close to the ventricular ependyma, such as the periventricular somatostatin cells, and that systemically administered GABA acts on cell bodies located outside the blood-brain-barrier, such as the arcuate GRF neurons, leading to decreased GH release (see Fiók et al., 1984).

VIII. Cellular Modes of Action

After binding to the somatostatin receptor in the anterior pituitary (Enjalbert et al., 1982), somatostatin causes a rapid, dose-dependent decrease in the intracellular concentrations of cyclic AMP (Bourgeat et al., 1974; Vale et al., 1975). Evidence exists that somatostatin inhibits Ca^{2+} influx into the cell and reduces levels of intracellular Ca^{2+}, thereby preventing stimulated hormone release from the cell (Bicknell and Schofield, 1976; Kraicer and Chow, 1982; Schlegel et al., 1984; Drouva et al., 1988). Somatostatin suppresses GRF-stimulated GH secretion in a noncompetitive, dose-dependent fashion (Bilezikjian and Vale, 1983; Vale et al., 1983).

GRF also initiates the cellular processes leading to increased GH release by binding to specific receptors located on the surface of the somatotrophs (Seifert et al., 1985), resulting in a rapid elevation of intracellular cyclic AMP with an accompanied increased release of GH (Brazeau et al., 1982c; Bilezikjian and Vale, 1983; Culler et al., 1984; Spada et al., 1984). Furthermore, GRF stimulates transcription of the GH gene and increases GH mRNA levels in the pituitary (Barinaga et al., 1983; Gick et al., 1984), leading to increased synthesis of GH. Intracellular Ca^{2+} levels are of fundamental importance for GH release. Increased Ca^{2+} activity is necessary for exocytocis of GH. GRF elevates the concentrations of cytosolic free Ca^{2+} in the somatotrophs (Schöfl et al., 1987), presumably via influx from the extracellular space, since Ca^{2+} channel blockers inhibit GRF-induced GH release (R. W. Millard et al., 1982; Bilezikjian and Vale, 1983). The mechanisms by which GRF modifies Ca^{2+} fluxes are at present unclear.

In addition to the stimulation of GH release and biosynthesis, GRF also acts as a growth factor (Billestrup et al., 1986). In cultures of rat anterior pituitary cells, GRF induces expression of the c-*fos* protooncogene as well as the synthesis of c-*fos* protein. This suggests that GRF regulates the mitotic activity of somatotrophs (see Billestrup et al., 1987).

Glucocorticoids have a role in modifying GH secretion at the pituitary level. They enhance GH release in response to GRF both *in vivo* and *in vitro* (Vale et al., 1983; Wehrenberg et al., 1983) and conversely, adrenalectomy reduces the amount of GH released in response to

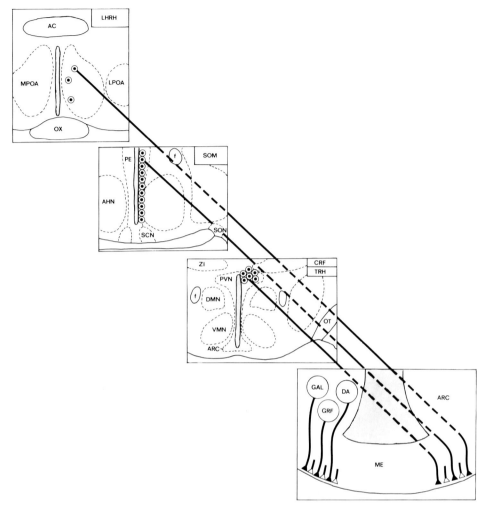

Figure 30. Schematic drawing of different levels of the hypothalamus, illustrating different pathways to the median eminence (ME) containing the main hypothalamic hormones. Luteinizing hormone-releasing hormone (LHRH)-containing neurons are located in the medial preoptic area, somatostatin (SOM)-containing neurons are located in the anterior hypothalamic periventricular nucleus, corticotropin-releasing factor (CRF)- and thyro-tropin-releasing factor (TRH)-containing neurons are located in the parvocellular part of the paraventriclular nucleus, and dopamine (DA), galanin (GAL), and growth hormone-releasing factor (GRF)-containing neurons are located in the arcuate nucleus. AC, Anterior commissure; AHN, anterior hypothalamic nucleus; ARC, arcuate nucleus; DMN, dorsomedial nucleus; f, fornix; LPOA, lateral preoptic area; MPOA, medial preoptic area; OT, optic tract; OX, optic chiasm; PE, periventricular nucleus; PVN, paraventricular nucleus; SCN, suprachiasmatic nucleus; SON, supraoptic nucleus; ventromedial nucleus.

GRF (Wehrenberg et al., 1983). These effects may be due to enhanced GRF receptor capacity in somatotrophs after glucocorticoid treatment (Seifert et al., 1985).

IX. Summary

The secretion of GH from the somatotrophs is primarily regulated by inhibitory soma-tostatin synthesized in the anterior periventricular nucleus, and by stimulatory GRF produced in neurons located in the ventral part of the arcuate nucleus (Figure 30). Both cell groups release their peptide product at the level of the median eminence into the pericapillary space to reach the somatrophs via the portal vascular plexus (Figure 30). Somatostatin has, apart from its hypothalamic localization, a wide distribution in the nervous system and is also found in endocrine and endocrine-like cells, whereas GRF has a very limited neuronal distribution but has been identified in some peripheral tissues. The somatostatin neurons in the periventricular nucleus have so far not been demonstrated to contain any cotransmitter, whereas several different neurotransmitters and neuropeptides have been localized in GRF neurons in the arcuate nucleus. These coexisting messenger molecules may have a role by interacting with GRF or somatostatin in the regulation of GH secretion. One of these comessengers, galanin, has been shown to stimulate GH secretion, presumably via a direct or indirect effect on the GRF neuron. Anatomical and physiological evidence suggests that the GRF and somatostatin systems may interact and regulate each other's activity. Both the somatostatin- and GRF-containing neurons receive inputs from several other brain areas containing classical transmitters as well as neuropeptides that regulate/modulate their secretory activity. Further studies remain to reveal the detailed organization of the somatostatin and GRF neuronal systems, with emphasis on transmitter-identified afferent pathways.

Acknowledgments

This study was supported by grants from the Swedish Medical Research Council (04X-2887), Marianne and Marcus Wallenbergs Stiftelse Tore Nilsons Fond, Magnus Bergvalls Stiftelse and Stiftelsen Sigurd and Elsa Goljes Minne.

References

Abe, H., Kato, Y., Chihara, K., Ohgo, S., Iwasaki Y., and Imura, H., Growth hormone release by gamma-aminobutyric acid (GABA) and gamma-amino-γ-hydroxybutyric acid in the rat, *Endocrinol. Jpn.*, 24, 229, 1977.

Abe, H., Molitch, M. E., Van Wyk, J. J., and Underwood, L. E., Human growth hormone and somatomedin C suppress the spontaneous release of growth hormone in unanesthetized rats, *Endocrinology*, 113, 1319, 1983.

Aguila, M. C. and McCann, S. M., Stimulation of somatostatin release *in vitro* by synthetic growth hormone-releasing factor by a nondopaminergic mechanism, *Endocrinology*, 117, 762, 1985.

Arentzen, R., Baldino, F., Davis, L. G., Higgins, G. A., Lin, Y., Manning, R. W., and Wolfson, B., In situ hybridization of putative somatostatin mRNA within hypothalamus of the rat using synthetic oligonucleotide probes, *J. Cell Biochem.*, 27, 415, 1985.

Arimura, A. and Culler, M. D., Regulation of growth hormone secretion, in *The Pituitary Gland*, Imura, H., Ed., Raven Press, New York, 1985, 221.

Arimura, A. and Fishback, J. B., Somatostatin: regulation of secretion, *Neuroendocrinology*, 33, 246, 1981.

Arimura, A., Sato, H., Dupont, A., Nishi, N., and Schally, A. V., Somatostatin: abundance of immunoreactive hormone in rat stomach and pancreas, *Science*, 189, 1007, 1975.

Arnold, M. A. and Fernstrom, J. D., Administration of anti-somatostatin serum to rats reverses the inhibition of pulsatile growth hormone secretion produced by injection of metergoline but not yohimbine, *Neuroendocrinology*, 31, 194, 1980.

Baird, A., Wehrenberg, W. B., and Ling, N., Ontogeny of the response to growth hormone-releasing factor, *Regul. Peptides,* 10, 23, 1984.

Baird, A., Wehrenberg, W. B., Böhlen, P., and Ling, N., Immunoreactive and biologically active growth hormone-releasing factor in the rat placenta, *Endocrinology*, 117, 1598, 1985.

Baird, A., Wehrenberg, W. B., and Ling, N., Relative potencies of human, rat, bovine/caprine, porcine and ovine hypothalamic growth hormone-releasing factor by the rat anterior pituitary in vitro, *Neuroendocrinology*, 42, 2273, 1986.

Baldino, F., Fitzpatrick-McElligott, S., O'Kane, T. M., and Gozes, I., Hormonal regulation of somatostatin messenger RNA, *Synapse*, 2, 317, 1988.

Bansal, S., Lee, L. A., and Woolf, P. D., Dopaminergic regulation of growth hormone (GH) secretion in normal man: correlation of L-dopa and dopamine levels with the GH response, *J. Clin. Endocrinol. Metab.*, 53, 301, 1981.

Barinaga, M., Yamonoto, G., Rivier, C., Vale, W., Evans, R., and Rosenfeld, M. G., Transcriptional regulation of growth hormone gene expression by growth hormone-releasing factor, *Nature (London)*, 306, 84, 1983.

Bauer, F. E., Ginsberg, L., Venetikou, M., MacKay, D. J., Burrin, J. H., and Bloom, S. R., Growth hormone release in man induced by galanin, a new hypothalamic peptide, *Lancet* ii, 192, 1986.

Beauvillain, J. C., Tramu, G., and Mazzuca, M., Fine structural studies of growth hormone-releasing factor (GRF)-immunoreactive neurons and their synaptic connections in the guinea-pig arcuate nucleus, *J. Comp. Neurol.*, 255, 110, 1987.

Bennet-Clarke, C., Romagnano, M. A., and Joseph, S. A., Distribution of somatostatin in the rat brain: telencephalon and diencephalon, *Brain Res.*, 188, 472, 1980.

Benoit, R., Ling, N., Alford, B., and Guillemin, R., Seven peptides derived from prosomatostatin in rat brain, *Biochem. Biophys. Res. Commun.*, 107, 944, 1982.

Berelowitz, M., Hudson, A., Pimstone, B., Kronheim, S., and Bennet, G., Subcellular localization of growth hormone release inhibiting hormone in rat hypothalamus, cerebral cortex, striatum, and thalamus, *J. Neurochem.*, 31, 751, 1978.

Berelowitz, M., Szabo, M., Frohman, L. A., Firestone, S., Chu, L., and Hintz, R. L., Somatomedin C mediates growth hormone negative feedback by effects on both the hypothalamus and the pituitary, *Science*, 212, 1279, 1981a.

Berelowitz, M., Firestone, S. L., and Frohman, L. A., Effects of growth hormone excess and deficiency on hypothalamic somatostatin content and release and on tissue somatostatin distribution, *Endocrinology*, 109, 714, 1981b.

Berry, S. A. and Pescovitz, O. H., Identification of a rat GHRH-like substance and its messenger RNA in rat testis, *Endocrinology*, 123, 661, 1988.

Bicknell, R. J. and Schofield, J. G., Mechanism of action of somatostatin: inhibition of the ionophore A23187-induced release of growth hormone from dispersed bovine pituitary cells, *FEBS Lett.*, 68, 23, 1976.

Bilezikjian, L. M. and Vale, W. W., Stimulation of adenosine $3',5'$-monophosphate production by growth hormone-releasing factor and its inhibition by somatostatin in anterior pituitary cells *in vitro*, *Endocrinology*, 113, 1726, 1983.

Billestrup, N., Swanson, L. W., and Vale, W., Growth hormone-releasing factor stimulates proliferation of somatotrophs *in vitro*, *Proc. Natl. Acad. Sci. U.S.A.*, 83, 6854, 1986.

Billestrup, N., Bilezikjian, L. M., Struthers, S., Seifert, H., Montminy, M., and Vale, W., Cellular actions of growth hormone releasing factor and somatostatin, in *Growth Hormone — Basic and Clinical Aspects,* Isaksson, O., Binder, C., Hall, K., and Hökfelt, B., Eds., Elsevier, Amsterdam, 1987, 55.

Björklund, A. and Lindvall, O., Dopamine-containing systems in the CNS, in *Handbook of Chemical Neuroanatomy,* Vol. 2, Classical Transmitters in the CNS, Björklund, A. and Hökfelt, T., Eds., Elsevier, Amsterdam, 1984, 55.

Blackard, W. G. and Heidingsfelder, S. A., Adrenergic receptor control mechanism for growth hormone secretion, *J. Clin. Invest.*, 47, 1407, 1968.

Bloch, B., Brazeau, P., Ling, N., Böhlen, P., Esch, F., Wehrenberg, W. B., Benoit, R., Bloom, F., and Guillemin, R., Immunohistochemical detection of growth hormone-releasing factor in brain, *Nature (London)*, 301, 607, 1983a.

Bloch, B., Brazeau, P., Bloom, F., and Ling, N., Topographical study of the neurons containing hpGRF immunoreactivity in monkey hypothalamus, *Neurosci. Lett.*, 37, 23, 1983b.

Bloch, B., Ling, N., Benoit, R., Wehrenberg, W. B., and Guillemin, R., Specific depletion of immunoreactive growth hormone-releasing factor by monosodium glutamate in rat median eminence, *Nature (London)*, 307, 2272, 1984.

Bohannon, N. J., Figlewicz, D. P., Corp, E. S., Wilcox, B. J., Porte, D., and Baskin, D. G., Identification of binding sites for an insulin-like growth factor (IGF-I) in the median eminence of the rat brain by quantitative autoradiography, *Endocrinology*, 119, 943, 1986.

Böhlen, P., Brazeau, P., Bloch, B., Ling, N., Gaillard, R., and Guillemin, R., Human hypothalamic growth hormone releasing factor (GRF): evidence for two forms identical to tumor derived GRF-44-NH$_2$ and GRF-40, *Biochem. Biophys. Res. Commun.*, 114, 930, 1983a.

Böhlen, P., Esch, F., Brazeau, P., Ling, N., and Guillemin, R., Isolation and characterization of the porcine growth hormone-releasing factor, *Biochem. Biophys. Res. Commun.*, 116, 726, 1983b.

Bosman, F. T., Van Asche, C., Nieuwenhuyzen, A. C., Jackson, S., and Lowry, P. J., Growth hormone-releasing factor (GRF) immunoreactivity in human and rat gastrointestinal tract and pancreas, *J. Histochem. Cytochem.*, 32, 1139, 1984.

Bourgeat, P., Labrie, F., Drouin, J., Belanger, A., Immer, H., Sestanj, K., Nelson, V., Gotz, M., Schally, A. V., Coy, D. H., and Coy, E. J., Inhibition of adenosine-3',5'-monophosphate accumulation in anterior pituitary gland *in vitro* by growth hormone release-inhibiting hormone, *Biochem. Biophys. Res. Commun.*, 56, 1052, 1974.

Brazeau, P., Vale, W., Burgus, R., Ling, N., Butcher, M., Rivier, J., and Guillemin, R., Hypothalamic polypeptide that inhibits the secretion of immunoreactive pituitary growth hormone, *Science*, 179, 77, 1973.

Brazeau, P., Ling, N., Böhlen, P., Esch, F., Ying, S.-Y., and Guillemin, R., Growth hormone-releasing factor, somatocrinin, releases pituitary growth hormone *in vitro*, *Proc. Natl. Acad. Sci. U.S.A.*, 79, 7909, 1982a.

Brazeau, P., Guillemin, R., Ling, N., van Wyk, J., and Humbel, R., Inhibition par les somatomédines de la sécrétion de l'hormone de croissance stimulée par le facteur hypothalamique somatocrinine (GRF) ou le peptide de synthése hpGRF, *C.R. Seances Acad. Sci. (Paris) Serie III*, 295, 651, 1982b.

Brazeau, P., Ling, N., Esch, F., Böhlen, P., Mougin, C., and Guillemin, R., Somatocrinin (growth hormone releasing factor) in vitro bioactivity; Ca^{++} involvement, cAMP mediated action and additivity of effect with PGE$_2$, *Biochem. Biophys. Res. Commun.*, 109, 588, 1982c.

Brazeau, P., Böhlen, P., Esch, F., Ling, N., Wehrenberg, W. B., and Guillemin, R., Growth hormone releasing factor from ovine and caprine hypothalamus: isolation, sequence analysis and total synthesis, *Biochem. Biophys. Res. Commun.*, 125, 606, 1984.

Brecha, N, Retinal neurotransmitters: histochemical and biochemical studies, in *Chemical Neuroanatomy*, Emson, P. C., Ed., Raven Press, New York, 1983, 85.

Bresson, J. L., Clavequin, M. C., Fellmann, D., and Bugnon, C., Ontogeny of the neuroglandular system revealed with hpGRF-44 antibodies in human hypothalamus, *Neuroendocrinology*, 39, 68, 1984.

Breton, C., Fellmann, D., and Bugnon, C., Cloning and sequence analysis of cDNA of common precursors of three hypothalamic neuropeptides immunologically related to human somatocrinin 1-37, alpha melanotropin and salmon melanin-concentrating hormone, *C.R. Acad. Sci.*, 309, 749, 1989.

Brownstein, M. J., Arimura, A., Sato, H., Schally, A. V., and Kizer, J. S., The regional distribution of somatostatin in the rat brain, *Endocrinology*, 96, 1456, 1975.

Brownstein, M. J., Arimura, A., Fernandez-Durango, R., Schally, A. V., Palkovits, M., and Kizer, J. S., The effect of hypothalamic deafferentiation on somatostatin-like activity in rat brain, *Endocrinology*, 100, 246, 1977.

Bruhn, T. O., Mason, R. T., and Vale, W. W., Presence of growth hormone-releasing factor in the rat duodenum, *Endocrinology*, 117, 1710, 1985.

Bruhn, T.O., Anthony, E. L. P., Wu, P., and Jackson, I. M. D., GRF immunoreactive neurons in the paraventricular nucleus of the rat: an immunohistochemical study with monoclonal and polyclonal antibodies, *Brain Res.*, 424, 290, 1987.

Bugnon, C., Gouget, A., Fellmann, D., and Clavequin, M. C., Immunocytochemical demonstration of a novel peptidergic neuron system in cat brain with an anti-growth hormone-releasing factor serum, *Neurosci. Lett.*, 38, 131, 1983.

Camanni, F., Massara, F., Belforte, L., and Molinatti, G. M., Changes in plasma growth hormone levels in normal and acromegalic subjects following administration of 2-bromo-α-ergocryptine, *J. Clin. Endocrinol. Metab.*, 40, 363, 1975.

Camanni, F., Massara, F., Belforte, L., Rosaletto, A., and Molinatti, G. M., Effects of dopamine on plasma growth hormone and prolactin levels in normal and acromegalic subjects, *J. Clin. Endocrinol. Metab.*, 44, 465, 1977.

Casanueva, F. F., Villanueva, L., et al., Atropine blockade of growth hormone (GH)-releasing hormone-induced GH secretion in man is not exerted at pituitary level, *J. Endocrinol. Metab.*, 62(1), 186—191, 1986.

Ceda, G. P., Hoffman, A. R., Silverberg, G. D., Wilson, D. M., and Rosenfeld, R. G., Regulation of GH release from cultured human pituitary adenomas by somatomedins and insulin, *J. Endocrinol. Metab.*, 60, 1204, 1985.

Ceda, G. P., Davis, R. G., Rosenfeld, R. G., and Hoffman, A. R., The growth hormone GH-releasing hormone (GHRH)-GH-somatomedin axis: evidence for rapid inhibition of GHRH-elicited GH release by insulin-like growth factors I and II, *Endocrinology*, 120, 1658, 1987.

Cella, S. G., Locatelli, V., De Gennaro, V., Puggioni, R., Pintor, C., and Müller, E. E., Human pancreatic growth hormone (GH)-releasing hormone stimulates GH synthesis and release in infant rats: an *in vivo* study, *Endocrinology*, 110, 1018, 1985.

Cella, S.G., Locatelli, V., De Gennaro, V., Bondiolotti, G. P., Pintor, C., Loche, S., Provezza, M., and Müller, E. E., Epinephrine mediates the growth hormone-releasing effect of galanin in infant rats, *Endocrinology*, 122, 855, 1988.

Chihara, K., Arimura, A., Kubli-Garfias, C., and Schally, A. V., Enhancement of immunoreactive somatostatin release into hypophysial portal blood by electrical stimulation of the preoptic area in the rat, *Endocrinology*, 105, 1416, 1979.

Chihara, K., Minamitani, N., Kaji, H., Arimura, A., and Fujita, T., Intraventricularly injected growth hormone stimulates somatostatin release into rat hypophysial portal blood, *Endocrinology*, 109, 2279, 1981.

Chihara, K., Minamitani, N., Kaji, H., Kodama, H., Kita, T., and Fujita, T., Noradrenergic modulation of human pancreatic growth hormone-releasing factor (hp GHRF 1-44)-induced growth hormone release in conscious male rabbits: involvement of endogenous somatostatin, *Endocrinology*, 114, 1402, 1984.

Chomczynski, P., Downs, T. R., and Frohman, L. A., Feed-back regulation of growth hormone (GH)-releasing factor gene expression by GH in rat hypothalamus, *Mol. Endocrinol.*, 2, 236, 1988.

Chowen-Breed, J. A., Steiner, R. A., and Clifton, D. K., Sexual dimorphism and testosterone-dependent regulation of somatostatin-gene expression in the periventricular nucleus of the rat brain, *Endocrinology*, 125, 357, 1989.

Cintra, A., Fuxe, K., Härfstrand, A., Agnati, L. F., Wikström, Λ.-C., Vale, W., and Gustafsson, J.-Å., Evidence for the presence of glucocorticoid receptor immunoreactivity in corticotropin-releasing factor and in growth hormone-releasing factor immunoreactive neurons of the rat di- and telencephalon, *Neurosci. Lett.*, 76, 269, 1987.

Ciofi, P., Croix, D., and Tramu, G., Coexistence of hGHRF and NPY immunoreactivities in neurons of the arcuate nucleus of the rat, *Neuroendocrinology*, 45, 425, 1987.

Ciofi, P., Croix, D., and Tramu, G., Colocalization of GHRF and NPY immunoreactivities in neurons of the infundibular area of the human brain, *Neuroendocrinology*, 47, 469, 1988.

Ciofi, P., Tramu, G., and Bloch, B., Comparative immunohistochemical study of the distribution of neuropeptide Y, growth hormone-releasing factor and the carboxy terminus of precursor protein GHRF in the human hypothalamic infundibular area, *Neuroendocrinology*, 51, 429, 1990.

Clark, R. G., Carlsson, L. M. S., Rafferty, B., and Robinson, I. C. A. F., The rebound release of growth hormone (GH) following somatostatin infusion in rats involves hypothalamic GH-releasing factor release, *J. Endocrinol.*, 119, 397, 1988.

Cocchi, D., Casanueva, F., Locatelli, V., Apud, J., Martinez-Campos, A., Civati, C., Racagni, G., and Müller, E. E., GABAergic mechanisms in the control of PRL and GH release, in *GABA and Benzodiazepine Receptors*, Costa, E., Di Chihara, G., and Gessa, G. L., Eds., Raven Press, New York, 1981, 247.

Critchlow, V., Rice, R. W., Abe, K., and Vale, W., Somatostatin content of the median eminence in female rats with lesion-induced disruption of the inhibitory control of growth hormone secretion, *Endocrinology*, 103, 817, 1978.

Critchlow, V., Abe, K., Urman, S., and Vale, W., Effects of lesions in the periventricular nucleus of the preoptic anterior hypothalamus on growth hormone and thyrotropin secretion and brain somatostatin, *Brain Res.*, 222, 267, 1981.

Crowley, W. R. and Terry, L. C., Biochemical mapping of somatostatinergic systems in rat brain: effects of periventricular and medial basal amygdaloid lesions on somatostatin-like immunoreactivity in discrete brain nuclei, *Brain Res.*, 200, 283, 1980.

Culler, M.D., Kenjo, T., Obara, N., and Arimura, A., Stimulation of pituitary cAMP accumulation by human pancreatic GH-releasing factor (1-44), *Am. J. Physiol.*, 247, E609, 1984.

Daikoku, S., Hisano, S., Kawano, H., Okamura, Y., and Tsuruo, Y., Ontogenetic studies on the topographical heterogeneity of somatostatin-containing neurons in rat hypothalamus, *Cell Tissue Res.*, 23, 347, 1983.

Daikoku, S., Kawano, H., Noguchi, M., Nakanishi, J., Tokuzen, M., Chihara, K., Haruhiko, S., and Shibasaki, T., Ontogenetic appearance of immunoreactive GRF-containing neurons in the rat hypothalamus, *Cell Tissue Res.*, 242, 511, 1985.

Daikoku, S., Kawano, H., Noguchi, M., Nakanishi, J., Tokuzen, M., Chihara, K., and Nagatsu, I., GRF neurons in the rat hypothalamus, *Brain Res.*, 399, 250, 1986.

Daikoku, S., Hisano, S., Kawano, H., Chikamori-Aoyama, M., Kagotani, Y., Ahang, R., and Chihara, K., Ultrastructural evidence for neuronal regulation of growth hormone secretion, *Neuroendocrinology*, 47, 405, 1988.

Davis, T. M. E., Burrin, J. M., and Bloom, S. R., Growth hormone (GH) release in response to GH-releasing hormone in man is 3-fold enhanced by galanin, *J. Clin. Endocrinol. Metab.*, 65, 1248, 1987.

Delitala, G., T. Frulio, Pacificio, A., and Maioli, M., Participation of cholinergic muscarinic receptors in glucagon- and arginine-mediated growth hormone secretion in man, *J. Clin. Endocrinol. Metab.*, 55, 1231, 1982.

Delitala, G., Maioli, M., Pacificio, A., Brianda, S., Palermo, M., and Mannelli, M., Cholinergic receptor control mechanisms for L-dopa apomorphine, and clonidine-induced growth hormone secretion in man, *J. Clin. Endocrinol. Metab.*, 57, 1145, 1983.

Deuben, R. R. and Meites, J., Stimulation of pituitary growth hormone release by hypothalamic extracts in vitro, *Endocrinology*, 74, 4408, 1964.

Dhariwal, A. P. S., Krulich, L., and McCann, S. M., Purification of growth hormone-inhibiting factor (GIF) from sheep hypothalami, *Neuroendocrinology*, 4, 282, 1969.

Drouva, S. V., Rerat, E., Bihoreau, C., Laplante, E., Rasolonjanahary, R., Clauser, H., and Kordon, C., Dihydropyridine-sensitive calcium channel activity related to prolactin, growth hormone, and luteinizing hormone release from anterior pituitary cells in culture: interactions with somatostatin, dopamine, and estrogens, *Endocrinology*, 123, 2762, 1988.

Dubois, M. P., Immunoreactive somatostatin is present in discrete cells of the endocrine pancreas, *Proc. Natl. Acad. Sci. U.S.A.*, 72, 1340, 1975.

Dubois, M. P., Barry, J., and Leonardelli, J., Mise en évidence par immunofluorescence et répartition de la somatostatine (SRIF) dans l'éminence médiane des vertébrés (mammifères, oiseaux, amphibiens, poissons), *C.R. Hebd. Séanc. Acad. Sci. Paris*, 279, 1899, 1974.

Durand, D., Martin, J. B., and Brazeau, P., Evidence for a role of α-adrenergic mechanisms in regulation of episodic growth hormone secretion in the rat, *Endocrinology*, 100, 722, 1977.

Elde, R. P. and Parsons, J. A., Immunocytochemical localization of somatostatin in cell bodies of the rat hypothalamus, *Am. J. Anat.*, 144, 541, 1974.

Enjalbert, A., Tapia-Arancibia, L., Rieutort, M., Brazeau, P., and Kordon, C., Somatostatin receptors on rat anterior pituitary membranes, *Endocrinology*, 110, 1634, 1982.

Epelbaum, J., Brazeau, P., Tsang, D., Brawer, J., and Martin, J. B., Subcellular distribution of radioimmunoassayable somatostatin in rat brain, *Brain Res.*, 126, 309, 1977.

Epelbaum, J., Moyse, E., Tannenbaum, G. S., Kordon, C., and Baudet, A., Combined autoradiographic and immunohistochemical evidence for an association of somatostatin binding sites with growth hormone-releasing factor-containing nerve cell bodies in the rat arcuate nucleus, *J. Neuroendocrinol.,* 1, 109, 1989.

Esch, F., Böhlen, P., Ling, N., Brazeau, P., and Guillemin, R., Isolation and characterization of bovine growth hormone-releasing factor, *Biochem. Biophys. Res. Commun.,* 117, 772, 1983a.

Esch, F., Böhlen, P., Ling, N. C., Brazeau, P. E., Wehrenberg, W. B., and Guillemin, R., Primary structure of three human pancreatic peptides with growth hormone-releasing activity, *J. Biol. Chem.,* 258, 1806, 1983b.

Everitt, B.J., Meister, B., Hökfelt, T., Melander, T., Terenius, L., Rökaeus, Å., Theodorsson-Norheim, E., Dockray, G., Edwardson, J., Cuello, C., Elde, R., Goldstein, M., Hemmings, H., Ouimet, C., Walaas, I., Greengard, P., Vale, W., Weber, E., Wu, J. Y., and Chang, K. J., The hypothalamic arcuate nucleus-median eminence complex: immunohistochemistry of transmitters, peptides and DARPP-32 with special reference to coexistence in dopamine neurons, *Brain Res. Rev.,* 11, 97, 1986.

Fellmann, D., Bugnon, C., and Lavry, G. N., Immunohistochemical demonstration of a new neuron system in rat brain using antibodies against human growth hormone-releasing factor (1-37), *Neurosci. Lett.,* 58, 91, 1985.

Fellmann, D., Bugnon, C., Verstegen, J., and Lawry, G. N., Coexpression of human growth hormone-releasing factor 1-37-like and α-melanotropin-like immunoreactivities in neurones of the rat lateral dorsal hypothalamus, *Neurosci. Lett.,* 68, 122, 1986.

Fellmann, D., Bugnon, C., and Risold, P. Y., Unrelated peptide immunoreactivities coexist in neurons of the rat dorsal hypothalamus: human growth hormone-releasing factor-37-, salmon melanin-concentrating hormone- and α-melanotropin-like substances, *Neurosci. Lett.,* 74, 275, 1987.

Fellmann, D., Bresson, J. L., Breton, C., Bahjaouni, M., Rouillon, A., Gouget, A., and Bugnon, C., Cloning of cDNAs encoding a rat neuropeptide immunologically related to salmon melanin-concentrating hormone, *Neurosci. Lett.,* 106, 23, 1989.

Ferland, L., Labrie, F., and Jobin, M., Physiological role of somatostatin in the control of growth hormone and thyrotropin secretion, *Biochem. Biophys. Res. Commun.,* 68, 149, 1976.

Finley, J. C. W., Maderdrut, J. L., Roger, L. J., and Petrusz, P., The immunocytochemical localization of somatostatin-containing neurons in the rat central nervous system, *Neuroscience,* 6, 2173, 1981.

Fiók, J., Ács, Z., Makara, G. B., and Erdö, S. L., Site of γ-aminobutyric acid (GABA)-mediated inhibition of growth hormone secretion in the rat, *Neuroendocrinology,* 39, 510, 1984.

Fitzpatrick-McElligott, S., Card, J. P., Lewis, M. E., and Baldino, F., Neuronal localization of prosomatostatin mRNA in the rat brain with in situ hybridization histochemistry, *J. Comp. Neurol.,* 273, 558, 1988.

Foster, G. A. and Johansson, O., Ultrastructural morphometric analysis of somatostatin-like immuno-reactive neurones in the central nervous system after labelling with colloidal gold, *Brain Res.,* 342, 117, 1985.

Froesch, E. R., Schmid, C., Schwander, J., and Zapf, J., Actions of insulin-like growth factors, *Annu. Rev. Physiol.,* 47, 443, 1985.

Frohman, L. A. and Bernardis, L. L., Growth hormone and insulin levels in weanling rats with ventromedial hypothalamic lesions, *Endocrinology,* 82, 1125, 1968.

Frohman, L. A. and Jansson, J.-O., Growth hormone-releasing hormone, *Endocrine Rev.,* 7, 223, 1986.

Frohman, L. A., Bernardis, L. L., and Kant, K. J., Hypothalamic stimulation of growth hormone secretion, *Science,* 162, 580, 1969.

Frohman, M. A., Downs, T. R., Chomczynski, P., and Frohman, L. A., Cloning and characterization of mouse growth hormone-releasing factor (GRH) complemenary DNA: increased GRH messenger RNA levels in the growth hormone-deficient *lit/lit* mouse, *Mol. Endocrinol.,* 3, 1529, 1989.

Furness, J. B. and Costa, M., *The Enteric Nervous System,* Churchill Livingstone, Edinburgh, 1987.

Fuxe, K., Agnati, L. F., Zini, I., Merlo Pich, E., Cintra, A., Kitayama, I., Härfstrand, A., von Euler, G., Vale, W., Toffano, G., and Goldstein, M., Evidence for selective changes in peptide and monoamine synapses and their interactions in the aging rat brain. Possible loss of homeostatic responses and of trophic signals, in *New Trends in Aging Research,* Vol. 15, Fidia Research Series, Pepeu, G., Tomlinson, B., and Wischik, C. M., Eds., Livana Press, Padova, 1988, 3.

Gabriel, S. M., Milbury, C. M., Nathanson, J. A., and Martin, J. B., Galanin stimulates rat pituitary growth hormone secretion *in vitro, Life Sci.,* 42, 1981, 1988.

Gabriel, S. M., Kaplan, L. M., Martin, J. B., and Koenig, J. I., Tissue-specific sex differences in galanin-like immunoreactivity and galanin mRNA during development in the rat, *Peptides,* 10, 369, 1989.

Gabriel, S. M., Koenig, J. I., and Kaplan, L. M., Galanin-like immunoreactivity is influenced by estrogen in prepubertal and adult rats, *Neuroendocrinology,* 51, 168, 1990.

Gaymann, W. and Falke, N., Galanin lacks binding sites in the porcine pituitary and has no detectable effect on oxytocin and vasopressin release from rat neurosecretory endings, *Neurosci. Lett.,* 112, 114, 1990.

Gerich, J. E., Somatostatin, in *Handbook of Diabetes Mellitus,* Vol. 1, Brownlee, M., Ed., Garland STPM Press, New York, 1980, 297.

Gick, G. G., Zeytin, F. N., Barzeau, P., Ling, N. C., Esch, F., and Bancroft, C., Growth hormone-releasing factor regulates growth hormone mRNA in primary cultures of rat pituitary cells, *Med. Sci.,* 81, 1553, 1984.

Goodman, R. H., Aron, D. C., and Roos, B. A., Rat-preprosomatostatin: structure and processing by microsomal membranes, *J. Biol. Chem.,* 258, 5570, 1983.

Goodyer, C. C., De Stephano, L., Guyda, H. J., and Posner, B. I., Effects of insulin-like growth factor on adult male rat pituitary function, *Endocrinology,* 115, 1568, 1984.

Gordin, A., Lamberg, B., Pelkonen, R., and Almqvist, S., Somatostatin inhibits the pentagastrin-induced release of serum calcitonin in medullary carcinoma of the thyroid, *Clin. Endocrinol.,* 8, 289, 1978.

Gubler, U., Monahan, J. J., Lomedico, P. T., Bhatt, R. S., Collier, K. J., Hoffman, B. J., Böhlen, P., Esch, F., Ling, N., Zeytin, F., Brazeau, P., Poonian, M. S., and Gage, L. P., Cloning and sequence analysis of cDNA for the precursor of human growth hormone-releasing factor, somatocrinin, *Proc. Natl. Acad. Sci. U.S.A.,* 80, 4311, 1983.

Guillemin, R., Brazeau, P., Böhlen, P., Esch, F., Ling, N., and Wehrenberg, W. B., Growth hormone-releasing factor from a human pancreatic tumour that caused acromegaly, *Science,* 218, 5585, 1982.

Hall, K. and Sara, V. R., Growth and the somatomedins, *Vitam. Horm.,* 40, 175, 1983.

Harmar, A. J., Pierotti, A. R., and Lightman, S. L., Somatostatin, in *Neuroendocrinology,* Everitt, B. J. and Lightman, S. L., Eds., Blackwell Scientific, London, 1986, 389.

Harris, G. W., *Neural Control of the Pituitary Gland,* Edward Arnold, London, 1955.

Hökfelt, T., Efendic, S., Johansson, O., Luft, R., and Arimura, A., Immunohistochemical localization of somatostatin (growth hormone release-inhibiting factor) in the guinea pig brain, *Brain Res.,* 80, 165, 1974.

Hökfelt, T., Efendic, S., Hellerström, C., Johansson, O., Luft, R., and Arimura, A., Cellular localization of somatostatin in endocrine-like cells and neurons of the rat with special reference to the A_1-cells of the pancreatic islets and to the hypothalamus, *Acta Endocrinol. Suppl.,* 200, 1, 1975.

Hökfelt, T., Elfvin, L.-G., Elde, R., Schultzberg, M., Goldstein, M., and Luft, R., Occurrence of somatostatin-like immunoreactivity in some peripheral sympathetic noradrenergic neurons, *Proc. Natl. Acad. Sci. U.S.A.,* 74, 3587, 1977.

Hökfelt, T., Holets, V. R., Staines, W., Meister, B., Melander, T., Schalling, M., Melander, T., Schultzberg, M., Freedman, J., Björklund, H., Olson, L., Lindh, B., Elfvin, L. G., Lundberg, J. M., Lindgren, J. Å., Samuelsson, B., Pernow, B., Terenius, L., Post, C., Everitt, B., and Goldstein, M., Coexistence of neuronal messengers — an overview, *Prog. Brain Res.,* 68, 33, 1986.

Horváth, S. and Palkovits, M., Synaptic interconnections among growth hormone-releasing hormone (GHRH)-containing neurons in the arcuate nucleus of the rat hypothalamus, *Neuroendocrinology,* 48, 471, 1988.

Horváth, S., Palkovits, M., Görcs, T., and Arimura, A., Electron microscopic immunocytochemical evidence for the existence of bidirectional synaptic connections between growth hormone-releasing hormone- and somatostatin-containing neurons in the hypothalamus of the rat, *Brain Res.*, 481, 8, 1989a.

Horváth, S., Mezey, E., and Palkovits, M., Partial coexistence of growth hormone-releasing hormone and tyrosine hydroxylase in paraventricular neurons in rats, *Peptides*, 10, 791, 1989b.

Hulting, A. L., Meister, B., Grimelius, L., Wersäll, J., Änggård, A., and Hökfelt, T., Production of a galanin-like peptide by a human pituitary adenoma: immunohistochemical evidence, *Acta Physiol. Scand.*, 137, 561, 1989.

Hunt, S., Cytochemistry of the spinal cord, in *Chemical Neuroanatomy*, Emson, P. C., Ed., Raven Press, New York, 1983, 53.

Ibata, I., Okamura, H., Makino, S., Kawakami, F., Morimoto, N., and Chihara, K., Light and electron microscopic immunocytochemistry of GRF-like immunoreactive neurons and terminals in the rat hypothalamic arcuate nucleus and median eminence, *Brain Res.*, 370, 136, 1986.

Imura, H., Nakai, Y., and Hoshimi, T., Effect of 5-hydroxytryptophan (5-HTP) on growth hormone and ACTH release in man, *J. Clin. Endocrinol. Metab.*, 36, 204, 1973.

Inagaki, S., Shiosaka, S., Takatsuki, K., Iida, H., Sakanaka, M., Senba, E., Hara, Y., Matsuzaki, T., Kawai, Y., and Tohyama, M., Ontogeny of somatostatin-containing system of the rat cerebellum including its fiber connections: an experimental and immunohistochemical analysis, *Dev. Brain Res.*, 3, 509, 1982.

Inagaki, S., Shiosaka, S., Sikitani, M. M., Noguchi, K., Shimada, S., and Takagi, H., *In situ* hybridization analysis of the somatostatin-containing neuron system in developing cerebellum of rats, *Mol. Brain Res.*, 6, 298, 1989.

Isaksson, O. G. P., Lindahl, A., Nilsson, A., and Isgaard, J., Mechanism of the stimulatory effect of growth hormone on longitudinal bone growth, *Endocrine Rev.*, 8, 426, 1987.

Ishikawa, K., Katakami, H., Jansson, J.-O., and Frohman, L. A., Ontogenesis of growth hormone-releasing hormone neurons in the rat hypothalamus, *Neuroendocrinology*, 43, 537, 1986.

Ishikawa, K., Taniguchi, Y., Kurosumi, K., Suzuki, M., and Shinoda, M., Immunohistochemical identification of somatostatin-containing neurons projecting to the median eminence of the rat, *Endocrinology*, 121, 94, 1987.

Jacobowitz, D. M., Schulte, H., Crousos, G. P., and Loriaux, D. L., Localization of GRF-like immunoreactive neurons in the rat brain, *Peptides*, 4, 521, 1983.

Jansson, J.-O., Edén, S., and Isaksson, O., Sexual dimorphism in the control of growth hormone secretion, *Endocrine Rev.*, 6, 128, 1986.

Jansson, J.-O., Ishikawa, K., Katakami, H., and Frohman, L. A., Pre- and postnatal developmental changes in hypothalamic content of rat growth hormone-releasing factor, *Endocrinology*, 120, 525, 1987.

Johansson, O., Hökfelt, T., and Elde, R. P., Immunohistochemical distribution of somatostatin-like immunoreactivity in the central nervous system of the adult rat, *Neuroscience*, 13, 265, 1984.

Jones, E. G. and Hendry, S. H. C., Colocalization of GABA and neuropeptides in neocortical neurons, *TINS*, 9, 71, 1986.

Jones, B. J. and Moore, R. Y., Ascending projections of the locus coeruleus in the rat. II. Autoradiographic study, *Brain Res.*, 127, 23, 1977.

Jósza, R., Korf, H.-W., and Merchenthaler, I., Growth hormone-releasing factor (GRF)-like immunoreactivity in sensory ganglia of the rat, *Cell Tissue Res.*, 247, 441, 1987.

Kaplan, L. M., Spindel, E. R., Isselbacher, K. J., and Chin, W.W., Tissue-specific expression of the rat galanin gene, *Proc. Natl. Acad. Sci. U.S.A.*, 85, 1065, 1988a.

Kaplan, L. M., Gabriel, S. M., Koenig, J. I., Sunday, M. E., Spindel, E. R., Martin, J. B., and Chin, W. W., Galanin is an estrogen-inducible, secretory product of the rat anterior pituitary, *Proc. Natl. Acad. Sci. U.S.A.*, 85, 7408, 1988b.

Katakami, H., Kato, Y., Matsushita, N., and Imura, H., Possible involvement of γ-aminobutyric acid in growth hormone release induced by a Met[5]-enkephalin analog in conscious rats, *Endocrinology*, 109, 1033, 1981.

Katakami, H., Arimura, A., and Frohman, L. A., Growth hormone releasing hormone stimulates hypothalamic somatostatin release: an inhibitory feedback effect on growth hormone secretion, *Endocrinology*, 118, 1872, 1986.

Katz, S. H., Molitch, M., and McCann, S. M., Effects of hypothalamic implants of GH on anterior pituitary weight and GH concentration, *Endocrinology*, 85, 725, 1969.

Kawano, H. and Daikoku, S., Somatostatin-containing neurons systems in the rat hypothalamus: retrograde tracing and immunohistochemical studies, *J. Comp. Neurol.*, 271, 293, 1988.

Kawano, H., Daikoku, S., and Saito, S., Immunohistochemical studies of intrahypothalamic somatostatin-containing neurons in rat, *Brain Res.*, 242, 227, 1982.

Keast, J. R., Furness, J. B., and Costa, M., Somatostatin in human enteric nerves: distribution and characterization, *Cell Tissue Res.*, 237, 299, 1984.

Knobil, E., Meyer, V., and Schally, A. V., Hypothalamic extracts and the secretion of growth hormone in the rhesus monkey, in *Growth Hormone*, Pecile, A. and Müller, E. E., Eds., Excerpta Medica, Amsterdam, 1968, 226.

Koshiyama, H., Kato, Y., Shimatsu, A., Katakami, H., Yanaihara, N., and Imura, H., Central galanin stimulates pituitary prolactin secretion in rats: possible involvement of hypothalamic vasoactive intestinal polypeptide, *Neurosci. Lett.*, 75, 49, 1987.

Kraicer, J. and Chow, A. E. H., Release of growth hormone from purified somatotrophs: use of perifusion system to elucidate interrelations among Ca^{++}, adenosine-3',5'-monophosphate, and somatostatin, *Endocrinology*, 111, 1173, 1982.

Krulich, L. and McCann, S. M., Influence of growth hormone (GH) on content of GH in the pituitaries of normal rats, *Proc. Soc. Exp. Biol. Med.*, 121, 1114, 1966.

Krulich, L., Dhariwal, A. P. S., and McCann, S. M., Stimulatory and inhibitory effects of purified hypothalamic extracts on growth hormone release from rat pituitary *in vitro*, *Endocrinology*, 83, 783, 1968.

Krulich, L., Illner, C., Fawcell, C. P., Quijada, M., and McCann, S.M., Dual hypothalamic regulation of growth hormone secretion, in *Growth and Growth Hormone*, Pecile, A. and Müller, E. E., Eds., Excerpta Medica, Amsterdam, 1972, 306.

Krulich, L., Mayfeld, M. A., Steele, M. K., McMillen, B. A., McCann, S. M., and Koenig, J. I., Differential effects of pharamacological manipulations of central α-1- and α-2-adrenergic receptors on the secretion of thyrotropin and growth hormone in male rats, *Endocrinology*, 110, 796, 1982.

Laemle, L. K., Feldman, S. C., and Lichtenstein, F., Somatostatin-like immunoreactivity in the central visual pathway of the prenatal rat, *Brain Res.*, 251, 365, 1982.

Lal, S., Martin, J. B., De La Vega, C., and Friesen, H. G., Comparison of the effect of apomorphine and L-dopa on serum growth hormone levels in man, *J. Clin. Endocrinol. Metab.*, 41, 227, 1975a.

Lal, S., Tolis, G., Martin, J. B., Brown, G. M., and Guyda, H., Effect of clonidine on growth hormone, prolactin, luteinizing hormone, follicle-stimulating hormone in the serum of normal men, *J. Clin. Endocrinol. Metab.*, 41, 827, 1975b.

Leblanc, H., Lachelin, G. C. L., Abu-Fadil, S., and Yen, S. S. C., Effects of dopamine infusion on pituitary hormone secretion in humans, *J. Clin. Endocrinol. Metab.*, 43, 688, 1976.

Lechan, R. M., Nestler, J. L., and Jacobson, S., The tuberoinfundibular system of the rat as demonstrated by immunohistochemical localization of retrogradely transported wheat germ agglutinin (WGA) from the median eminence, *Brain Res.*, 245, 1, 1982.

Lechan, R. M., Lin, H. D., Ling, N., Jackson, I. M. D., Jacobson, S., and Reichlin, S., Distribution of immunoreactive growth hormone-releasing factor(1-44)NH2 in the tuberoinfundibular system of the rhesus monkey, *Brain Res.*, 309, 55, 1984.

Ling, N., Esch, F., Böhlen, P., Wehrenberg, W. B., and Guillemin, R., Isolation, primary structure, and synthesis of human hypothalamic somatocrinin: growth hormone-releasing factor, *Proc. Natl. Acad. Sci. U.S.A.*, 81, 4302, 1984.

Ling, N., Zeytin, F., Böhlen, P., Esch, F., Brazeau, P., Wehrenberg, W. B., Baird, A., and Guillemin, R., Growth hormone releasing factors, *Annu. Rev. Biochem.*, 54, 403, 1985.

Liposits, Z., Merchenthaler, I., Paull, W. K., and Flerkó, B., Synaptic communication between somatostatinergic axons and growth hormone-releasing factor (GRF) synthesizing neurons in the arcuate nucleus of the rat, *Histochemistry*, 89, 247, 1988.

Loche, S., Cella, S. G., Puggioni, R., Stabilini, L., Pintor, C., and Müller, E. E., The effects of galanin on growth hormone secretion in children of normal and short stature, *Ped. Res.*, 26, 316, 1989.

Luft, R., Efendic, S., Hökfelt, T., Johansson, O., and Arimura, A., Immunohistochemical evidence for the localization of somatostatin-like immunoreactivity in a cell population of the pancreatic islets, *Med. Biol.*, 52, 428, 1974.

Luft, R., Efendic, S., and Hökfelt, T., Somatostatin — both hormone and neurotransmitter? *Diabetologica*, 14, 1, 1978.

Lumpkin, M. D. and McDonald, J. K., Blockade of growth hormone-releasing factor (GRF) activity in the pituitary and hypothalamus of the concious rat with a peptidic GRF antagonist, *Endocrinology*, 124, 1522, 1989.

Lumpkin, M. D., Mulroney, S. E., and Haramati, A., Inhibition of pulsatile growth hormone (GH) secretion and somatic growth in immature rats with a synthetic GH-releasing factor antagonist, *Endocrinology*, 124, 1154, 1989.

MacLeod, R. M. and Abad, A., On the control of prolactin and growth hormone synthesis in rat pituitary glands, *Endocrinology*, 83, 799, 1968.

Maiter, D. M., Hooi, S. C., Koenig, J. I., and Martin, J. B., Galanin is a physiological regulator of spontaneous pulsatile secretion of growth hormone in the male rat, *Endocrinology*, 126, 1216, 1990.

Makara, G. B., Palkovits, M., Antoni, F. A., and Kiss, J. Z., Topography of the somatostatin-immunoreactive fibers to the stalk-median eminence of the rat, *Neuroendocrinology*, 37, 1, 1983.

Marcovitz, S., Goodyer, C. G., Guyda, H., Gardiner, R. J., and Hardy, J., Comparative study of human fetal, normal adult, and somatotropic adenoma pituitary function in tissue culture, *J. Clin. Endocrinol. Metab.*, 54, 6, 1982.

Martin, J. B., Plasma growth hormone (GH) responses to hypothalamic or extrahypothalamic electrical stimulation, *Endocrinology*, 91, 107, 1972.

Martin, J. B., Durand, D., Gurd, W., Gaille, G., Audet, J., and Brazeau, P., Neuropharmacological regulation of episodic growth hormone and prolactin secretion in the rat, *Endocrinology*, 102, 106, 1978a.

Martin, J. B., Brazeau, P., Tannenbaum, G. S., Willoughby, J. O., Epelbaum, J., Terry, L.C., and Durand, D., Neuroendocrine organization of growth hormone regulation, in *The Hypothalamus*, Reichlin, S., Baldessarini, R. J., and Martin, J. B., Eds., Raven Press, New York, 1978b, 329.

Mayo, K. E., Vale, W., Rivier, J., Rosenfeld, M. G., and Evans, R. M., Expression-cloning and sequence of a cDNA encoding human growth hormone-releasing factor, *Nature (London)*, 306, 86, 1983.

Mayo, K. E., Cerelli, G. M., Rosenfeld, M. G., and Evans, R. M., Characterization of cDNA and genomic clones encoding the precursor to rat hypothalamic growth hormone-relcasing factor, *Nature (London)*, 314, 464, 1985a.

Mayo, K. E., Cerelli, G. M., Lebo, R. V., Bruce, B. D., Rosenfeld, M. G., and Evans, R. M., Gene encoding human growth hormone-releasing factor precursor: structure, sequence, and chromosomal assignment, *Proc. Natl. Acad. Sci. U.S.A.*, 62, 63, 1985b.

Meigan, G., Sasaki, A., and Yoshinaga, K., Immunoreactive growth hormone-releasing factor in rat placenta, *Endocrinology*, 123, 1098, 1988.

Meister, B. and Hökfelt, T., Peptide- and transmitter-containing neurons in the mediobasal hypothalamus and their relation to GABAergic systems: possible roles in control of prolactin and growth hormone secretion, *Synapse*, 2, 585, 1988.

Meister, B. and Hulting, A.-L., Influence of coexisting hypothalamic messengers on growth hormone secretion from rat anterior pituitary cells *in vitro*, *Neuroendocrinology*, 46, 387, 1987.

Meister, B., Hökfelt, T., Vale, W., and Goldstein, M., Growth hormone-releasing factor and dopamine coexist in hypothalamic arcuate neurons, *Acta Physiol. Scand.*, 124, 133, 1985.

Meister, B., Hökfelt, T., Vale, W. W., Sawchenko, P. E., Swanson, L. W., and Goldstein, M., Coexistence of tyrosine hydroxylase and growth hormone-releasing factor in a subpopulation of tubero-infundibular neurons of the rat, *Neuroendocrinology*, 42, 237, 1986.

Meister, B., Hökfelt, T., Johansson, O., and Hulting, A.-L., Distribution of growth hormone-releasing factor, somatostatin and coexisting messengers in the brain, in *Growth Hormone — Basic and Clinical Aspects,* Isaksson, O., Binder, C., Hall, K., and Hökfelt, B., Eds., Elsevier, Amsterdam, 1987a, 29.

Meister, B., Hökfelt, T., Brown, J., Joh, T. H., and Goldstein, M., Dopaminergic cells in the caudal A13 cell group express somatostatin-like immunoreactivity, *Exp. Brain Res.,* 67, 441, 1987b.

Meister, B., Hökfelt, T., Steinbusch, H. W. M., Skagerberg, G., Lindvall, O., Geffard, M., Joh, T. H., Cuello, A. C., and Goldstein, M., Do tyrosine hydroxylase-immunoreactive neurons in the ventrolateral arcuate nucleus produce dopamine or only L-dopa? *J. Chem. Neuroanat.,* 1, 59, 1988.

Meister, B., Ceccatelli, S., Hökfelt, T., Andén, N.-E., Andén, M., and Theodorsson, E., Neurotransmitters, neuropeptides and binding sites in the rat mediobasal hypothalamus, effects of monosodium glutamate (MSG) lesions, *Exp. Brain Res.,* 76, 343, 1989.

Meister, B., Scanlon, M. F., and Hökfelt, T., Occurrence of galanin-like immunoreactivity in growth hormone-releasing factor(GRF)-containing neurons of the monkey (*Macaca fascicularis*) infundibular nucleus and median eminence, *Neurosci. Lett.,* 119, 136, 1990.

Melander,T., Rökaeus, Å., and Hökfelt, T., Distribution of galaninlike immunoreactivity in the rat central nervous system, *J. Comp. Neurol.,* 248, 475, 1986.

Melander, T., Fuxe, K., Härfstrand, A., Eneroth, P., and Hökfelt, T., Effects of intraventricular injections of galanin on neuroendocrine functions in the male rat: possible involvement of hypothalamic catecholamine nerve terminal systems, *Acta Physiol. Scand.,* 131, 25, 1987.

Melander, T., Köhler, C., Nilsson, S., Hökfelt, T., Brodin, E., Theodorsson, E., and Bartfai, T., Autoradiographic quantitation and anatomical mapping of ^{125}I-galanin binding sites in the rat central nervous system, *J. Chem. Neuroanat.,* 1, 213, 1988.

Mendelsohn, W. B., Sitaram, N., Wyatt, R. J., Gillin, J. C., and Jacobs, L. S., Methscopolamine inhibition of sleep-related growth hormone secretion, *J. Clin. Invest.,* 61, 1683, 1978.

Merchenthaler, I., Vigh, S., Schally, A. V., and Petrusz, P., Immunocytochemical localization of growth hormone-releasing factor in the rat hypothalamus, *Endocrinology,* 144, 1082, 1984a.

Merchenthaler, I., Thomas, C. R., and Arimura, A., Immunocytochemical localization of growth hormone-releasing factor (GHRF) in the rat brain using anti-rat GHRF serum, *Peptides,* 5, 1071, 1984b.

Merchenthaler, I., Csontos, C., Kallo, I., and Arimura, A., The hypothalamo-infundibular growth hormone-releasing hormone (GH-RH) system of the rat, *Brain Res.,* 378, 2297, 1986.

Merchenthaler, I., Setalo, G., Csontos, C., Petrusz, P., Flerko, B., and Negro-Vilar, A., Combined retrograde tracing and immunocytochemical identification of luteinizing hormone-releasing hormone- and somatostatin-containing neurons projecting to the median eminence of the rat, *Endocrinology,* 125, 2812, 1989.

Mesguich, P., Benoit, R., Dubois, P. M., and Morel, G., Somatostatin-28- and somatostatin-14-like immunoreactivities in the rat pituitary gland, *Cell Tissue Res.,* 252, 419, 1988.

Miki, N., Ono, M., and Shizume, K., Evidence that opiatergic and α-adrenergic mechanisms stimulate rat growth hormone release via growth hormone-releasing factor (GRF), *Endocrinology,* 114, 1950, 1984.

Millard, R. W., Lathrop, D. A., Grupp, G., Ashraf, M., Grupp, I. L., and Schwartz, A., Differential cardiovascular effects of calcium channel blocking agents: potential mechanisms, *Am. J. Cardiology,* 49, 499, 1982.

Millard, W. J., Martin, J. B., Jr., Audet, J., and Martin, J. B., Evidence that reduced growth hormone secretion observed in monosodium glutamate-treated rats is the result of a deficiency in growth hormone-releasing factor, *Endocrinology,* 110, 540, 1982.

Miller, R. E., Pancreatic neuroendocrinology: peripheral neural mechanisms in the regulation of the islet of Langerhans, *Endocrine Rev.,* 2, 471, 1981.

Miller, R. J., PHI and GRF: two new members of the glucagon/secretin family, *Med. Biol.,* 62, 159, 1984.

Molitch, M. E., Neuroendocrine aspects of growth hormone regulation., in *Clinical Neuroendocrinology,* Chapter 7, Collu, R., Brown, G. M., and Van Loon, G. R., Eds., Blackwell, Boston, 1988, 145.

Moore, R. Y., The reticular formation: monoamine neuron system, in *The Reticular Formation Revisited: Specifying Function for a Nonspecific System,* IBRO Series, Vol. 6, Raven Press, New York, 1980, 67.

Morel, G., Mesguich, P., Dubois, M. P., and Dubois, P. M., Ultrastructural evidence for endogenous growth hormone-releasing factor-like immunoreactivity in the monkey pituitary glands, *Neuroendocrinology,* 38, 123, 1984.

Morimoto, N., Kawakami, F., Makino, S., Chihara, K., Hasegawa, M., and Ibata, Y., Age-related changes in growth hormone releasing factor and somatostatin in the rat hypothalamus, *Neuroendocrinology,* 47, 459, 1988.

Mugnaini, E. and Oertel, W. H., An atlas of the distribution of GABAergic neurons and terminals in the rat CNS as revealed by GAD immunohistochemistry, in *Handbook of Chemical Neuroanatomy,* Vol. 4, (Part 1, GABA and Neuropeptides in the CNS), Björklund, A. and Hökfelt, T., Eds., Elsevier, Amsterdam, 1985, 456.

Mulroney, S. E., Lumpkin, M. D., and Haramati, A., Antagonist to GH-releasing factor inhibits growth and renal reabsorption of P_i in immature rats, *Am. J. Physiol.,* 257, F29, 1989.

Murakami, Y., Kato, Y., Kabayama, Y., Tojo, K., Inoue, T., and Imura, H., Involvement of growth hormone-releasing factor on growth hormone secretion induced by γ-aminobutyric acid in conscious rats, Endocrinology, 117, 787, 1985.

Murakami, Y., Kato, Y., Koshiyama, H., Inoue, T., Yanaihara, N., and Imura, H., Galanin stimulates growth hormone (GH) secretion via GH-releasing factor (GRF) in conscious rats, *Eur. J. Pharmacol.,* 136, 415, 1987a.

Murakami, Y., Kato, Y., Kabayama, Y., Inoue, T., Koshiyama, H., and Imura, H., Involvement of hypothalamic growth hormone (GH) releasing factor in GH secretion induced by intracerebroventricular injection of somatostatin in rats, *Endocrinology,* 120, 311, 1987b.

Murakami, Y., Kato, Y., Shimatsu, A., Koshiyama, H., Hattori, N., Yanaihara, N., and Imura, H., Possible mechanism involved in growth hormone secretion induced by galanin in the rat, *Endocrinology,* 124, 1224, 1989.

Mutt, V., Gastrointestinal hormones, *Adv. Metab. Disorders,* 11, 1988.

Nahon, J. L., Presse, F., Bittencourt, J. C., Sawchenko, P. E., and Vale, W., The rat melanin-concentrating hormone messsenger ribonucleic acid encodes multiple neuropeptides coexpressed in the dorsolateral hypothalamus, *Endocrinology,* 125, 2056, 1989.

Nakai, Y., Imura, H., Sakurai, H., Kurahachi, H., and Yoshimi, T., Effect of cyproheptadine on human growth hormone secretion, *J. Clin. Endocrinol. Metab.,* 38, 446, 1974.

Naus, C. C. G., Miller, F. D., Morrison, J. H., and Bloom, F. E., Immunohistochemical and *in situ* hybridization analysis of the development of the rat somatostatin-containing neocortical neuronal system, *J. Comp. Neurol.,* 269, 448, 1988.

Negro-Vilar, A., Ojeda, S. R., Arimura, A., and McCann, S. M., Dopamine and norepinephrine stimulate somatostatin release by median eminence fragments in vitro, *Life Sci.,* 23, 1493, 1978.

Niimi, M., Takahara, J., Sato, M., and Kawanishi, K., Sites of origin of growth hormone-releasing factor-containing neurons projecting to the stalk-median eminence of the rat, *Peptides,* 10, 605, 1989.

Niimi, M., Takahara, J., Sato, M., and Kawanishi, K., Immunohistochemical identification of galanin and growth hormone-releasing factor-containing neurons projecting to the median eminence of the rat, *Neuroendocrinology,* 51, 572, 1990.

Nissley, S. P. and Rechler, M. M., Insulin-like growth factors: biosynthesis, receptors, and carrier proteins, in *Hormonal Proteins and Peptides,* Vol. XII, (Chapter 4), Academic Press, New York, 1984, 127.

Noe, B. D., Andrews, P. C., Dixon, J. E., and Spiess, J., Cotranslational and posttranslational proteolytic processing of preprosomatostatin-I in intact islet tissue, *J. Cell Biol.,* 103, 1205, 1987.

Nordström, Ö., Melander, T., Hökfelt, T., Bartfai, T., and Goldstein, M., Evidence for an inhibitory effect of the peptide galanin on dopamine release from the rat median eminence, *Neurosci. Lett.,* 73, 21, 1987.

Okamura, H., Murakami, S., Chihara, K., Nagatsu, I., and Ibata, Y., Coexistence of growth hormone-releasing factor-like and tyrosine hydroxylase-like immunoreactivities in neurons of the rat arcuate nucleus, Neuroendocrinology, 41, 177, 1985.

Olney, J. W., Brain lesions, obesity, and other disturbances in mice treated with monosodium glutamate, Science, 164, 719, 1969.

Orci, L., Baetens, D., Dubois, M. P., and Rufener, C., Evidence for the D-cell of the pancreas secreting somatostatin, Horm. Metab. Res., 7, 400, 1975.

Ottlecz, A., Samson, W. K., and McCann, S. M., Galanin: evidence for a hypothalamic site of action to release growth hormone, Peptides, 7, 51, 1985.

Ottlecz, A., Snyder, G. D., and McCann, S. M., Regulatory role of galanin in control of hypothalamic pituitary function, Proc. Natl. Acad. Sci. U.S.A., 85, 9861, 1988.

Pagesy, P., Li, J. Y., Rentier-Delerue, F., Le Bouc, Y., Martial, J. A., and Peillon, F., Evidence of pre-prosomatostatin mRNA in human normal and tumoral anterior pituitary gland, Mol. Endocrinol., 3, 1289, 1989.

Parnavelas, J. G. and McDonald, J. K., The cerebral cortex, in Chemical Neuroanatomy, Emson, P. C., Ed., Raven Press, New York, 1983, 505.

Parnavelas, J. G., Dinoupolos, A., and Davies, S. W., The central visual pathways, in Handbook of Chemical Neuroanatomy, Vol. 7, (Part II, Integrated systems of the CNS), Björklund, A., Hökfelt, T., and Swanson, L.W., Eds., Elsevier, Amsterdam, 1989, 1.

Parsons, J. A., Erlandsen, S. L., Hegre, O. D., McEvoy, R., and Elde, R. P., Central and peripheral localization of somatostatin. Immunoenzyme immunocytochemical studies, Trans. Am. Neurol. Assoc., 102, 90, 1976.

Patel, Y. C., Growth hormone stimulates hypothalamic somatostatin, Life Sci., 24, 1589, 1979.

Patel, Y. C., Hoyte, K., and Martin, J. B., Effect of anterior hypothalamic lesions on neurohypophyseal and peripheral tissue concentrations of somatostatin in the rat, Endocrinology, 105, 712, 1979.

Pelletier, G., Désy, L., Coté, J., Lefèvre, G., and Vaudry, H., Light-microscopic immunocytochemical localization of growth hormone-releasing factor in the human hypothalamus, Cell Tissue Res., 245, 461, 1986.

Pierotti, A. R. and Harmar, A. J., Multiple forms of somatostatin-like immunoreactivity in the hypothalamus and amygdala of the rat: selective localisation of somatostatin-28 in the median eminence, J. Endocrinol., 105, 383, 1985.

Plotsky, P. M. and Vale, W., Patterns of growth hormone-releasing factor and somatostatin secretion into the hypophysial-portal circulation of the rat, Science, 230, 461, 1985.

Polonsky, K., Jaspan, J., Berelowitz, M., Pugh, W., Moossa, A., and Ling, N., The in vivo metabolism of somatostatin 28: possible relationship between diminished metabolism and enhanced biological action, Endocrinology, 111, 1698, 1982.

Pradayrol, L., Somatostatin-28, Adv. Metab. Disorders, 11, 457, 1988.

Reichlin, S., Growth and the hypothalamus, Endocrinology, 67, 760, 1960.

Reichlin, S., Regulation of somatotropic hormone secretion, in Handbook of Physiology, Vol. 4 (Part 2), Knobil, E. and Sawyer, W. H., William & Wilkins, Baltimore, 1974, 405.

Reichlin, S., Somatostatin, in Brain Peptides, Chapter 29, Krieger, D. T., Brownstein, M. J., and Martin, J. B., Eds., John Wiley & Sons, New York, 1983, 711.

Reichlin, S., Neuroendocrinology, in Textbook of Endocrinology, Chapter 17, Wilson, J. D., and Foster, D. W., Eds., W. B. Saunders, Philadelphia, 1985, 492.

Reubi, J. C. and Maurer, R., Autoradiographic mapping of somatostatin receptors in the rat central nervous system and pituitary, Neuroscience, 15, 1183, 1985.

Reubi, J. C., Cortés, R., Maurer, R., Probst, A., and Palacios, J. M., Distribution of somatostatin receptors in the human brain: an autoradiographic study, Neuroscience, 18, 329, 1986.

Richardson, S. B., Hollander, C. S., D'Eletto, R., Greenleaf, P. W., and Thaw, C., Acetylcholine inhibits the release of somatostatin from rat hypothalamus in vitro, Endocrinology, 117, 122, 1980.

Richardson, S., Twente, S., and Audhya, T., GHRF causes biphasic stimulation of SRIF secretion from rat hypothalamic cells, Am. J. Physiol., 255, E829, 1988.

Rivier, J., Spiess, J., Thorner, M. O., and Vale, W., Characterization of a growth hormone-releasing factor from a pancreatic islet tumor, *Nature (London)*, 300, 276, 1982.

Robinson, I. C. A. F. and Clarke, R. G., The secretory pattern of GH and its significance for growth in the rat, in *Growth Hormone — Basic and Clinical Aspects*, Isaksson, O., Binder, C., Hall, K., and Hökfelt, B., Eds., Elsevier, Amsterdam, 1987, 109.

Rogers, K. V., Vician, L., Steiner, R. A., and Clifton, D. K., The effect of hypophysectomy and growth hormone administration on pre-prosomatostatin messenger ribonucleic acid in the periventricular nucleus of the rat hypothalamus, *Endocrinology*, 122, 586, 1988.

Rökaeus, Å., Galanin: a newly isolated biologically active neuropeptide, *TINS*, 10, 158, 1987.

Rökaeus, Å. and Brownstein, M., Construction of a porcine adrenal medullary cDNA library and nucleotide sequence analysis of two clones encoding a galanin precursor, *Proc. Natl. Acad. Sci. U.S.A.*, 83, 6287, 1986.

Rökaeus, Å. and Carlquist, M., Nucleotide sequence analysis of cDNAs encoding a bovine galanin precursor protein in the adrenal medulla and chemical isolation of bovine gut galanin, *FEBS Lett.*, 234, 400, 1988.

Romagnano, M. A., Pilcher, W. H., Bennet-Clarke, C., Chafel, T. L., and Joseph, S. A., Distribution of somatostatin in the mouse brain, effects of neonatal MSG treatment, *Brain Res.*, 234, 387, 1982.

Sakaue, M., Saito, N., Taniguchi, H., Baba, S., and Tanaka, C., Immunohistochemical localization of γ-aminobutyric acid in the rat pituitary gland and related hypothalamic regions, *Brain Res.*, 46, 343, 1988.

Sandman, J., Arimura, A., and Schally, A. V., Stimulation of growth hormone release by anterior pituitary perfusion in the rat, *Endocrinology*, 90, 1315, 1972.

Sawchenko, P. E. and Swanson, L. W., Growth hormone releasing hormone, in *The Handbook of Chemical Neuroanatomy*, Vol. 9, Part II, Björklund, A., Hökfelt, T., and Kuhar, M., Eds., Elsevier, Amsterdam, 1990, 131.

Sawchenko, P. E., Swanson, L. W., Rivier, J., and Vale, W. W., The distribution of growth hormone-releasing factor (GRF) immunoreactivity in the central nervous system of the rat: an immunohistochemical study using antisera directed against rat hypothalamic GRF, *J. Comp. Neurol.*, 237, 100, 1985.

Schally, A. V., Dupont, A., Arimura, A., Redding, T. W., Nishi, N., Linthicum, G. L., and Schlesinger, D., Isolation and structure of somatostatin from porcine hypothalami, *Biochemistry*, 15, 509, 1976.

Schlegel, W., Wuarin, F., Wollheim, C. B., and Zahnd, G. R., Somatostatin lowers the cytosolic free Ca^{2+} concentration in clonal rat pituitary cells (GH_3 cells), *Cell Calcium*, 5, 223, 1984.

Schöfl, C., Sandow, J., and Knepel, W., GRF elevates cytosolic free calcium concentration in rat anterior pituitary cells, *Am. J. Physiol.*, 253, E591, 1987.

Schultzberg, M. and Lindh, B., Transmitters and peptides in autonomic ganglia, in *Handbook of Chemical Neuroanatomy*, Vol. 6 (The peripheral nervous system), Björklund, A., Hökfelt, T., and Owman, C., Eds., Elsevier, Amsterdam, 1988, 297.

Seifert, H., Perrin, M., Rivier, J., and Vale, W., Binding sites for growth hormone releasing factor on rat anterior pituitary cells, *Nature (London)*, 313, 487, 1985.

Shen, L.-P. and Rutter, W. J., Sequence of the human somatostatin I gene, *Science*, 224, 168, 1984.

Shen, L.-P., Pictet, R. L., and Rutter, W. J., Human somatostatin I: sequence of the cDNA, *Proc. Natl. Acad. Sci. U.S.A.*, 79, 4575, 1982.

Shiosaka, S., Takatsuki, K., Skanaka, M., Inagaki, S., Takagi, H., Senba, E., Kawai, Y., Minagawa, H., and Tohyama, M., New somatostatin containing sites in the diencephalon of the neonatal rat, *Neurosci. Lett.*, 25, 69, 1981a.

Shiosaka, S., Takatsuki, K., Sakanaka, M., Inagaki, S., Takagi, H., Senba, E., Kawai, Y., Minagawa, H., and Tohyama, M., Ontogeny of somatostatin-containing neuron systems of the rat: immunohistochemical observations. I. Lower brain stem, *J. Comp. Neurol.*, 203, 173, 1981b.

Shiosaka, S., Takatsuki, K., Sakanaka, M., Inagaki, S., Takagi, H., Senba, E., Kawai, Y., Iida, H., Minagawa, H., Hara, Y., Matzusaki, T., and Tohyama, M., Ontogeny of somatostatin-containing neuron systems of the rat: immunohistochemical observations. II. Forebrain and diencephalon, *J. Comp. Neurol.*, 204, 211, 1982.

Sizer, A. R., Rökaeus, Å., and Foster, G. A., Analysis of the ontogeny of galanin in the rat central nervous system by immunohistochemistry and radioimmunoassay, *Int. J. Devl. Neurosci.*, 8, 81, 1990.

Skofitsch, G. and Jacobowitz, D. M., Quantitative distribution of galanin-like immunoreactivity in the rat central nervous system, *Peptides*, 7, 609, 1985a.

Skofitsch, G. and Jacobowitz, D. M., Immunohistochemical mapping of galanin-like neurons in the rat central nervous system, *Peptides*, 6, 509, 1985b.

Skofitsch, G., Sills, M. A., and Jacobowitz, D. M., Autoradiographic distribution of ^{125}I-galanin binding sites in the rat central nevous system, *Peptides*, 7, 1029, 1986.

Smith, R. M., Howe, P. R. C., Olivier, J. R., and Willoughby, J. O., Growth hormone-releasing factor immunoreactivity in rat hypothalamus, *Neuropeptides*, 4, 109, 1984.

Sorenson, R. L. and Elde, R. P., Dissociation of glucose stimulation of somatostatin and insulin release from glucose inhibition of glucose release in the isolated perfused rat pancreas, *Diabetes*, 32, 561, 1983.

Spada, A., Vallar, L., and Giannattasio, G., Presence of an adenylate cyclase dually regulated by somatostatin and human pancreatic growth hormone (GH)-releasing factor in GH-secreting cells, *Endocrinology*, 115, 1203, 1984.

Spiess, J., Rivier, J., and Vale, W., Characterization of rat hypothalamic growth hormone-releasing factor, *Nature (London)*, 303, 532, 1983.

Srikant, C. B. and Patel, Y. C., Receptor binding of somatostatin-28 is tissue specific, *Nature (London)*, 294, 259, 1981.

Sundler, F. and Håkanson, R., Peptide hormone-producing endocrine/paracrine cells in the gastro-entero-pancreatic region, in *Handbook of Chemical Neuroanatomy*, Vol. 6 (The peripheral nervous system), Björklund, A., Hökfelt, T., and Owman, C., Eds., Elsevier, Amsterdam, 1988, 219.

Swanson, L. W., The hypothalamus, in *Handbook of Chemical Neuroanatomy*, Vol. 5 (Part I, Integrated systems in the CNS), Björklund, A., Hökfelt, T., and Swanson, L. W., Eds., Elsevier, Amsterdam, 1987, 1.

Szabo, M. and Cuttler, L., Differential responsiveness of the somatotroph to growth hormone-releasing factor during early neonatal development in the rat, *Endocrinology*, 118, 69, 1986.

Szentagothai, J., Flerkó, B., Mess, B., and Halasz, B., Hypothalamic control of the anterior pituitary, *Akademiai Kiado (Budapest)*, 1972.

Takahara, J., Yunoki, S., Hosogi, H., Yakushiji, W., Yama, J., and Ofuji, T., Concomitant increases in serum growth hormone and hypothalamic somatostatin in rats after injection of γ-aminobutyric acid, aminooxyacetic acid, or γ-hydroxybutyric acid, *Endocrinology*, 106, 343, 1980.

Takatsuki, K., Sakanaka, M., Shiosaka, S., Inagali, S., Takagi, H., Senba, E., Hara, Y., Kawai, Y., Minigawa, H., Lida, H., and Tohyama, M., Pathways and terminal fields of the cochlear fugal somatostatin tracts of very young rats, *Dev. Brain Res.*, 3, 613, 1982.

Tallo, D. and Malarkey, W. B., Adrenergic and dopaminergic modulation of growth hormone and prolactin secretion in normal and tumor-bearing human pituitaries in monolayer culture, *J. Clin. Endocrinol. Metab.*, 53, 1278, 1981.

Tannenbaum, G. S., Somatostatin as a physiological regulator of pulsatile growth hormone secretion, *Horm. Res.*, 23, 70, 1988.

Tannenbaum, G. S. and Ling, N., The interrelationship of growth hormone (GH)-releasing factor and somatostatin in generation of the ultradian rythm of GH secretion, *Endocrinology*, 115, 1952, 1984.

Tannenbaum, G. S and Martin, J. B., Evidence for an endogenous rhythm governing growth hormone secretion in the rat, *Endocrinology*, 98, 562, 1976.

Tannenbaum, G. S., Guyda, H. J., and Posner, B. I., Insulin-like growth factors: a role in growth hormone negative feedback and body weight regulation via brain, *Science*, 220, 77, 1983.

Tatemoto, K., Rökaeus, Å., Jörnvall, H., McDonald, T. J., and Mutt, V., Galanin — a novel biologically active peptide from porcine intestine, *FEBS Lett.*, 164, 124, 1983.

Terry, L. C. and Martin, J. B., Evidence for α-adrenergic regulation of episodic growth hormone and prolactin secretion in the undisturbed male rat, *Endocrinology*, 108, 1869, 1981.

Thorner, M. O., Vance, M. L., Rogol, A. D., Blizzard, R. M., Klingensmith, G., Najjar, J., Brook, C. G., Smith, P., Reichlin, S., Rivier, J., and Vale, W., Some physiological and therapeutic considerations of GHRH in the regulation of growth, in *Growth Hormone — Basic and Clinical Aspects,* Isaksson, O., Binder, C., Hall, K., and Hökfelt, B., Eds., Elsevier, Amsterdam, 1987, 153.

Toivola, P. T. K. and Gale, C. C., Stimulation of growth hormone release by microinjection of norepinephrine into hypothalamus of baboons, *Endocrinology,* 90, 895, 1972.

Torres, I., Guaza, C., Fernandez-Durango, R., Borrell, J., and Charo, A. L., Evidence for a modulatory role of catecholamines on hypothalamic somatostatin in the rat, *Neuroendocrinology,* 35, 159, 1982.

Tramu, G., Beauvillain, J. C., Pillez, A., and Mazzuca, M., Présence d'une substance immunologiquement apparentée à la somatolibérine extraite d'une tumeur pancréatique humaine (hpGRF) dans des neurones de l'aire hypophysiotrope du Cobaye et du Rat, *C.R. Acad. Sci., Paris,* 297, 435, 1983.

Tran, V. T., Uhl, G. R., Perry, D. C., Manning, D. C., Vale, W. W., Perrin, M. H., Rivier, J. E., Martin, J. B., and Snyder, S. H., Autoradiographic localization of somatostatin receptors in rat brain, *Eur. J. Pharmacol.,* 101, 307, 1984.

Tran, V. T, Beal, M. F., and Martin, J. B., Two types of somatostatin receptors differentiated by cyclic somatostatin analogs, *Science,* 228, 492, 1985.

Uhl, G. R. and Sasek, C. A., Somatostatin mRNA: regional variation in hybridization densities in individual neurons, *J. Neurosci.,* 6, 3258, 1986.

Uhl, G. R., Tran, V., Snyder, S. H., and Martin, J. B., Somatostatin receptors: distribution in rat central nervous system and human frontal cortex, *J. Comp. Neurol.,* 240, 288, 1985.

Uvnäs-Wallensten, K., Luminal secretion of gut peptides, *Clin. Gastroenterol.,* 9, 545, 1980.

Vale, W., Brazeau, P., Grant, G., Nussey, A., Burgus, R., Rivier, J., Ling, N., and Guillemin, R., Premières observations sur le mode d'action de la somatostatin, un facteur hypothalamique qui inhibe le sécrétion de l'hormone de croissance, *C.R. Hebd. Séance Acad. Sci. Paris,* 275, 2913, 1972.

Vale, W., Brazeau, P., Rivier, C., Brown, M., Boss, B., Rivier, J., Burgus, R., Ling, N., and Guillemin, R., Somatostatin, *Rec. Prog. Horm. Res.,* 31, 365, 1975.

Vale, W., Vaughan, J., Yamamoto, G., Spiess, J., and Rivier, J., Effects of synthetic human pancreatic (tumor) GH releasing factor and somatostatin, triiodothyronine and dexamethasone on GH secretion *in vitro, Endocrinology,* 112, 1553, 1983.

VandePol, C. J., Leidy, J. W., Finger, T. E., and Robbins, R. J., Immunohistochemical localization of GRF-containing neurons in rat brain, *Neuroendocrinology,* 42, 143, 1986.

Van Wyk, J. J., The somatomedins: biological actions and physiologic control mechanisms, in *Hormonal Proteins and Peptides,* Vol. XII, Chapter 3, Academic Press, New York, 1984, 82.

Vigas, M., Malatinsky, J., Nemeth, J., and Jurcivicova, J., Alpha-adrenergic control of growth hormone release during surgical stress in man, *Metabolism,* 26, 399, 1977.

Villar, M. J., Hökfelt, T., and Brown, J. C., Somatostatin expression in the cerebellar cortex during postnatal development, *Anat. Embryol.,* 179, 257, 1989.

Vincent, S. R., McIntosh, C. H. S., Buchan, A. M. J., and Brown, J. C., Central somatostatin systems revealed with monoclonal antibodies, *J. Comp. Neurol.,* 238, 169, 1985.

Voogt, J. L., Clemens, J. A., Negro-Vilar, A., Welsch, C., and Meites, J., Pituitary GH and hypothalamic GHRF after median eminence implantation of ovine or human GH, *Endocrinology,* 88, 1363, 1971.

Vrontakis, M. E., Peden, L. M., Duckworth, M. L., and Friesen, H. G., Isolation and characterization of a complementary DNA (galanin) clone from estrogen-induced pituitary tumor messenger RNA, *J. Biol. Chem.,* 262, 16755, 1987.

Vrontakis, M. E., Yamamoto, T., Schroedter, I. C., Nagy, J. I., and Friesen, H. G., Estrogen induction of galanin synthesis in the rat anterior pituitary gland demonstrated by in situ hybridization and immunohistochemistry, *Neurosci. Lett.,* 100, 59, 1989.

Wakabayashi, T., Miyazawawa, H., Kanda, M., Demura, H., and Shizume, K., Stimulation of immunoreactive somatostatin release from hypothalamic synaptosomes by high K^+ and dopamine, *Endocrinol. Jpn.,* 24, 601, 1977.

Wehrenberg, W. B., Ling, N., Brazeau, P., Esch, F., Böhlen, P., Baird, A., Ying, S., and Guillemin, R., Somatocrinin, growth hormone-releasing factor, stimulates secretion of growth hormone in anesthetized rats, *Biochem. Biophys. Res. Commun.*, 109, 382, 1982a.

Wehrenberg, W. B., Brazeau, P., Luben, R., Böhlen, P., and Guillemin, R., Inhibition of the pulsatile secretion of growth hormone by monoclonal antibodies to the hypothalamic growth hormone releasing factor, GRF, *Endocrinology*, 111, 2147, 1982b.

Wehrenberg, W. B., Ling, N., Böhlen, P., Esch, F., Brazeau, P., and Guillemin, R., Physiological roles of somatocrinin and somatostatin in the regulation of growth hormone secretion, *Biochem. Biophys. Res. Commun.*, 109, 562, 1982c.

Wehrenberg, W. B., Baird, A., and Ling, N., Potent interaction between glucocorticoids and growth hormone-releasing factor *in vivo*, *Science*, 221, 556, 1983.

Wehrenberg, W. B., Bloch, B., and Phillips, B. J., Antibodies to growth hormone-releasing factor inhibit somatic growth, *Endocrinology*, 115, 1218, 1984.

Werner, H., Koch, Y., Baldino, F., and Gozes, I., Steroid regulation of somatostatin mRNA in the rat hypothalamus, *J. Biol. Chem.*, 263, 7666, 1988.

Wiegand, S. J. and Price, J. L., Cells of origin of the afferent fibers to the median eminence in the rat, *J. Comp. Neurol.*, 192, 1, 1980.

Wilber, J. F., Nagel, T., and White, W. F., Hypothalamic growth hormone releasing activity (GRH): characterization by the in vitro rat pituitary and radioimmunoassay, *Endocrinology*, 89, 1419, 1971.

Willoughby, J. O. and Martin, J. B., The suprachiasmatic nucleus synchronizes growth hormone secretory rhythms with the light-dark cycle, *Brain Res.*, 151, 413, 1978.

Willoughby, J. O., Brogan, M., and Kapoor, R., Hypothalamic interconnections of somatostatin and growth hormone releasing factor neurons, *Neuroendocrinology*, 50, 584, 1989.

Wilson, J. T. and Frohman, L. A., Concomitant association between high plasma levels of growth hormone and low hepatic mixed function activity in the young rat, *J. Pharmacol. Exp. Ther.*, 189, 255, 1974.

Woolf, P. D. and Lee, L., Effect of the serotonin precursor, tryptophan, on pituitary hormone secretion, *J. Clin. Endocrinol. Metab.*, 45, 123, 1977.

Zaborsky, L., Afferent connections to the medial basal hypothalamus, *Adv. Anat. Embryol. Cell Biol.*, 69, 1982.

10

Thyrotropin-Releasing Hormone Neuronal Systems in the Central Nervous System

RONALD M. LECHAN AND ROBERTO TONI*
Department of Medicine
Division of Endocrinology, Diabetes, Metabolism and Molecular Medicine
New England Medical Center Hospitals
Boston, Massachusetts

I. Introduction

For more than a decade following the chemical characterization of thyrotropin-releasing hormone (TRH) (Burgus et al., 1970; Nair et al., 1970), anatomical studies on the distribution of TRH in the CNS were remarkably limited when compared to a rapidly expanding literature on numerous other peptidergic systems in the brain (Hökfelt et al., 1975, 1979; Choy and Watkins, 1977). This difficulty was due to technical problems, partly due to the loss of this highly soluble peptide during processing, since TRH lacks a free amino group that would permit its immobilization in tissue by conventional fixatives (Figure 1). In addition, as most antisera raised against TRH require that the NH_2-terminal pyroglutamyl ring and COOH-terminal amide be intact for immunologic reactivity, any alteration of the antigenic determinants by the fixation steps could also result in the loss of immunoreactivity. With the use of a novel fixative capable of reacting with the imidazole group of the antigenically silent histidine residue of TRH (King et al., 1983), detailed information on the immunocytochemical localization of TRH neuronal processes and perikarya in the central nervous system (Lechan and Jackson, 1982; Lechan et al., 1983a) was more readily obtained.

Further advances in the elucidation of the anatomy of TRH neuronal systems in the brain have been facilitated by characterizing the structure of the TRH prohormone, first from frog skin by Richter et al. (1985) and then from rat hypothalamus by our group (Lechan et al., 1986b). As illustrated in Figure 2, proTRH (molecular weight approximately 26,000) contains five Gln-His-Pro-Gly progenitor sequences for TRH, each flanked by potential cleavage sites. Glycine is necessary for carboxyl-terminal amidation of the proline residue in mature TRH (Bradbury et al., 1982) and further posttranslational modification to TRH occurs by converting the N-terminal glutaminyl residue into pyroglutamyl by the enzyme glutaminyl cyclase (Fischer and Speiss, 1987). In addition to the sequences coding for TRH, the prohormone contains five spacer peptides and N and C terminal-flanking peptides. Since the N-terminal peptide also contains a potential cleavage site in addition to TRH, seven nonTRH peptides could conceivably be generated from enzymatic cleavage at all paired basic residues by carboxypeptidase B-like endopeptidases (Docherty and Steiner, 1982). Chromatographic analysis

* Current address: Instituto di Anatomia Umana Normale, University of Bologna, Bologna, Italy.

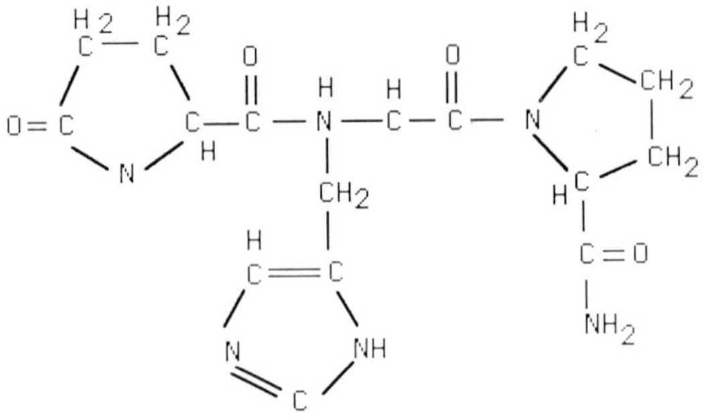

Figure 1. Structure of mature TRH (pyroglutamic acid-histidine-proline-amide).

```
                                        TCCTTGGATTCGGGAGTATTGCAAACTCTAC
CCAGCCAGTTTGCACTCTTCAGCTCAGCATCTTGGAAAGCTCTGCAGAGTCTCCACTTCGCAGACTCCAGG 102

ATG CCG GGA CCT TGG TTG CTG CTG GCT CTG GCT TTG ATC TTC ACC CTA ACT GGT
1 Met-Pro-Gly-Pro-Trp-Leu-Leu-Leu-Ala-Leu-Ala-Leu-Ile-Phe-Thr-Leu-Thr-Gly
------------------------------------------------------------------------

ATC CCT GAA TCC TGC GCC TTG CCG GAG GCA GCC CAG GAG GAA GGT GCA GTG ACT 210
Ile-Pro-Glu-Ser-Cys-Ala-Leu-Pro-Glu-Ala-Ala-Gln-Glu-Glu-Gly-Ala-Val-Thr
----------------------------

CCT GAC CTT CCT GGC CTG GAG AAT GTT CAG GTC CGG CCA GAA CGT CGA TTC TTG
37 Pro-Asp-Leu-Pro-Gly-Leu-Glu-Asn-Val-Gln-Val-Arg-Pro-Glu-Arg-Arg-Phe-Leu

TGG AAA GAC CTC CAG CGG GTG AGA GGG GAC CTC GGT GCT GCC TTA GAC TCC TGG 318
Trp-Lys-Asp-Leu-Gln-Arg-Val-Arg-Gly-Asp-Leu-Gly-Ala-Ala-Leu-Asp-Ser-Trp

ATC ACA AAA CGC CAG CAT CCA GGC AAA AGG GAG GAG GAG GAA AAA GAC ATT GAA
73 Ile-Thr-Lys-Arg-Gln-His-Pro-Gly-Lys-Arg-Glu-Glu-Glu-Glu-Lys-Asp-Ile-Glu

GCT GAA GAG AGG GGA GAC TTG GGA GAA GGG GGA GCC TGG AGA CTC CAC AAA CGA 426
Ala-Glu-Glu-Arg-Gly-Asp-Leu-Gly-Glu-Gly-Gly-Ala-Trp-Arg-Leu-His-Lys-Arg

CAG CAC CCC GGC CGA CGT GCC AAC CAG GAC AAG TAT TCA TGG GCA GAT GAG GAG
109 Gln-His-Pro-Gly-Arg-Arg-Ala-Asn-Gln-Asp-Lys-Tyr-Ser-Trp-Ala-Asp-Glu-Glu

GAC AGT GAC TGG ATG CCA CGG TCC TGG TTA CCA GAT TTC TTT CTG GAT TCC TGG 534
Asp-Ser-Asp-Trp-Met-Pro-Arg-Ser-Trp-Leu-Pro-Asp-Phe-Phe-Leu-Asp-Ser-Trp

TTC TCA GAT GTC CCC CAA GTC AAG CGG CAG CAC CCT GGC AGG CGA TCC TTC CCC
145 Phe-Ser-Asp-Val-Pro-Gln-Val-Lys-Arg-Gln-His-Pro-Gly-Arg-Arg-Ser-Phe-Pro

TGG ATG GAG TCT GAT GTC ACC AAG AGG CAA CAT CCA GGC CGG AGG TTC ATA GAT 642
Trp-Met-Glu-Ser-Asp-Val-Thr-Lys-Arg-Gln-His-Pro-Gly-Arg-Arg-Phe-Ile-Asp

CCC GAG CTC CAA AGA AGC TGG GAA GAA AAA GAG GGA GAG GGT GTC TTA ATG CCT
181 Pro-Glu-Leu-Gln-Arg-Ser-Trp-Glu-Glu-Lys-Glu-Gly-Glu-Gly-Val-Leu-Met-Pro

GAG AAA CGC CAG CAT CCT GGC AAA AGG GCA TTG GGT CAT CCC TGT GGG CCC CAG 750
Glu-Lys-Arg-Gln-His-Pro-Gly-Lys-Arg-Ala-Leu-Gly-His-Pro-Cys-Gly-Pro-Gln

GGG ACT TGT GGT CAA ACA GGC CTG CTC CAG CTT CTA GGT GAC CTG AGC AGG GGT
217 Gly-Thr-Cys-Gly-Gln-Thr-Gly-Leu-Leu-Gln-Leu-Leu-Gly-Asp-Leu-Ser-Arg-Gly

CAG GAG ACC CTG GTG AAG CAA AGC CCA CAA GTG GAA CCC TGG GAC AAG GAA CCT 858
Gln-Glu-Thr-Leu-Val-Lys-Gln-Ser-Pro-Gln-Val-Glu-Pro-Trp-Asp-Lys-Glu-Pro

CTG GAG GAG TAAGGCCAGAGTCAGGCTTTAGGTCTAGGATGATGTAAGCCCTGTATTCCCTATCCTGT
253 Leu-Glu-Glu ***

TCCCTTCACTAGCTGTCCTCTCTTAGATGCTAACCCTGGGCCCTCTGTACATCGTCCACCCAAACCCCTTC 997
CTTACCGACTTCAGAGACTTTAGAAAGCCAGTCAGGAAGTTAAAACCCTACTTATCCCTTCAAGCAAGGGG
GTGGGAGTCACACCCCTTCAGCACTGGCCAAGATGGTTCTTTCACACCTTCTAAGGGACCTCCTCAGAAAG
GAAGGGTAGAATTGAAATGTTTTGGTGTTAAAAACTTCTGTAATCTGCCCCATGTGGTAAGACTGACCTGGT
ATAGCTTCAGCGCATCCTCCAAGGTTGGGGTCCCTGAGCAGTTTGGGAGATGTTTAGATATGTCCTTGGGG 1201
TGGGGGGTCGCATCTTGTATATAACCCTGCTCTTGGGAAT
```

Figure 2. Nucleotide and predicted amino acid sequence of preproTRH. Arg-Arg residues contained in the amino-terminal flanking peptide of the prohormone and the repeating progenitor sequences of TRH and flanking dibasic amino acids are underlined. The stop codon is designated by three asterisks. The region underlined by dashes designates the predicted signal region.

of the processed forms of proTRH indicates that all five TRH progenitor sequences are, in fact, processed in the CNS, giving rise to five copies of the mature prohormone as well as each of the potential nonTRH peptides (Bulant et al., 1988; Wu et al., 1987; Wu and Jackson, 1988). The physiological significance of these nonTRH peptides remains uncertain, although evidence for differential processing of proTRH in certain regions of the brain (Lechan et al., 1987; Wu et al., 1987; Wu and Jackson, 1988; Bulant et al., 1988) suggests potential biological importance. In addition, preproTRH- (160—169) may have potent TSH-releasing activity (Carr and Wessendorf, 1988; Roussell et al., 1989; Bulant et al., 1990).

Only a single TRH gene has been found in the rat genome (Lee et al., 1988); its nucleotide sequence is schematically illustrated in Figure 3. The human TRH gene has also been isolated by Yamada et al. (1989) and although homologous to the rat nucleotide sequence, it contains a sixth copy of the TRH coding sequence at its C-terminal end. The rat TRH transcriptional unit extends 2.6 kilobases (kb) and includes three exons interrupted by two introns. Exon 1 encodes the 5'-untranslated region of the mRNA, exon 2 encodes the signal sequence and the majority of the amino-terminal peptide, and exon 3 encodes the remainder of the translated sequence of proTRH.

The development of specific antisera against proTRH, extended forms of TRH, and a number of the non-TRH proTRH-derived sequences has allowed new insight into the organization of TRH neuronal systems in the brain and processing of its prohormone. In contrast to TRH, these peptides are less water soluble and appear to retain their antigenicity with conventional fixatives (Lechan et al., 1986a, 1987). Immunoreactive intact or partially processed proTRH is confined to the Golgi apparatus and to immature secretory granules, giving the appearance of packets, closely juxtaposed to the nucleus and leaving the rest of the cytoplasm and axonal processes devoid of immunoreactivity (Jackson et al., 1985; Lechan et al., 1986a) (Figure 4A and B). This contrasts to the appearance of immunoreactive TRH, which is associated with mature, dense-core vesicles and fills perikarya and processes (Figures 5 and

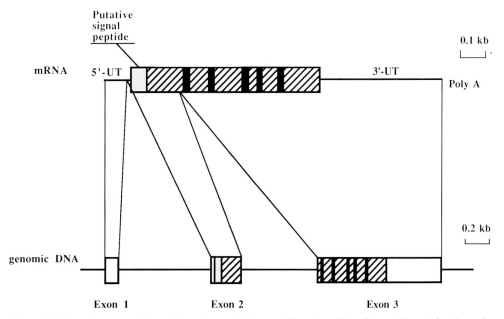

Figure 3. Schematic representation of the rat preproTRH gene. (From Lee, S. L., Stewart, K., and Goodman, R. H., *J. Biol. Chem.*, 263, 16604, 1988. With permission.)

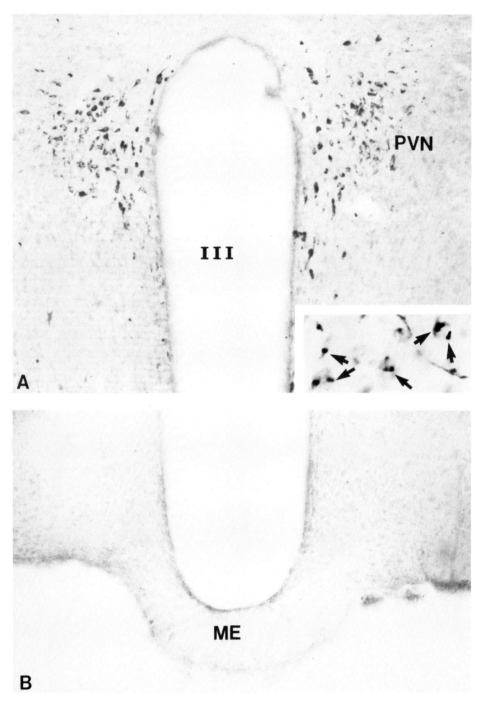

Figure 4. (A) Immunolocalization of proTRH in neuronal perikarya of the hypothalamic paraventricular nucleus (PVN). Peroxidase-positive material is restricted to a subcompartment in the cytoplasm, closely juxtaposed to the nucleus (arrows in inset). (B) No immunoreaction product is present in the median eminence (ME). III, Third ventricle.

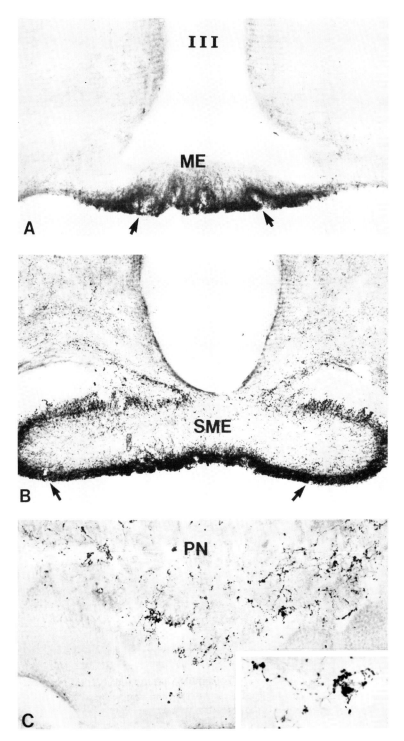

Figure 5. Coronal sections through the (A) median eminence (ME) and (B) stalk median eminence (SME), showing the presence of TRH immunoreactivity in the external zone in close association with portal capillaries (arrowheads). (C) Some fibers extend distally to innervate the posterior pituitary (PN) Branching axons terminate in characteristic grapelike swellings (inset). III, Third ventricle.

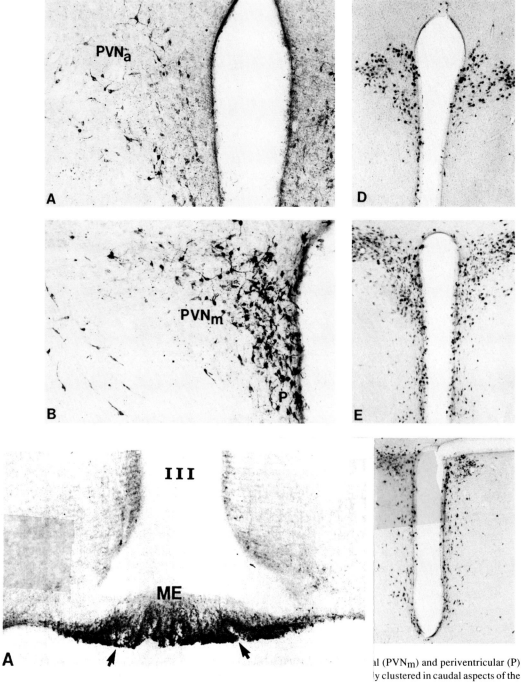

al (PVN_m) and periventricular (P)
ly clustered in caudal aspects of the
PVN_m. (D to F) Distribution of neurons accumulating the retrogradely transported marker substance, wheat germ agglutinin, after injection into the median eminence. Note similarities in distribution when compared to TRH.

6) (Johansson et al., 1980; Liposits et al., 1987). These observations indicate that proTRH is rarely transported in axons and that initial processing occurs rapidly in neuronal perikarya rather than during axonal transport as described for propressophysin, the precursor to vasopressin (Gainer et al., 1977).

II. TRH Neuronal Systems

A.   Anatomy of the TRH-Hypothalamic Tuberoinfundibular System

As anticipated for a hypothalamic releasing hormone involved in the regulation of anterior pituitary thyroid-stimulating hormone (TSH) and prolactin secretion, TRH is present in great abundance in axons terminating in the median eminence (Choy and Watkins, 1977; Hökfelt et al., 1975; Lechan et al., 1983a; Lechan and Jackson, 1982), the neural-hemal contact zone of the tuberoinfundibular system. Immunoreactive axon terminals are found primarily in the midregion of the external zone throughout the rostral-caudal extent of the median eminence and in close apposition to the portal capillary system (Figure 5A and B). Some axons extend further distally to terminate in the posterior pituitary in a characteristic grape-like cluster of immunoreactive material (Figure 5C). This potentially provides an alternative route by which TRH can regulate anterior pituitary secretion through vascular channels that connect the two structures (Porter et al., 1978).

Neuronal perikarya that give rise to TRH axon terminals in the median eminence originate in the hypothalamic paraventricular nucleus, a region contained within the classic "thyrotropic" area described by Greer (1952). The paraventricular nucleus is composed of two major components, including magnocellular and parvocellular divisions. The magnocellular division can be further divided into at least three subdivisions and the parvocellular division into five subdivisions (Swanson and Kuypers, 1980). TRH-containing neurons are located exclusively within small to medium-sized cells in the parvocellular division, primarily in anterior, medial, and periventricular subdivisions (Figure 6A to C). The densest populations of immunopositive neurons are located in medial and periventricular parvocellular subdivisions, organized in a triangular configuration, symmetric to the dorsal aspect of the third ventricle (Figure 6B and C), whereas the anterior parvocellular subdivision neurons are more dispersed (Figure 6A). This distribution is highly reminiscent of the organization of tuberoinfundibular neurons in the paraventricular nucleus, visualized after the injection of retrogradely transported marker substances into the median eminence (Lechan et al., 1980, 1982; Weigand and Price, 1980) (Figure 6D to F).

Not all TRH-containing neurons in the paraventricular nucleus project to the median eminence. After injection of horseradish peroxidase (HRP) into the median eminence, Ishikawa et al. (1988a) identified doubly-labeled cells (TRH and HRP) in medial and periventricular subdivision neurons. Fewer doubly-labeled cells in the anterior parvocellular subdivision would indicate that they are not part of the TRH-tuberoinfundibular system, although technical difficulties cannot be excluded. The medial and periventricular TRH-parvocellular subdivisions appear functionally diverse from anterior TRH-parvocellular neurons, however, as suggested by the striking differences in the concentration of proTRH mRNA in these cell groups (Segerson et al., 1987a) and the selective increase in proTRH mRNA exclusively in medial and periventricular subdivisions in hypothyroid animals (Segerson et al., 1987b) (Figure 7A to D). Similar conclusions have been reached by Nishiyama et al. (1985) on the basis of morphologic studies in hypothyroid animals.

Although many neurons in the PVN have been shown to contain more than one peptide, TRH-containing neurons are unique in being almost always unassociated with any other known coexistant peptide (Ceccatelli et al., 1989). Only rare cells have been noted to co-contain corticotropin-releasing factor and neurotensin. Earlier reports from our laboratory of the coexistence of a growth hormone-like material in TRH neurons (Lechan et al., 1983) were due to the recognition of an epitope in human growth hormone that is homologous with a portion of the TRH prohormone, as hypothesized in our original studies. Similarly, the report of the coexistence of proctolin in these neurons is most likely due to the presence of a cross-reacting material and not the authentic pentapeptide (Holets et al., 1987; Hökfelt et al., 1989). In the bullfrog, however, TRH coexists with mesotocin in axon terminals in the pars nervosa (Shioda et al., 1989). Outside the hypothalamus, TRH is colocalized with substance P and serotonin (see later).

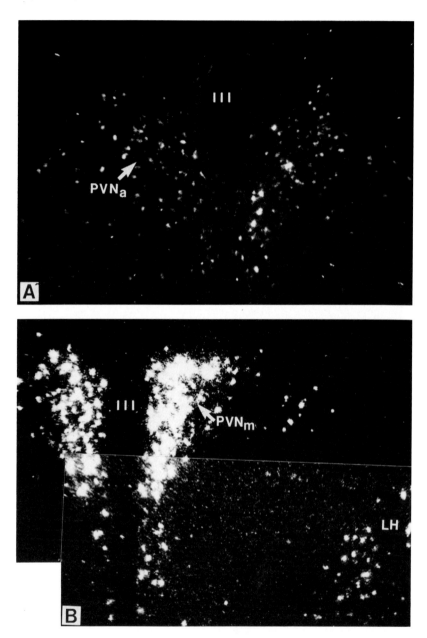

Figure 7. *In situ* hybridization autoradiogram (^{32}P labeled) of proTRH mRNA in the (A) anterior and (B) medial and periventricular parvocellular subdivisions of the paraventricular nucleus (dark-field microscopy). High-power bright-field micrographs of (C) hybridized anterior parvocellular subdivision neurons show fewer silver grains accumulating over neurons when compared to (D) medial parvocellular neurons. LH, Lateral hypothalamus; III, third ventricle.

Projections from TRH-producing neuronal perikarya in the paraventricular nucleus to the median eminence proceed primarily through the lateral retrochiasmatic area (Palkovits et al., 1982) after extending laterally from paraventricular nucleus (PVN) neurons dorsal to the fornix and arching toward the medial basal hypothalamus (Figure 8A). It is likely, therefore, that earlier studies recognizing a marked reduction of TRH in the hypothalamus after complete hypothalamic deafferentation with Halasz knife cuts (Brownstein et al., 1975), was due to transection of these descending fibers and not due to neurons originating outside the hypotha-

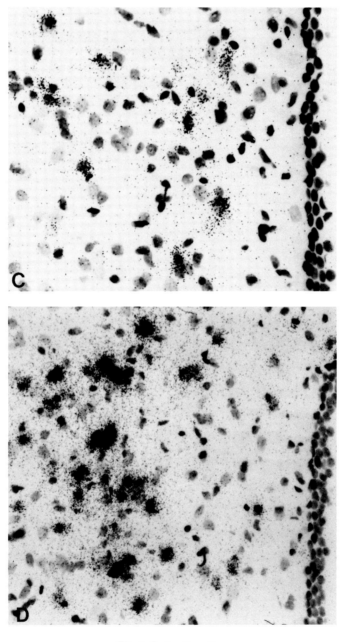

Figure 7. (continued).

lamic islands. Axons from TRH neurons also descend along the wall of the third ventricle in the subependymal neuropil to the medial eminence (Nishiyama et al., 1985) but these contribute only minimally to the total TRH-tuberoinfundibular input (Palkovits et al., 1982). Some fibers may also enter the stria terminalis and ascend to innervate midline thalamic groups (Figure 8B).

B.   Regulation of TRH-Tuberoinfundibular Neurons by Thyroid Hormone

TRH-synthesis in neurons of the medial and periventricular parvocellular subdivisions of the PVN is regulated by thyroid hormone (Segerson et al., 1987; Dyess et al., 1988). Hypothyroidism, induced surgically by thyroidectomy or by the oral administration of thioamines, causes an increase in the concentration of proTRH mRNA extracted from a micropunch of the paraventricular nucleus (Figure 9A and B). After 3 weeks of hypothyroidism, proTRH mRNA increases from approximately 469 attomoles (amol) ±85 SEM in euthyroid animals to 914 amol ±126 SEM in the hypothyroid animals (Segerson et al., 1987b). This response follows the fall in serum L-thyroxine (T_4) to undetectable levels and parallels a gradual rise in serum TSH (Figure 9C). Changes in proTRH mRNA are not mediated by TSH; proTRH mRNA is increased in animals made hypothyroid by hypophysectomy, a preparation in which the plasma TSH is undetectable (Lechan and Segerson, 1989). Similar conclusions have been reached by Zoeller et al. (1988). Conversely, the administration of pharmacologic doses of T_4 inhibits the hypothyroid-induced rise in proTRH mRNA (Segerson et al., 1987b; Koller et al., 1987), while supraphysiological levels cause an even further decline below euthyroid levels, establishing an inverse relationship between circulating thyroid hormone and paraventricular nucleus proTRH mRNA concentrations. This effect is sharply limited to TRH-containing neurons in the medial and periventricular PVN and not anterior parvocellular neurons or TRH-containing neurons in

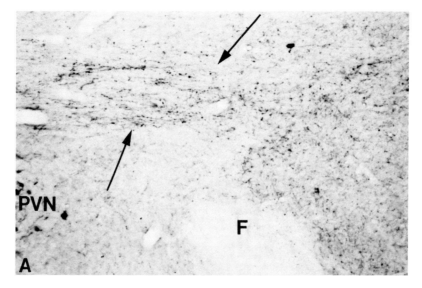

Figure 8. (A) Axonal projections (arrows) of TRH-synthesizing, medial parvocellular neurons of the paraventricular nucleus (PVN) *en route* to the median eminence. (B) Other fibers ascend in the thalamus to enter the (C) stria terminalis (arrows). BNST, bed nucleus of the stria terminalis; F, fornix; III, third ventricle.

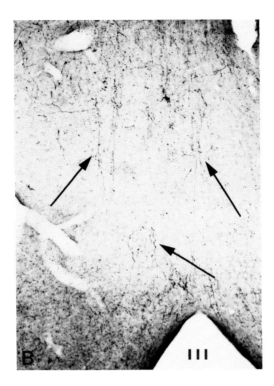

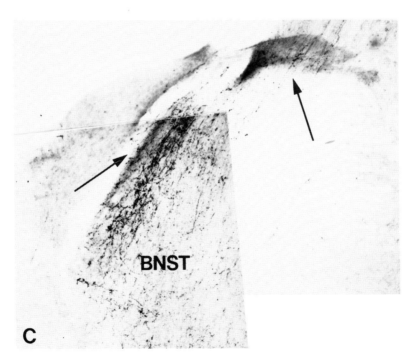

Figure 8. (continued).

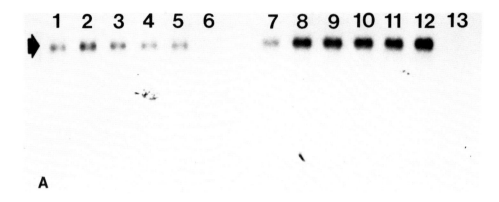

A

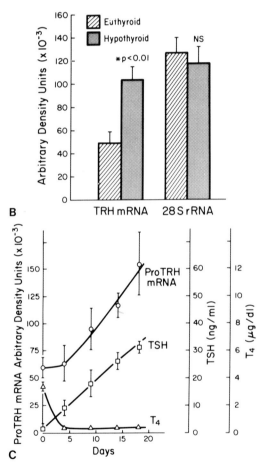

B

C

Figure 9. (A) Northern blot of proTRH mRNA from euthyroid (lanes 1 to 6) and hypothyroid (lanes 7 to 13) rats, extracted from the paraventricular nucleus. A hybridizing band of approximately 1.6 kb (arrowhead) is present in paraventricular nucleus extracts (lanes 1 to 5, 7 to 12) but not in cerebral cortex extracts (lanes 6 and 13). (B) Graphic representation of hybridized bands above as analyzed by computer densitometry. A significant increase in proTRH mRNA occurs in hypothyroid animals. Normalization of RNA samples is confirmed by the absence of a significant difference in ribosomal RNA in the two groups of extracts. (C) Effect of hypothyroidism on serum T_4, TSH, and paraventricular nucleus proTRH mRNA. T_4 falls rapidly after thioamide treatment, followed by a gradual rise in both serum TSH and proTRH mRNA.

other regions of the diencephalon (Figure 10). Since the immunocytochemical staining characteristics also change in parallel with the content of proTRH mRNA (Segerson et al., 1987b), we have proposed that thyroid hormone controls both transcription and translation of the TRH prohormone in the paraventricular nucleus. As the set point for TSH secretion is determined by TRH (Martin et al.,1970; Kaplan et al., 1986), the normal set point for TSH secretion may be dynamically regulated by the effects of thyroid hormone on the transcription of proTRH mRNA in the paraventricular nucleus.

The central regulation of proTRH mRNA in paraventricular nucleus neurons by thyroid

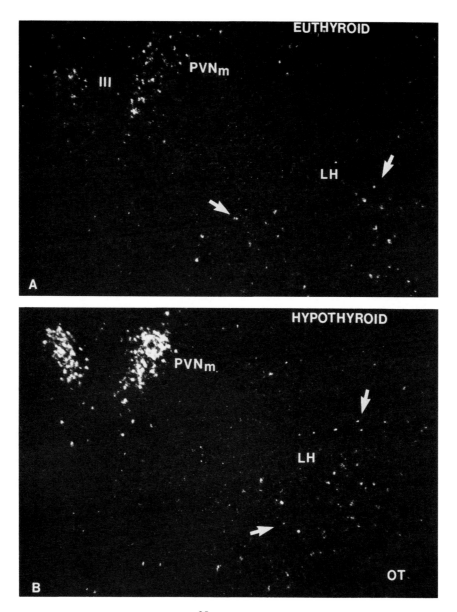

Figure 10. *In situ* hybridization autoradiogram (^{35}S labeled, dark-field illumination) of paraventricular nucleus proTRH mRNA (medial parvocellular subdivision, PVN$_m$) in (A) euthyroid and (B) hypothyroid animals. A marked increase in silver grain accumulation over neurons in the hypothyroid animal is seen. No change in hybridization density occurs over TRH neurons in the lateral hypothalamus (LH; arrows).

hormone appears to be mediated by direct effects rather than by long tract afferent input to these neurons (Dyess et al., 1988). Stereotaxic placement of crystalline triiodothyronine (T_3), but not the relatively inactive diiodothyronine (T_2) into hypothyroid animals adjacent to one side of the paraventricular nucleus, causes marked suppression of the content of proTRH mRNA on that side (Figure 11). Since the paraventricular nucleus lacks the enzyme that converts T_4 to its active metabolite, T_3 (type II deiodinase; Riskind et al., 1987), it would appear that feedback regulation of TRH gene expression is mediated by T_3 rather than by intracellular conversion of T_4 to T_3.

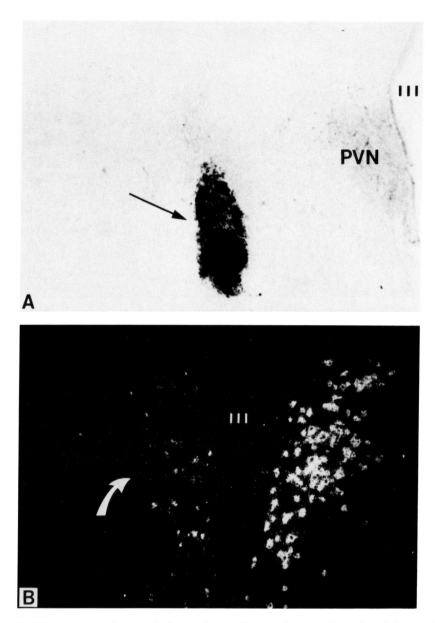

Figure 11. (A) Appearance of stereotaxically placed crystalline material (arrow) in the hypothalamus, adjacent to one side of the paraventricular nucleus (PVN). (B) Marked diminution of proTRH mRNA in paraventricular neurons on the same side of an implant of T_3 (curved arrow, *in situ* hybridization histochemistry, dark-field illumination). No reduction is seen in neurons on the opposite side or (C) after unilateral implants of the relatively inactive T_2. III, Third ventricle.

C.   Regulation of TRH-Tuberoinfundibular Neurons by Afferent Input

TRH-containing neurons in the PVN are in a strategic position to be regulated by a number of neuroendocrine factors. The nucleus is crowded with neurons producing numerous neuropeptides adjacent to TRH cells and the PVN receives rich afferent inputs from other regions of the diencephalon, the telencephalon, and brainstem (Ricardo and Koh, 1978; Saper and Loewy, 1980; Tribollet and Dreifuss, 1981; Sawchenko and Swanson, 1982, 1983; Cunningham

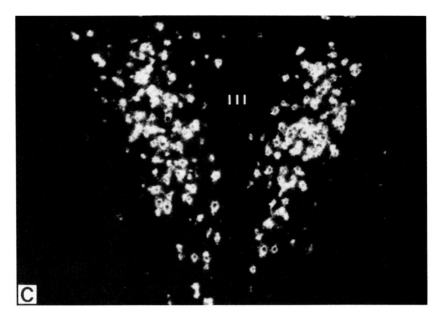

Figure 11. (continued).

and Sawchenko, 1988). The origin and content of axons in presynaptic contact with TRH-synthesizing neurons in the paraventricular nucleus are under intense study with catecholamines, neuropeptide Y, and TRH already having been described (see below).

1.   Catecholamines

Recent studies by Shioda et al. (1986) and Liposits et al. (1987) have provided morphologic evidence for the presence of catecholaminergic axons in synaptic association with TRH neurons in the PVN. Using antiserum to the catecholamine-synthesizing enzymes, dopamine β-hydroxylase (DBH) and phenylethanolamine N-methyltransferase (PNMT) as markers for norepinephrine- and epinephrine-containing axons, respectively, the paraventricular nucleus can be seen to receive a dense innervation in medial and parvocellular subdivisions (Figure 12A and B). Some of these axon terminals make multiple contacts with both cell bodies and dendrites of TRH-producing neurons (Figure 12B). On the basis of tract tracing and immuno-cytochemical studies of noradrenergic inputs to the PVN (Sawchenko and Swanson, 1982; Cunningham and Sawchenko, 1988), hypophysiotropic TRH neurons appear to be innervated by ascending catecholamine projections mainly of medullary origin. In confirmation of the anatomical findings, discrete electrical stimulation of brainstem A_1 and A_2 noradrenergic cell groups is capable of activating antidromically identified tuberoinfundibular neurons of the PVN (Day et al., 1985).

The role of epinephrine and norepinephrine in TRH secretion is likely stimulatory. Numerous studies, including the early work of Annunziato et al. (1977), Krulich et al. (1977), and Montoya et al. (1979), suggest that catecholamine antagonists inhibit TSH secretion and agonists increase TSH secretion through an α-adrenergic mechanism and that norepinephrine can stimulate TRH release in culture (Hirooka et al., 1978). Using quantitative microfluorimetry to measure catecholamine levels and utilization in the PVN and median eminence, Andersson and Enroth (1987) have confirmed this view, but also proposed an inhibitory role for dopamine, probably by influencing the secretion of TRH-containing axon terminals in the median eminence. In contrast, attempts to elucidate a specific role for serotonin in the regulation of

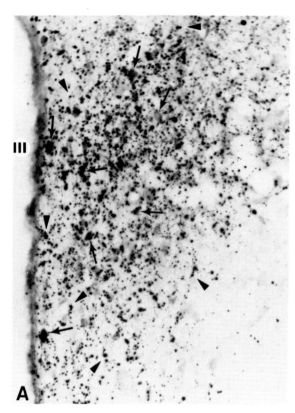

Figure 12. (A) Association of catecholaminergic fibers (PNMT immunoreactive) with TRH neurons (arrows) in the paraventricular nucleus. Note numerous terminals in medial and periventricular parvocellular subdivisions. (B) Innervation of a TRH-containing neuron in the paraventricular nucleus by catecholaminergic axon terminals (arrows). Contacts are present both on the cell body (asterisk) and dendrites (arrowhead). III, Third ventricle. (From Liposits, Zs., Paull, W. K., Wu, P., Jackson, I. M. D., and Lechan, R. M., *Histochemistry,* 88, 1, 1987. With permission.)

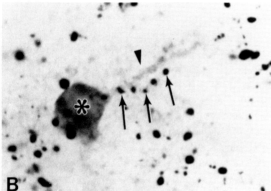

tuberoinfundibular TRH have been controversial as both stimulatory and inhibitory effects on TSH secretion have been seen (Krulich, 1982).

2. Neuropeptide Y

Other than the catecholamines, several neuropeptides may regulate the biosynthesis and/or secretion of hypophysiotropic TRH. Neuropeptide Y (NPY) (Tatemoto et al., 1982) is present in axon terminals that heavily innervate the PVN (Gray and Morley, 1986) and has been shown to induce a fall in serum TSH levels after central administration (Harfstrand, 1987).

NPY fibers appear to innervate TRH-containing neurons in all subdivisions of the PVN,

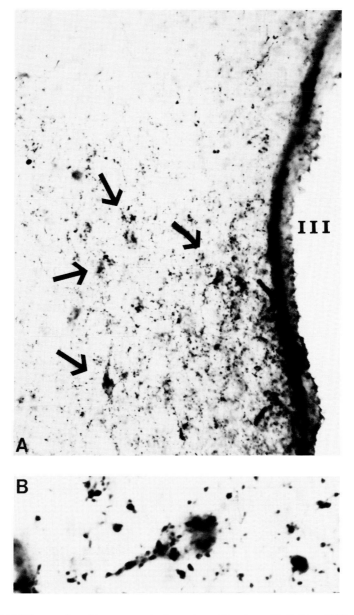

Figure 13. (A) NPY innervation of the paraventricular nucleus (silver intensified). Many NPY-containing axon terminals are in close proximity to TRH-containing neurons (arrows). This is clearly seen under high magnification in (B). (C) A synaptic association between NPY-containing axon terminals (arrows) and TRH-containing neuronal perikarya is established by double-labeling, ultrastructural immunocytochemistry. III, third ventricle.

contacting both perikarya and dendrites (Figure 13A). Some cells are inundated with NPY-immunopositive boutons, receiving multiple contacts on the cell surface (Figure 13B) (Toni et al., 1990a). Not all contacts show typical synaptic specializations (Figure 13C), however, with many NPY-containing axon terminals seen only in close juxtaposition to the perikaryal membrane of TRH cells. Whether the latter type of association is functional in the PVN is unknown but similar types of interactions have been observed in the median eminence where they may regulate neuropeptide and/or transmitter release into the portal capillary system (Buma, 1989).

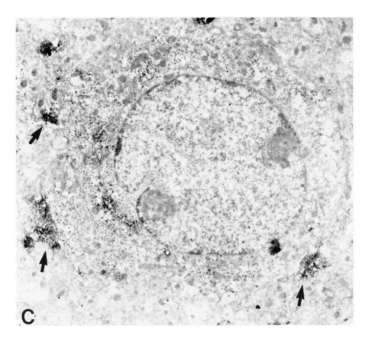

Figure 13. (continued).

As many of the NPY-containing axon terminals in the PVN co-contain catecholamines and originate from catecholamine-producing neurons in the lower brainstem (Sawchenko et al., 1985), it is intriguing to speculate that NPY may modulate (inhibit) the facilitory adrenergic and noradrenergic influences on TRH-synthesizing neurons. This would be in keeping with recent observations that NPY can reduce catecholaminergic outflow in the hypothalamus (Ciarleglio et al., 1988). Not all NPY-immunoreactive fibers in the PVN derive from catecholamine-containing brainstem neurons, however, as demonstrated by a marked reduction in the concentration of NPY in the PVN after pharmacologic ablation of the arcuate nucleus (Kerkerian and Pelletier, 1986). This suggests a greater complexity to NPY regulation of TRH PVN neurons that will require further elucidation.

3.   TRH

The availability of antisera that recognize cryptic portions of proTRH has provided new anatomical tools to study the possibility of ultrashort feedback regulation by TRH of its own secretion. As opposed to antiserum to TRH, these immunocytochemical probes readily identify TRH-synthesizing neuronal perikarya in normal animals, allowing for rich anatomical detail of TRH axons in the PVN, unimpeded by reagents, such as colchicine, that inhibit axonal transport. Using this approach and a novel immunocytochemical method providing rich anatomical detail of peptide-containing neuronal systems (Toni and Lechon, 1990b), immunoreactive boutons are found in close proximity to TRH-synthesizing neurons in the PVN (Figure 14A) (Toni et al., 1990c). At the ultrastructural level, axodendritic and axosomatic TRH-TRH synaptic interactions were recognized (Figure 14B). Synaptic interactions have also been described for neurons containing luteinizing hormone-releasing hormone (LHRH) (Leranth et al., 1985; Pelletier, 1987) and somatostatin (Epelbaum et al., 1986)-containing neurons and may serve to regulate their own set point for secretion (Richardson and Twente, 1986; Zanisi et al., 1987). Alternatively, TRH-synthesizing neurons may receive projections from TRH-synthesizing neurons outside the PVN and utilize TRH, processed forms of

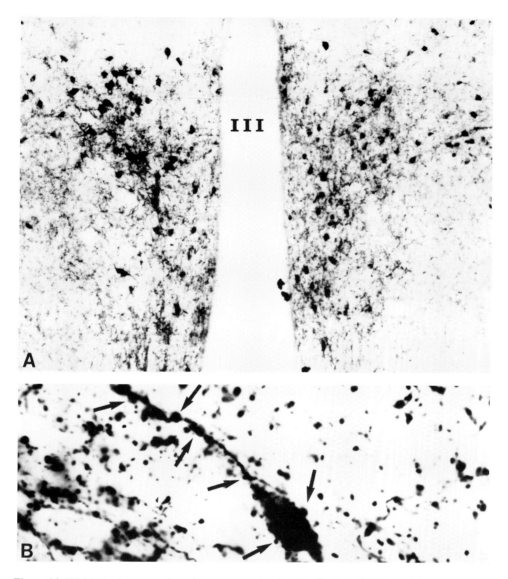

Figure 14. (A) Light microscope view of immunocytochemical distribution of TRH-containing perikarya and fibers in the hypothalamic paraventricular nucleus (silver intensified), using antiserum recognizing the N-terminal-flanking peptide of proTRH. (B) Close apposition of immunopositive TRH boutons and fibers (arrows) to TRH-immunopositive cell body is shown. (C) Electron micrograph labeled with immunogold showing contacts between TRH-containing axon terminal (A) and TRH-containing perikarya (P).

proTRH, or coexistent peptides or neurotransmitters to influence the secretion of hypophysiotropic TRH.

4.   Other

A preliminary report by Toni et al. (1989) has suggested that somatostatin-containing axon terminals innervate some TRH-producing neurons in the PVN, consistent with the observations by Hirooka et al. (1978) that somatostatin inhibits TRH secretion from isolated hypothalamic fragments. In addition, a number of reports have implicated other neurotransmitters and peptides in the regulation of TRH secretion but tend to be contradictory, and no anatomic

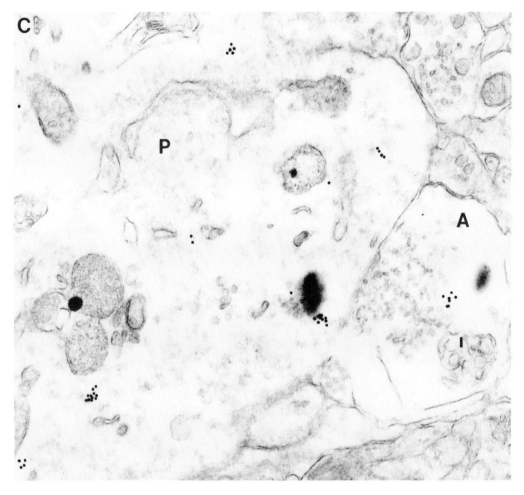

Figure 14. (continued).

evidence to substantiate a true physiologic role is yet available. Histamine was demonstrated by Joseph-Braveo et al. (1979) to stimulate TRH release from hypothalamic explants but Mitsuma et al. (1979) found inhibition of TRH release. γ-Aminobutyric acid (GABA) (Vijayan and McCann, 1979; Roussel et al., 1988), oxytocin (Frawley et al., 1985), vasopressin (Lumpkin et al., 1983), substance P (Vijayan and McCann, 1980), and cholecystokinin (Vijayan et al., 1979) have all been shown to influence TSH secretion but their effects may be primarily directly on the anterior pituitary or other neuromodulators of TSH secretion such as somatostatin and dopamine. TRH-containing neurons also reside in a region inundated with axon terminals containing galanin (Melander et al., 1986; Levin et al., 1987), adrenocortico-tropic hormone (ACTH) (Pelletier and Leclerc, 1979), and cortocotropin-releasing factor (Merchenthaler et al., 1982) but their potential effects on TRH secretion are unknown. The presence of an endogenous, neuronal cytokine system in the mammalian hypothalamus (Breder et al., 1988; Lechan et al., 1990) has raised the possibility that interleukin-1 (IL-1) may also be involved in the regulation of hypophysiotropic TRH. This is suggested by early findings by Kasting and Martin (1982) that bacterial endotoxin suppresses plasma concentrations of TSH and that the systemic administration of IL-1 β causes a rapid decline in thyroid function and fall in TSH. Furthermore, preliminary studies by Lee et al. (personal communication) have shown that the addition of IL-1 β to dispersed cultures of hypothalamic neurons is associated with a reduction in TRH mRNA.

D.   Other Hypothalamic TRH Neuronal Systems

In addition to the paraventricular nucleus, TRH-containing neurons are present in many other regions of the hypothalamus (Table 1). This was anticipated from the presence of radioimmunoassayable TRH in microdissected nuclei of the hypothalamus (Brownstein et al., 1974) and has now been verified by several immunocytochemical studies (Hökfelt et al., 1979; Johansson et al., 1980; Lechan and Jackson, 1982; Lechan et al., 1983a, 1987; Jackson et al., 1985; Tsuruo et al., 1987; Merchenthaler et al., 1988, 1989). As these populations of neurons have no known projections to the median eminence (Lechan et al., 1980, 1982; Weigand and Price, 1980), it is presumed that they do not subserve a direct hypophysiotropic function.

The largest concentrations of TRH-containing neurons outside of the PVN are found in the dorsomedial nucleus, lateral hypothalamus, and preoptic areas (Figure 15A to D), including medial, periventricular, suprachiasmatic nuclei, and the sexual dimorphic nucleus of the preoptic area. Smaller collections of neurons encircle the fornix and arch through the anterior and lateral hypothalamus and can be found in posterior portions of the arcuate nucleus (Figure 15E). Occasional cells are also found in the supraoptic nuclei, posterior hypothalamus, and premammillary nuclei (Lechan et al., 1987). Although TRH-containing neurons outside of the PVN comprise a very substantial portion of hypothalamic TRH and are well characterized anatomically, very little is known of their afferent or efferent projections and physiological significance.

1.   Hypothalamic-Septal Connections

Ishikawa et al. 1986 have indicated that TRH neurons in the lateral hypothalamus, perifornical group, and lateral preoptic area project to the lateral septum, a region heavily inundated with TRH-containing axon terminals. Numerous unlabeled somata in the intermediate and ventral portions of the lateral septal nucleus are outlined by punctate densities, suggesting a synaptic relationship between TRH-containing axon terminals and septal neurons (Figure 16). As injections of HRP into the lateral septum will also retrogradely label cells in the suprachiasmatic subdivision of the preoptic area, bed nucleus of the stria terminalis, and anterior commissural nucleus (Ishikawa et al., 1986), regions that also contain TRH-synthesizing neurons (Lechan et al., 1986a, 1987), it is possible that these neurons also contribute to septal TRH. This would be consistant with general observations by Simerly and Swanson (1988) that neurons in the medial preoptic nucleus have massive projections to the ventral part of the lateral septal nucleus.

The significance of the TRH hypothalamic-septal projection system may be seen in light of reports that one of the most sensitive sites for the analeptic effects of TRH is the septum (Kalivas and Horita, 1980). The reduction of pentobarbital-induced sleeping time or ethanol-induced narcosis by TRH or TRH analogs (Breese et al., 1975; Cott et al., 1976; Yamamoto and Shimizu, 1989), however, may not be a direct effect of TRH but rather mediated through acetylcholine. Atropine completely blocks the analeptic actions of TRH (Breese et al., 1975; Nagai et al., 1980) and carbachol is able to excite most of the same septohippocampal neurons excited by TRH (Lamour et al., 1985). Indeed, evidence for the interaction of TRH with cholinergic neurons has been shown in several loci in the CNS (Yarborough, 1983), indicating that this may be a common mechanism by which the behavorial effects of TRH are mediated. This view is not universally accepted, however, as other studies have proposed that the

Table 1
TRH Distribution in the CNS

	Perikarya	Fibers
Diencephalon		
Anterior hypothalamus	+	+
Arcuate nucleus	+	+
Dorsomedial nucleus	+	+
Lateral habenula		+
Lateral hypothalamus	+	+
Median eminence		+
Medial nucleus, thalamus	+	
OVLT		+
Paratenial nucleus, thalamus		+
Paraventricular nucleus, hypothalamus	+	+
Paraventricular nucleus, thalamus		+
Perifornical region	+	
Premammillary nuclei		+
Preoptic area	+	+
Reticular nucleus, thalamus		+
Subfornical organ		+
Supraoptic nucleus	+	
Ventromedial nucleus		+
Telencephalon		
Anterior olfactory nucleus	+	
Accessory olfactory bulb		+
Bed nucleus, anterior commissure	+	
Bed nucleus, stria terminalis	+	+
Caudate-putamen	+	+
Central and medial nuclei, amygdala	+	+
Diagonal band of B roca	+	+
Entorhinal cortex	+	
External plexiform layer, olfactory bulb	+	
Glomerular layer, olfactory bulb	+	+
Hilus, dentate gyrus	+	
Hippocampal pyramidal layer (CA2/CA3)	+	
Internal plexiform layer, olfactory bulb	+	
Medial and lateral septum		+
Nucleus accumbens		+
Pyriform cortex	+	
Stratum oriens, hippocampus		+
Mesencephalon and metencephalon		
Locus coeruleus		+
Motor nucleus V		+
Oculomotor nucleus		+
Parabrachial nuclei		+
Periaqueductal gray	+	+
Pontine nuclei	+	
Red nuclei		+
Substantia nigra, pars lateralis	+	
Trochlear nucleus		+
Myelencephalon		
Cochlear nucleus	+	
Dorsal motor nucleus, vagus	+	+
External cuneate nucleus	+	
Facial nucleus		+

Table 1 (continued)

	Perikarya	Fibers
Hypoglossal nucleus		+
Inferior olive		+
Lateral reticular nucleus	+	
Nucleus ambiguus		+
Nucleus tractus solitarius		+
Raphe nuclei	+	+
Reticular formation		+
Spinal cord		
Anterior funiculus		+
Central canal		+
Dorsal horn (laminae II and III)	+	+
Intermediolateral column		+
Lateral funiculus		+
Ventral horn (lamina IX)		+

excitatory behaviors induced by TRH may be mediated by enhancing the release of dopamine (Miyamoto and Nagawa, 1977; Hirooka et al., 1978; Joseph-Bravo et al., 1979; Maeda and Frohman, 1980). The likelihood that analeptic effects of TRH can occur at several loci in addition to the septum, including the caudate putamen (Heal and Green, 1979; Nagai et al., 1980) and hypothalamic ventromedial nucleus (Lin et al., 1987), may explain these findings.

2. Role of Medial Preoptic Nucleus TRH in Temperature Regulation

In addition to the contribution of TRH-containing preoptic neurons to the septum to mediate some of the analeptic actions of TRH, it is likely that other preoptic neurons are involved in thermoregulation. TRH attenuates the hypothermic effects of pentobarbital, ethanol, and several peptides (Breese et al., 1975; Prange et al., 1975; Bissete et al., 1976; Brown et al., 1977) and induces a rise in body temperature after central administration (Boschi and Rips, 1981), particularly when injected into the preoptic region. In addition, microiontophoretic injection of TRH into the preoptic area decreases the activity of warm-sensitive neurons (that normally elicit heat loss responses) and increases the activity of cold-sensitive neurons (that normally elicit heat retention responses) (Hori et al., 1988), providing evidence for direct, local effects of the tripeptide.

The role of TRH in heat generation, however, appears to be far more diverse than actions exclusively on the preoptic nucleus and may involve the coordinated activity of several central TRH systems in different regions of the brain. The administration of TRH to animals with lesions in the preoptic area still shows antagonism to the hypothermic effects of pentobarbital (Ishikawa and Suzuki, 1986), suggesting a second locus for the thermogenic effects of TRH. In addition, in some animal species, acute cold exposure induces thyroid thermogenesis by stimulating the secretion of TSH from the anterior pituitary (Krulich, 1982). This is presumably due to activation of the hypothalamic TRH-tuberoinfundibular system, originating in the paraventricular nucleus (see above), to increase the secretion of TRH.

Since yohimbine, phentolamine, and propranolol can reduce the hypothermic response of TRH (Chi and Lin, 1983) and the hypophysiotropic response to cold exposure is dependent on the central noradrenergic system (Krulich, 1982), catecholamines appear to be important mediators of this response. Studies by Lin et al. (1989) have also shown that the injection of pyrogen into the hypothalamus is associated with an elevation of hypothalamic TRH, raising the possibility that thermogenic TRH neurons in the preoptic nucleus could be regulated by cytokines.

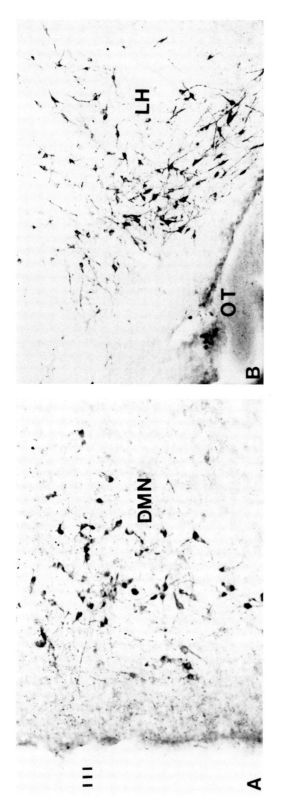

Figure 15. Immunoreactive TRH in the (A) dorsomedial nucleus (DMN), (B) lateral hypothalamus (LH), (C) preoptic nucleus (PON), (D) sexual dimorphic nucleus (arrow), and (E) arcuate nucleus (ARC). IR, Infundibular recess; OC, optic chiasm; OT, optic tract; SR, supraoptic recess; III, third ventricle.

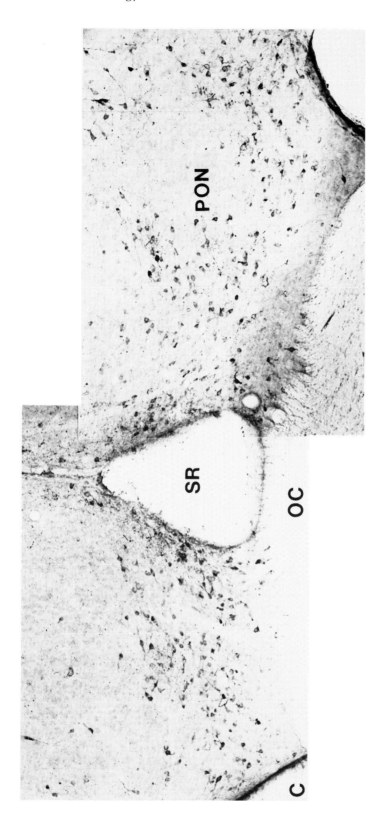

Figure 15. (continued).

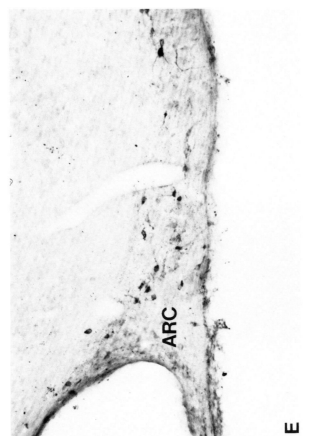

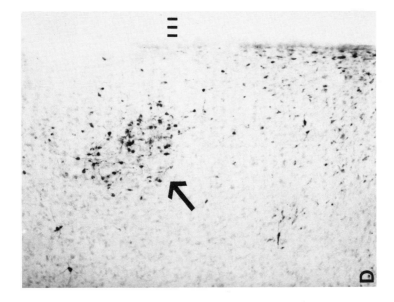

Figure 15. (continued).

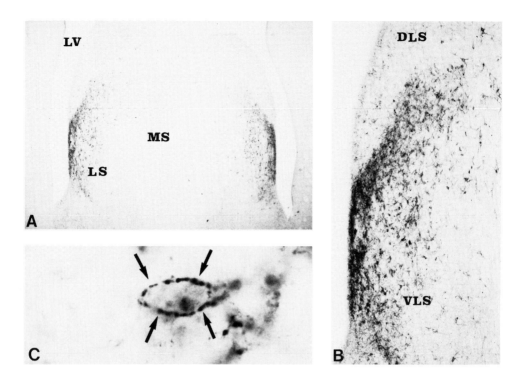

Figure 16. (A) Distribution of TRH-containing axon terminals in the lateral septum (LS). (B) Fibers terminate primarily in ventral portions of the lateral septum (VLS) and are often seen to (C) envelop nonreactive neuronal perikarya (arrows). LV, lateral ventricle; DLS, dorsal portions of lateral septum; MS, medial septum.

E.   Thalamus

Of the several brain areas in which proTRH mRNA is present, the thalamus is unique in that no TRH perikarya have been identified in any region. Intense hybridization to TRH mRNA is present in the reticular nucleus of the thalamus by *in situ* hybridization histochemistry (Segerson et al., 1987a), however, accentuating its characteristic crescent shape (Figure 17). As these neurons also immunostain with antiserum to the TRH prohormone (Lechan et al., 1986, 1987; Merchanthaler et al., 1988), and N terminal-flanking peptides of proTRH (Lechan et al., 1987), we have proposed that proTRH may be processed differently to components other than TRH in this nucleus, compared to other regions of the diencephalon. As the reticular nucleus exerts an inhibitory effect on sensory input delivered to the dorsal thalamus from somatic sensory receptive fields in the periphery, *en route* to the cortex (Yen et al., 1985), it is conceivable that N-terminal peptides of proTRH may act as one of its peptide mediators. Since the majority of reticular nucleus neurons also contain GABA and somatostatin (Houser et al., 1980; Oertel et al., 1983), proTRH-derived peptides could also be involved in an intricate, intrinsic, neuroregulatory system involving several substances.

III. Telencephalon

A.   Olfactory System

The presence of large quantities of immunoreactive TRH in the olfactory lobes was

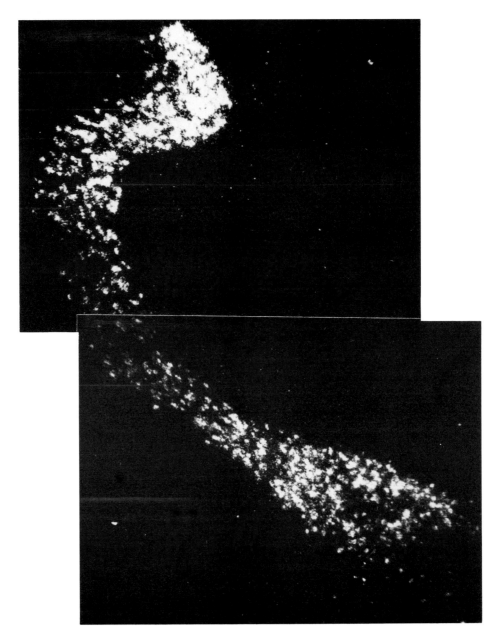

Figure 17. *In situ* hybridization histochemistry of proTRH mRNA in the reticular nucleus of the thalamus (dark-field microscopy).

recognized by Krieder et al. (1981) nearly a decade ago but the distribution of TRH-immuno-reactive elements in this structure has only recently been elucidated. Most (if not all) of olfactory lobe TRH appears to arise exclusively from neurons intrinsic to the olfactory lobes, as deafferentation of the bulbs is not followed by any reduction in TRH content (Krieder et al., 1982). Similarly, bulbectomy causes little reduction in TRH receptors in the bulb whereas injection of kaininc acid into the bulb results in a marked reduction in TRH receptor-binding capacity (Sharif, 1988). These data indicate that TRH is synthesized locally in the olfactory

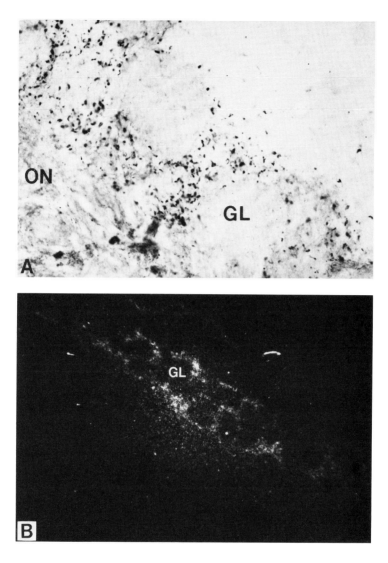

Figure 18. (A) Immunoperoxidase staining of proTRH and (B) *in situ* hybridization histochemistry of proTRH mRNA in the olfactory lobes. Note labeled cells in the glomerular (GL) layer. ON, Olfactory nerve layer.

bulb for local use in neurons largely intrinsic to the bulb. Since a 35% reduction in TRH receptors in the bulb is also achieved by local injection of 6-hydroxydopamine, Sharif (1988) has proposed that TRH may also have an effect in modulating the release of dopaminergic or noradrenergic neurons in this structure.

Immunoreactive neurons have been identified using antiserum recognizing proTRH or proTRH-derived peptides (Lechan et al., 1986, 1987) in the glomerular and external plexiform layers of the olfactory bulb with processes extending into the glomeruli (Figure 18A). A similar distribution has been seen by *in situ* hybridization histochemistry (Segerson et al., 1987) using a proTRH cRNA probe (Figure 18B). Tsuruo et al. (1988) have shown in addition the presence of TRH immunoreactivity in neurons in the mitral cell body, granule cell, and internal plexiform layers and an extensive fiber network in the accessory olfactory bulb. The presence of some immunoreactive fibers in a longitudinal bundle coursing with the intrabulbar

Figure 19. ProTRH-immunoreactive neuronal perikarya in pyramidal cells of CA3 layer of the hippocampus.

portion of the anterior commissure (Lechan et al., 1987) suggests that some olfactory cells could also project outside of this structure.

B.   Hippocampus

The hippocampal TRH-neuronal system has recently been described by Kubek and associates (Kubek and Sattin, 1984; Kubek et al., 1985, 1989; Sattin et al., 1987), using a sensitive radioimmunoassay (RIA) for TRH. The immunocytochemical delineation of hippocampal TRH neurons, however, awaited the development of antisera to proTRH (Lechan et al., 1986a, 1987; Merchenthaler et al., 1989) and more sensitive methods for immobilizing TRH *in situ* (Tsuruo et al., 1987). Immunoreactive neurons have now been identified in pyramidal layers CA3 and CA2 of the hippocampus proper, as well as in the stratum radiatum and hilus of the dentate (Figure 19). Since lesions of the fornix result in a 60.6% reduction in radioimmunoassayable TRH in the hippocumpus (Kubek et al., 1989), a portion of hippocampal TRH could originate from an extrinsic source. As few or no TRH fibers have been seen in the fornix, however, afferent input to the hippocampus may simply exert a neuromodulatory or trophic effect on what is otherwise an intrinsic TRH system. Hippocampal TRH is not reduced following lesions of the perforant pathway (Low et al., 1989), indicating that TRH neurons in the entorhinal cortex (Lechan et al., 1987; Tsuruo, 1987) do not contribute to hippocampal TRH.

Since electrical- or chemical-induced seizure activity causes a significant increase in the content of TRH, and TRH and TRH analogs have dose-dependent anticonvulsant effects on seizure activity (Ogawa et al., 1985; Sato et al., 1984) and have been used therapeutically in human epilepsy (Ogawa et al., 1985), Kubek et al. (1989) have proposed that hippocampal TRH may modulate seizure activity and be involved in the pathology of epilepsy. Another potential physiological role for hippocampal TRH may be facilitation of memory, possibly by activating cholinergic neurons (Horita et al., 1989).

C.   Other

Other than in areas discussed previously, TRH-synthesizing neurons have been identified by immunocytochemistry or *in situ* hybridization histochemistry in neuronal perikarya in the central and medial nuclei of the amygdala, anterior commissural nucleus, and pyriform cortex (Lechan et al., 1986a, 1987; Merchenthaler et al., 1988; Tsuruo et al., 1988). The presence of TRH in the amygdala and its sustained elevations after electroconvulsive shock (Sattin et al.,

1987) have raised the possibility that TRH may contribute to the successful outcome of electroconvulsive shock in depressive illness. TRH has also been reported to be deficient in the amygdala of depressed patients (Biggins et al., 1983). Efforts to treat depression in humans with massive intravenous, subcutaneous, or oral doses of TRH, however, have not been beneficial (Prange et al., 1978) but it is unclear whether adequate central levels of TRH were achieved in these studies.

The presence of TRH-producing neurons in the cerebral cortex is somewhat controversial. Immunoreactive proTRH has been identified in a sausage-shaped inclusion in some cerebral cortical neurons in our original study (Lechan et al., 1986a) and by Merchenthaler et al. (1989). As we have not been able to demonstrate proTRH mRNA in the cerebral cortex by *in situ* hybridization histochemistry or Northern hybridization or with other antisera to fragments of proTRH (Lechan et al., 1987; Segerson et al., 1987), we are concerned that this may be a cross-reacting material and not authentic proTRH.

IV. Brainstem

The brainstem has been recognized to be a rich source of TRH, with 36 of 40 brainstem nuclei shown to contain radioimmunoassayable TRH by Eskay et al. (1983). In many of these areas, TRH has also been visualized by immunocytochemistry in neuronal perikarya, fibers or both (Hökfelt et al., 1975; Lechan et al., 1983a, 1986a, 1987; Tsuruo et al., 1987; Merchenthaler et al., 1988, 1989) and is summarized in Table 1. Within the medulla, Kubek et al. (1983) have observed that 65% of the total radioimmunoassayable TRH content is present in nuclei associated with the vagal complex, including the dorsal motor nucleus of the vagus, nucleus ambiguus, and nucleus tractus solitarius. The dorsal motor nucleus and nucleus ambiguus give rise to vagal preganglionic neurons that terminate in the gastrointestinal tract, heart, and lungs (Takayama et al., 1982; Shapiro and Miselis, 1985; Bieyer and Hopkins, 1987) and the nucleus solitarius is a major relay nucleus that conveys information traveling from the facial, glossopharyngeal, and vagus nerves to the CNS (Ricardo and Koh, 1978). Other brainstem areas that contain significant amounts of TRH are the midbrain periaqueductal gray and medullary raphe. The anatomy and potential significance of TRH in the dorsal vagal complex and periaqueductal gray are discussed below; TRH in the medullary raphe is discussed in Section V.

A.   Vagal Complex

TRH-immunoreactive fibers are present in high concentration in the nucleus tractus solitarius as well as in the nucleus intercalatus and commissuralis, caudal extensions of the nucleus tractus solitarius (Figure 20A and B). The dorsal motor nucleus of the vagus is also inundated with TRH fibers but fewer fibers are present in the nucleus ambiguus. Collectively, these fibers arise primarily from TRH-containing perikarya in the medullary raphe (see below under Spinal Cord and Figure 22C) as demonstrated by the loss of TRH immunostaining in the vagal complex after transection of ascending axons from the raphe (Palkovits et al., 1986). Although the oxytocin innervation of the nucleus tractus solitarius arises from the hypothalamic paraventricular nucleus (Milaner et al., 1980; Sofroniew and Schrell, 1981), the paraventricular nucleus does not appear to contribute to the TRH innervation of the dorsal vagal complex. Neither bilateral electrolytic ablation of the hypothalamic paraventricular nucleus (Lechan et al., 1983b; Siaud et al., 1987) nor transection of descending hypothalamic axons at the diencephalon-midbrain border cause any reduction in TRH content in this area (Palkovits et

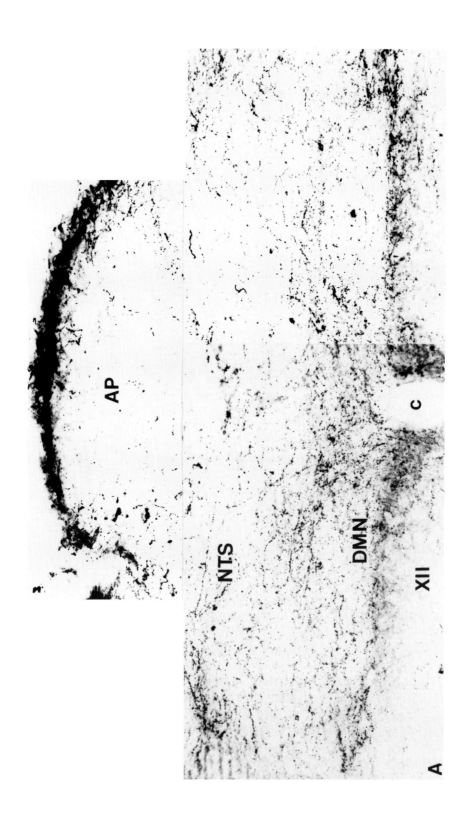

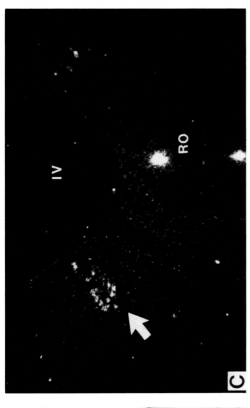

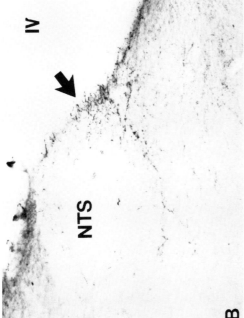

Figure 20. (A) TRH immunoreactivity throughout the nucleus commissuralis of the nucleus tractus solitarius (NTS) and dorsal motor nucleus of the vagus (DMN) in the caudal brainstem. (B) Immunoreactive fibers (arrow) are also present in the medial aspect of the NTS proper in more rostral regions. (C) Perikarya containing proTRH mRNA are present in the DMN. AP, Area postrema; c, central canal; RO, raphe obscurus; IV, fourth ventricle; XII, nucleus of cranial nerve XII.

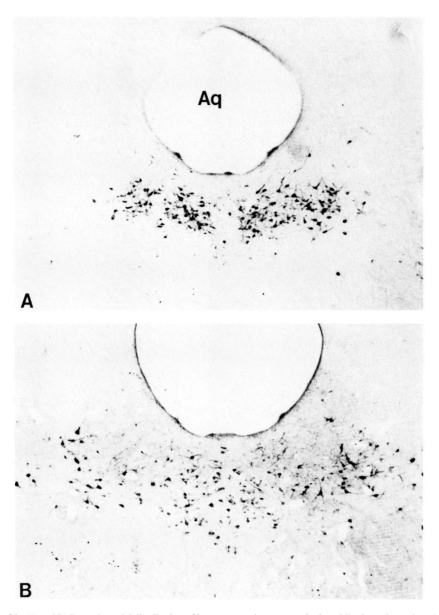

Figure 21. (A and B) Rostral-caudal distribution of immunoreactive neurons in the midbrain periaqueductal gray (PAG) using antiserum to the N-terminal-flanking peptide of proTRH (colchicine pretreated). Peroxidase-positive cells are confined primarily to the rostral two thirds of the ventrolateral PAG. (C) Immunoreactive processes in the ventrolateral PAG extend laterally toward the reticular formation (arrows). Aq, Cerebral aqueduct.

al., 1986). More recent studies using antiserum recognizing proTRH (Lechan et al., 1986a, 1987) and *in situ* hybridization histochemistry (Segerson et al., 1987a) have demonstrated the presence of a population of TRH neurons in the dorsal motor nucleus, itself (Figure 20C), suggesting a second, intrinsic source for TRH innervation of the dorsal vagal complex.

One of the potential roles for TRH in the dorsal vagal complex may be to influence gastrointestinal function via the vagus nerve, recently reviewed by Tache et al. (1989). Using anatomical tracing techniques and immunocytochemistry, TRH-containing axon terminals in

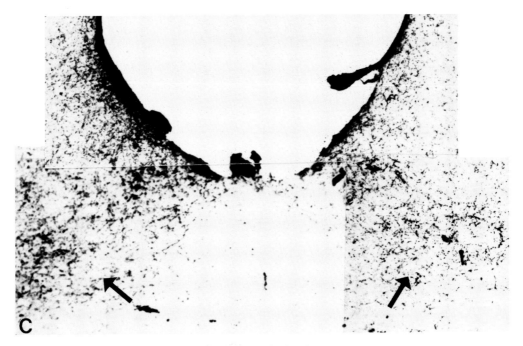

Figure 21. (continued).

the dorsal motor nucleus have been seen in close proximity to preganglionic neurons accumulating a retrogradely transported marker substance after its injection into the greater curvature and pyloris of the stomach (Hornby et al., 1989). Microinjection of small doses (1 to 10 pmol) of TRH or TRH analogs into the dorsal vagal complex activates parasympathetic outflow to stimulate gastric acid secretion and increase gastrointestinal motility in the rat and cat (Ishikawa et al., 1988b; Stephens et al., 1988; Hornby et al., 1989; Raybould et al., 1989), a response that can be prevented by bilateral vagotomy. Furthermore, TRH elicits a marked vasodilation in the gastrointestinal tract and pancreas of the rat, a response that also appears to be vagally mediated (Koskinen, 1989). Although intracerebroventricular TRH causes an increase in intestinal motility (Tonoue and Nomoto, 1979), this does not appear to be mediated through the dorsal vagal complex but rather through forebrain structures, including the medial septum and anterior hypothalamus (Carino and Horita, 1987).

TRH innervation of the nucleus tractus solitarius may also have an important neuromodulatory role in the control of respiration. Dekin et al. (1985) have shown that *in vitro* application of TRH to a brainstem slice preparation results in rhythmic bursting activity of neurons in the nucleus tractus solitarius. In addition, microinjection of TRH into medial portions of the nucleus tractus solitarius, particularly in the caudal medulla but not other regions of the brainstem, causes shortening of inspiratory time (McCown et al., 1986). TRH also may be involved in control of motor outflow to the diaphragm through its innervation of phrenic nerve motor neurons in the spinal cord at C_5 (Holtman et al., 1984).

B.   Periaqueductal Gray

A discrete population of immunoreactive neurons has been identified in the periaqueductal gray (PAG) using antiserum that recognizes proTRH (Lechan et al., 1986a) or non-TRH peptides derived from proTRH (Lechan et al., 1987; Van den Bergh et al., 1988b) (Figure 21A and B). These neurons are organized in a symmetrical butterfly configuration in the ventrolateral PAG, primarily in its rostral two thirds. Dense networks of immunoreactive fibers are also present in the PAG encircling the aqueduct and extend laterally outside of the PAG at its ventrolateral margin (Figure 21C). These neurons also contain proTRH mRNA (Figure 21C) as revealed by *in situ* hybridization histochemistry and Northern blot hybridization (Segerson et al., 1987).

The unique location of the TRH-PAG neurons, distinct from all other described peptides and neurotransmitter substances in this region (Van den Bergh et al., 1988), is of interest since

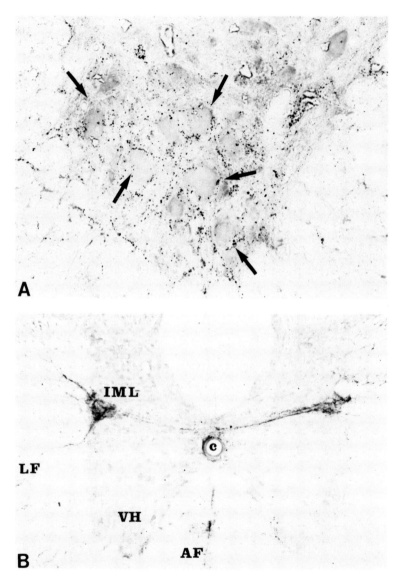

Figure 22. TRH immunoreactivity in the (A) ventral horn (VH) and (B) intermediolateral column (IML) of the spinal cord. Note close proximity of axon terminals with unstained motoneurons (arrows) in (A). (C) These fibers arise from TRH-containing neurons in the medullary raphe (RO and RP) and peripyramidal cell groups (arrow). (Bright-field *in situ* hybridization autoradiogram proTRH mRNA.) AF, Anterior funiculus; c, central canal; LF, lateral funiculus; RO, raphe obscurus; RP, raphe pallidus; PY, pyramidal tracts.

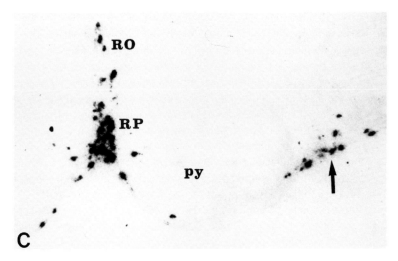

Figure 22. (continued).

the PAG has been recognized as a critical center for the regulation of the pain control system (Basbaum and Fields, 1984). Electrical stimulation or injection of morphine into the ventrolateral subdivision of the PAG, more so than any other region of the PAG, produces analgesia and inhibits the responses to noxious stimuli (Yeung et al., 1977; Gebhart and Toleikis, 1978; Fardin et al., 1984; Oliveras et al., 1979). Although opiate peptides are one of the recognized mediators of the pain response in the PAG, naloxone, a specific opiate antagonist, only partly reverses antinociception produced by electrical stimulation (Osbahr et al., 1981), indicating that there are other nonopioid mediators of the pain response in the PAG.

The role of TRH as an endogenous modulator of pain has been somewhat controversial. Most studies, however, have indicated that TRH has antinociceptive effects as judged by footshock, hot plate, and acid writhing tests (Cuenca et al., 1978; Boschi et al., 1983; Webster et al., 1983; Fardin et al., 1984; Kawamura et al., 1985) and its ability to potentiate swim analgesia (Butler and Bodnar, 1987). The presence of TRH-synthesizing neurons in the PAG in a location implicated in stimulation and chemically induced analgesia, therefore, suggests that they may be part of a nociceptive modulating system, either as interneurons or through descending projections to the rostral-ventral medulla. Since TRH is also present in the dorsal horn of the spinal cord and raphe magnus (see below), other integral components of the pain control system (Basbaum and Fields, 1984), as well as in the reticular nucleus of the thalamus (see above), TRH or TRH-derived peptides may have actions at multiple levels of the neuroaxis to modulate the pain response.

V. Spinal Cord

One of the highest concentrations of TRH in the CNS is in the spinal cord, where levels closely compare to that in the hypothalamus (Jeffcoate et al., 1976; Kardon et al., 1977). The authenticity of this material has been established chromatographically (Jackson, 1980; Spindel and Wurtman, 1980), dispelling earlier concerns that this represents a cross-reacting material (Youngblood et al., 1978). Spinal cord TRH has now been demonstrated in a number of different animal species, including human (Young et al., 1985; Wilber et al., 1976; Lechan et al., 1984; Mitsuma et al., 1984; Harkness and Brownfield, 1986; Jackson et al., 1986; Gibson et al., 1988; Chung et al., 1989).

As opposed to most neuropeptides in the cord, which are confined to the substantia gelatinosa of the dorsal horn, TRH is found mainly in the ventral horn and intermediolateral column. In the ventral horn, immunoreactive material is present exclusively in axon terminals, closely apposed to the perikarya and dendrites of motor neurons in lamina IX of Rexed (Figure 22A). This distribution is not uniform, however, suggesting that TRH could preferentially regulate only certain muscle groups (Lechan et al., 1984). In the rhesus monkey, for example, motoneurons in the ventrolateral subdivision of lamina IX that supply proximal muscle groups of the extremities, lumbar epiaxial muscles, and some of the perineal muscles are more densely innervated by TRH than are dorsolateral and retrodorsolateral motor subdivisions that supply distal muscles of the extremities and intrinsic muscles of the hands and feet. In addition, TRH-containing fibers have not been identified in Onuf's nucleus (Gibson et al., 1988), a motor cell group that supplies the external urethral sphincter and muscles in the perineum.

Within the intermediolateral column, TRH-containing fibers are highly concentrated and present in close association with sympathetic and parasympathetic preganglionic perikarya (Figure 22B). In addition, immunoreactive fibers are found in the intermediate gray of lamina VII (nucleus intercalatus spinalis), dorsal to the central canal in lamina X (dorsal commissural nucleus), and in the lateral funiculus, regions that also contain preganglionic sympathetic neurons. This suggests that TRH may have diffuse effects on the preganglionic neurons of the autonomic nervous system, in contrast to the sharply circumscribed localization of oxytocin and neurophysin (Swanson and McKellar, 1979).

The origin of neuronal perikarya that give rise to TRH-containing axon terminals in the ventral horn and intermediolateral column is the medullary raphe, including the raphe magnus, obscurus, pallidus, and peripyramidal and periolivar accessory groups (Figure 22C). These neurons send axons that descend primarily in the dorsolateral funiculus, close to the pial margin, to innervate spinal cord structures (Figure 23). Axons in the thoracic and upper portions of the lumbar cord often can be seen to extend medially through the substance of the lateral funiculus to supply the intermediolateral column and then continue medially through the intermediate gray, dorsal to the central canal, to innervate the contralateral intermediolateral cell column (Figure 21B).

The majority of medullary raphe-TRH cells co-contain serotonin (Johansson et al., 1981; Bowker et al., 1982; Gilbert et al., 1982, Marsden et al., 1982), dramatically demonstrated by the profound reduction in spinal cord TRH after pharmacologic ablation of serotonin-containing axons with the neurotoxin, 5,7-dihydroxytryptamine (5,7-DHT) (Table 2). Other raphe neurons have been shown to co-contain TRH and substance P or all three substances (Johansson et al., 1981). Not all spinal cord TRH immunoreactivity disappears after treatment with 5,7-DHT, however, particularly in the intermediolateral cell column (Gilbert et al., 1982; Van den Bergh et al., 1987), consistant with the observation that some neurons in the medullary raphe contain only TRH (Johansson et al., 1981). Although Swanson and McKellar (1979) have demonstrated long tract projections from vasopressin- and oxytocin-containing cells of the hypothalamic paraventricular nucleus to the intermediolateral cell column, it is not likely that any of the cell groups in the PVN contribute to the TRH innervation of the spinal cord. Complete electrolytic ablation of the paraventricular nucleus (Harkness and Brownfield, 1986) did not change the TRH content of spinal cord, in contrast to marked diminution in median eminence TRH. Chung et al. (1989) described TRH-containing neurons in Clarke's column but this has not been observed in other studies (Jackson et al., 1986; Gibson et al., 1988).

Recent work by Coffield et al. (1986) and Harkness and Brownfield (1986) has also observed TRH-immunoreactive fibers in the dorsal horn of the spinal cord in lamina II and superficial lamina III. These fibers are not thought to originate from neurons in the medullary raphe as 5,7-DHT does not diminish immunostaining characteristics or content of TRH in this

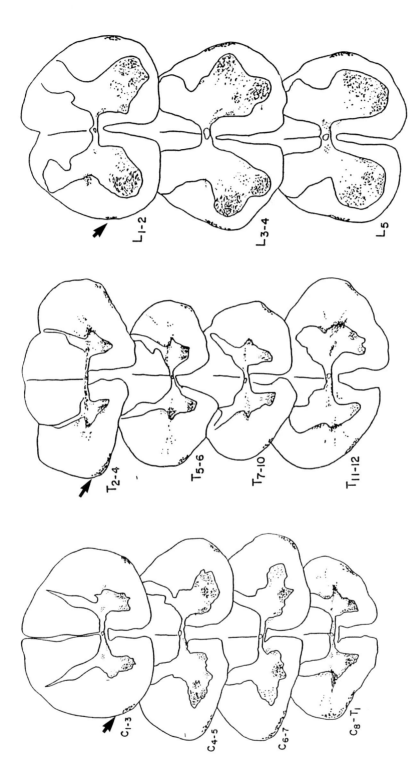

Figure 23. Schematic representation of TRH innervation to the human spinal cord. Note that the majority of fibers descending from the raphe proceed at the pial margin in the lateral funiculus (arrows).

Table 2

TRH and 5-HT Content in Rat Spinal Cord 11 Weeks after
Intracerebroventricular Injection of 5,7-DHT or Vehicle

Spinal cord level	Substance injected	TRH (pg/mg protein)	5-HT (pg/mg protein)
Cervical	Vehicle	1043 ± 161	2641 ± 362
	5,7-DHT	222 ± 34	518 ± 111
Thoracic	Vehicle	3311 ± 247	3873 ± 329
	5,7-DHT	392 ± 44	601 ± 46
Lumbosacral	Vehicle	3200 ± 416	6720 ± 362
	5,7-DHT	161 ± 54	464 ± 74

Adapted from Van den Bergh, P., Kelly, J. J., Adelman, L., Munsat, T., Jackson, I. M.
D., and Lechan, R. M., *Muscle Nerve*, 10, 397, 1987.

region. Rather this material may arise from small interneurons within the dorsal horn itself
(Harkness and Brownfield, 1986) or from neurons in the dorsal root ganglia (Schoenen et al.,
1989).

TRH in the spinal cord probably has several functions, in keeping with its varied
anatomical distribution in regions associated with motor, autonomic, and sensory function.
TRH is capable of depolarizing motoneurons in spinal cord preparations (Nicoll, 1977; Cooper
and Boyer, 1978; Barbeau and Bedard, 1981; Ono and Fukuda, 1982; Takahashi, 1985),
augments the synthesis of serotonin (Fone et al., 1989), and stimulates the release of norepinephrine from catecholamine terminals in the ventral horn (Bennett et al., 1989), thus indicating that it may act as a neuromodulator to facilitate the excitability of motoneurons in the spinal
cord. However, TRH may have an antagonistic action to serotonin-induced motoneuron
excitability when the two are administered simultaneously and, therefore, may not be important
in maintaining enhanced excitability of motoneurons in the intact cord (Oka and Fukuda, 1984;
White et al., 1989).

A trophic role for TRH on motoneurons of the spinal cord has been claimed. TRH
stimulates the growth of neuronal processes and choline acetyltransferase in cultured ventral
horn neurons (Schmidt-Ackert et al., 1984; Banda et al., 1985; Iwasaki et al., 1989), augments
the growth of spinal cord transplants *in oculo* (Henschen et al., 1988), and is necessary to
permit complete reinnervation of muscles functionally denervated by botulinum toxin (Van
den Bergh et al., 1988a). Therapeutic trials of TRH have been carried out in spinal muscular
atrophy (Sobue, 1986) and TRH has been extensively tested in the treatment of amyotrophic
lateral sclerosis (Brooks, 1989; Engel, 1989; Guiloff, 1989; Munsat et al., 1989). Unfortunately, only minor or transient benefits have been found (Brooke, 1989). The reduction in the
content of spinal cord TRH that occurs in this disease (Mitsuma et al., 1984) is proportional to
the loss of motoneurons and does not appear to be primary to the disease process (Jackson et
al., 1986).

Intrathecal administration of TRH to humans or experimental animals results in a number
of responses, including piloerection, tremor, hypertension, tachycardia, and diaphoresis (Reichlin,
1986), that have been attributed to actions on autonomic preganglionic neurons in the
intermediolateral column and accessory groups. The protective effects of TRH in experimental
animals following spinal trauma (Faden et al., 1989), is thought to occur through effects on the
spinal cord microcirculation to increase regional blood flow. Wet dog shakes, a characteristic
behavioral response to TRH in animals, is likely mediated by effects of TRH on the brainstem
rather than the spinal cord (Fone et al.,1989).

TRH can also modify the excitability of dorsal horn neurons either directly or by
facilitating the action of other neurotransmitters such as glutamate (Jackson and White, 1988),

but its functional significance is still unknown. Intrathecal or intracerebroventricular adminis-tration of TRH produces short-lasting analgesia (Boschi et al., 1983; Kawamura et al., 1985; Yakish et al., 1985; Coffield et al., 1986; Watkins et al., 1986; Butler and Bodnar, 1987), suggesting an antinociceptive action of the tripeptide. This is consistent with observations by Engel (1986) that high doses of TRH administered to patients with amyotrophic lateral sclerosis reduces chronic pain. The location of TRH in small interneurons at the border of lamina II/III, however, has led Coffield et al. (1986) to propose that TRH may also be involved in nonnociceptive somatosensory transmission. Indeed, Fone et al. (1989) have speculated that the characteristic behavioral response of forepaw licking after intrathecal administration of TRH analogs in rats may be due to the action of TRH on dorsal horn neurons and the functional correlate of warmth and tingling observed in humans.

VI. Conclusion

A dramatic advancement in the knowledge of TRH neuronal systems in the brain has followed the chemical characterization of TRH 2 decades ago and has revolutionized thinking about the neurobiology of the tripeptide. Although an important role in the regulation of TSH secretion from anterior pituitary thyrotropes has been clearly established, the wide distribution of TRH in the CNS originating from neurons outside of the hypothalamic tuberoinfundibular system suggests a much more versatile physiologic role for this peptide. In addition, the demonstration that TRH derives from a larger precursor protein raises the intriguing possibility that proTRH-derived peptides other than TRH could exert independent biologic functions. This may be particularly important in regions of the brain where processing of proTRH may be primarily to its nonTRH components, such as the reticular nucleus of the thalamus. This extensive distribution helps to explain the widespread actions of TRH on autonomic, motor, sensory, and limbic systems, arousal, seizure threshold, thermoregulation, appetite regulation, and gastrointestinal function.

Acknowlegments

The authors wish to express their sincere appreciation to Dr. Seymour Reichlin for his critical review of this manuscript.

References

Andersson, K. and Enroth, P., Thyroidectomy and central catecholamine neurons of the male rat, *Neuroendocrinology*, 45, 14, 1987.

Annunziato, L., DiRenzo, G., Lombardi, G., Scopacasa, F., Schettini, G., Preziosi, P., and Scapagnini, U., The role of central noradrenergic neurons in the control of thyrotropin secretion in the rat, *Endocrinology*, 100, 738, 1977.

Banda, R., Means, E., and Samaha, F. J., Trophic effect of thyrotropin-releasing hormone on murine ventral horn neurons in culture, *Ann. Neurol.*, 35, 93, 1985.

Barbeau, H. and Bedard, P., Similar motor effects of 5-HT and TRH in rats following chronic spinal transection and 5,7-dihydroxytryptamine injections, *Neuropharmacology*, 20, 477, 1981.

Basbaum, A. I. and Fields, H. L., Endogenous pain control systems: brainstem spinal pathways and endorphin circuitry, *Annu. Rev. Neurosci.*, 7, 309, 1984.

Bennett, G. W., Nathan, P. A., Wong, K. K., and Marsden, C. A., Regional distribution of immunore-active-thyrotropin releasing hormone and substance P and indolamines in human spinal cord, *J. Neurochem.,* 46, 1718, 1986.

Bennett, G. W., Marsden, C. A., Fone, K. C. F., Johnson, J. V., and Heal, D. J., TRH-catecholamine interactions in brain and spinal cord, *Ann. N.Y. Acad. Sci.,* 553, 106, 1989.

Bieyer, D. and Hopkins, D. A., Viserotopic representation of the upper alimentary tract in the medulla oblongata in the rat: the nucleus ambiguus, *J. Comp. Neurol.,* 262, 546, 1987.

Biggins, J. A., Perry, E. K., McDermott, J. R., Smith, I. A., Perry, R. H., and Edwardson, J. A., Postmortem levels of thyrotropin-releasing hormone and neurotensin in the amygdala in Alzheimer's disease, schizophrenia and depression, *J. Neurol. Sci.,* 58, 117, 1983.

Bissette, G., Nemeroff, C. B., Loosen, P. T., Prange, A. J., Jr., and Lipton, M.A., Hypothermia and intolerance to cold induced by intracisternal administration of the hypothalamic peptide neurotensin, *Nature (London)*, 262, 607, 1976.

Boschi, G. and Rips, R., Effects of thyrotropin releasing hormone injections into different loci of rat brain on core temperature, *Neurosci. Lett.,* 23, 93, 1981.

Boschi, G., Desiles, M., Reny, V., Rips, S., and Wrigglesworth, S., Antinociceptive properties of thyrotropin releasing hormone in mice: comparison with morphine, *Br. J. Pharmacol.,* 79, 85, 1983.

Bowker, R. M., Westlund, K. W., Sullivan, M. C., Wilber, J. F., and Coulter, J. D., Transmitter of the raphe-spinal complex: immunocytochemical studies, *Peptides,* 3, 291, 1982.

Bradbury, A. F., Finnie, M. D. A., and Smythe, D. G., Mechanism of C-terminal amide formation by pituitary enzymes, *Nature (London),* 298, 686, 1982.

Breder, C. D., Dinorello, C. A., and Saper, C. B., Interleukin-1 immunoreactive innervation of the human hypothalamus, *Science,* 240, 321, 1988.

Breese, G. R., Cott, J. M., Cooper, B. R., Prange, A. J., Jr., Lipton, M. A., and Plotnikoff, N. P., Effects of thyrotropin-releasing hormone (TRH) on the actions of pentobarbital and other centrally acting drugs, *J. Pharmacol. Exp. Ther.,* 193, 11, 1975.

Brooke, M. H., Thyrotropin-releasing hormone in ALS, *Ann. N.Y. Acad. Sci.,* 553, 422, 1989.

Brooks, B. R., A summary of the current position of TRH in ALS therapy, *Ann. N.Y. Acad. Sci.,* 553, 431, 1989.

Brown, M., Rivier, J., and Vale, W., Bombesin: potent effects on thermoregulation in the rat, *Science,* 196, 998, 1977.

Brownstein, M. J., Palkovits, M., Saavedra, J. M., Bassiri, R. M., and Utiger, R. D., Thyrotropin-releasing hormone in specific nuclei of rat brain, *Science,* 185, 267, 1974.

Brownstein, M. J., Utiger, R. D., Palkovits, M., and Kizer, J. S., Effect of hypothalamic deafferentation on thyrotropin-releasing hormone levels in rat brain, *Proc. Natl. Acad. Sci. U.S.A.,* 72, 4177, 1975.

Bulant, M., Delfour, A., Vaudry, H., and Nicholas, P., Processing of thyrotropin-releasing hormone prohormone (Pro-TRH) generates pro-TRH-connecting peptides, *J. Biol. Chem.,* 263, 17189, 1988.

Bulant, M., Roussell, J.-P., Astier, H., Nicholos, P., and Vandry, H., Processing of thyrotropin-releasing hormone (pro-TRH) generates a biologically active peptide, prepro-TRH-(160-169), which regulates TRH-induced thyrotropin secretion, *Proc. Natl. Acad. Sci. U.S.A.,* 87, 4439, 1990.

Buma, P., Synaptic and nonsynaptic release of neuromediators in the central nervous system, *Acta Morphol. Neerl. Scand.,* 26, 81, 1989.

Burgus, R., Dunn, T. F., DeSiderio, D., Ward, D. W., Vale, W., and Guillemin, R., Characterization of ovine hypothalamic hypophysiotropic TSH-releasing factor, *Nature (London),* 226, 321, 1970.

Butler, P. D. and Bodnar, R. J., Neuromodulatory effects of TRH upon swim and cholinergic analgesia, *Peptides,* 8, 299, 1987.

Carino, M. A. and Horita, A., Localization of TRH-sensitive sites in rat brain mediating intestinal transit, *Life Sci.,* 41, 2663, 1987.

Carr, F. E. and Wessendorf, M., A pre-prothyrotropin-releasing hormone fragment is a more potent stimulator that thyrotropin-releasing hormone (TRH) of thyrotropin beta-subunit (TSHB) gene, *Endocrinology,* 123 (Suppl.), T-56, 1988.

Ceccatelli, S., Eriksson, M., and Hökfelt, T., Distribution and coexistence of corticotropin-releasing factor-, neurotensin-, enkephalin-, cholecystokinin-, galanin- and vasoactive intestinal polypep-tide/peptide histidine isoleucine-like peptides in the parvocellular part of the paraventricular nucleus, *Neuroendocrinology,* 49, 309, 1989.

Chi, M. L. and Lin, M. T., Involvement of adrenergic receptor mechanisms within hypothalamus in the fever induced by amphetamine and thyrotropin-releasing hormone in the rat, *J. Neurol. Trans.*, 58, 213, 1983.

Choy, V. J. and Watkins, W. B., Immunohistochemical localization of thyrotropin-releasing factor in the rat median eminence, *Cell Tissue Res.*, 177, 371, 1977.

Chung, K., Briner, R. P., Carlton, S. M. and Westlund, K. N., Immunohistochemical localization of seven different pepides in the human spinal cord, *J. Comp. Neurol.*, 280, 158, 1989.

Ciarleglio, A. E., Beingeld, M. C., and Westfall, T. C., Release of neuropeptide Y-like activity (NPY-LI) from the hypothalamus, in *Abstracts of the 18th Annual Meeting of the Society for Neuroscience*, Toronto, Ontario, 1988, 873.

Cockle, S. M. and Smyth, D. G., Specific processing of the thyrotropin-releasing hormone prohormone in rat brain and spinal cord, *Eur. J. Biochem.*, 165, 693, 1987.

Coffield, J. A., Miletic, V., Zimmerman, E., Hoffert, M. J., and Brooks, B. R., Demonstration of thyrotropin-releasing hormone immunoreactivity in neurons of the mouse spinal dorsal horn, *J. Neurosci.*, 6, 1194, 1986.

Cooper, B. R. and Boyer, C. E., Stimulant action of thyrotropin releasing hormone on cat spinal cord, *Neuropharmacology*, 17, 153, 1978.

Cott, J. M., Breese, G. R., Cooper, B. R., Barlow, S., and Prange, A. J., Jr., Investigations into the mechanism of reduction of ethanol sleep by thyrotropin-releasing hormone (TRH), *J. Pharmacol. Exp. Ther.*, 196, 594, 1976.

Cuenca, E., Serrano, M. I., Gilbert-Rahola, J., Carrasco, M. S., and Esteban, J. M., The analgesic activity of TRH and MSH, *Arch. Pharmacol. Toxicol.*, 4, 71, 1978.

Cunningham, E. T. and Sawchenko, P. E., Anatomical specificity of noradrenergic inputs to the paraventricular and supraoptic nuclei of the rat hypothalamus, *J. Comp. Neurol.*, 274, 60, 1988.

Day, T. A., Ferguson, A. V., and Renaud, L. P., Noradrenergic afferents facilitate the activity of tuberoinfundibular neurons of the hypothalamic paraventricular nucleus, *Neuroendocrinology*, 41, 17, 1985.

Dekin, M. S., Richerson, G. B., and Getting, P. A., Thyrotropin-releasing hormone induces rhythmic bursting in neurons of the nucleus tractus solitarius, *Science*, 229, 67, 1985.

Docherty, K. and Steiner, D. F., Post-translational proteolysis in polypeptide hormone biosynthesis, *Annu. Rev. Physiol.*, 44, 625, 1982.

Dyess, E. M., Segerson, T. P., Liposits, Zs., Paull, W. K., Kaplan, M. M., Wu, P., Jackson, I. M. D., and Lechan, R. M., Triiodothyronine exerts direct cell-specific regulation of thyrotropin-releasing hormone gene expression in the hypothalamic paraventricular nucleus, *Endocrinology*, 123, 2291, 1988.

Engel, W. K., High-dose thyrotropin releasing hormone (TRH) can reduce chronic pain: does it have a normal anti-nociceptive role?, *Muscle Nerve*, 9, 113, 1986.

Engel, W. K., High-dose TRH treatment of neuromuscular diseases: summary of mechanisms and critique of clinical studies, *Ann. N.Y. Acad. Sci.*, 553, 462, 1989.

Epelbaum, J., Tapia-Arancibia, L., Alonso, G., Astier, H., and Kardon, C., The anterior periventricular hypothalamus is the site of somatostatin inhibition of its own release: an *in vitro* and immunocyto-chemical study, *Neuroendocrinology*, 44, 255, 1986.

Eskay, R. L., Long, R. T., and Palkovits, M., Localization of immunoreactive thyrotropin releasing hormone in the lower brainstem of the rat, *Brain Res.*, 277, 159, 1983.

Faden, A. I., Vink, R., and McIntosh, T. K., Thyrotropin-releasing hormone and central nervous system trauma, *Ann. N.Y. Acad. Sci.*, 553, 380, 1989.

Fardin, V., Oliveras, J. L., and Besson, J. M., A reinvestigation of analgesic effects induced by stimulation of the periaqueductal gray matter in the rat. I. The production of behavioral side effects together with analgesia, *Brain Res.*, 306, 105, 1984.

Fischer, W. H. and Speiss, J., Identification of a mammalian glutaminyl cyclase converting glutaminyl into pyroglutamyl peptides, *Proc. Natl. Acad. Sci. U.S.A.*, 84, 3628, 1987.

Fone, K. C. F., Johnson, J. V., Marsden, C. A., and Bennett, G. W., Comparative behavioral and biochemical effects of repeated intrathecal administration of thyrotropin-releasing hormone (TRH) or two analogues of TRH in adult rats, *Neuropharmacology*, 28, 867, 1989a.

Fone, K. C. F., Johnson, J. V., Bennett, G. W., and Marsden, C. A., Involvement of 5-HT$_2$ receptors in the behaviors produced by intrathecal administration of selected 5-HT agonists and the TRH analogue (CG 3509) to rats, *Br. J. Pharmacol.*, 96, 599, 1989b.

Frawley, L. S., Leong, D. A., and Neill, J. D.,Oxytocin attenuates TRH-induced TSH release from rat pituitary cells, *Neuroendocrinology,* 40, 201, 1985.

Gainer, H., Sarne, Y., and Brownstein, M. J., Neurophysin biosynthesis: conversion of a putative precursor during axonal transport, *Science*, 195, 1354, 1977.

Gebhart, G. F. and Toleikis, T. R., An evaluation of stimulation-produced analgesia in the cat, *Exp. Neurol.,* 62, 570, 1978.

Gibson, S. J., Polak, J. M., Katagiri, T., Su, H., Weller, R. O., Brownell, D. B., Hollard, S., Hughes, J. T., Kikuyama, S., Ball, J., Bloom, S. R., Steiner, T. J., deBelleroche, J., and Clifford, R. F., A comparison of the distribution of eight peptides in spinal cord from normal controls and cases of motor neuronal disease with special reference to Onuf's nucleus, *Brain Res.,* 474, 255, 1988.

Gilbert, R. F. T., Emson, P. C., Hunt, S. P., Bennett, G. W., and Verhosfstad, J., The effect of monamine neurotoxin on peptides in the rat spinal cord, *Neuroscience*, 7, 69, 1982.

Gray, T. S. and Morley, J. E., Neuropeptide Y: anatomical distribution and possible function in mammalian nervous system, *Life Sci.,* 38, 389, 1986.

Greer, M. A., Role of the hypothalamus in control of thyroid function, *J. Clin. Endocrinol.,* 12, 1259, 1952.

Griffiths, E. C., Rothwell, N. J., and Stock, M. J., Thermogenic effects of thyrotropin-releasing hormone and its analogues in the rat, *Experientia*, 44, 40, 1988.

Guiloff, R. J., Use of TRH analogues in motoneurone disease, *Ann. N.Y. Acad. Sci.,* 553, 399, 1989.

Harfstrand, A., Brain neuropeptide Y mechanisms. Basic aspects and involvement in cardiovascular and neuroendocrine regulation, *Acta Physiol. Scand.*, 131, 565, 1987.

Harkness, D. H. and Brownfield, M. S., A thyrotropin-releasing-hormone-containing system in rat dorsal horn separate from serotonin, *Brain Res.,* 384, 323, 1986a.

Harkness, D. H. and Brownfield, M. S., Segmental distribution of thyrotropin releasing hormone in rat spinal cord, *Brain Res. Bull.,* 17, 11, 1986b.

Heal, D. J. and Green, A. R., Administration of thyrotropin releasing hormone (TRH) to rats releases dopamine in the n. accumbens but not in n. caudatus, *Neuropharmacology*, 18, 23, 1979.

Henschen, A., Zerbe, G., Nadzan, A. M., McKelvy, J. F., Olson, L., and Hoffer, B., Thyrotropin releasing hormone augments growth of spinal cord transplants *in oculo, Exp. Neurol.,* 102, 125, 1988.

Hirooka, Y., Hollander, C. S., Suzuki, S., Ferdinand, P., and Juan, S., Somatostatin inhibits release of thyrotropin releasing factor from organ cultures in rat hypothalamus, *Proc. Natl. Acad. Sci. U.S.A.,* 75, 4508, 1978.

Hökfelt, T., Fuxe, K., Johansson, O., Jeffcoate, S., and White, N., Distribution of thyrotropin-releasing hormone (TRH) in the central nervous system as revealed by immunocytochemistry, *Eur. J. Pharmacol.*, 34, 389, 1975.

Hökfelt, T., Elde, R., Fuxe, K., Johansson, O., Ljungdahl, A., Goldstein, M., Luft, R., Efendic, S., Nilsson, G., Terenius, L., Ganten, D., Jeffcoate, S.L., Rehfeld, J., Said, S., Perez de la Mora, M., Possani, L., Tapia, R., Teran, K., and Palacios, R., Aminergic and peptidergic pathways in the nervous system with special reference to the hypothalamus, in *The Hypothalamus*, Reichlin, S., Baldessarini, R. J., and Martin, J. B., Eds., Raven Press, New York, 1979, 69.

Hökfelt, T., Tsuruo, Y., Ulfhake, B., Cullheim, S., Arvidsson, U., Foster, G. A., Schultzberg, M., Schalling, M., Arborelius, L., Freedman, J., Post, C., and Visser, T., Distribution of TRH-like immunoreactivity with special reference to coexistence with other neuroactive compounds, *Ann. N.Y. Acad. Sci.,* 553, 76, 1989.

Holets, V. R., Hökfelt, T., Ude, J., Eckert, M., Penzlir, H., Verhofstad, A. A. J., and Visser, T. J., A comparative study of the immunohistochemical localization of a presumptive proctolin-like peptide, thyrotropin-releasing hormone and 5-hydroxytryptamine in the rat central nervous system, *Brain Res.,* 408, 141, 1987.

Holtman, J. R., Jr., Norman, W. P., Skirboll, L., Dretchen, K. L., Cuello, C., Visser, T. J., Hökfelt, T., and Gillis, R. A., Evidence for 5-hydroxytryptamine, substance P, and thyrotropin-releasing hormone in neurons innervating the phrenic motor nucleus, *J. Neurosci.*, 4, 1064, 1984.

Hori, T., Yamasaki, M., Asami, T., Koya, H., and Kiyobara, T., Responses of anterior hypothalamic-preoptic thermosensitive neurons to thyrotropin releasing hormone and cyclo(His-Pro), *Neuropharmacology*, 27, 895, 1988.

Horita, A., Carino, M. A., Zabawska, J., and Lai, H., TRH analog MK-771 reverses neurochemical and learning deficits in medial septal-lesioned rats, *Peptides*, 10, 121, 1989.

Hornby, P. J., Rossiter, C. D., Pineo, S. V., Norman, W. P., Friedman, E. K., Benjamin, S., and Gillis, R. A., TRH: immunocytochemical distribution in vagal nuclei of the cat and physiological effects of microinjection, *Am. J. Physiol.*, 257, G454, 1989.

Houser, C. R., Vaughn, J. E., Barber, R. P., and Roberts, E., GABA neurons are the major cell type of the nucleus reticularis thalami, *Brain Res.*, 200, 341, 1980.

Ishikawa, K. and Suzuki, M., Antagonism by thyrotropin-releasing hormone (TRH) of pentobarbital-induced hypothermia in rats with brain lesions, *Experientia*, 42, 1029, 1986.

Ishikawa, K., Taniguchi, Y., Kurosumi, K., and Suzuki, M., Origin of septal thyrotropin-releasing hormone in the rat, *Neuroendocrinology*, 44, 54, 1986.

Ishikawa, K., Taniguchi, Y., Inoue, K., Kurosumi, K., and Suzuki, M., Immunocytochemical delineation of thyrotrophic area: origin of thyrotropin-releasing hormone in the median eminence, *Neuroendocrinology*, 47, 384, 1988.

Ishikawa, K., Inoue, K., Tosaka, H., Shimada, O., and Suzuki, M., Immunohistochemical characterization of thyrotropin-releasing hormone-containing neurons in rat septum, *Neuroendocrinology*, 39, 448, 1989.

Ishikawa, T., Yang, H., and Tache, Y., Medullary sites of action of the TRH analogue, RX 77368, for stimulation of gastric acid secretion in the rat, *Gastroenterology*, 95, 1470, 1988.

Iwasaki, Y., Kinoshita, M., Ikeda, K., Takamiya, K., and Shiojima, T., Trophic effect of various neuropeptides on the cultured ventral spinal cord of rat embryo, *Neurosci. Lett.*, 101, 316, 1989.

Jackson, D. A. and White, S. R., Thyrotropin releasing hormone (TRH) modifies excitability of spinal cord dorsal horn cells, *Neurosci. Lett.*, 92, 171, 1988.

Jackson, I. M. D., TRH in the rat nervous system: identity with synthetic TRH in high performance liquid chromatography following affinity chromatography, *Brain Res.*, 210, 245, 1980.

Jackson, I. M. D. and Reichlin, S., Thyrotropin-releasing hormone (TRH): distribution in hypothalamic and extrahypothalamic brain tissues of mammalian and submammalian chordates, *Endocrinology*, 95, 854, 1974.

Jackson, I. M. D., Wu, P., and Lechan, R. M., Immunohistochemical localization in rat brain of the precursor for thyrotropin-releasing hormone, *Science*, 229, 1097, 1985.

Jackson, I. M. D., Adelman, L. S., Munsat, T. L., Forte, S., and Lechan, R. M., Amyotrophic lateral sclerosis, thyrotropin-releasing hormone and histidyl proline diketopiperazine in the spinal cord and cerebrospinal fluid, *Neurology*, 36, 1218, 1986.

Jeffcoate, S. L., White, N., Hökfelt, T., Fuxe, K., and Johansson, O., Localization of thyrotropin releasing hormone in the spinal cord of the rat by immunohistochemistry and radioimmunoassay, *J. Endocrinol.*, 69, 9P, 1976.

Johansson, O., Hökfelt, T., Jeffcoate, S. L., White, N., and Sternberger, L. A., Ultrastructural localization of TRH-like immunoreactivity, *Exp. Brain Res.*, 38, 1, 1980.

Johansson, O., Hökfelt, T., Pernow, B., Jeffcoate, S. L., White, N., Steinbusch, H. W. M., Verhofstad, A. A. J., Emson, P. C., and Spindel, E., Immunohistochemical support for three putative transmitters in one neuron: coexistence of 5-hydroxytryptamine, substance P- and thyrotropin releasing hormone-like immunoreactivity in medullary neurons projecting to the spinal cord, *Neuroscience*, 6, 1857, 1981.

Joseph-Bravo, P., Charli, J. L., Palacios, J. M., and Kardon, C., Effect of neurotransmitters on the *in vitro* release of immunoreactive thyrotropin-releasing hormone from the medial basal hypothalamus, *Endocrinology*, 104, 80, 1979.

Kalivas, P. W. and Horita, A., Thyrotropin-releasing hormone: neurogenesis of actions in the pentobarbital narcotized rat, *J. Pharmacol. Exp. Ther.*, 212, 203, 1980.

Kaplan, M. M., Taft, J. A., Reichlin, S., and Munsat, T. L., Sustained rises in serum thyrotropin, thyroxine and triiodothyronine during long term, continuous thyrotropin-releasing hormone treatment in patients with amyotrophic lateral sclerosis, *J. Clin. Endocrinol. Metab.*, 63, 808, 1986.

Kardon, F. C., Winokur, A., and Utiger, R. D., Thyrotropin-releasing hormone (TRH) in rat spinal cord, *Brain Res.*, 122, 578, 1977.

Kasting, N. W. and Martin, J. B., Altered release of growth hormone and thyrotropin induced by endotoxin in the rat, *Am. J. Physiol.*, 243, E332, 1982.

Kawamura, S., Sakurada, S., Sakurada, T., Kisara, K., Sasaki, Y., and Suzuki, K., The antinociceptive effects of histidyl-proline diketopiperazine and thyrotropin-releasing hormone in the mouse, *Eur. J. Pharmacol.*, 112, 287, 1985.

Kerkerian, L. and Pelletier, G., Effects of monosodium L-glutamate administration on neuropeptide Y-containing neurons in the rat hypothalamus, *Brain Res.*, 369, 388, 1986.

King, J. C., Lechan, R. M., Kugel, G., and Anthony, E. L. P., Acrolein: a fixative for immunocytochemical localization of peptides in the CNS, *J. Histochem. Cytochem.*, 31, 62, 1983.

Koller, K. J., Wolff, R. S., Warden, M. K., and Zoeller, R. T., Thyroid hormones regulates levels of thyrotropin-releasing hormone mRNA in the paraventricular nucleus, *Proc. Natl. Acad. Sci. U.S.A.*, 84, 7329, 1987.

Koskinen, L.-O.D., Cerebral and peripheral blood flow effects of TRH in the rat — a role of vagal nerves, *Peptides*, 10, 933, 1989.

Krieder, M. S., Winokur, A., and Krieger, N. R., The olfactory bulb is rich in TRH immunoreactivity, *Brain Res.*, 217, 69, 1981.

Krieder, M. S., Knight, P., Winokur, A., and Krieger, N. R., TRH concentration in rat olfactory bulb is undiminished by deafferentation, *Brain Res.*, 241, 351, 1982.

Krulich, L., Neurotransmitter control of thyrotropin secretion, *Neuroendocrinology*, 35, 139, 1982.

Krulich, L., Giachetti, A., Marchlewska-Koj, A., Hefco, E., and Jameson, H. E., On the role of the central noradrenergic and dopaminergic systems in the regulation of TSH secretion in the rat, *Endocrinology*, 100, 496, 1977.

Kubek, M. J. and Sattin, A., Effect of electroconvulsive shock on the content of thyrotropin-releasing hormone in rat brain, *Life Sci.*, 34, 1149, 1984.

Kubek, M. J., Rea, M. A., Hodes, Z. I., and Aprison, M. H., Quantitation and characterization of thyrotropin-releasing hormone in vagal nuclei and other regions of the medulla oblongata of the rat, *J. Neurochem.*, 40, 1307, 1983.

Kubek, M. J., Meyerhoff, J. L., Hill, T. G., Norton, J. A., and Sattin, A., Effects of subconvulsive and repeated electroconvulsive shock on thyrotropin-releasing hormone in rat brain, *Life Sci.*, 36, 315, 1985.

Kubek, M. J., Low, W. C., Sattin, A., Morzorati, S. L., Meyerhoff, J. L., and Larsen, S. H., Role of TRH in seizure modulation, *Ann. N.Y. Acad. Sci.*, 553, 286, 1989.

Lamour, Y., Dutar, P., and Jobert, A., Effects of TRH, cyclo-(His-Pro) and, (3-Me-His$_2$) TRH on identified septohippocampal neurons in the rat, *Brain Res.*, 331, 343, 1985.

Lechan, R. M. and Jackson, I. M. D., Immunohistochemical localization of thyrotropin-releasing hormone in the rat hypothalamus and pituitary, *Endocrinology*, 111, 55, 1982.

Lechan, R. M. and Segerson, T. P., Pro-TRH gene expression and precursor peptides in rat brain: observations by hybridization analysis and immunocytochemistry, *Ann. N.Y. Acad. Sci.*, 553, 29, 1989.

Lechan, R. M., Nestler, J. L., Jacobson, S., and Reichlin, S., The hypothalamic "tuberoinfundibular" system of the rat as demonstrated by horseradish peroxidase (HRP) microiontophoresis, *Brain Res.*, 195, 13, 1980.

Lechan, R. M., Nestler, J. L., and Jacobson, S., The tuberoinfundibular system of the rat as demonstrated by immunohistochemical localization of retrogradely transported wheat germ agglutinin (WGA) from the median eminence, *Brain Res.*, 245, 1, 1982.

Lechan, R. M., Molitch, M. E., and Jackson, I. M. D., Distribution of immunoreactive human growth hormone-like material and thyrotropin-releasing hormone in the rat central nervous system: evidence for their coexistence in the same neurons, *Endocrinology*, 112, 877, 1983a.

Lechan, R. M., Snapper, S. B., and Jackson, I. M. D., Evidence that spinal cord thyrotropin-releasing hormone is independent of the paraventricular nucleus, *Neurosci. Lett.*, 43, 61, 1983b.

Lechan, R. M., Snapper, S. B., Jacobson, S., and Jackson, I. M. D., The distribution of thyrotropin-releasing hormone (TRH) in the rhesus monkey spinal cord, *Peptides*, 5, 185, 1984.

Lechan, R. M., Wu, P., and Jackson, I. M. D., Immunolocalization of the thyrotropin-releasing hormone prohormone in the rat central nervous system, *Endocrinology*, 119, 1210, 1986a.

Lechan, R. M., Wu, P. W., Jackson, I. M. D., Wolf, H., Cooperman, S., Mandel, G., and Goodman, R., Thyrotropin-releasing hormone precursor: characterization in rat brain, *Science*, 231, 159, 1986b.

Lechan, R. M., Wu, P., and Jackson, I. M. D., Immunocytochemical distribution in rat brain of putative peptides derived from thyrotropin-releasing hormone prohormone, *Endocrinology*, 121, 1879, 1987.

Lechan, R. M., Toni, R., Clark, B. O., Cannon, J. G., Shaw, A. P., Dinorello, C. A., and Reichlin, S., Immunoreactive interleukin-1β localization in the rat forebrain, *Brain Res.*, 514, 135, 1990.

Lee, S. L., Stewart, K., and Goodman, R. H., Structure of the gene encoding rat thyrotropin releasing hormone, *J. Biol. Chem.*, 263, 16604, 1988.

Leranth, Cs., Segura, I. M. G., Palkovits, M., MacLusky, N. J., Skanabrough, M., and Naftolin, F., The LH-RH-containing network in the preoptic area of the rat: demonstration of LHRH-containing nerve terminals in synaptic contact with LH-RH neurons, *Brain Res.*, 345, 332, 1985.

Levin, M. C., Sawchenko, P. E., Howe, P. R. C., Bloom, S. R., and Polak, J. M., Organization of galanin-immunoreactive inputs to the paraventricular nucleus with special reference to their relationship to catecholaminergic afferents, *J. Comp. Neurol.*, 261, 568, 1987.

Lin, L. S., Chiu, W. T., Shih, C. J., and Lin, M. T., Involvement of both opiate and catecholaminergic receptors of ventromedial hypothalamus in the locomotor stimulant action of thyrotropin-releasing hormone, *J. Neurol.*, 68, 217, 1987.

Lin, M. T., Wang, P. S., Chuang, J., Fan. L. J., and Won, S. J., Cold stress of a pyrogenic substance elevates thyrotropin-releasing hormone levels in the rat hypothalamus and induces thermogenic reactions, *Neuroendocrinology*, 50, 177, 1989.

Liposits, Zs., Paull, W. K., Wu, P., Jackson, I. M. D., and Lechan, R. M., Hypophysiotrophic thyrotropin releasing hormone (TRH) synthesizing neurons: ultrastructure, adrenergic innervation and putative transmitter action, *Histochemistry*, 88, 1, 1987.

Low, W. C., Farber, S. D., Hill, T. G., Sattin, A., and Kubek, M. J., Evidence for extrinsic and intrinsic sources of thyrotropin-releasing hormone (TRH) in the hippocampal formation as determined by radioimmunoassay and immunocytochemistry, *Ann. N.Y. Acad. Sci.*, 553, 574, 1989.

Lumpkin, M. D., Samson, W. K., and McCann, S. M., Arginine vasopressin releases thyroid stimulating hormone *in vitro* and *in vivo*, *Fed. Proc.*, 42, 973, 1983.

Maeda, K. and Frohman, L. A., Release of somatostatin and thyrotropin-releasing hormones from rat hypothalamic fragments *in vitro*, *Endocrinology*, 106, 1837, 1980.

Marsden, C. A., Bennett, G. W., Irons, J., Gilbert, R. F. T., and Emson, P. C., Localization and release of 5-hydroxytryptamine, thyrotropin releasing hormone and substance P in rat ventral spinal cord, *Comp. Biochem. Physiol.*, 72C, 263, 1982.

Martin, J. B., Boshans, R., and Reichlin, S., Feedback regulation of TSH secretion in rats with hypothalamic lesions, *Endocrinology*, 87, 1032, 1970.

Matsuishi, T., Yano, E., Inanaga, K., Terasawa, K., Isihara, O., Shiotsuki, Y., Katafuchi, Y., Aoki, N., and Yamashita, F., A pilot study on the anticonvulsant effects of thyrotropin releasing hormone analogue in intractable epilepsy, *Brain Dev.*, 5, 421, 1983.

McCown, T. J., Hedner, J. A., Towle, A. C., Breese, G. R., and Mueller, R. A., Brainstem localization of a thyrotropin-releasing hormone-induced change in respiratory function, *Brain Res.*, 373, 189, 1986.

Melander, T., Hökfelt, T., and Rokaeus, A., Distribution of galanin-like immunoreactivity in the rat central nervous system, *J. Comp. Neurol.*, 248, 475, 1986.

Merchenthaler, I., Vigh, S., Petrusz, P., and Schally, A. V., Immunocytochemical localization of corticotropin releasing factor (CRF) in the rat brain, *Am. J. Anat.*, 165, 385, 1982.

Merchenthaler, I., Csernus, V., Csontos, C., Petrusz, P., and Bela, M., New data on the immunocyto-chemical localization of thyrotropin-releasing hormone in the rat, *Am. J. Anat.*, 181, 359, 1988.

Merchenthaler, I., Meeker, M., Petrusz, P., and Kizer, J. S., Identification and immunocytochemical localization of a new thyrotropin-releasing hormone presursor in rat brain, *Endocrinology*, 124, 1888, 1989.

Milaner, G., Zimmerman, E. A., Wilkins, J., Michaels, J., Hoffman, D., and Silverman, A. J., Magnocellular hypothalamic projections to the lower brainstem and spinal cord of the rat, *Neuroendocrinology*, 30, 150, 1980.

Mitsuma, T., Nogimori, T., Sun, D. H., and Chaya, M., Effects of histamine and related compounds on thyrotropin secretion in rats, *Horm. Res.*, 23, 99, 1979.

Mitsuma, T., Nogimori, T., Adachi, K., Mukoyama, M., and Andok, K., Concentrations of immuno-reactive TRH in spinal cord of patients with amyotrophic lateral sclerosis, *Am. J. Med. Sci.*, 287, 34, 1984.

Miyamoto, M. and Nagawa, Y., Mesolimbic involvement in the locomotor stimulant action of thyrotropin-releasing hormone (TRH) in rats, *Eur. J. Pharmacol.*, 44, 143, 1977.

Montoya, E., Wilber, J. F., and Lorincz, M., Catecholaminergic control of thyrotropin secretion, *J. Lab. Med.*, 93, 887, 1979.

Munsat, T. L., Lechan, R., Taft, J. M., Jackson, I. M. D., and Reichlin, S., TRH and diseases of the motor system, *Ann. N. Y. Acad. Sci.*, 553, 388, 1989.

Nagai, Y., Narumi, S., Nagawa, Y., Sakurada, O., Ueno, H., and Ishii, S., Effect of thyrotropin-releasing hormone (TRH) on local cerebral glucose utilization by the autoradiographic 2-deoxyglucose method in conscious and pentobarbitalized rats, *J. Neurochem.*, 35, 963, 1980.

Nair, R. M. G., Barrett, J. F., Bowers, C. Y., and Schally, A. V., Structure of porcine thyrotropin releasing hormone, *Biochemistry*, 9, 1103, 1970.

Nicoll, R. A., Excitatory action of TRH on spinal motoneurons, *Nature (London)*, 265, 242, 1977.

Nishiyama, T., Kawano, H., Tsuruo, Y., Masahiko, M., Hisano, S., Adachi, T., Daikoku, S., and Suzuki, M., Thyrotropin-releasing hormone (TRH)-containing neurons involved in the hypothalamic-hypophysial-thyroid axis. Light microscopic immunohistochemistry, *Brain Res.*, 345, 205, 1985.

Oertel, W. H., Graybiel, A. M., Mugaini, E., Elde, R. P., Schmechel, D. E., and Kopin, I. J., Coexistence of glutamic acid decarboxylase- and somatostatin-like immunoreactivity in neurons of the feline nucleus reticularis thalami, *J. Neurosci.*, 3, 1322, 1983.

Ogawa, N., Hirose, Y., Mori, A., Kajita, S., and Sato, M., Involvement of thyrotropin-releasing hormone (TRH) neural systems of the brain in pentylenetetrazol-induced seizures, *Regul. Peptides*, 12, 249, 1985.

Oka, J.-I. and Fukuda, H., Properties of the depolarization induced by TRH in the isolated frog spinal cord, *Neurosci. Lett.*, 46, 167, 1984.

Oliveras, J. L., Besson, J. M., Guilbaud, G., and Liebskind, J. C., Behavioral and electrophysiological evidence of pain inhibition from midbrain stimulation in the cat, *Exp. Brain Res.*, 20, 32, 1979.

Ono, H. and Fukuda, H., Ventral root depolarization and spinal reflex augmentation by a TRH analogue in rat spinal cord, *Neuropharmacology*, 21, 739, 1982.

Osbahr, A. J., Nemeroff, C. B., Luttinger, D., Mason, G. A., and Prange, A. J., Jr., Neurotensin-induced antinociception in mice: antagonism by thyrotropin-releasing hormone, *J. Pharmacol. Exp. Ther.*, 217, 645, 1981.

Palkovits, M., Eskay, R. L., and Brownstein, M. J., The course of thyrotropin releasing hormone fibers to the median eminence in rats, *Endocrinology*, 110, 1526, 1982.

Palkovits, M., Mezy, E., Eskay, R. L., and Brownstein, M. J., Innervation of the nucleus of the solitary tract and the dorsal vagal nucleus by thyrotropin-releasing hormone-containing raphe neurons, *Brain Res.*, 373, 246, 1986.

Pelletier, G., Demonstration of contacts between neurons staining for LHRH in the preoptic area of the rat brain, *Neuroendocrinology*, 46, 457, 1987.

Pelletier, G. and Leclerc, R., Immunohistochemical localization of adrenocorticotropin in the rat brain, *Endocrinology*, 104, 1426, 1979.

Porter, J. C.. Kamberi, I. A., and Grazia, Y. R., Pituitary blood flow and portal vessels, in *Frontiers in Neuroendocrinology,* Martini, L. and Ganong, W., Eds., Oxford University Press, London, 1978, 145.

Prange, A. J., Jr., Breese, G. R., Jahnke, G. D., Martin, B. R., Cooper, B. R., Cott, J. M., Wilson, I. C., Alltop, L. B., Lipton, M. A., Bissette, G., Nemeroff, C. B., and Loosen, P. T., Modification of pentobarbital effects by natural and synthetic polypeptides: dissociation of brain and pituitary effects, *Life Sci.,* 16, 1907, 1975.

Prange, A. J., Jr., Nemeroff, C. B., Loosen, P. T., Bissette, G., Osbahr, A. J., Wilson, I. C., and Lipton, M. A., Behavioral effects of thyrotropin-releasing hormones in animals and man: a review, in *Central Nervous System Effects of Hypothalamic Hormones and Other Peptides,* Collu, R., Barbeau, A., Ducharme, J. R., Rochefort, J.-G., Eds., Raven Press, New York, 1978, 75.

Raybould, H. E., Jakobsen, L. J., Novin, D., and Tache, Y., TRH stimulation and L-glutamic acid inhibition of proximal gastric motor activity in the rat dorsal vagal complex, *Brain Res.,* 495, 319, 1989.

Reichlin, S., Neural functions of TRH, *Acta Endocrinol.,* 276, 21, 1986.

Ricardo, J. A. and Koh, E. T., Anatomical evidence of direct projections from the nucleus of the solitary tract to the hypothalamus, amygdala, and other forebrain structures in the rat, *Brain Res.,* 153, 1, 1978.

Richardson, S. B. and Twente, S., Inhibition of rat hypothalamic somatostatin release by somatostatin: evidence for somatostatin ultrashort loop feedback, *Endocrinology,* 118, 2076, 1986.

Richter, K., Kawashima, E., Egger, R., and Kreil, G., Structure of porcine thyrotropin releasing hormone, *Biochemistry,* 9, 1103, 1970.

Riskind, P. N., Kolodny, J. M., and Larsen, P. R., The regional hypothalamic distribution of type II 5'-monodeiodinase in euthyroid and hypothyroid rats, *Brain Res.,* 420, 194, 1987.

Roussel, J. P., Tapia-Aranciba, L., Jourdan, J., and Astier, H., Effect of norfloxacin, a new quinolone, on GABA modulation of TRH-induced TSH release from perifused rat pituitaries, *Acta Endocrinol.,* 119, 481, 1988.

Roussel, J. P., Bulant, M., Nicholas, P. Vaudry, H., and Astier, H., A pre-pro-thyrotropin-releasing hormone (preproTRH) fragment causes potentiation of TRH-induced TSH release from perifused rat pituitaries, *Annules D'Endocrinologie,* 50, 148, 1989.

Saper, C. B. and Loewy, A. D., Efferent connections of the parabrachial nucleus in the rat, *Brain Res.,* 197, 198, 1980.

Sato, M., Morimoto, K., and Wada, J. A., Antiepileptic effects of thyrotropin-releasing hormone and its new derivative, DN-1417, examined in feline amygdaloid kindling preparation, *Epilepsia,* 15, 537, 1984.

Sattin, A., Hill, T. G., Meyerhoff, J. L., Norton, J., and Kubek, M. J., The prolonged increase in thyrotropin-releasing hormone in rat limbic forebrain regions following electrcoconvulsont shock, *Regul. Peptides,* 19, 13, 1987.

Sattom, A., Hill, T. G., Meyerhoff, J. L., Norton, J. A., and Kubek, M. J., The prolonged increase in thyrotropin-releasing hormone in rat limbic forebrain regions following electroconvulsive shock, *Regul. Peptides,* 19, 13, 1987.

Sawchenko, P. E. and Swanson, L. W., The organization of noradrenergic pathways from the brainstem to the paraventricular and supraoptic nuclei in the rat, *Brain Res. Rev.,* 4, 275, 1982.

Sawchenko, P. E. and Swanson, L. W., The organization of forebrain afferents to the paraventricular and supraoptic nuclei of the rat, *J. Comp. Neurol.,* 218, 121, 1983.

Sawchenko, P. E., Swanson, L. W., Grzanna, R., Howe, P. R. C., Bloom, S. R., and Polak, J. M., Co-localization of neuropeptide Y immunoreactivity in brainstem catecholaminergic neurons that project to the paraventricular nucleus of the hypothalamus, *J. Comp. Neurol.,* 241, 138, 1985.

Schmidt-Ackert, K. M., Askanas, V., and Engel, W. K., Thyrotropin-releasing hormone enhances choline acetyltransferase and creatine kinase in cultured spinal ventral horn neurons, *J. Neurochem.,* 43, 586, 1984.

Schoenen, J., Delree, P., Leprince, P., and Moonen, G., Neurotransmitter phenotype plasticity in cultured dissociated adult rat dorsal root ganglia: an immunohistochemical study, *J. Neurosci. Res.,* 22, 473, 1989.

Segerson, T. P., Hoefler, H., Childers, H., Wolfe, H. J., Wu, P., Jackson, I. M. D., and Lechan, R. M., Localization of thyrotropin-releasing hormone prohormone messenger ribonucleic acid in rat brain by *in situ* hybridization, *Endocrinology*, 121, 98, 1987a.

Segerson, T. P., Kauer, J., Wolfe, H. C., Mobtaker, H., Wu, P., Jackson, I. M. D., and Lechan, R. M., Thyroid hormone regulates TRH biosynthesis in the paraventricular nucleus of the rat hypothalamus, *Science*, 238, 78, 1987b.

Shapiro, R. E. and Miselis, R. R., The central organization of the vagus nerve innervating the stomach of the rat, *J. Comp. Neurol.*, 238, 473, 1985.

Sharif, N. A., Chemical and surgical lesions of the rat olfactory bulb: changes in thyrotropin-releasing hormone and other systems, *J. Neurochem.*, 50, 388, 1988.

Shioda, S., Nakai, Y., Sato, A., Sunayama, S., and Shimoda, Y., Electron-microscopic cytochemistry of the catecholaminergic innervation of TRH neurons in the rat hypothalamus, *Cell Tissue Res.*, 245, 247, 1986.

Shioda, S., Nakai, Y., Imai, C., and Sunayama, H., Co-existence of TRH with mesotocin in the same axon terminals of the bullfrog pars nervosa as revealed by double labeling immunocytochemistry, *Neurosci. Lett.*, 98, 25, 1989.

Siaud, P., Tapia-Arancibia, L., Szafarczy, A., and Alonso, G., Increase of thyrotropin-releasing hormone immunoreactivity in the nucleus of the solitary tract following bilateral lesions of the hypothalamic paraventricular nuclei, *Neurosci. Lett.*, 79, 47, 1987.

Simerly, R. B. and Swanson, L. W., Projections of the medial preoptic nucleus: a *phaseolus vulgaris* leucoagglutinin anterograde tract-tracing study in the rat, *J. Comp. Neurol.*, 270, 209, 1988.

Sobue, I., *TRH and Spinocerebellar Degeneration*, Elsevier, Amsterdam, 1986.

Sofroniea, M. V. and Schrell, U., Evidence for a direct projection from oxytocin and vasopressin neurons in the hypothalamic paraventricular nucleus to the medulla oblongata: immunocytochemical visualization of both the horseradish peroxidase transported and the peptide produced by the same neurons, *Neurosci. Lett.*, 22, 211, 1981.

Spindel, E. and Wurtman, R. J., TRH immunoreactivity in rat brain regions, spinal cord and pancreas: validation by high-pressure liquid chromatography and thin-layer chromatography, *Brain Res.*, 201, 279, 1980.

Stephens, R. L., Ishikawa, T., Weiner, H., Novin, D., and Tache, Y., TRH analogue, RX 77368, injected into dorsal vagal complex stimulates gastric secretion in rats, *Am. J. Physiol.*, 254, G639, 1988.

Swanson, L. W. and McKellar, S., The distribution of oxytocin and neurophysin-stained fibers in the spinal cord of the rat and monkey, *J. Comp. Neurol.*, 188, 87, 1979.

Swanson, L. W. and Kuypers, H. G. J. M., The paraventricular nucleus of the hypothalamus, cytoarchitectonic subdivisions and organization of projections to the pituitary, dorsal vagal complex and spinal cord as demonstrated by retrograde fluorescence double-labeling methods, *J. Comp. Neurol.*, 194, 555, 1980.

Tache, Y., Stephens, R. L., Jr., and Ishikawa, T., Central nervous system action of TRH to influence gastrointestinal function and ulceration, *Ann. N.Y. Acad. Sci.*, 553, 269, 1989.

Takayama, K., Ishikawa, N., and Miura, N., Sites of origin and termination of gastric vagus preganglionic neurons: an HRP study in the rat, *J. Auton. Nerv. Syst.*, 6, 211, 1982.

Takahashi, T., Thyrotropin-releasing hormone mimics descending slow synaptic potentials in rat spinal motoneurons, *Proc. R. Soc. Lond. Ser. B*, 225, 391, 1985.

Tatemoto, K., Cariquist, M., and Mutt, V., Neuropeptide Y — a novel peptide with structural similarities to peptide YY and pancreatic polypeptide, *Nature (London)*, 296, 659, 1982.

Toni, R., Jackson, I. M. D., and Lechan, R. M., Neuropeptide Y-immunoreactive innervation of thyrotropin-releasing hormone-synthesizing neurons in the rat hypothalamic paraventricular nucleus, *Endocrinology*, 126, 2444, 1990a.

Toni, R. and Lechan, R. M., 1-Naphthol-pyronin B as a novel substrate for silver intensification: application to light and electron microscopic immunocytochemistry of neuroendocrine systems, *J. Histochem. Cytochem.*, 38, 1209, 1990b.

Toni, R., Jackson, I. M. D., and Lechan, R. M., Thyrotropin-releasing-hormone-immunoreactive innervation of thyrotropin-releasing-hormone tuberoinfundibular neurons in rat hypothalamus: anatomical basis to suggest ultrashort feedback regulation, *Neuroendocrinology*, 52, 422, 1990c.

Toni, R., Jackson, I. M. D., and Lechan, R. M., Somatostatinergic innervation of TRH neurons in the rat hypothalamic paraventricular nucleus (PVN): evidence for unique specialization of contacts with thyroid hormone-responsive cells, *Abstr. Endocrine Soc.*, 1989.

Tonoue, T. and Nomoto, T., Effect of intracerebroventricular administration of thyrotropin-releasing hormone upon the electroenteromyogram of rat duodenum, *Eur. J. Pharmacol.*, 58, 369, 1979.

Tribollet, E. and Dreifuss, J. J., Localization of neurons projecting to the hypothalamic paraventricular nucleus area of the rat: a horseradish peroxidase study, *Neuroscience*, 6, 1315, 1981.

Tsuruo, Y., Hokfelt, T., and Visser, T., Thyrotropin releasing hormone (TRH)-immunoreactive cell groups in the rat central nervous system, *Exp. Brain Res.*, 68, 213, 1987.

Tsuruo, Y., Hökfelt, T., and Visser, T. J., Thyrotropin-releasing hormone (TRH)-immunoreactive neuron populations in the rat olfactory bulb, *Brain Res.*, 447, 183, 1988.

Van den Bergh, P., Kelly, J. J., Adelman, L.,Munsat, T., Jackson, I. M. D., and Lechan, R. M., Effects of spinal cord TRH deficiency on lower motoneuron function in the rat, *Muscle Nerve*, 10, 397, 1987.

Van den Bergh, P., Kelly, J. J., Jr., Soule, N., Munsat, T. L., Jackson, I. M. D., and Lechan, R. M., Spinal cord TRH deficiency is associated with incomplete recovery of denervated muscle in the rat, *Neurology*, 38, 452, 1988a.

Van den Bergh, P., Wu, P., Jackson, I. M. D., and Lechan, R. M., Neurons containing a N-terminal sequence of the TRH-prohormone (PreproTRH$_{53-74}$) are present in a unique location of the midbrain periaqueductal gray of the rat, *Brain Res.*, 461, 53, 1988b.

Vijayan, E. and McCann, S. M., Blockade of dopamine (DA) receptors with pimozide and pituitary hormone release in response to intraventricular injection of γ-aminobutyric acid (GABA) in conscious ovariectomized rats, *Brain Res.*, 162, 69, 1979.

Vijayan, E. and McCann, S. M., Effects of substance P and neurotensin on growth hormone and thyrotropin release *in vivo* and *in vitro.*, *Life Sci.*, 26, 32, 1980.

Vijayan, E., Samson, W. K., and McCann, S. M., *In vivo* and *in vitro* effects of cholecystokinin on gonadotrophin, prolactin, growth hormone and thyrotropin in the rat, *Brain Res.*, 172, 295, 1979.

Watkins, L. R., Suberg, S. N., Thurston, C. L., and Culhane, E. S., Role of spinal cord neuropeptides in pain sensitivity and analgesia: thyrotropin releasing hormone and vasopressin, *Brain Res.*, 362, 308, 1986.

Webster, V. A. D., Griffiths, E. C., and Slater, P., Antinociceptive effects of thyrotropin-releasing hormone and its analogues in the rat periaqueductal grey region, *Neurosci. Lett.*, 42, 67, 1983.

Weigand, S. J. and Price, J. L., Cells of origin of the afferent fibers to the median eminence in the rat, *J. Comp. Neurol.*, 192, 1, 1980.

White, S. R., A comparison of the effects of serotonin, substance P and thyrotropin-releasing hormone on excitability of rat spinal motoneurons *in vivo*, *Brain Res.*, 335, 63, 1985.

White, S. R., Crane, G. K., and Jackson, D. A., Thyrotropin-releasing hormone (TRH) effects on spinal cord neural excitability, *Ann. N.Y. Acad. Sci.*, 553, 327, 1989.

Wilber, J. F., Montoya, E., Plotnikoff, N. P., White, W. F., Gendrich, R., Renaud, L., and Martin, J. E., Gonadotropin releasing hormone and thyrotropin releasing hormone: distribution and effects in the central nervous system, *Recent Prog. Horm. Res.*, 32, 117, 1976.

Wu, P. and Jackson, I. M. D., Post-translational processing of thyrotropin-releasing hormone precursor in rat brain: identification of 3 novel peptides derived from proTRH, *Brain Res.*, 456, 22, 1988.

Wu, P., Lechan, R. M., and Jackson, I. M. D., Identification and characterization of thyrotropin releasing hormone precursor peptides in rat brain, *Endocrinology*, 121, 108, 1987.

Yakish, T. L., Dirksen, R., and Harty, G., Antinociceptive effects of intrathecally injected cholinomimetic drugs in the rat and the cat, *Eur. J. Pharmacol.*, 117, 81, 1985.

Yamada, M., Rudovick, S., Wondisford, F. E., Nakayama, Y., Weintraub, B. O., and Wilber, J. F., Cloning and structure of human genomic DNA and hypothalamic cDNA encoding human preprothyrotropin-releasing hormone, *Mol. Endocrinol.*, 4, 551, 1990.

Yamamoto, M. and Shimizu, M., Effects of a new analogue of thyrotropin-releasing hormone on pentobarbital-induced sleeping time in rodents, *Neuropharmacology*, 28, 863, 1989.

Yarbrough, G. G., Thyrotropin releasing hormone and CNS cholinergic neurons, *Life Sci.*, 33, 111, 1983.

Yen, C. T., Conley, M., Hendry, S. H. C., and Jones, E. G., The morphology of physiologically identified GABAergic neurons in the somatic sensory part of the thalamic reticular nucleus in the cat, *J. Neurosci.*, 5, 2254, 1985.

Yeung, J., Yakisn, T., and Rudy, J., Concurrent mapping of brain sites for sensitivity to the direct application of morphine and focal electrical stimulation in the production of antinociception in the rat, *Pain*, 4, 23, 1977.

Young, L. J., Winokur, A., and Selzer, M. E., Thyrotropin-releasing hormone in lamprey central nervous system, *Brain Res.*, 338, 177, 1985.

Young, R. A. and Davis, R. W., Yeast RNA polymerase II genes: isolation with antibody probes, *Science*, 222, 778, 1983.

Youngblood, W. W., Lipton, M. A., and Kizer, J. S., TRH-like immunoreactivity in urine, serum and extrahypothalamic brain: non-identity with synthetic pyroGlu-His-ProNH$_2$ (TRH), *Brain Res.*, 151, 99, 1978.

Zanisi, M., Messi, M., Motta, M., and Martini, L., Ultrashort feedback control of luteinizing hormone-releasing hormone secretion *in vitro, Endocrinology*, 121, 2199, 1987.

Zoeller, R. T., Wolff, R. S., and Koller, K. J., Thyroid hormone regulation of messenger ribonucleic acid encoding thyrotropin (TSH)-releasing hormone is independent of the pituitary gland and TSH, *Mol. Endocrinol.*, 2, 248, 1988.

Section III
Behavioral Neuroendocrinology

George F. Koob, Section Editor

11

Effects of the Steroid/Thyroid Hormone Family on Neural and Behavioral Plasticity

BRUCE S. McEWEN
Laboratory of Neuroendocrinology
Rockefeller University
New York, New York

I. Introduction

The term *neuroendocrinology* originally described the production of hormones by nerve cells and then came to encompass the feedback control of this hormone production by circulating hormones such as those of the gonads, adrenals, and thyroid gland (Meites et al., 1975). However, the current definition of neuroendocrinology recognizes the important behavioral and other neural actions of the circulating hormone products. Steroid hormone effects on behavior have been known from the studies of Berthold (1849), showing the effects of the testes on sexual, aggressive, and vocal behaviors in roosters. In this experiment, considered the first in the field of endocrinology, testes transplanted into the abdominal cavity of castrated roosters restored the behaviors that had disappeared as a result of castration. Because the transplanted testes were not reinnervated and were highly vascularized, Berthold correctly concluded that a blood-borne substance must be responsible for the changes and must be acting on the brain, among other organs. Subsequently, the pioneering studies of the late Frank Beach, W. C. Young, and Daniel Lehrman began to establish systematically the relationships between sex hormones and reproductive behaviors in a variety of animals (Beach, 1948; Young et al., 1964; Lehrman, 1964).

That steroid hormones act on the brain to produce their behavioral and neuroendocrine effects is a more recent finding, and it derives from experiments showing that crystalline sex steroid implants in the brain stimulate sexual behaviors and from the demonstration that the brain contains receptors for steroid hormones (McEwen et al., 1979). These receptors are of the type that interacts with the genome to alter expression of genetic information, and they mediate the long-term effects of steroids on behavior and brain structure and function. Recently attention has been directed at actions of steroids on the membranes of cells, leading to more rapid and direct effects on cellular function and neuronal activity. Furthermore, the brain appears capable of making certain steroids independently of the adrenals and gonads, and these so-called "neurosteroids" may have a unique role in the brain (Robel et al., 1987). Both membrane and genomic effects of steroids are increasingly seen as being involved in the alteration of behavioral states. This chapter will describe the receptors that mediate genomic effects and indicate what is known about the receptors that mediate membrane steroid effects. It will also describe the categories of genomic and nongenomic steroid effects on neural tissue

333

and give specific examples. Finally, there will be a discussion of the role of steroids in regulating integrated physiological and behavioral states.

II. Receptors That Act on the Genome

Around 1960, high specific activity tritiated steroids and iodinated thyroid hormone were synthesized, which allowed the detection of protein-binding sites in extracts of various tissues. Biophysical measurements and biochemical analysis established the binding proteins as putative receptor sites, with the property of binding to DNA (Jensen et al., 1982). Cell fractionation studies and autoradiography demonstrated that the cell nuclei are the ultimate destination of the labeled hormone in the cell (see Figure 1). Moreover, the cell nuclear sites constitute a limited number of the soluble receptors that have been transformed to enhance their DNA-binding properties. The recent cloning of steroid and thyroid hormone receptors has shown them to belong to a superfamily of DNA-binding proteins that regulate gene expression (Evans, 1988).

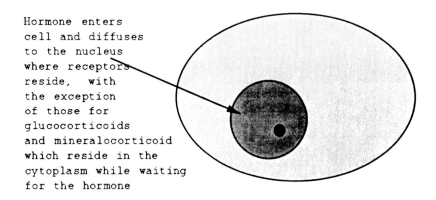

Receptors which are members of family

Estrogen	Glucocorticoid	Thyroid hormone
Androgen	Mineralocorticoid	Retinoic Acid
Progesterone	Vitamin D	

Hormone enters cell and diffuses to the nucleus where receptors reside, with the exception of those for glucocorticoids and mineralocorticoid which reside in the cytoplasm while waiting for the hormone

Structural domains of receptors which act as gene regulators

| N- | Modulator | DNA binding | Hormone binding | -C |

Figure 1. Receptors for steroid and thyroid hormones are members of a family of DNA-binding proteins that have a structure consisting of a DNA-binding domain, a hormone-binding domain, and a modulatory domain of less clear function. Hormone binding to the receptor leads to a conformational change in receptor structure (activation) that exposes the DNA-binding domain so that it can find the enhancer elements (short DNA sequences) in regulatable genes. Binding of the activated receptor to the enhancer with the aid of factors under control of the modulatory domain leads to enhancement of transcription. Most of the receptors in this family reside in the cell nucleus in the presence or absence of hormone, with the exception of the glucocorticoid and mineralocorticoid receptors, which appear to translocate to the cell nuclei when hormone is attached.

The brain contains receptors for all six classes of steroid hormones (androgens, estrogens, progestins, glucocorticoids, mineralocorticoids, and vitamin D) as well as thyroid hormone (Figure 1). These receptors have been demonstrated in brain tissue by direct binding assays, including autoradiography; by immunocytochemistry; and very recently by *in situ* hybridization histochemistry (McEwen et al., 1991). Each type of steroid receptor has a unique distribution in the brain, in neurons, and sometimes also in glial cells. In some cases these receptors interact with each other. For example, estradiol induces receptors for progesterone in cells of the uterus, pituitary, and hypothalamus. In other cases, steroid-metabolizing enzymes play an important role in governing access of steroids to particular types of receptors. For example, the aromatization of testosterone to estradiol is a property of neurons in the hypothalamus, but not of cells in the pituitary, with the consequence that testosterone-derived estradiol in male animals occupies hypothalamic estradiol receptor sites (McEwen et al., 1982).

III. Long-Term Effects of Steroid and Thyroid Hormone on Brain Cells

Genomic receptors for steroid and thyroid hormones mediate changes in gene expression, which are generally slow processes that last over many hours or even days. These changes affect many aspects of brain function, including such processes as inducing new synaptic structures and changing the amount of myelin, altering the biosynthetic capacity to make neurotransmitters, or increasing the number of neurotransmitter receptors in discrete brain regions. In some instances, these hormones affect the survival of neurons or accelerate their destruction. Many of these effects occur in the adult nervous system, but there exists a subset of hormone actions that occur during critical periods of early development. The following sections classify and describe some of these effects.

A. Protection and Destruction of Neurons

The hippocampus is particularly rich in receptors for adrenal steroids and contains two types, type I (high affinity for glucocorticoids and also for mineralocorticoids) and type II (lower affinity, also glucocorticoid specific). These receptors participate in the various effects of adrenal steroids on brain function and behavior, as will be discussed below. In addition, they mediate protective and destructive effects of adrenal steroids during a variety of natural or experimental conditions, such as ischemia, seizures, and aging (Table 1). The hippocampus, especially the subiculum and CA1 region of Ammon's horn, is vulnerable to neuronal loss as a result of ischemia, whereas it is the CA3 region that is especially sensitive to damage resulting from seizures and during the aging process. In spite of the disparate character of these events, a common denominator is the high levels of excitatory amino acids used as transmitters in the

Table 1
Damage to the Hippocampus

Cause	Regions most affected
Ischemia	CA1, subiculum
Seizures	CA3
Aging	CA3
High corticosterone	CA3
Stress	CA3
Adrenalectomy	Dentate gyrus

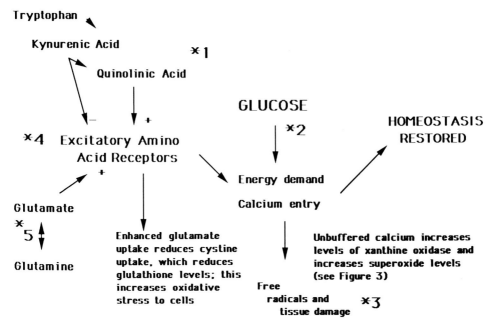

Figure 2. Schematic summary of the interactions between excitatory amino acids and cytotoxicity, showing control points at which glucocorticoids have been shown to exert positive or negative effects on cytotoxicity: (1) glucocorticoid treatment reduces quinolinic acid levels in brain; (2) glucocorticoids reduce glucose uptake, particularly in hippocampus. Note that if sufficient energy is supplied via glucose, the cell is able to re-establish calcium homeostasis, thus reducing the deleterious effects of unbuffered calcium ions; (3) glucocorticoids retard cellular damage related to lipid peroxidation, an effect that is mainly true of synthetic steroids like prednisolone; (4) glucocorticoids reduce levels of recognition sites for glutamate, particularly in hippocampus; (5) glucocorticoids induce glutamine synthetase, and glutamine is a sink for excess glutamate and at the same time a substance able to potentiate the effects of glutamate action via NMDA receptors. (For details, see McEwen, B. S. and Gould, E., *Biochem. Pharmacol.,* in press. Reproduced with permission.)

hippocampus. Moreover, it appears that glucocorticoids may play a key role in accelerating damage related to all three of these processes, possibly through interacting with the excitatory amino acid neurotransmitters and their effects on Ca^{2+} balance (McEwen and Gould, 1990).

What is the mechanism behind these glucocorticoid effects? One possibility is that energy supplies are rate limiting and that glucocorticoids inhibit glucose uptake sufficiently to disrupt the supply of ATP necessary to restore calcium ion homeostasis that is disrupted by high levels of excitatory amino acids (see Figure 2). Indeed, glucocorticoids inhibit glucose uptake in cultures of hippocampal neurons and even in hippocampal glial cells and do not appear to have such effects in other brain regions. Further support for this notion is provided by evidence that metabolizable sugars such as glucose can reduce the damage produced by excitatory amino acids in both the intact nervous system and cultured hippocampal neurons (Sapolsky, 1990).

Why is the CA3 region particularly sensitive to aging and seizure-related damage, as well as to high doses of glucocorticoids (Table 1)? Within 3 weeks, daily treatment with excess glucocorticoids initially causes the apical dendrites of CA3 neurons to shrink and atrophy and yet is without effect on CA1 pyramidal neurons. Perhaps, then, it is the input from the dentate granule cells, whose mossy fiber system innervates CA3 and does not innervate the CA1 region. What is the effect of glucocorticoids on the dentate gyrus? Absence of glucocorticoids after bilateral adrenalectomy causes dentate granule neurons to shrink in size and causes many granule neurons to die. It therefore appears likely that excess glucocorticoids may be maintaining the dentate gyrus neurons in a hyperactive state, while at the same time exacerbating the damage that their excitatory amino acids produce on the apical dendrites when released from the mossy fiber system (McEwen and Gould, 1990) (see Figure 3). It is interesting to note that the protective effect of glucocorticoids on survival of dentate granule neurons is also seen developmentally and may play a role in the development of the dentate gyrus (Gould et al., 1990).

The atrophy and death of CA3 neurons as a result of excess glucocorticoids may also occur as a result of severe and prolonged stress, as recent studies of vervet monkeys indicate (Uno et al., 1989). Death related to severe social stress in subordinate male vervets was accompanied by loss of neurons in the CA3 regions of Ammon's horn. Tantalizing as these results are, much more work is required to systematically set forth the conditions and time course under which stress affects neuronal plasticity. For example, recent work on catecholamine innervation of the cerebral cortex indicates that 1 hr/day restraint stress over 14 days causes increased innervation, whereas 6 hr/day of the same stress causes atrophy of catecholamine innervation (Sakaguchi and Nakamura, 1990).

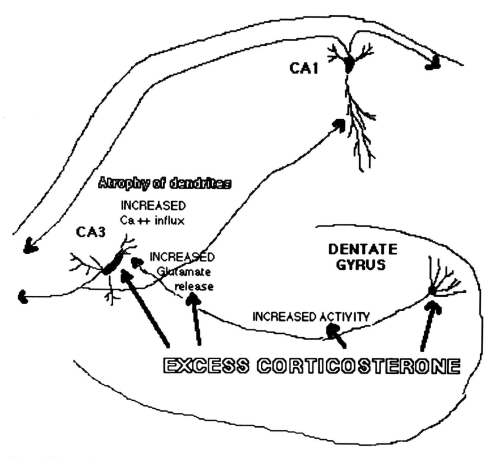

Figure 3. Schematic representation of a possible mechanism whereby chronic corticosterone (CORT) administration could affect adversely CA3 pyramidal neurons by altering dentate gyrus (DG) granule cell activity. Excess glucocorticoids could increase the release of glutamate (Glu) onto their CA3 target neurons, and the increased Glu acting on CA3 pyramidal neurons would result in increased Ca^{2+} influx, which would result in pyramidal neuron degeneration. (From McEwen, B. S. and Gould, E., *Biochem. Pharmacol.*, in press. With permission.)

B. Plasticity of Dendrites and Synapses

Not all of the effects of steroids are disruptive to brain morphology. Steroids also cause synaptic and dendritic plasticity, and some of this plasticity can be seen in naturally occurring endocrine cycles (Frankfurt et al., 1990; Woolley et al., 1991). Spines on dendrites of neurons in the ventromedial hypothalamus and the CA1 regions of the hippocampus undergo cyclic changes in density during the estrous cycle of the female rat, and estrogen replacement of ovariectomized female rats induces increased density of dendritic spines (see Figure 4). Electron microscopic evidence supports the notion that new spines are accompanied by new synapses. Thus synaptic and dendritic plasticity is a natural and cyclic phenomenon in the adult brain and is not relegated to early development.

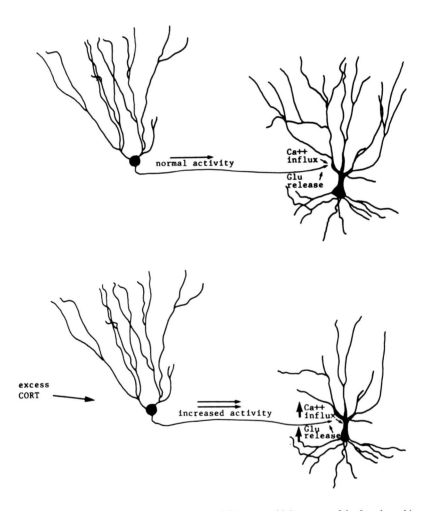

Figure 4. Camera lucida drawings of the apical dendrites of CA1 pyramidal neurons of the female rat hippocampus. (A) Control, ovariectomized rats; (B) estrogen-primed, ovariectomized rats. Note the increase in (B) in the number of dendritic spines with pronounced heads. Scale bar = 10 μm. (From Gould, E., Woolley, C. S., Miller, D. J., Begany, G. M., Brinton, R. E., and McEwan, B. S., *Abstr. Soc. Neurosci.*, 16, No. 144.17, 328, 1990. With permission.)

C. Hormonal Control of Neuropeptide Gene Expression

Steroid and thyroid hormone effects on gene expression are responsible for the regulation of neuropeptide gene expression in some brain regions or pituitary gland, as summarized in Table 2. Notable examples include the huge induction of galanin mRNA in pituitary by estradiol (Kaplan, 1988) and the negative regulation of pituitary proopiomelanocortin mRNA by glucocorticoids (Roberts et al., 1982). Corticotropin-releasing hormone (CRH) mRNA is also under negative control by glucocorticoids in the paraventricular nuclei of the hypothalamus (PVN), and the expression of vasopressin mRNA in CRH-producing parvocellular neurons of the PVN increases to detectable levels after adrenalectomy (for review, see Sawchenko, 1987). Preproenkephalin (PPK) mRNA is under positive control by estrogens in the ventromedial nuclei of the hypothalamus (Romano et al., 1989), whereas glucocorticoids regulate its level in the striatum and adrenal medulla (Chao and McEwen, 1990; LaGamma and Adler, 1987). Preprotachykinin (PPTK) mRNA is positively regulated in the striatum by glucocorticoids (Chao and McEwen, 1991). In the striatum, glucocorticoid regulation of the PPK mRNA and PPTK mRNA is superimposed on top of a diurnal rhythm, which persists to some degree after adrenalectomy, pointing to other controlling mechanisms (Chao and McEwen, 1990, 1991). Oxytocin gene expression can be regulated by estrogens because there is an estrogen regulatory element in the promotor region of the gene (Richard and Zingg, 1990); moreover, oxytocin mRNA levels are also positively regulated in some hypothalamic neurons by estradiol (Chung and Pfaff, 1990). Presumably, these hypothalamic neurons contain estrogen receptors.

D. Plasticity of Neurotransmitter Receptors

Steroid hormones induce increases and decreases in receptors for a number of neurotransmitters (McEwen et al., 1991). The following examples may be but a few of a larger array of effects of hormones on neurotransmitter receptor levels in the central nervous system. The induction by androgens of 5-HT1A receptors for serotonin in the male rat preoptic area may be a key regulatory step in the facilitation of male sexual behavior, because 5-HT1A agonists applied to this brain region stimulate this behavior. In a like manner, oxytocin receptors are induced by estradiol not only in the female reproductive tract but also in the ventromedial nuclei of the hypothalamus (VMN). The induction in VMN is of particular interest because of the role of the VMN in female sexual behavior in the rat and because progesterone has an effect of promoting an increase in the area of oxytocin receptors in the area surrounding the VMN. These phenomena will be described below. In neither of these two examples is it clear yet

Table 2
Steroid Hormone Regulation of Neuropeptide Gene
Expression

Neuropeptide	Known steroid regulators
Oxytocin	Estradiol
Vasopressin	Glucocorticoids
Corticotrophin releasing hormone	Glucocorticoids
Enkephalin	Estradiol, glucocorticoids
Galanin	Estradiol
Proopiomelanocortin	Glucocorticoids
Thyrotropin releasing hormone	Thyroid hormone

whether the hormone regulates the transcription of the gene for the neurotransmitter receptors. Such studies require the development of probes for the mRNA for each receptor type.

GABAa receptors are regulated by estrogens, and these effects are in opposite direction in hippocampus from the regulation seen in the hypothalamus and midbrain (Schumacher and McEwen, 1989). One reason for this difference might be the existence of multiple forms of the GABAa receptor subunits coded by different genes. The regulation of different receptor subunits by estrogens may differ in magnitude and even in the direction of the effect, although this possibility has not yet been demonstrated.

E. Developmental Influences and Sex Differences

Steroid and thyroid hormones act during critical periods of early development to trigger permanent changes in cellular differentiation and morphology within the brain. Thyroid hormone levels are tightly regulated, and deviations above or below these levels are associated with abnormalities in development of normal brain structure and function (Nunez, 1984). Testosterone, on the other hand, is secreted in males, but not in females, during perinatal development and is responsible for differentiation of male secondary sex characteristics as well as structures and processes within the brain. Permanent, developmentally programmed sex differences in the brain were first detected in painstaking electron microscopic studies by Raisman and Field (1972) and then were subsequently found at the light microscopic level as well as in the realm of biochemistry (for review, see Arnold and Gorski, 1984). Examples of neural sex differences are now very plentiful, and one of them will be illustrated below in discussing the hormonal control of feminine sexual behavior in the rat.

Thyroid hormone excess or deficiency in the developing brain results in disordered neural development that is only partially reversible by subsequent correction of the endocrine defect. For example, early neonatal hyperthyroidism in the rat pup causes permanent alterations within the basal forebrain cholinergic neurons as well as the hippocampal formation and leads to less efficient learning of spatial tasks (McEwen et al., 1991). Hyperthyroidism causes increased cholinergic cell number and content in the septum of male, but not female, rats. It also causes dendrites of hippocampal CA3 pyramidal neurons to be larger and more extensively branched, with more dendritic spines. These features persist in the adult brain.

IV. Steroid Metabolism

Steroids are metabolized by brain tissue as well as by other tissues of the body. Some structural formulae for steroids and their metabolites are shown in Figure 5. Testosterone is converted (aromatized) to estradiol, whereas testosterone, progesterone, and deoxycorticosterone are reduced in the A ring to form 5α and 5β steroid derivatives, and these derivatives are subject to further metabolism; e.g., the reduction of the 3-keto groups to an alcohol. Such steroid metabolism plays a major role in genomic as well as nongenomic effects of steroids: e.g., estradiol and 5α-dihydrotestosterone are potent ligands for genomic effects, whereas 5α and 5β derivatives of progesterone and desoxycorticosterone are potent ligands for direct membrane effects (see below).

V. Rapid Effects of Steroids on Brain Cells

Although steroids are now thought of primarily as affecting genomic activity via intracel-

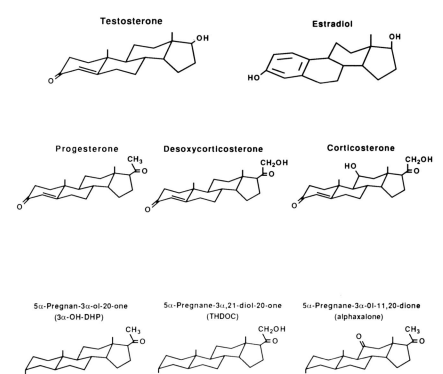

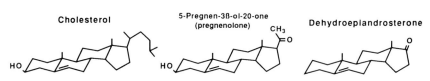

Figure 5. Some representative structures of steroids.

lular receptors, they were originally recognized for their rapid effects on the membrane. For example, the anesthetic properties of steroids were recognized and studied by the late Hans Selye (1942). There has been a resurgence of interest in such membrane actions of steroids, and the progestogenic steroids have led the way, particularly in relation to the GABA-benzodiazepine receptor system.

A. The GABAa Receptor

The GABAa receptor is one example of a receptor that forms and gates an ion channel, other examples being the nicotinic acetylcholine receptor and the N-methyl-D-aspartate (NMDA) receptor. As shown in Figure 6, the chloride channel of the GABAa-benzodiazepine receptor complex is highly sensitive to A ring-reduced metabolites of progesterone, such as 3α-hydroxy-5α-dihydroprogesterone, which are generated by enzymes in various parts of the body, including the brain, as well as to the A ring-reduced adrenal steroid metabolite, 5α-tetrahydrodesoxycorticosterone (THDOC). For structural formulas of these steroids, see Figure 5. Levels of THDOC are increased in stress and this leads to the concept that adrenal steroid metabolites may have inhibitory neural effects by potentiating activation of the GABAa-benzodiazepine receptor complex, and steroids that are active on the GABAa receptor have anesthetic, antiepileptic, and anxiolytic effects, which are potentially important physiologically as well as pharmacologically (Simmonds, 1990; McEwen, 1991).

Recent cloning of the various subunits of the GABAa-benzodiazepine receptor complex has revealed the existence of as many as 8 to 10 isoforms with the designations of α, β, γ, and δ. Expression of these cloned subunits in oocytes or kidney cells has led to the finding that pharmacological and physiological features depend on which isoforms are expressed. For example, the benzodiazepine sensitivity is conferred by the presence of the γ isoform together with α and β isoforms. Moreover, steroid sensitivity is associated most clearly with the coexpression of α, β, and γ subunits. What this means is that the drug or steroid sensitivity of these receptors is a feature conferred on the expressing cell by the protein structure, even though it is likely that membrane lipids play an important role in determining the final conformation and function of the expressed receptors (for review, see McEwen, 1991).

B. Calcium Ion Flux

Membrane actions of certain steroids lead to mobilization of calcium ions in neural and nonneural cells (McEwen, 1991). Progesterone, and several of its metabolites, which differ from those described above, activate Ca⁺ entry and mobilization in oocytes as well as in spermatozoa, leading to their functional maturation. Progesterone also facilitates release of a number of neurotransmitters, such as dopamine in the striatum and luteinizing hormone-releasing hormone (LHRH) in the hypothalamus, and it is possible that these effects also involve Ca^{2+} mobilization. Estradiol has also been reported to alter Ca^{2+} levels in endometrial cells. It is presently not clear how progesterone or estradiol interact with the membrane to alter calcium mobilization, whether by a cell surface receptor or receptor located within the cytoplasm where Ca^{2+} is sequestered.

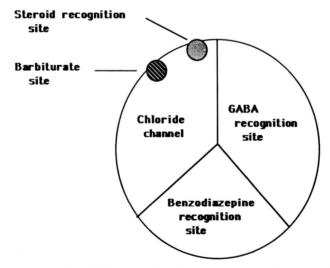

Figure 6. Functional divisions of the GABAa-benzodiazepine receptor complex, showing that the barbiturate and steroid regulatory sites are believed to be separate and to reside on the chloride channel domain.

C. Membrane Receptors

Many pharmacologists would prefer to study receptors by their binding properties, rather than by relying on characterizing just the response (Simmonds, 1990; McEwen, 1991). (It should be noted, however, that a binding site without a functional endpoint is not sufficient to be classified as a receptor.) Membrane receptors for steroids are difficult to demonstrate by direct binding assays because of the problem of nonspecific binding due to the stickiness of the membrane. Steroids immobilized on macromolecular supports have been used successfully in a few instances to demonstrate binding sites as well as to separate cells with steroid receptors on their surfaces. Recent work in an amphibian brain has demonstrated a binding site for corticosterone that is linked to a rapid, steroid-mediated suppression of mating behavior (Orchinik et al., 1990).

D. Rapid Electrophysiological Effects

One of the oldest and best means of characterizing membrane effects of steroids has been via their effects on electrical activity (Simmonds, 1990; McEwen, 1991). The more rapid the response, the more likely that it is a direct membrane effect rather than genomically mediated, particularly when the steroid is applied by pressure ejection or iontophoresis from a pipette next to the cell being recorded. Rapid electrophysiological effects have been described for estradiol, corticosteroids, and progesterone and some of its metabolites. Of particular interest are rapid effects of estrogens on neurons and on pituitary cells, as well as effects of estrogens on the response to excitatory amino acids and progestins on the response to glycine. Such effects strongly suggest that membrane actions of steroids are quite numerous and suggest that they may subserve a variety of physiological roles.

E. Neurosteroids

The steroids pregnenolone and dehydroepiandrosterone are found in brain tissue in both the sulfated and unsulfated forms and do not disappear from neural tissue after adrenalectomy or gonadectomy (Robel et al., 1987). Oligodendroglial cells convert cholesterol to pregnenolone and further to progesterone, indicating that the brain is capable of a limited degree of steroid formation (Jung-Testas et al., 1989). Yet the amount and type of steroids produced is not sufficient to substitute for those produced by the gonads and adrenals, and they must have some other role. The functional significance of neurosteroids is unclear, although effects have been described for these steroids, when exogenously administered, on memory and on aggressive behavior. Whatever their function, it is clear that the brain still depends to a very large extent on circulating steroid hormones for their major behavioral and neuroendocrine feedback effects.

VI. Integration of Hormone Actions to Regulate Behavioral States

One of the most visible consequences of the neural actions of the steroid/thyroid hormone family is the coordination of behavioral states with other events in the body. The behavioral changes that are produced and their coordination with nonneural processes is most evident in the case of reproduction, where sexual behavior is coordinated with fertility, and it is also evident in the diurnal cycle of sleep and activity, where metabolism is coordinated with food seeking and other behaviors related to the active state. This section will briefly describe examples of this coordination by concentrating on the influence of hormones at the neural level.

A. Sequential Actions of Estradiol and Progesterone on Feminine Sexual Behavior in the Rat

Estradiol and progesterone act synergistically during the 4-day estrous cycle of the female rat to activate reproductive behavior, referred to as lordosis behavior because of the concave arching of the back during receptivity caused by the mounting attempts of the male (McEwen et al., 1991). Hormone implant studies have revealed that the ventromedial nuclei of the hypothalamus (VMN) are the primary sites for the actions of estradiol and progesterone. Neurons in the ventrolateral VMN contain estrogen receptors and show induction of progestin receptors after estrogen priming. Giving estradiol to an ovariectomized female rat induces a rapid morphological and biochemical response in hormone-sensitive VMN neurons, beginning with decondensation of chromatin in cell nuclei and followed by enlargements of nucleolar, cell nuclear, and cell soma volume. Within a few hours there is more ribosomal RNA and an increased capacity for protein formation. Within 18 to 48 hr, the timeframe for the induction of lordosis, VMN neurons develop increased numbers of dendritic spines and with that new synapses as well. In addition, as shown in Figure 7, oxytocin receptors are induced in the VMN and spread laterally over 12 to 48 hr along the path where the VMN dendrites project. Estrogen priming brings about other changes in the VMN in GABAa receptors and muscarinic cholin-ergic receptors, as well as in the mRNA for enkephalin. However, it is the actions of progesterone that lead to the expression of the lordosis behavior, and these actions are rapid, taking as little as 30 min to 1 hr to be manifested. The effects of progesterone to activate lordosis in estrogen-primed female rats involve both protein synthetic mechanisms and local membrane actions. The protein synthesis inhibitor, anisomycin, blocks progestin activation of lordosis. However, the effects of progesterone on oxytocin receptors apparently do not involve protein synthetic mechanisms (see below). Thus both genomic and nongenomic mechanisms appear to be involved in the control of lordosis behavior.

B. Interactions Between Genomic and Nongenomic Mechanisms in the Control of Lordosis Behavior

Some membrane effects of steroids are independent of priming by circulating hormones, while other effects, such as the rapid electrical effects of iontophoretically applied estradiol in the preoptic area, are dependent on the stage of the ovarian cycle. Local membrane actions of

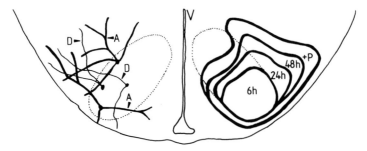

Figure 7. Schematic diagram showing the time course of spread of the oxytocin receptor field as a function of up to 48 hr of estrogen priming, as well as the effects of progesterone treatment in estrogen-primed animals, which induces further spread of the receptor field within 1 hr. (Based on Schumacher et al., 1990.)

progesterone on the oxytocin receptors of the VMN become evident after estrogen priming has induced a four- to fivefold increase in receptor density over a time course consistent with a genomic action (McEwen et al., 1991). As shown in Figure 7, the progesterone effects lead to an increase in the area occupied by the oxytocin receptors as if receptors are either moving along dendrites of VMN neurons or else are rapidly activated from a low- to a high-affinity state. These effects can be seen *in vivo* and can be duplicated by progesterone applied *in vitro* to sections prepared for the autoradiographic labeling of oxytocin receptors (Schumacher et al., 1990).

C. Sexual Differentiation in the Ventromedial Nuclei of the Hypothalamus

Because of its key role in feminine sexual behavior, which is sexually dimorphic in the rat, the ventromedial nuclei of the hypothalamus (VMN) have been studied extensively for morphological and neurochemical sex differences (McEwen et al., 1991). Synapses on dendritic spines and shafts are more numerous in males than in females in the VMN, and yet the estrogenic induction of spines, and presumably new synapses, on VMN dendrites occurs in females and not in males; in other words, the female has spine synapses that are more regulatable than the male, but the male appears to have more synaptic connections of both the spine and nonspine variety than the female. An analogous situation applies as far as the spread of oxytocin receptors in the area lateral to the VMN in response to progesterone, in that progesterone induces spread in the caudal VMN of the female but not in the male. However, it should be noted that the male has a larger area of oxytocin receptors in the area lateral to the VMN than the female after the estrogen priming but before progesterone treatment. The lack of a progesterone-induced spread of receptors in males fits with the almost total lack of male sensitivity to progesterone with regard to showing female-like sexual behavior, and it is also consistent with the lesser degree of induction of intracellular progestin receptors in male VMN compared to female VMN.

Thus estrogen induction of progestin receptors and of spines on dendrites is much greater in the VMN of gonadectomized females than in gonadectomized males, whereas estrogen induction of oxytocin receptors is not deficient in males. How are we to understand these differences? As shown in Figure 8, one possibility is that the estrogen-controlled events occur in different cell types in the VMN, each of which can be affected differently by the process of sexual differentiation. The other possibility is that these events occur in the same cells, with each effect involving a different set of transcriptional regulators that can be independently sexual differentiated.

D. Adrenal Steroids as Coordinators of Activity-Sleep Cycles and Ingestive Behaviors

Adrenal steroids are key participants in maintaining salt and water homeostasis (mineralocorticoids); in diurnal rhythms of sleeping, waking, and consuming and metabolizing food (glucocorticoids); and in restoring homeostasis after stress (glucocorticoids). Many of these effects appear to involve the type I and type II adrenal steroid receptors that were described earlier (McEwen et al., 1990).

With regard to salt appetite, there are three types: (1) adrenalectomy induced, (2) aldosterone induced, and (3) sodium depletion induced. Whereas 1 and 2 are unlikely to occur naturally, type 3 is a physiopathological response, since there are natural conditions that can cause sodium depletion. This form of salt appetite appears to involve the synergistic interaction between aldosterone and angiotensin somewhere within the confines of the blood-brain

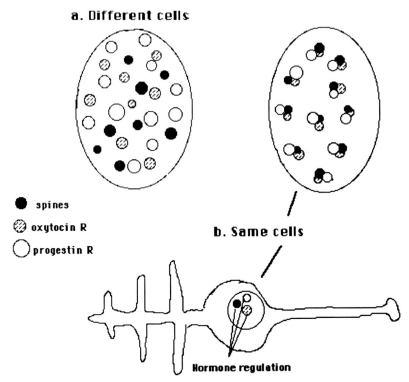

Figure 8. Two possible schemes for understanding sex differences in estrogen regulation of spine density, oxytocin receptors, and progestin receptors in the ventromedial hypothalamus (VMN) of the rat brain. (a) Estrogen-regulated characteristics may reside in different cells in the VMN; (b) estrogen-regulated characteristics may reside in the same, or at least overlapping, population of cells, in which case the basis of the sex differences or lack thereof would be at the genomic level.

barrier. The specific type I receptor blocker, Ru28318, blocks this appetite, when applied intracranially, and angiotensin receptor antagonists also block the appetite (Sakai et al., 1986). Studies are currently underway to identify which type I receptors may be involved. This is an important question, because type I receptors have the same affinity for the natural glucocorticoid, corticosterone, as they do for aldosterone, and corticosterone is present in 100- to 1000-fold excess over aldosterone. Nevertheless, in the kidney there is a mechanism by which type I receptors bind aldosterone, and a search is underway for a similar mechanism in the brain. In the kidney, the enzyme, 11β-hydroxysteroid dehydrogenase (11-DH), metabolizes corticosterone and not aldosterone, thus allowing aldosterone access to the type I receptors (Funder et al., 1988; Edwards et al., 1988). The brain also has 11-DH, but it is still not proved that 11-DH does the same thing that it does in the kidney.

Type I receptors are also implicated in effects of adrenal steroids to maintain normal food intake and body weight, and in the increases in body weight that occur in rats with lesions of the VMN and paraventricular nucleus (PVN) (King, 1988; Devenport et al., 1989). Other actions of adrenal steroids on feeding are related to the wake-sleep cycle, and the adrenal steroid peak always precedes the waking period and appears to act as a "wake-up" call, increasing locomotor activity and food-seeking behavior. In fact, food deprivation is one of the most powerful signals to increase corticosterone levels, and rats can have their diurnal corticosterone rhythms "food shifted" by providing access to food for only several hours per day (Krieger, 1974). Under these conditions, the corticosterone peak shifts to precede the expected time of food presentation. Corticosterone is also implicated in the diurnal rhythm of neurochemical events within the PVN, where noradrenergic activity stimulates feeding behavior. α_2-Adrenergic receptors show a diurnal rhythm that correlates with the peak of corticosterone, and corticosterone treatment of adrenalectomized rats increases α_2-adrenergic receptor density in the PVN (Jhanwar-Uniyal et al., 1986) (see Figure 9).

E. The Pathological Aspects of Glucocorticoid Action

Adrenal steroids participate in protective as well as damaging effects on the organism related to the adaptation to stress and the consequences of repeated stress. As shown in Figure 10, too much or too little glucocorticoid in the circulation can have deleterious consequences for the organism. One way of viewing the protective actions of adrenal steroids is as a buffer against the primary response of many physiological systems to stressful challenge (Munck et al., 1984). For example, inflammation is counteracted by the anti-inflammatory actions of glucocorticoids; and swelling and edema are counteracted by glucocorticoids. In the brain,

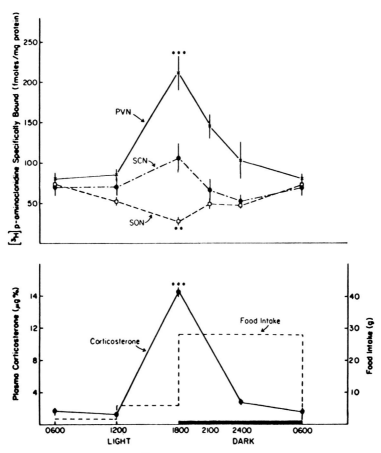

Figure 9. Diurnal variation of the binding of [³H]p-aminoclonidine to α2-adrenergic receptors in the paraventricular (PVN), suprachiasmatic (SCN), and supraoptic (SON) nuclei of the rat hypothalamus. Also shown are the plasma corticosterone levels (mean μg% ± SEM) at five time points during the course of 24 h, as well as food intake during the light and dark periods. Solid horizontal bars represent the dark phase of the 12:12 light:dark cycle. **, $p < 0.01$; ***, $p < 0.001$, as compared to values at preceding and succeeding time points. (From Jhanwar-Uniyal, M., Roland, C., and Leibowitz, S., *Life Sci.,* 38, 473, 1986. With permission.)

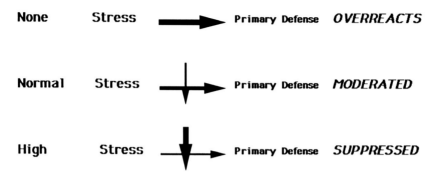

Figure 10. Glucocorticoids are involved in both protection of the organism and damage. Normal levels of glucocorticoids moderate the primary responses of the body and brain to stressful challenge and buffer them against large or prolonged responses. Lack of glucocorticoids allows the primary responses to stressful challenge to go unchecked, whereas high levels of glucocorticoids suppress the primary responses to such a degree that the body and brain are adversely affected by the stressful challenge.

glucocorticoids secreted in stress reduce the postsynaptic responsiveness of the noradrenergic system in the cerebral cortex. Why then is stress damaging? Apparently, it is so because glucocorticoid secretion must be shut off after stress in order to avoid deleterious effects of prolonged exposure, such as the neuronal death described above or the well-known phenomenon of immunosuppression. When glucocorticoid secretion is shut off efficiently after stress, then glucocorticoids can have their protective action with minimal negative consequences (McEwen et al., 1990).

What shuts off glucocorticoid secretion? Apparently, this is accomplished by neural control in which the hippocampus plays a significant role. The old idea that glucocorticoid negative feedback is the shut-off signal has been replaced by the notion that the diurnal rhythm of glucocorticoids primes the brain to efficiently shut off adrenocorticotropic hormone (ACTH) secretion after stress, even in the absence of a rise in circulating glucocorticoids (Jacobson et al., 1988). It is not clear which part of the brain maintains these interactions. However, lesions of the hippocampus lead to glucocorticoid hypersecretion during and after stress, and hippocampal damage in aging rats is associated with inefficient shut-off of the pituitary-adrenal stress response (McEwen et al., 1990). Moreover, fimbria-fornix transection leads to elevated levels of CRH mRNA in the PVN, and the output pathway for this effect seems to involve the bed nucleus of the stria terminalis as a way station. Thus the hippocampus is an important part of the regulation of pituitary-adrenal function and is also vulnerable to the damaging effects of a number of agents, many of which produce effects that are exacerbated by elevated circulating glucocorticoid levels.

What determines the set point for operation of the pituitary adrenal axis during the lifetime and thus influences the degree to which stress and glucocorticoids may impact on the brain? Figure 11 summarizes our current understanding of the continuing interactions between the environment and the brain during the life span, emphasizing that the developmental process is a cascade of events that alter the state of the neuroendocrine system and brain to respond to later challenges. More specifically, it has been shown that unpredictable prenatal stress in rats produces a permanent increase in emotionality and pituitary-adrenal reactivity, whereas postnatal handling of rat pups produces the opposite developmental effect (Wakshlak and Weinstock, 1990). Indeed, postnatal handling can wipe out the effects of prenatal stress on emotionality (Wakshlak and Weinstock, 1990). One consequence of handling is that the aging process is slowed down, at least in terms of hippocampal neuronal degeneration (Meaney et al., 1988). It is attractive to think of this slowing down as the result of the lower levels of circulating

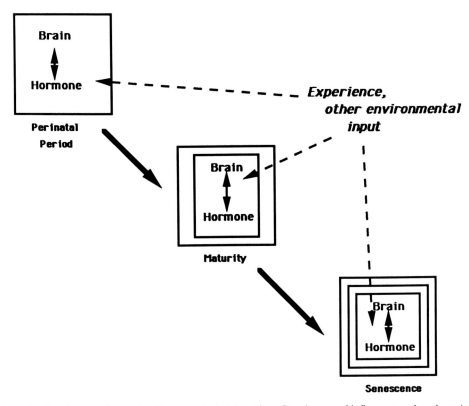

Figure 11. Developmental cascade of hormone-brain interactions. Developmental influences, such as the actions of sex hormones to promote sexual differentiation or the effects of prenatal stress or postnatal experience, shape the development of the brain, making it respond differently to environmental input in the mature state. Different set points of operation of neuroendocrine systems as a result of events early in life determine not only the operation of the mature neuroendocrine system but also the impact of environmental factors on the aging of the brain.

glucocorticoids produced during and in the aftermath of stress in the handled animals because of their more efficient shut-off mechanism. It has not yet been established whether random prenatal stress has the opposite consequence on the rat as hippocampal aging.

A final cautionary note is in order. Because glucocorticoids exacerbate the effects of a variety of neuropathological insults on hippocampal morphology, it is attractive to wonder whether neurodegenerative diseases like Alzheimer's disease can be caused or at least exacerbated by stress. Stress is not a likely cause of Alzheimer's disease, although it is possible that it may be a factor in the rate of pathogenesis in susceptible individuals whose disease is precipitated by other causes. Moreover, the question of whether repeated stress can cause brain damage and has been reported so far in only one opportunistic study (Uno et al., 1989), and much more systematic work is in order to establish the connection between stress and changes in brain morphology and neurochemistry.

References

Arnold, A. and Gorski, R.A., Gonadal steroid induction of structural sex differences in the central nervous system, *Annu. Rev. Neurosci.*, 7, 413, 1984.

Beach, F., *Hormones and Behavior: a Study of Interrelationships between Endocrine Secretions and Patterns of Overt Response*, Paul B. Hoeber, New York, 1948.

Berthold, A. A., Transplantation der Hoden, *Arch. Anat. Physiol. Wiss. Med.,* 16, 42, 1849.

Chao, H. and McEwen, B. S., Glucocorticoid regulation of preproenkephalin messenger ribonucleic acid in the rat striatum, *Endocrinology,* 126, 3124, 1990.

Chao, H. and McEwen, B. S., Glucocorticoid regulation of neuropeptide mRNAs in the rat striatum, *Mol. Brain Res.,* 9, 307, 1991.

Chung, S. K. and Pfaff, D. W., Estrogen influences on oxytocin mRNA expression in preoptic and anterior hypothalamic regions studied by *in situ* hybridization, *Abstr. Soc. Neurosci.,* 16, No. 526.1, 1990.

Devenport, L., Knehans, A., Sundstrom, A., and Thomas, T., Corticosterone's dual metabolic actions, *Life Sci.,* 45, 1389, 1989.

Edwards, C., Burt, D., McIntyre, M., DeKloet, R., Stewart, P., Brett, L., Sutanto, W., and Monder, C., Localization of 11-beta-hydroxysteroid dehydrogenase-tissue specific protector of the mineralo-corticoid receptor, *Lancet,* ii, 986, 1988.

Evans, R., The steroid and thyroid hormone receptor superfamily, *Science,* 240, 889, 1988.

Frankfurt, M., Gould, E., Woolley, C., and McEwen, B. S., Gonadal steroids modify dendritic spine density in ventromedial hypothalamic neurons: a Golgi study in the adult rat, *Neuroendocrinology,* 51, 530, 1990.

Funder, J., Pierce, P., Smith, R., and Smith, A., Mineralocorticoid action: target tissue specificity is enzyme, not receptor, mediated, *Science,* 242, 583, 1988.

Gould, E., Woolley, C. S., Miller, D. J., Begany, G. M., Brinton, R. E., and McEwen, B. S., The stress non-responsive period permits naturally occurring cell death in the developing dentate gyrus, *Abstr. Soc. Neurosci.,* 16, No. 144.17, 328, 1990.

Jacobson, L., Akana, S., Cascio, C., Shinsako, J., and Dallman, M., Circadian variations in plasma corticosterone permit normal termination of adrenocorticotropin responses to stress, *Endocrinology,* 122, 1343, 1988.

Jensen, E., Greene, G., Closs, L., DeSombre, E., and Nadji, M., Receptors reconsidered: a 20-year perspective, *Recent Prog. Horm. Res.,* 38, 1, 1982.

Jhanwar-Uniyal, M., Roland, C., and Leibowitz, S., Diurnal rhythm of alpha-2-noradrenergic receptors in the paraventricular nucleus and other brain areas: relation to circulating corticosterone and feeding behavior, *Life Sci.,* 38, 473, 1986.

Jung-Testas, I., Hu, Z., Baulieu, E., and Robel, P., Neurosteroids: biosynthesis of pregnenolone and progesterone in primary cultures of rat glial cells, *Endocrinology,* 125, 2083, 1989.

Kaplan, L., Galanin is an estrogen-inducible, secretory product of rat anterior pituitary, *Proc. Natl. Acad. Sci. U.S.A.,* 85, 7408, 1988.

King, B., Glucocorticoids and hypothalamic obesity, *Neurosci. Biobehav. Rev.,* 12, 29, 1988.

Krieger, D., Food and water restriction shifts corticosterone, temperature, activity and brain amine periodicity, *Endocrinology,* 95, 1195, 1974.

LaGamma, E. and Adler, J., Glucocorticoids regulate adrenal opiate peptides, *Mol. Brain Res.,* 2, 125, 1987.

Lehrman, D., The reproductive behavior of ring doves, *Sci. Am.,* 211, 48, 1964.

McEwen, B. S., Steroids affect neural activity by acting on the membrane and the genome, TIPS, in press.

McEwen, B. S. and Gould, E., Adrenal steroid influences on the survival of hippocampal neurons, *Biochem. Pharmacol.,* 40, 2393, 1990.

McEwen, B. S., Davis, P., Parsons, B., and Pfaff, D., The brain as target for steroid hormone action, *Annu. Rev. Neurosci.,* 2, 65, 1979.

McEwen, B. S., Biegon, A., Davis, P., Krey, L., Luine, V., McGinnis, M., Paden, C., Parsons, B., and Rainbow, T., Steroid hormones: humoral signals which alter brain cell properties and functions, *Recent Prog. Brain Res.,* 38, 41, 1982.

McEwen, B. S., Brinton, R., Chao, H., Coirini, H., Gould, E., O'Callaghan, J., Spencer, R., Sakai, R., and Woolley, C., The hippocampus: a site for modulatory interactions between steroid hormones, neurotransmitters and neuropeptides, in *Neuroendocrine Perspectives,* Muller, E. and MacLeod, R., Eds., Springer-Verlag, New York, 1990, 99.

McEwen, B. S., Coirini, H., Danielsson, A., Frankfurt, M., Gould, E., Mendelson, S., Schumacher, M., Segarra, A., and Woolley, C., Steroid and thyroid hormones modulate a changing brain, *J. Steroid Biochem.,* 40, 1, 1991.

Meaney, M., Aitken, D., van Berkel, C., Bhatnagar, S., and Sapolsky, R., Effect of neonatal handling on age-related impairments associated with the hippocampus, *Science,* 239, 766, 1988.

Meites, J., Donavan, B. T., and McCann, S. M., Eds., *Pioneers in Neuroendocrinology,* Plenum Press, New York, 1975, 327.

Munck, A., Guyre, P., and Holbrook, N., Physiological functions of glucocorticoids in stress and their relation to pharmacological actions, *Endocrine Rev.,* 5, 25, 1984.

Nunez, J., Effects of thyroid hormones during brain differentiation, *Mol. Cell. Endocrinol.,* 37, 125, 1984.

Orchinik, M., Murray, T. F., and Moore, F. L., Novel steroid binding site on synaptic membranes may mediate stress-induced inhibition of sexual behaviors, *Abstr. Soc. Neurosci.,* 16, No. 315.12, 1990.

Raisman, G. and Field, P., Sexual dimorphism in the neuropil of the preoptic area of the rat and its dependence on neonatal androgen, *Brain Res.,* 54, 1, 1973.

Richard, S. and Zingg, H. H., The human oxytocin gene promotor is regulated by estrogens, *J. Biol. Chem.,* 265, 6098, 1990.

Robel, P., Bourreau, E., Corpechot, C., Dang, D., Halberg, F., Clarke, C., Haug, M., Schlegel, M., Synguelakis, M., Vourch, C., and Baulieu, E., Neuro-steroids: 3beta-hydroxy-gamma5-derivatives in rat and monkey brain, *J. Steroid Biochem.,* 27, 649, 1987.

Roberts, J., Chen, C.-L., Eberwine, J., Evinger, M., Gee, C., Herbert, E., and Schachter, B., Glucocorticoid regulation of proopiomelanocortin gene expression in rodent pituitary, *Prog. Horm. Res.,* 38, 227, 1982.

Romano, G., Mobbs, C., Howells, R., and Pfaff, D., Estrogen regulation of proenkephalin gene expression in the ventromedial hypothalamus of the rat: temporal qualities and synergism with progesterone, *Mol. Brain Res.,* 5, 51, 1989.

Sakaguchi, T. and Nakamura, S., Duration-dependent effects of repeated restraint stress on cortical projections of locus coeruleus neurons, *Neurosci. Lett.,* 118, 193, 1990.

Sakai, R., Nicolaidis, S., and Epstein, A., Salt appetite is suppressed by interference with angiotensin II and aldosterone, *Am. Physiol. Soc.,* R762, 1986.

Sapolsky, R., Glucocorticoid hippocampal damage and the glutamatergic synapse, *Prog. Brain Res.,* 86, 13, 1990.

Sawchenko, P., Evidence for a local site of action for glucocorticoids in inhibiting CRF and vasopressin expression in the paraventricular nucleus, *Brain Res.,* 403, 213, 1987.

Schumacher, M. and McEwen, B. S., Steroid and barbiturate modulation of the GABAa receptor, *Mol. Neurobiol.,* 3, 275, 1989.

Schumacher, M., Coirini, H., and McEwen, B. S., Behavioral effects of progesterone associated with rapid modulation of oxytocin receptors, *Science,* 250, 691, 1990.

Selye, H., Correlations between chemical structure and the pharmacological actions of the steroids, *Endocrinology,* 30, 437, 1942.

Simmonds, M., Ed., *Steroids and Neuronal Activity,* CIBA Foundation Symposium, John Wiley & Sons, London, 1990.

Uno, H., Ross, T., Else, J., Suleman, M., and Sapolsky, R., Hippocampal damage associated with prolonged and fatal stress in primates, *J. Neurosci.,* 9, 1705, 1989.

Wakshlak, A. and Weinstock, M., Neonatal handling reverses behavioral abnormalities induced in rats by prenatal stress, *Physiol. Behav.,* 48, 289, 1990.

Woolley, C., Gould, E., Frankfurt, M., and McEwen, B. S., Naturally occurring fluctuation in dendritic spine density on adult hippocampal pyramidal neurons, *J. Neurosci.,* 10, 4035, 1990.

Young, W., Goy, R., and Phoenix, C., Hormones and sexual behavior. Broad relationships exist between the gonadal hormones and behavior, *Science,* 143, 212, 1964.

12

The Behavioral Neuroendocrinology of Corticotropin-Releasing Factor, Growth Hormone-Releasing Factor, Somatostatin, and Gonadotropin-Releasing Hormone

GEORGE F. KOOB
Department of Neuropharmacology
The Scripps Research Institute
La Jolla, California

I. Introduction

The hypothalamic releasing factors corticotropin-releasing factor, growth hormone-releasing factor, somatostatin, and gonadotropin-releasing hormone all have prominent roles in controlling pituitary adrenal function. Corticotropin-releasing factor (CRF) stimulates the release of adrenocorticotropin (ACTH) and β-endorphin from the anterior pituitary. ACTH, in turn, stimulates the adrenal cortex to secrete glucocorticoids, which have widespread effects on metabolism, such as gluconeogenesis, increased insulin secretion, lysis of lymphoid tissue, increased gastric secretions, and reduced inflammatory and antibody responses. Indeed, the activation of this hypothalamic-pituitary-adrenal axis has long been considered one of the major indications of the existence of a state of stress.

Growth hormone-releasing factor (GRF) stimulates the release of growth hormone from the anterior pituitary. Growth hormone acts to produce continuous growth and enlarge cartilage during development. Growth hormone stimulates the synthesis of somatomedins in the liver, which also help regulate growth. Growth hormone also is important for the metabolism of proteins, fats, and carbohydrates with a major role to promote conservation of carbohydrate stores. As such, growth hormone produces increases in blood sugar, increases muscle glycogen, and inhibits the action of insulin. Growth hormone shifts the source of energy for the body to fats from carbohydrates.

Somatostatin inhibits the release of growth hormone secretion from the anterior pituitary. Somatostatin, however, also inhibits secretion in a variety of endocrine and exocrine glands. For example, somatostatin inhibits secretion of insulin and glucagon in the endocrine pancreas. Somatostatin also suppresses most gastrointestinal secretions, including gastrin, secretin, cholecystokinin, and vasoactive intestinal peptide. Somatostatin produces these effects by binding to receptors on the surface of target cells and activating second messenger systems.

Gonadotropin-releasing hormone (GnRH) is also known as luteinizing hormone-releasing hormone and controls the secretion of both follicle-stimulating hormone (FSH) and luteinizing hormone (LH). Endogenous GnRH is pulsatilely secreted from the hypothalamus, and GnRH secretion itself is controlled by feedback from the sex steroids. Administration of GnRH produces a rapid elevation of FSH and LH, which in turn stimulates increased secretion of gonadal steroids. Continued administration of GnRH for 2 to 4 weeks will desensitize GnRH receptors in the pituitary, producing a suppression of both gonadotropins and gonadal steroids; however, the regular pulsatile administration of GnRH does not desensitize the pituitary. GnRH antagonists act as competitive inhibitors at GnRH receptors, which are located on the cell surface of pituitary gonadotrophs.

These releasing factors that control the function of the anterior pituitary also are located in the brain, outside the hypothalamus, and are thought to play neurotropic roles in the central nervous system in addition to their classical roles as hypothalamic releasing factors. From a biological perspective, the function of these neuropeptides in the brain may be related to their classic hormonal action (Iversen, 1981). An excellent example of this possible homology of function is exemplified by the central nervous system action of corticotropin-releasing factor.

II. Corticotropin-Releasing Factor

Corticotropin-releasing factor has been localized in the central nervous system in the hypothalamus. A 41-amino acid polypeptide, CRF stimulates *in vitro* and *in vivo* ACTH and β-endorphin. It is thought to be the long sought-after hypothalamic factor with the specific function of releasing ACTH from the anterior pituitary (Vale et al., 1981). Cell bodies for CRF are localized to the paraventricular nucleus and project a dense fiber plexus to the median eminence. Subsequent work has revealed an extensive extrahypothalamic distribution of CRF cell bodies and fibers. CRF-stained cells are found in the central nucleus of the amygdala, bed nucleus of the stria terminalis, parabrachial nucleus, laterodorsal tegmental nucleus, substantia innominata, and some neocortical areas, and a few cells are observed in the hippocampus. The most densely stained CRF fibers are seen in the median eminence and neurohypophysis. High-density staining is also seen in the medial preoptic area, central and dorsal medial nuclei of the amygdala, the substantia innominata, and the parabrachial nuclei. Thus, the majority of CRF-stained cell groups and pathways is associated predominantly with the hypothalamus and brainstem and with limbic parts of the telencephalon (Figure 1). A system of CRF pathways appears to interrelate several systems in the basal forebrain, pons, and medulla that could be involved in the integration of autonomic and neuroendocrine responses (Swanson et al., 1983).

When CRF is directly administered into the central nervous system it produces an activation of CNS function. CRF administered intracerebroventricularly produces a long-lasting activation of the electroencephalogram. CRF also produces a depolarization and excitation of hippocampal pyramidal cells, and increases the firing rate of cells within the locus coeruleus. The locus coeruleus is a brain system thought to be of importance for attention to changes in internal and external events.

The cellular activation produced by central administration of CRF is accompanied by a dose-dependent behavioral activation. CRF produces a locomotor stimulation in rats that appears to be independent of direct mediation by the pituitary adrenal system. This activation is still observed in rats that have been hypophysectomized or pretreated with a synthetic steroid to shut off the pituitary adrenal activation. CRF administered centrally also potentiates the acoustic startle response. The acoustic startle reflex is an easily quantifiable muscular contraction in response to an intense acoustic stimulus. CRF increases startle amplitude, an effect that can be reversed by the benzodiazepine chlordiazepoxide.

More importantly for the homology of function hypothesis, CRF appears to potently

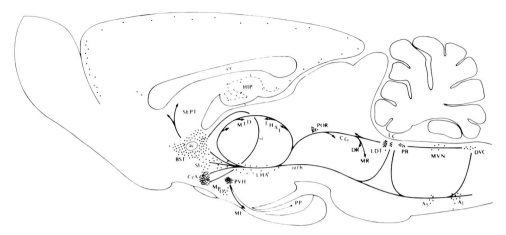

Figure 1. Major CRF-stained cell groups (dots) and fiber systems in the rat brain. cc, Corpus callosum; HIP, hippocampus; SEPT, septal region; ac, anterior commissure; BST, bed nucleus of the stria terminalis; SI, substantia innominata; CeA, central nucleus of the amygdala; MPO, medial preoptic area; PVH, paraventricular nucleus of hypothalamus; ME, medial eminence; PP, posterior pituitary; LHA, lateral hypothalamic area; mfb, medial forebrain bundle; MID THAL, midline thalamic nuclei; st, stria terminalis; POR, perioculomotor nucleus; CG, central gray; DR, dorsal raphe; MR, median raphe; LDT, laterodorsal tegmental nucleus; LC, locus coeruleus; PB, parabrachial nucleus; MVN, medial vestibular nucleus; DBC, dorsal vagal complex; A5, A1, noradrenergic cell groups. Arrows indicate potential terminal fields. (From Swanson, et al., *Neuroendocrinology*, 36, 165, 1983. With permission of S. Karger, Basel.)

exaggerate behavioral responses to stress (Koob, 1990). CRF decreases exploration in a variety of open field situations and decreases feeding in a novel open field, both characteristics of an enhanced stress response. CRF further enhances the suppression in behavior associated with conflict situations and conditioned fear. It also enhances fear-induced freezing in rats. However, these changes in response to anxiety and stress are not accompanied by changes in pain threshold.

At high doses, CRF can disrupt organized behavior. Rhesus monkeys, when injected intracerebroventricularly with CRF, showed behavioral withdrawal similar to the separation response. CRF can also, at high doses, suppress sexual behavior, feeding, and operant performance. Finally, CRF itself injected intracerebroventricularly is aversive. Animals will avoid places and tastes previously associated with intracerebroventricular administration of CRF. For a summary of the behavioral actions of centrally administered CRF, see Table 1.

Further support for a role for brain CRF in behavioral responses to stress comes from studies using a CRF antagonist, α-helical CRF. α-Helical CRF_{9-41}, a competitive antagonist for the brain CRF receptor, will reverse the behavioral effects of exogenously administered CRF and has some actions in non-CRF-treated animals. For example, the CRF antagonist administered intracerebroventricularly in rats reverses stress-induced suppression of feeding, blocks the development of stress-induced fighting, reverses stress-induced changes in exploratory behavior and freezing, blocks inhibition associated with a novel environment, blocks fear-potentiated startle, and blocks the acquisition of a conditioned emotional response (Table 2).

CRF administered directly into the brain also produces a variety of physiological effects that reflect stresslike activation of the body. CRF produces a prolonged elevation of plasma norepinephrine, epinephrine, glucagon, and glucose and also increases heart rate and blood pressure. The metabolic and cardiovascular changes are reversed by chlorisonadamine, an autonomic ganglionic blocker. The effects of CRF on sympathetic outflow and on the adrenal medulla appear to be mediated at a central site, since CRF-induced increases in plasma

Table 1

Summary of Behavioral Effects of Corticotropin-Releasing Factor

1. CRF injected intracerebroventricularly increases locomotor activity in a familiar photocell environment
2. CRF facilitates the acoustic startle response
3. CRF produces increased responsiveness to "stress" in an open field test
4. CRF has an "anxiogenic-like" effect in the operant conflict test
5. CRF produces enhanced suppression of responding in conditioned emotional response test
6. CRF produces a dose-dependent facilitation of stress-induced fighting
7. CRF produces an "anxiogenic-like" response in the plus maze
8. CRF produces a dose-dependent taste aversion and place aversion

Table 2

Summary of Behavioral Effects of CRF Antagonist, α-Helical CRF

1. CRF antagonist reverses CRF and stress-induced suppression of feeding
2. CRF antagonist blocks development of stress-induced fighting in rats
3. CRF antagonist reverses stress-induced changes in exploratory behavior in mice
4. CRF antagonist attenuates stress-elicited freezing in the rat
5. CRF antagonist blocks fear-potentiated startle
6. CRF antagonist blocks defensive withdrawal and reverses inhibition associated with a novel environment
7. CRF antagonist reverses "anxiogenic-like" effects of ethanol withdrawal
8. CRF antagonist blocks the acquisition of a conditioned emotional response

catecholamine concentrations are comparable in animals pretreated with intravenous anti-CRF serum. Also, these effects are not blocked by hypophysectomy or adrenalectomy.

The hypothesis that CRF has a direct neurotropic action in activating the sympathetic nervous system is supported by the observation that the CRF antagonist injected into the central nervous system attenuates the increases in plasma epinephrine levels produced by stressors such as hemorrhage, hypoglycemia, and ether exposure. The CRF antagonist injected into the central nervous system also attenuates the increases in arterial pressure and heart rate produced by treadmill running, suggesting that CRF is involved physiologically in mediating stress-induced cardiovascular responses (Fisher, 1989). The exact central nervous system CRF receptors responsible for these physiological actions of CRF are not yet known.

CRF inhibits gastric acid secretion and prevents gastric ulcerations produced by cold-restraint. It also inhibits gastric and small intestinal contractility and inhibits gastric emptying of a nonnutrient solution. Interestingly, stress-related changes in gastrointestinal (GI) function, such as inhibition of GI transit, are similar to those of central CRF administration in rats, and these effects also are not dependent on activation of the pituitary adrenal axis. The CRF antagonist, α-helical CRF_{9-41}, can prevent stress-induced inhibition of gastric emptying. The data suggest a role for endogenous central nervous system CRF in mediating stress-induced changes in GI function (Tache et al., 1990) (Figure 2).

Evidence suggests that the locomotor activation induced by CRF may depend on forebrain CRF receptors since obstruction of the cerebral aqueduct blocks the increases in locomotor activity produced by cisterna magna injections of CRF, but not the increases in locomotor activity induced by lateral ventricle injections. Other results show that local injections of low doses of CRF into the norepinephrine-containing system of the locus coeruleus in the pons can produce decreases in exploratory behavior, and the stress-inducing effects of CRF can be blocked by blockade of the central norepinephrine system. Thus the behavioral activation produced by CRF may involve forebrain CRF receptors, while the stresslike effects, both behavioral and physiological, may involve activation of norepinephrine systems in the pons and hindbrain.

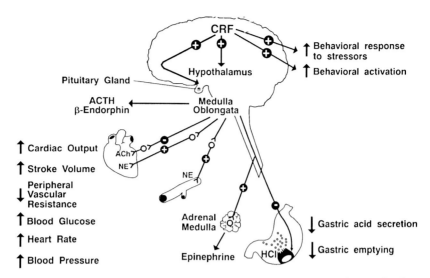

Figure 2. Schematic diagram depicting the classic hormonal function of corticotropin-releasing factor and its various neurotropic actions in the central nervous system.

III. Growth Hormone-Releasing Factor

Growth hormone-releasing factor (GRF) neurons are located in the arcuate nucleus of the hypothalamus with fibers extending to the median eminence. The terminals are located near the capillaries that drain into the hypophysial portal system, and it is through this system that GRF stimulates the release of growth hormone from the anterior pituitary.

However, as with CRF, there is evidence of a GRF neuronal system present in sites outside of the median eminence-hypophysial portal system (Sawchenko et al., 1985). CRF cell bodies are located in the caudal aspects of ventromedial hypothalamus and fibers project throughout the hypothalamus and adjoining parts of the basal telencephalon. These terminal sites include the anterior, periventricular, dorsomedial, paraventricular, suprachiasmatic, and premammillary nuclei of the hypothalamus as well as the medial preoptic, lateral preoptic, and lateral hypothalamic areas (Figure 3).

Administration of GRF directly into the brain stimulates food intake in rats and sheep. The observation that peripheral injection of either GRF or growth hormone itself does not induce feeding suggests that this also is a centrally mediated effect. Intracerebroventricular GRF increases feeding in both food-deprived and free-feeding rats. This feeding response to GRF appears to be dependent on photopcriod in that GRF facilitated feeding only during the light period but not during the dark. Further work has shown that GRF injected directly into the suprachiasmatic nucleus/medial preoptic area increases food intake dose dependently by increasing meal length and increasing the rate of eating. GRF also appears to increase the motivation to obtain food in that GRF increases operant responding for food reward. This motivational effect is consistent with the observation that GRF-induced feeding can be blocked by opioid antagonists (Vaccarino, 1990).

Perhaps more importantly, a GRF antibody injected directly into the suprachiasmatic nucleus/medial preoptic area decreased feeding associated with the onset of the active dark-phase feeding response in rats (Vaccarino et al., 1990). Together these results suggest that GRF may play a role in the central nervous system that may be functionally homologous to the role of growth hormone in the periphery to promote growth and protein synthesis (Figure 4). Thus, central nervous system GRF may have a role in the central regulation of hunger motivation and

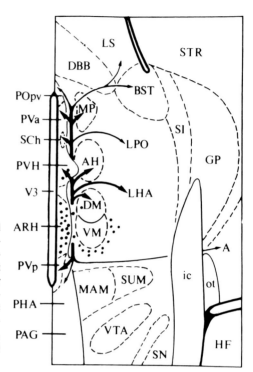

Figure 3. A drawing of a horizontal view of the basal forebrain of the rat to show the organization of rhGRF-stained neurons (dots) and extrahypophysiotropic projections (arrows). Thicker arrows represent more prominent projections. Abbreviations: A, amygdala; AH, anterior hypothalamic area; DM, dorsomedial nucleus (hypothalamus); HF, hippocampal formation; MP, medial preoptic area; STR, striatum; VM, ventromedial nucleus (hypothalamus). (From Sawchenko et al., *J. Comp. Neurol.,* 237, 100, 1985. With permission from Alan R. Liss, Inc.)

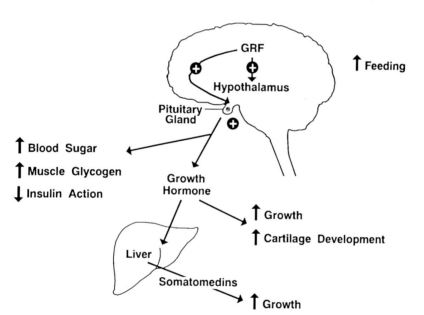

Figure 4. Schematic diagram depicting the classic hormonal function of growth hormone-releasing factor and its neurotropic action in the central nervous system.

thus be functionally compatible with the stimulation of growth produced by the GRF-GH connection.

IV. Somatostatin

As noted above, somatostatin has powerful physiological effects in inhibiting growth hormone release from the pituitary, and somatostatin is found in high concentrations in the basal hypothalamus. Most somatostatin (< 90%), however, is found outside the hypothalamus in the central nervous system. There are somatostatin neurons in the amygdala, midbrain neocortex, and hippocampus. Terminals have been seen in the extrapyramidal system as well as in the cortex, amygdala, and spinal cord (Figure 5).

When injected directly into the brain, somatostatin produces a variety of behavioral effects. Somatostatin increases motor activation and grooming and prolongs pentobarbital sleeping time, suggesting mild stimulant-like effects. Somatostatin also decreases food intake acutely but appears to increase food intake with chronic administration. There are reports of analgesic effects of somatostatin, but these apparently occur only at doses that cause toxic effects. At high doses, somatostatin can induce a toxic motor response in rats called barrel

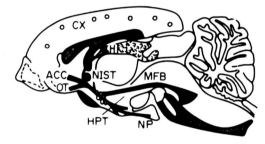

Figure 5. Diagrams representing distribution of somatostatin-containing neuronal systems. *Above:* sagittal representation. *Below:* coronal representation. ACC, Accumbens; CX, cortex; CP, caudate-putamen; F, fornix; HI, hippocampus; HPT, hypothalamus; MB, mamilary bodies; MFB, median forebrain bundle; NIST, nucleus interstitialis stria terminalis; NPE, periventricular hypothalamic nucleus; NPO, preoptic nucleus; NP, neurohypophysis; NVM, ventromedian nucleus; OT, olfactory tubercle; TO, olfactory tracts. (From Epelbaum, J., *Prog. Neurobiol.*, 27, 63, 1986. With permission from Pergamon Journals, Ltd.)

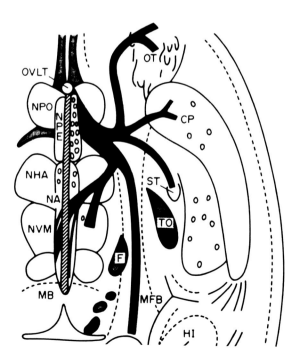

rolling, in which the animal loses equilibrium and rolls spontaneously. The continuous infusion of somatostatin and a long-acting somatostatin analog into the subarachnoid space of nonhuman primates produces dramatic neurotoxic effects, such as truncal ataxia, severe hypokinesia, and even some catatonia (Leblanc et al., 1988).

Somatostatin brain levels are decreased dramatically in patients with senile dementia (Alzheimer's disease). Somatostatin is also significantly decreased in patients with major affective disorders. Consistent with a possible role for somatostatin in cognitive function, somatostatin has been shown to improve performance in several learning tasks and to attenuate experimentally induced amnesia. In support of this hypothesis, depletion of central nervous system somatostatin using the drug cysteamine can produce deficits in learning of both appetitively and aversively motivated learning. A role for somatostatin in behavioral arousal, and as such, learning/memory, might be consistent with its role in the pituitary to reduce secretion of growth hormone in that this may be a means of shifting energy from homeostatic function to more motivated activities (Figure 6).

V. Gonadotropin-Releasing Hormone

As discussed above, GnRH induces the release of both follicle-stimulating hormone (FSH) and luteinizing hormone (LH). The anatomical basis for these hormonal effects is a significant septo-preoptico-infundibular GnRH pathway with cell bodies in the medial-septal and preoptic-suprachiasmatic regions that projects to the median eminence. However, there is also a widespread distribution of extrahypothalamic GnRH systems. There are cell bodies located in the olfactory bulb and olfactory tubercle, the diagonal band of Broca, medial septum, medial preoptic area and suprachiasmatic nucleus, and anterior and lateral hypothalamus (Figure 7). Four GnRH pathways have been described. One pathway originates in the septal preoptic area and projects to the preoptic area. A second pathway originates in the preoptic-suprachiasmatic-medial-septal areas and projects to the organum vasculosum lamina terminalis and the median eminence. A third pathway originates in the periventricular hypo-

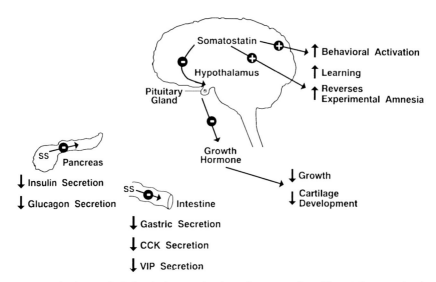

Figure 6. Schematic diagram depicting the hormonal actions of somatostatin and its putative neurotropic actions in the central nervous system.

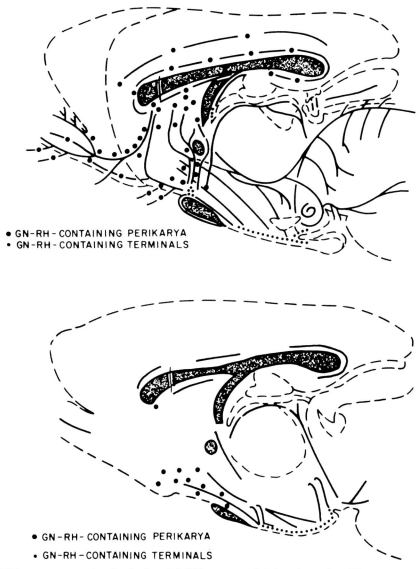

Figure 7. Diagrams representing distribution of GnRH neurons and their pathways in a 600-m*M* thick median-sagittal segment (top) and a 500-m*M* thick parasagittal segment (bottom) of the rat brain. (From Merchenthaler et al., *Cell Tissue Res.,* 237, 15, 1984. With permission from Springer-Verlag, New York.)

thalamus and projects to the median eminence, ventral tegmental area, and periaqueductal gray. A fourth pathway originates in the hippocampus and projects to the cingulum and cortex.

The presence of such a widespread distribution of GnRH neurons (Merchenthaler et al., 1984), and substantial physiological and behavioral evidence, suggest that GnRH may play a role in the coordination of reproductive processes with behavioral function. In the rat GnRH-induced release of luteinizing hormone is temporally linked to the onset of sexual heat in the female rat. Also, many of the same brain regions innervated by GnRH are implicated in the regulation of gonadotropin secretion and in the control of reproductive behavior.

In studies in rats, systemic administration of GnRH facilitates lordotic responsiveness in ovariectomized females primed with estrogen. The response is still observed in hypophysectomized or adrenalectomized rats, and even lower doses of GnRH directly injected into the medial preoptic area or arcuate nucleus of the hypothalamus facilitate lordotic responsiveness. More compelling evidence for a role of endogenous GnRH systems in behavior is the observation that antibodies to GnRH or GnRH antagonists infused into the lateral ventricle interferes with lordotic behavior in ovariectomized, estrogen-, progesterone-primed rats. Similar results are observed with injections of GnRH and anti-GnRH serum into the central gray. GnRH has also been shown to enhance sexual behavior in male rats. With a 2-hr pretreatment, GnRH decreased the latency to the first mounting response in male rats and decreased the latency to the first ejaculation. To summarize, there is some significant overlap of the brain sites involved in mating behavior, GnRH distribution, sites important for gonadotropin release, neurons that respond to GnRH electrophysiologically, and sites that concentrate estrogen (Moss et al., 1979) (Figure 8).

Recent work has shown that changes in the structure of the GnRH molecule can produce analogs that are very potent in modulating female sexual behavior but may not be active at enhancing LH release at the pituitary. A behaviorally active fragment of GnRH AC-LH-RH-(5-10) is effective in facilitating lordotic behavior when injected intraventricularly in ovariectomized, estrogen-primed rats but fails to alter LH release. This fragment also significantly enhances lordosis when infused bilaterally into the medial preoptic area, ventromedial hypothalamus, or midbrain central gray. These results suggest that only a part of the GnRH molecule may be required for behavioral activity and that some brain mechanism may exist to degrade GnRH to this and other possibly active metabolites (Dudley and Moss, 1988).

There is also evidence that GnRH may modulate the transmission of olfactory stimuli. GnRH-containing neurons are found in the olfactory bulb. Particularly intriguing is the presence of GnRH presynaptic elements in the accessory olfactory bulb of the Golden hamster; in the Golden hamster the accessory olfactory bulb is an important structure involved in the initiation of mating. Thus GnRH may play a role in coordinating physiological (gonadotropin secretion) and limbic aspects of reproductive function (olfaction and sexual behavior). As such

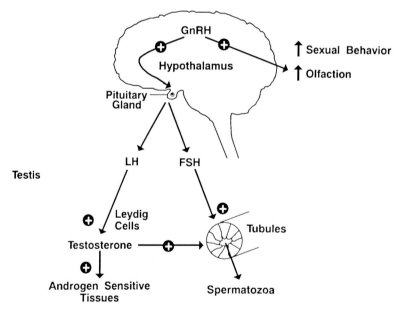

Figure 8. Schematic diagram depicting the hormonal actions of gonadotropin-releasing hormone and its neurotropic actions in the central nervous system.

the GnRH system provides a classic example of hypothesis of homology of function for a releasing factor involved in controlling hormonal function and a homologous behavioral function (Figure 8).

VI. Conclusions

Four hypothalamic-releasing factors have been discussed in terms of their classic physiological roles as inducers of hormone release from the anterior pituitary. Each of these factors is a peptide, and in addition to its hypothalamic infundibular connection has functional extrahypothalamic neuronal connections. For the most part, the functional significance of the extrahypothalamic projections of the peptides parallels their hormonal action. Corticotropin-releasing factor in the central nervous system produces behavioral and physiological activation and augments behavioral and physiological responses to stress. Growth hormone-releasing factor in the central nervous system induces hunger and facilitates feeding behavior. Somatostatin has some behavioral activating effects and facilitates performance in learning and memory tasks. Gonadotropin-releasing hormone induces sexual receptivity in female rats, may facilitate sexual behavior in male rats, and may have a role in mediating olfaction. From a biological perspective, the function of these neuropeptides in the brain may be an extension of their hormonal action and each neuropeptide may then be viewed as an integrator or coordinator of a major bodily function.

Acknowledgments

I thank the Molecular and Experimental Medicine Word Processing Center for their excellent help in manuscript preparation. Supported in part by a grant from The National Institute of Diabetes and Digestive and Kidney Diseases, DK26741. This is publication number 6599NP from the Research Institute of Scripps Clinic, La Jolla, California.

References

Dudley, C. A. and Moss, R. L., Facilitation of lordosis in female rats by CNS-site specific infusions of an LH-RH fragment AC-LH-RH-(5-10), *Brain Res.*, 44, 161, 1988.

Epelbaum, J., Somatostatin in the central nervous system: physiology and pathological modifications, *Prog. Neurobiol.*, 27, 63, 1986.

Fisher, L. A., Corticotropin-releasing factor: endocrine and autonomic integration of responses to stress, *Trends Pharmacol. Sci.*, 10, 189, 1989.

Iversen, S. D., Neuropeptides: do they integrate body and brain?, Nature (London), 291, 454, 1981.

Koob, G. F., Behavioral responses to stress-focus on corticotropin releasing factor, in *Neurobiology and Neuroendocrinology of Stress*, Brown, M. R., Rivier, C., and Koob, G., Eds., Marcel Dekker, New York, in press.

Leblanc, R., Gauthier, S., Gauvin, M., Quirion, R., Palmour, R., and Masson, H., Neurobehavioral effects of intrathecal somatostatinergic treatment in subhuman primates, *Neurology*, 38, 1887, 1988.

Merchenthaler, I., Gorcs, T., Sefalo, G., Petrusz, P., and Flerko, B., Gonadotropin-releasing hormone (GnRH) neurons and pathways in the rat brain, *Cell Tissue Res.*, 237, 15, 1984.

Moss, R. L., Riskind, P., and Dudley, C. A., Effects of LH-RH on sexual activities in animal and man, in *Central Nervous System Effects of Hypothalamic Hormones and Other Peptides*, Raven Press, New York, 1979, 345.

Sawchenko, P. E., Swanson, L. W., Rivier, J., and Vale, W. W., The distribution of growth hormone releasing factor (GRF) immunoreactivity in the central nervous system of the rat: an immunohistochemical study using antisera directed against rat hypothalamic GRF, *J. Comp. Neurol.*, 237, 100, 1985.

Swanson, L. W., Sawchenko, P. E., Rivier, J., and Vale, W. W., Organization of ovine corticotropin-releasing factor immunoreactive cells and fibers in the rat brain: an immunohistochemical study, *Neuroendocrinology*, 36, 165, 1983.

Tache, Y., Garrich, T., and Raybould, H., Central nervous system action of peptides to influence gastrointestinal motor function, *Gastroenterology*, 98, 517, 1990.

Vaccarino, F. J., Growth hormone releasing factor and feeding. Behavioral evidence for direct central actions, in *A Decade of Neuropeptides, Past, Present, and Future*, Koob, G. F., Sandman, C. A., and Strand, F., Eds., *Ann. N.Y. Acad. Sci.*, 579, 1990.

Vaccarino, F. J., Feifel, D., Rivier, J., and Vale, W., Antagonism of central growth hormone-releasing factor activity selectively attenuates dark-onset feeding in rats, *J. Neurosci.*, 11(12), 3924—3927, 1991.

Vale, W., Spiess, J., Rivier, C., and Rivier, J., Characterization of a 41-residue ovine hypothalamic peptide that stimulates the secretion of corticotropin and β-endorphine, *Science*, 213, 1394, 1981.

13

The Behavioral Neuroendocrinology of Arginine Vasopressin, Adrenocorticotropic Hormone, and Opioids

MICHEL LE MOAL, PIERRE MORMEDE, AND LUIS STINUS
INSERM Unit 259
University of Bordeaux II
Domaine de Carriere,
Bordeaux, France

I. Behavioral Neuroendocrinology of Vasopressin

A. Introduction

The principal physiological role of vasopressin (VP) is in the conservation of body water via its action on the kidney (for a review, see Sawyer and Manning, 1984). The pathological consequence of an impairment in vasopressin secretion is a pronounced and chronic diuresis (diabetes insipidus) (Hays, 1980). VP also has a vasopressor action, which is induced by hypovolemia and hypotension (Zerbe et al., 1982). Recent neuroendocrinological studies have extended these early physiological data. Central vasopressinergic circuits have been discovered, and this peptide is now a candidate on the growing list of neurotransmitters. More functional roles have been discovered for VP, including a role in the consolidation of memory, arousal, and central integrative processes.

B. Basic Anatomy and Physiology

Among the dozens of biologically active peptides discovered in neurons, vasopressin (VP) and oxytocin (OT) have a special position as they were the first to be synthesized, now more than 30 years ago (for a review, see Sawyer, 1964). Since then many structural analogs have been prepared, either as selective agonists, but devoid of one or other biological activity, or as antagonists acting selectively on one or other type of receptor, either peripherally or centrally. Over the past decade, the use of such analogs has provided much useful information on structure-activity relationships (Manning and Sawyer, 1984).

1. The Basic Structures of Endogenous Neurohypophysial Hormones and Their Relative Physiological Potencies

As shown in Table 1, although VP and OT differ only at positions 3 and 8, they differ sharply in their relative potencies in four classical physiological (Table 2) assays in the rat: (1)

Table 1

Basic Structures of Endogenous Neurohypophysial Hormones

Hormone	Amino acid position								
	1	2	3	4	5	6	7	8	9
Arginine vasopressin	Cys	Tyr	**Phe**	Glu	Asn	Cys	Pro	**Arg**	Gly(NH₂)
Oxytocin	Cys	Tyr	**Ile**	Glu	Asn	Cys	Pro	**Leu**	Gly(NH₂)
Vasotoxin	Cys	Tyr	**Ile**	Glu	Asn	Cys	Pro	**Arg**	Gly(NH₂)
Oxypressin	Cys	Tyr	**Phe**	Glu	Asn	Cys	Pro	**Leu**	Gly(NH₂)

Table 2

Relative Physiological Potencies of Four Neuropeptides

Peptide	Antidiuretic activity (U/mg)	Vasopressor activity (U/mg)	Oxytocic activity *in vitro* (U/mg)	Milk-ejecting activity (U/mg)
Vasopressin	323	369	14	70
Oxytocin	4	4	520	475
Vasotocin	230	300	112	270
Oxypressin	30	3	20	60

From Manning, M. and Sawyer, W. H., *TINS*, 7, 6, 1984.

Table 3

Typical Agonists for Different Receptors

Peptide	Antidiuretic activity (U/mg)	Vasopressor activity (U/mg)	Oxytocic activity *in vitro* (U/mg)	Milk-ejecting activity (U/mg)
dDAVP	1200	0.4	1.5	0.4
dVDAVP	1200	Antagonist	–8	Not tested
[Phe^2,Orn^8]OT	0.55	124	–1	7
[Thr^4,Gly^7]OT	0.002	<0.01	166	802

[a]dDAVP, 1-Deamino(8-arginine)vasopressin; dVDAVP, 1-deamino[4-valine, 8-D-arginine]vasopressin; [Phe2,Orn8]OT, [2-phenylalanine, 8-ornithine]oxytocin; [Thr4,Gly7]OT, [4-threonine, 7-glycine]oxytocin.

From Manning, M. and Sawyer, W. H., *TINS*, 7, 6, 1984.

an arginine in position 8 favors vasopressor and antidiuretic activities (cf. VP and vasotocin); (2) while an isoleucine in position 3 favors milk ejection and oxytocic activity (cf. OT and vasotoxin); and (3) oxypressin with no isoleucine or arginine is weakly active over the whole spectrum of the physiological actions of this family.

2. Specific Agonists and Antagonists: Discrimination of Different Receptor Classes

These structure-activity relationships indicated that VP and OT elicited their responses via different receptors. The use of agonists with specific activities has reinforced this idea. In particular, the development of agonists specific for vasopressor or antidiuretic activity suggested that the receptors for these pharmacological actions were different. Particularly good examples are dDAVP [1-deamino(8-arginine)vasopressin] and dVDAVP (1-deamino[4-valine,8-D-arginine]vasopressin), which are long-lasting potent antidiuretic agonists devoid of vasopressor action. The replacement of Glu in position 4 by Val in dDAVP to give dVDAVP increases the selectivity of action. These molecules have become drugs of choice in the treatment of central diabetes insipidus. Conversely, [Phe^2, Orn^8]OT has been shown to be a highly potent and specific vasopressor agonist, while [Thr^4, Gly^7]OT has selective oxytocic and milk-ejecting activity (Table 3). These findings and many others have led to the characterization of two types of vasopressin receptors: one, labeled as "V1", mediates glycogenolysis (in rat hepatocytes) and vasoconstriction (in vascular smooth muscle) and is not linked to activation of adenylate cyclase, while the second, labeled as "V2", mediates antidiuresis (in renal tubular cells) and is linked to adenylate cyclase.

3. Vasopressin Receptors Mediating Release of ACTH and Behavioral Responses in Brain

The identification of peripheral V1 and V2 receptors has been facilitated by the development of sensitive quantitative bioassays and agonists that are specific for these activities. Selective VP agonists have helped to characterize *in vivo* the receptors mediating the release of corticotropin from the adenohypophysis with respect to the so-called corticotropin-releasing factor (CRF)-like activity (Gillies and Lowry, 1979; Gillies et al., 1982). Although some studies have shown a similarity of these receptors with the V1 type, *in vitro* studies using VP agonists and antagonists have tended to show that the effect is not mediated by V1 or V2 receptors but by a third type. This third type is thought to be present in regions of the mammalian brain where vasopressin neurons and terminals have been identified. Interestingly, VP and various related moieties injected either peripherally or centrally (intracerebroventricularly, i.c.v.) have been found to enhance memory consolidation. It has been suggested that VP is more potent than dDAVP, tending to favor a V1-type receptor for this activity, but desglycinamide-AVP, which lacks vasopressor activity, is nevertheless claimed to be behaviorally active. Various metabolites of VP that are devoid of vasopressor action have also been reported to have behavioral activity. These findings, which remain to be replicated, may suggest the existence of central receptors different from the V2 type but more akin to the V1 type (Mormède et al. 1985).

4. The Use of Specific Antagonists in Physiological and Behavioral Studies

Additive modifications at positions 1, 2, 4, and 8, in VP and OT turn partial agonists into effective antagonists for one or other physiological responses, as shown for some selected molecules in Table 4 (Manning and Sawyer, 1984; Sawyer, 1964). Comparison of the relative potencies indicates that d(CH$_2$)$_5$[Tyr(Me)^2]AVP, for instance, is 100-fold more potent in blocking vasopressor than oxytocinergic responses, and it is a weak antidiuretic agonist; in other words this molecule can be regarded as a V1 receptor blocker. The same reasoning can be applied to the other molecules; for instance, d(CH$_2$)[D-Ile^2,Abu^4]AVP is an effective V2 antagonist. These antagonists have been shown to block the physiological actions of VP in the conscious animal, and they have been used to probe actions of endogenous VP on other systems such as the release of ACTH and even for the central action of VP on memory consolidation.

5. The Main Vasopressinergic Innervations: Central vs. Hypophysial Systems

Two main vasopressinergic systems are found in the central nervous system (CNS) and are to some extent independent; they are now divided into a hypothalamo-hypophysial system and a CNS innervation (Buijs, 1983; De Vries et al., 1985; Sofroniew and Weindl, 1978). The hypothalamic neurohypophysial hormones, synthesized in the paraventricular and supraoptic nuclei, are released into the bloodstream. The central extrahypothalamo-hypophysial vasopressinergic system (Figure 1) comprises different subsystems. An anterior system con-

Table 4

Typical Antagonists for Different Receptors

| | "Effective" antagonistic dose (nmol/kg)[a] | | |
| | Anti-
antidiuretic | Anti-
vasopressor | Anti-
oxytocic
(*in vivo*) |
Antagonists			
1. d(CH$_2$)$_5$[Tyr^{5}Me^2), Orn^8]OT	Agonist	0.80	4.2
2. dP[Tyr(Me)^2]AVP	Agonist	0.80	11
3. d(CH$_2$)$_5$[Tyr(Me)^2]AVP	Agonist	0.16	17
4. d(CH$_2$)$_5$[D-Ile^2,Abu^4]AVP	0.41	12	19

[a]The effective dose of an antagonist is defined as the dose, administered intravenously, that reduces the response observed to 2 units of agonist down to the response observed to 1 unit of agonist in the absence of antagonist. A nanomole of these peptides is equivalent to around 1.1 µg. The full names of these antagonists are as follows:

1. [1-β-mercapto-β,β-cyclopentamethylene-propionic acid), 2-*O*-methyl-ty-rosine, 8-ornithine]oxytocin.
2. [1-β-mercapto-β,β-dimethylpropionic acid), 2-*O*-methyltyrosine]arginine-vasopressin.
3. [1-β-mercapto-β,β-cyclopentamethylene-propionic acid), 2-*O*-methyltyrosine]arginine-vasopressin.
4. [1-β-mercapto-β,β-cyclopentamethylene-propionic acid), 2-D-isoleucine, 4-α aminobutyric acid]-arginine-vasopressin.

From Manning, M. and Sawyer, W. H., *TINS*, 7, 6, 1984.

tains fibers projecting from the bed nucleus of the stria terminalis to the lateral septum, diagonal band of Broca, olfactory tubercle, region of the basal nucleus of Meynert, as well as to the lateral habenula nucleus, periventricular central gray, dorsal raphe, and locus coeruleus, where VP cells are also found. A ventral system corresponding to the suprachiasmatic nucleus projects to the organum vasculosum of the laminae terminalis, the periventricular hypothalamic nucleus, paraventricular thalamic nucleus, and dorsomedial hypothalamic nucleus. A median system in the paraventricular nucleus projects through long fibers to the dorsal (dorsal parabrachial nucleus, dorsal vagal complex) and ventral (lateral reticular nucleus, ambiguus nucleus) midbrain, pons, and medulla oblongata. A central system whose cell bodies have not yet been fully identified projects to the hippocampus, ventral tegmental area, substantia nigra, and amygdala (where cell bodies have been localized in the medial nucleus). An interesting characteristic is that most of these projections disappear in male rats after castration (Figure 2), suggesting that VP projections from the bed nucleus, medial amygdala, and other regions require the presence of gonadal hormones (De Vries et al., 1984) since they are not lost if castrated rats are treated with testosterone (De Vries et al., 1985). Thus a major part of central VP innervation is implicated in functions influenced by gonadal steroids. However, sex differences in steroid-sensitive VP pathways depend on other factors besides circulating hormone levels during adulthood (De Vries and Al-Shamma, 1990).

C. VP and the Behavioral Neuroendocrinology of Learning and Memory

1. First Observations

In early behavioral work, De Wied and co-workers (De Wied, 1965) found that hypophysectomized rats were impaired in the acquisition and extinction of aversively motivated tasks. These deficiencies were reversed by administration of a raw pituitary extract, pitressin, and in later studies by subcutaneous injections of microgram quantities of lysine

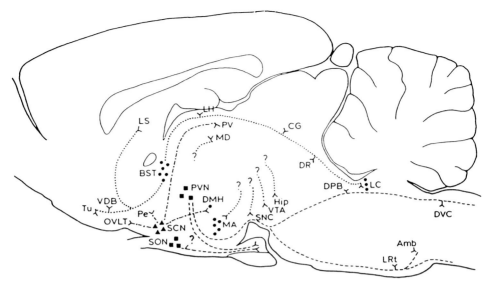

Figure 1. Major VP cell groups and pathways in the brain. ■, cells in the PVN and SON; •, cells in the BST, MA, and LC; ▲, cells in the SCN. (From De Vries, G. J., Buijs, R. M., Van Leeuwen, F. W., Caffé, A. R., and Swaab, D. F., *J. Comp. Neurol.*, 233, 236, 1985. With permission.)

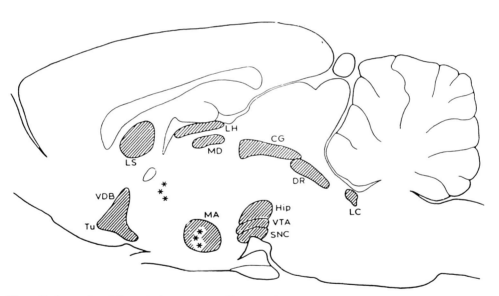

Figure 2. Areas where VP terminals were seen to disappear after castration. (From De Vries, G. J., Buijs, R. M., Van Leeuwen, F. W., Caffé, A. R., and Swaab, D. F., *J. Comp. Neurol.*, 233, 236, 1985. With permission.)

vasopressin (LVP). Such treatment by AVP or LVP given either systemically or intracerebroventricularly also (1) reversed the behavioral deficits observed in Brattleboro strain rats with congenital diabetes insipidus, as did DG-AVP, which is devoid of vasopressor activity, (2) delayed extinction in an active avoidance task in intact animals, and in passive (inhibitory) avoidance, and (3) enhanced retention of the passive avoidance response when injected subcutaneously (s.c.) either just after the training test (foot shock) or just before the retention test, but not at intermediate times. These results suggested a role for the peptide in both consolidation and retrieval (De Wied and Bohus, 1966; De Wied, 1976, 1984a, b; Van

Ree et al., 1978). Most of these findings have been replicated after both s.c. or i.c.v. administration (Le Moal et al., 1981, 1987; Koob et al., 1981; Koob, 1986), and have been extended using appetitively motivated tasks such as the one-trial, water-finding task (Ettenberg et al., 1983a, b) or an elevated eight-arm radial maze (Packard and Ettenberg, 1985). However, it was concluded that peripheral endocrinological responses were required to demonstrate memory-enhancing effects following peripheral administration of VP.

2. Reevaluation of the Role of VP Administered Peripherally in Learning and Memory

The use of more sophisticated behavioral techniques and selective VP antagonists have reopened some questions raised by the earlier observations (Saghal, 1984; De Wied, 1984a, b; Koob et al., 1989; Le Moal et al., 1984, 1987; Gash and Thomas, 1983, 1984). In 1981 (Le Moal et al., 1981; Koob et al., 1981) it was shown that the pressor antagonist dP[Tyr(Me)]AVP blocked the effects of VP injected peripherally (1 µg/rat, s.c.) on the prolongation of active avoidance (Figure 3). This antagonist had little effect on its own except at high doses, at which it facilitated extinction of active avoidance. Moreover, i.c.v. pretreatment with a VP antagonist did prevent the prolongation of extinction induced by s.c. injection of VP, at a dose (6 µg) that blocked the increase in systolic blood pressure induced by VP. When injected centrally, only the dose of VP antagonist that blocked the physiological actions of peripherally injected VP also blocked the behavioral actions of peripherally injected VP (Lebrun et al., 1985). Similar

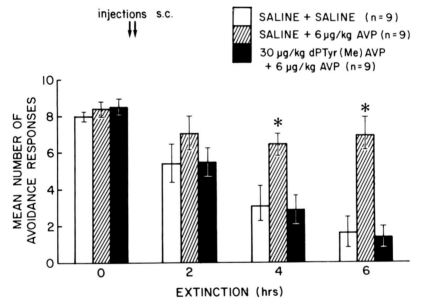

Figure 3. Effects of AVP and AVP plus dPTyr(Me)AVP on extinction of active avoidance behavior. After 3 days of training, rats were injected subcutaneously with saline (twice at 2.0-min intervals) or AVP plus saline or AVP plus dPTyr(Me)AVP immediately after the first set of 10 extinction trials on day 4. Rats receiving AVP showed persistent avoidance throughout the 6 hr of observation, when tested on 10 trials at each of the next three 2-hr intervals, whereas rats receiving either saline with no peptide or both peptides extinguished this active avoidance behavior at similar rates. Saline plus saline (open bars) ($N = 9$); saline plus AVP, 6 µg/kg (striped bars) ($N = 9$); dPTyr(Me)AVP, 30 µg/kg, plus AVP, 6 µg/kg (black bars). *, Significantly different from both the saline with no peptide and both peptide groups; $p < 0.05$, Newman-Keuls test following analysis of variance. (From Le Moal, M., Koob, G. F., Koda, L. Y., Bloom, F. E., Manning, M., Sawyer, W. H., and Rivier, J., *Nature (London)*, 291, 491, 1981. With permission.)

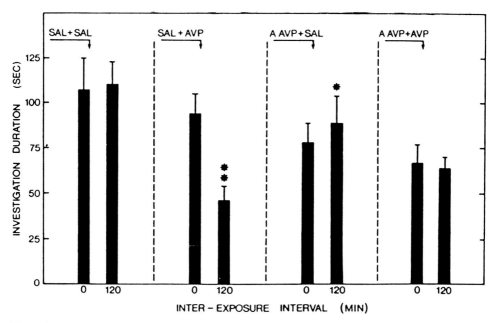

Figure 4. Effects of 30 µg/kg dPTyr(Me)AVP on retroactive facilitating effects of 6 µg/kg AVP on social memory. Means and SEM of social investigation times by adult male rat ($N = 7$) on first and second exposure to the same juvenile stimulus. Peptides were administered subcutaneously. Each group is identified by two terms describing the two treatments administered at 5-min intervals after the first exposure. AAVP, DP[Tyr(Me)]AVP. *, $p < 0.05$; **, $p < 0.01$ compared to time 0. (From Le Moal, M., Dantzer, R., Michaud, B., and Koob, G. F., *Neurosci. Lett.*, 77, 353, 1987b. With permission.)

results were obtained on the enhancement of retention in inhibitory (passive) avoidance, appetitively motivated tasks, and other approach or adaptive responses. For instance, i.c.v. infusion of an VP antagonist abolished the memory effect of VP in an appetitive water-finding task, but only at doses that prevented the aversive effects of peripherally administered VP.

Support for the data obtained from aversively motivated tasks was obtained in an appetitively motivated task sensitive to memory for past events, the so-called social memory task. This task involves an adaptive response in male rats where "memory" for a conspecific juvenile is measured by changes in the duration of investigation when the same juvenile is presented to the same individual at different times after the first exposure. Exposure of an adult male rat to a juvenile results in investigatory behavior that rapidly decreases with repeated exposures for short interexposure intervals (30 min), while longer interexposure intervals (120 min) produce reinvestigation with durations similar to or greater than the first investigation. VP injected s.c. into adult male rats immediately after investigation of the juvenile was found to reduce social investigation (Figure 4) of the same juvenile at a long (120 min) interexposure interval to levels comparable to those observed after a 30-min interexposure interval in untreated animals (Dantzer et al., 1987). This effect was also blocked by a V1-specific antagonist.

VP injected systemically does not appear to cross the blood-brain barrier (Deyo et al., 1986; Pardridge, 1983; Le Moal et al., 1987a, b). One possibility is that central and peripheral VP systems are able to act in a homologous manner to organize adaptive responses. In nearly all the reports on the behavioral effects of VP, the peptide was exogenous. Release of both plasma and central VP has been observed following various homeostatic challenges. It was thus of interest to find out whether the endogenous release of VP after physiological challenge could mediate behavioral responses. For example, injection of hypertonic saline, a potent

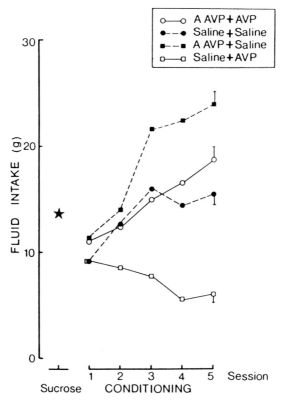

Figure 5. Effects of dPTyr(Me)AVP on conditioned taste aversion to AVP. The figure shows mean fluid intake during the last 2 days of sucrose presentation (star) and over repeated conditioning trials for groups treated with 10 μg/kg AVP or saline preceded by an injection of 50 μg/kg dPTyr(Me)AVP (AAVP) or saline, after milk presentation in a single bottle test. Each point is the mean of five rats. The standard error of each group mean is given for the last test session. (From Le Moal, M., Dantzer, R., Michaud, B., and Koob, G. F., *Neurosci. Lett.*, 77, 353, 1987b. With permission.)

peripheral osmotic stimulus, at doses known to release VP peripherally and centrally (in the septal region) has been shown to prolong extinction of active avoidance and facilitate passive avoidance. These effects were also blocked by peripheral pretreatment with a V1 receptor antagonist (Koob et al., 1985a, b; Lebrun et al., 1987).

Based on these observations, the behavioral effects of systematically administered VP were attributed to alterations in arousal, secondary to the visceral effects of the peptide (Le Moal et al., 1984; Saghal, 1984). It has been demonstrated that VP administered peripherally induces interoceptive signals with aversive and arousing properties. These properties have been investigated using the conditioned taste aversion (CTA) paradigm, in which a novelty-induced malaise or alteration in arousal serves as an unconditioned stimulus (Figure 5). It was shown that VP induced CTA via an interaction with V1-like receptors. Thus, the interoceptive cues responsible for the CTA appear to be related to the hypertensive action of the neuropeptide, and these peripheral arousing actions are essential components of the mechanism producing the improvement in memory (Bluthé et al., 1985a, b; Ettenberg, 1984). This effect also was blocked by a V1-specific antagonist.

3. Effects of VP in the Central Nervous System

VP also has behavioral effects when injected into the brain in nanogram quantities (De

Wied, 1971, 1976; Koob et al., 1981; Van Ree et al., 1978; Benjamini et al., 1968), doses that do not increase systemic blood pressure (Lebrun et al., 1985). It has been shown that local injection of VP into cerebral regions such as septum, dorsal hippocampus, or parafascicular nucleus facilitated retention in passive avoidance. The facilitory effect on learning was blocked by lesion of these regions or by lesion of their noradrenergic innervation. Moreover, a specific VP antiserum injected i.c.v. after training in inhibitory avoidance led to deficits in subsequent trials. These observations suggested that VP was involved in memory processes in the CNS (Ettenberg, 1984). Results similar to those described after s.c. administration of VP were also obtained in the social memory task in rats injected i.c.v. with doses of 0.5 to 0.2 ng of VP immediately after the initial investigation of the juvenile (Le Moal et al., 1987). These results suggested that increasing the availability of VP in CNS improves the consolidation of olfactory information about conspecific individuals in the rat. Moreover, VP injected directly into the lateral (0.1 ng) was found to facilitate social memory of adult male rats (Figure 6A), whereas local injection of the specific V1 antagonist, desGlyNH$_2$d(CH$_2$)$_5$[Tyr(Me)] AVP impaired (Figure 6B) this response (Dantzer et al., 1988). Consistent with anatomical studies demonstrating that part of the extrahypothalamic vasopressinergic innervation, especially the VP cells localized in the bed nucleus of the stria terminalis and projecting to the septum, of the rat brain is androgen dependent, recent work has shown that the effects of VP on social memory may also be androgen dependent (Bluthé et al., 1990). These workers found that (1) castrated male rats had a transient disruption of social memory when they were tested 1 week after surgery, while normal behavior was restored by more frequent daily testing, (2) s.c. administration of a vasopressor antagonist of VP (which crosses the blood-brain barrier) impaired social memory in normal rats, but was ineffective in castrated rats, and (3) in castrated rats testosterone restored the sensitivity of social memory to the VP antagonist. It is of interest in this respect that social recognition does not appear to involve VP neurotransmission in female rats. Relationships between central VP and learning performance have also been implicated in the differences in performance of a foot shock-motivated brightness discrimination task (Ermisch et al., 1986). Rats with high performance in this task were found to have higher levels of VP in the septum and posterior pituitary than those of the low performance group.

D. Other Central Integrative Processes

1. Rhythms, Seasonal Cycles, Homeostatic Functions, Aging

A considerable body of evidence implicates VP in complex physiological integrative actions (for a review see Doris, 1984). Brain VP is thought to be both anatomically and functionally compartmentalized for specific central actions (Reppert et al., 1981, 1987). Levels of VP in cerebrospinal fluid (CSF) and in the circulation have been determined in various free-moving animals. A central daily rhythm (Perlow et al., 1982) with a peak occurring during daylight hours was observed in CSF, but not in the circulation (Figure 7). The circadian regulation of VP in CSF appears to be insulated from the osmotic regulation of the peptide in blood. It probably involves a system separate from the classical hypothalamo-neurohypophysial system and the suprachiasmatic nuclei. A hypothalamic circadian pacemaker may underlie the circadian fluctuations in CSF VP. In animals with seasonal cycles and prone to hibernation, central VP follows the seasonal variations in weight of testes and plasma testosterone levels. Various observations suggest that, in addition to the sexually dimorphic part of the central VP innervation, the suprachiasmatic nucleus and VP are involved in the expression of seasonal functions (Hermes et al., 1989). For instance, in the wild European hamster, central VP is absent during hibernation. As a correlative function, VP in the lateral septum has been

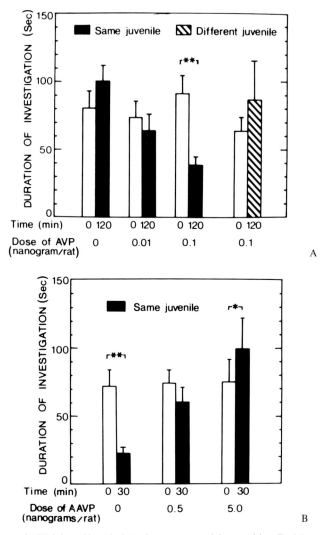

Figure 6. (A) Effects of AVP injected into the lateral septum on social recognition. Each bar represents the mean (±SEM) duration of investigation of the juvenile by adult rats on the first exposure (0) and on the second exposure test carried out 120 min later (120), for different doses of AVP. **, $p < 0.01$ by the least significant test. Black bars, same juvenile; striped bar, different juvenile. (B) Effects of the AVP antagonist (AAVP) injected in the lateral septum on social recognition. Each bar represents the mean (±SEM) duration of investigation of the juvenile by adult rats on the first exposure (0) and on the second exposure test carried out 30 min later (30), for different doses of AAVP. Black bars, same juvenile. * $p < 0.05$; **, $p < 0.01$ by the least significant test. (From Dantzer).

implicated in thermoregulation. In hamsters, as in rats, it is involved in the prevention of exaggerated responses of the brain to several environmental stimuli from the external or internal milieu, for instance by attenuating the impact of stressful events such as strong osmotic stimuli. This more general homeostatic function is now ascribed to central VP.

Finally, it has been shown that VP innervation in the male brain is decreased in senescence. This decrease is particularly pronounced in brain regions where VP fiber density is dependent on sex steroids. VP fiber density in senescent animals can be restored by administration of testosterone, which is indicative of a persistent plasticity in the central nervous system (Goudsmit et al., 1988).

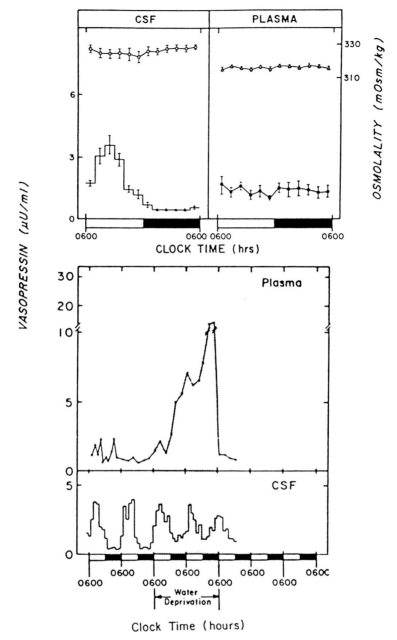

Figure 7. *Top:* Daily patterns of mean VP and osmolarity values in the blood and CSF of enhydrated cats (*N* = 6) studied in diurnal lighting. CSF was collected as 2-hr fractions; osmolarity data are plotted at the midpoint of each collection period. Plasma was obtained at the times indicated (°, osmolarity; •, plasma vasopressin). *Bottom:* patterns of VP in CSF and blood of one cat studied in diurnal lighting before, during, and after a 48-hr period of water deprivation. (From Reppert, S. M., Schwartz, W. J., and Uhl, G. R., *TINS*, 10, 76, 1987. With permission.)

In conclusion, VP in CSF is not derived from VP circulating in plasma. Peripheral administration of VP does not elevate VP levels in CSF in humans or animals, as demonstrated by the autonomous intrinsic daily cycle of VP in CSF, and the high levels of VP in CSF in patients with diabetes insipidus who have impaired VP secretion into plasma. Nevertheless, different populations of VP neurons may release their secretory products into both fluids since some stimuli induce elevations of VP in both plasma and CSF. Since memory processes are subject to temporal oscillations, the links between memory, circadian rhythms, and VP provide an intriguing challenge in assessing the role of hormonal neuromodulation in central integrative processes (see review in Doris, 1984).

2. VP and Body Temperature Regulation

Anatomical evidence suggests that central VP pathways from magnocellular neurons of the hypothalamus to the lateral septum and amygdala are involved in the regulation of body temperature (for a review, see Doris, 1984). Determination of endogenous VP release in the septal region by measuring VP in septal perfusates has revealed that VP and body temperature during fever are inversely related. VP release in the septum falls with increases in body temperature, and vice versa. The septal-amygdala VP system is activated in pregnant animals in the perinatal period. Fever induced by injection of bacterial endotoxin is suppressed in a dose-dependent fashion by infusion of VP into the septal region of nonpregnant ewes, although it is without effect in nonfebrile animals. Conversely, infusion of VP antiserum enhances fever responses in febrile animals. It has recently been reported that VP content in CSF and brain regions is altered during endotoxin-induced fever. Interestingly, i.c.v. administration of VP significantly reduces the fever induced by interleukins, while the antipyretic action of VP is blocked by a receptor antagonist of the V1 but not of the V2 type (Naylor et al., 1987).

3. VP and Central Cardiovascular Regulation

Cardiovascular baroreceptor afferent nerve fibers enter the medulla oblongata in the 9th and 10th cranial nerves and via the solitary tract, terminating in the nucleus tractus solitarius (NTS), a region rich in VP-containing terminals (Doris, 1984; Matshuguchi et al., 1982). Baroreceptor reflexes are an important concomitant of the long-term adjustments involved in the regulation of blood pressure. It has been shown that microinjection of VP in the NTS region produces dose-related increases in blood pressure and heart rate, probably by inhibiting vagal activity. Conversely, VP administered in the region of the vagal nuclei produces bradycardia. Spontaneously hypertensive rats have lower levels of VP in the brainstem, thereby reducing the sensitivity of the baroreflex. These findings suggest that the NTS and septal VP systems have separate integrative actions.

4. VP and Aggressive and Communicative Behaviors in Male Hamsters

Male golden hamsters display a pronounced and reproducible sequence of aggressive and communicative behaviors during repeated social interactions. Aggression diminishes as animals communicate their social status by rubbing pheromone-producing flank glands against objects in the environment, a stereotypic motor activity called flank marking, in which the dominant animal marks two to three times more than the submissive partner. Flank marking is employed to communicate social status and reduces aggression. This behavior is specifically triggered by microinjection of VP into the anterior hypothalamus in both males and females, and is mediated via V1-like VP receptors (Figure 8). Microinjection of a V1 receptor antagonist inhibits odor-induced flank marking and flank marking during paired agonistic encounters. It also temporarily reverses dominant-subordinate behavior with established social hierarchies, and blocks aggression (Ferris et al., 1984; Albers et al., 1986). The magnocellular neurons of the medial supraoptic nucleus appear to be involved, while the neighboring VP target cells and the lateral septum provide facilitory inputs. The central nucleus is activated during VP administration.

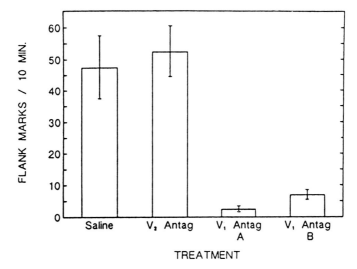

Figure 8. Inhibition of AVP-induced flank marking by pretreatment with selective V$_1$ pressor antagonists, but not by pretreatment with saline or a V$_2$ antidiuretic antagonist. Each group ($N = 5$) was injected with the AVP antagonist (100 ng in 100 nl saline). V$_2$ antagonist: [1-(β-mercapto-β,β-pentamethylenepropionic acid), 2-D-isoleucine, 4-isoleucine]8-arginine-vasopressin; V$_1$ antagonist B, [1-(β-mercapto-β,β-cyclopentamethylenepropionic acid), 2-(O-methyl)tyrosine]8-arginine-vasopressin or saline followed immediately by AVP (1 ng in 100 nl saline) except in the case of V$_1$ antagonist A [1-deaminopenicillamine-2-(O-methyl)-tyrosine]8-arginine-vasopressin. (From Albers, H. E., Pollock, J., Simmons, W. H., and Ferris, C. F., *J. Neurosci.*, 6, 2085, 1986. With permission.)

5. VP and Sexual Behavior in Females

VP influences other adaptive behaviors via its interaction with hypothalamic nuclei. The hypothalamic suprachiasmatic nuclei, a source of VP, has an inhibitory influence on sexual receptivity in estradiol-17P-treated ovariectomized rats during the light phase of the daily lighting cycle, and VP has been shown to inhibit sexual behavior (Södersten et al., 1983). The inhibition of sexual behavior in receptive rats by i.c.v. injection of VP (1 to 10 ng) is prevented by prior injection of an antiserum to VP. Interestingly, s.c. injection of VP (1 μg) has no behavioral action.

E. Conclusions

The findings discussed above support our general hypothesis that systemically and centrally administered VP can influence behavior in a homologous manner but via different mechanisms (Le Moal et al., 1987): (1) VP injected s.c. improves learning, but only at doses that induce physiological effects; (2) when these effects (increase in blood pressure) are blocked by a V1 antagonist, the behavioral action of AVP is also blocked; (3) central injections of VP at doses that do not act as aversive stimuli or alter systemic blood pressure improve learning. This effect is blocked by central administration of small doses and s.c. administration of high doses of V1 antagonist, suggesting that the central effects are mediated via receptors akin to the V1 type; (4) centrally administered VP acts by central mechanisms, and VP administered peripherally acts by peripheral mechanisms related to its physiological effects; (5) some of the central effects of VP require the permissive action of a peripheral hormone, testosterone. In the absence of testosterone, VP cell bodies disappear in the bed nucleus of the stria terminalis, and terminals disappear from the lateral system. VP modulates different functions in males and females. Two potential routes for the peripheral influences on neuropeptide function are via visceral afferent signals and steroid hormones; (6) VP acts centrally as a neurotransmitter, modulating the physiological processes integrated in the region to which the VP neurons project, for example, different adaptive processes that may be modulated in the pons, septum, amygdala, or hypothalamus.

Present in both the periphery and in the brain, VP is a good example of a messenger involved in the processing of information in both systems. Both VP systems, the pituitary and the CNS, may be involved in the generation of different types of arousal.

Finally, the dose-response relationship of many peptides such as VP show a U-shaped function. Mechanisms for this U-shaped function may be the same as those proposed to account for the notable relationship between performance and arousal (Saghal, 1984; Koob et al., 1989; Le Moal et al., 1987).

II. The Behavioral Neuroendocrinology of ACTH

A. Introduction

The hormone ACTH (adrenocorticotropic hormone) is a 39-amino acid polypeptide synthesized in and secreted by specialized cells of the anterior pituitary gland, the corticotrophs. It is released in the bloodstream under the influence of hypothalamic factors, principally CRF (corticotropin-releasing factor) and vasopressin, and reaches the anterior pituitary by the way of the hypothalamo-pituitary portal blood vessels. ACTH activates the synthesis of corticosteroid hormones by the adrenal cortex. This activation is characteristic of stress situations. Glucocorticoid hormones (cortisol or corticosterone) are the most sensitive to ACTH stimulation, and act on carbohydrate and protein metabolism to increase the availability of glucose, the most important energy metabolite. These actions help the organism to meet the metabolic requirements of the behavioral adaptive response to the threatening situation. Steroid hormones are highly lipophilic and readily cross the biological membranes (plasma cell membranes and blood-brain barrier, for instance). Therefore they also enter the brain and act on specific receptors to modulate neuroendocrine and behavioral output (feedback control of adrenocortical axis activity and regulation of food intake and "emotional" behaviors, for example) (De Kloet and Reul, 1987).

B. Synthesis and Structure

Like other peptides, ACTH is synthesized from a high molecular weight precursor. What is unique, however, is that this 265-amino acid precursor is multifunctional, and this function appears in the actions of a succession of biologically active peptides with opioid (endorphins), melanotropic (melanotropins or MSHs), and corticotropic (ACTH) properties (Nakanishi et al., 1979) (Figure 9). It was therefore labeled Proopiomelanocortin or POMC (Chrétien et al., 1979). This precursor is processed by enzymatic cleavage and trimming, producing several polypeptides that can be subsequently amidated at their carboxyl ends, acetylated at their amino termini, glycosylated, and phosphorylated. This processing differs throughout the various tissues where it takes place (Smith and Funder, 1988).

Indeed, the POMC gene is expressed in several cell types with different peptide contents and functional significance. In the adenohypophysis, the precursor is minimally processed and the major products are ACTH, the 16K N-terminal fragment, β-LPH, and β-endorphin, which reflects the involvement of the anterior pituitary in the adrenal gland function. In the interme-

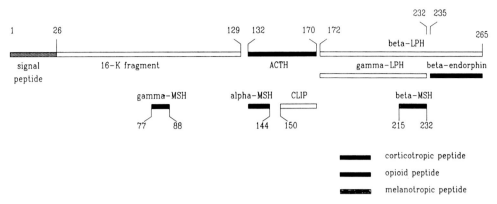

Figure 9. Peptides derived from the 265-amino acid precursor Pro-opiomelanocortin (POMC) under the action of peptidases. In the anterior pituitary corticotrophs, the major products are the 16K N-terminal fragment, the adrenocorticotropic hormone itself (ACTH), lipotropins (LPHs), and β-endorphin. In the intermediate lobe of the pituitary and in the brain, the processing is more complete and gives rise to the melanotropins (MSHs) and β-endorphin, which are also acetylated at their amino termini and amidated at their carboxyl ends. CLIP, Corticotropin-like intermediate peptide.

diate lobe of the pituitary, the processing is far more complete, with production of melanotropins and other acetylated small peptides with a different spectrum of activity dominated by the property of melanotropins to darken the skin of frogs and other animals. Finally, POMC is also expressed in the brain, mostly in cell bodies located in the arcuate nucleus of the hypothalamus. These neurons have long axons and innervate numerous brain regions: hypothalamic nuclei (paraventricular, dorsomedial, lateral, preoptic), nucleus of the diagonal band, thalamus (periventricular nucleus), limbic system (amygdala, septum, bed nucleus of the stria terminalis), reticular formation, periaqueductal gray, raphe dorsalis and parabrachial nucleus, and medulla. A few cell bodies are also present in the nucleus of the tractus solitarius (caudal medulla) (Figure 10, top) (Khachaturian et al., 1985). In these neurons, the processing is rather complete, although it can be different from one projection site to the other, where the various possible end-products are found in different combinations.

C. Neurotropic Effects of ACTH

In the early 1950s, it was found that, in addition to its neuroendocrine activity, ACTH also affected behavior (Mirsky et al., 1953). Most experimental data have been obtained in active avoidance conditioning tasks, in which the animal must emit an active behavioral response (bar press, shuttling, pole or bench jumping, for instance) to a buzzer to avoid an aversive stimulus, usually an electric shock. If the shock is disconnnected after completion of avoidance learning, the response progressively vanishes (extinction). It was initially shown that ACTH delays extinction of avoidance behavior in intact animals. Furthermore, the acquisition of the avoidance response is impaired after removal of the anterior pituitary gland and restored by either ACTH treatment or a combination of cortisone, testosterone, and thyroxine. It was not clear from these early experiments whether these effects of ACTH were related to its adrenal stimulating property or could result from an extraadrenal activity.

In an elegant series of experiments, De Wied and co-workers (reviewed in De Wied, 1977) clearly demonstrated that the effects of ACTH on avoidance behavior were completely independent from the adrenal. First, although ACTH retards the extinction of avoidance behavior, corticosteroids were shown to have the opposite effect, an acceleration of extinction.

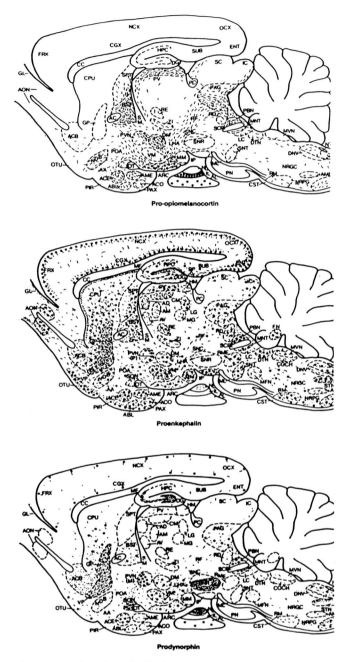

Figure 10. Schematic representation of the distribution of Pro-opiomelanocortin-, Pro-enkephalin-, and Pro-dynorphin-derived peptides in the rat CNS. (From Khachaturian, H., Lewis, M. E., Schafer, M. K.-H., and Watson, S. J., *Trends Neurosci.*, 8, 111, 1985. With permission.)

The second evidence came from structure-activity studies. When the ACTH polypeptide was shortened on both ends, it lost its corticotropic activity but retained its action on avoidance behavior. In that test, the heptapeptide ACTH$_{4-10}$ was fully active to delay extinction, when injected subcutaneously in microgram amounts. Still more surprising, the replacement of the phenylalanine residue at position 7 by its dextrorotatory analog produced a peptide [D-Phe[7]]ACTH$_{4-10}$ with opposite effects, which accelerated the extinction of active avoidance, suggesting that it behaved as an antagonist of an endogenous ACTH tone (van Nispen and Greven, 1982). This pioneering work has opened new avenues on the neurotropic effects of hormonal peptides and stimulated a considerable amount of work.

Selected effects of ACTH-related peptides are listed in Table 5. The behavioral actions that have received the most attention are the delay of extinction of active avoidance behavior, the facilitation of passive avoidance behavior, the reversal of the memory deficit induced by postlearning "amnesic" treatment like carbon dioxide, protein synthesis inhibitors, or electroconvulsive shock, and the induction of excessive grooming and a specific stretching and yawning syndrome when the peptide is administered into the cerebral ventricles.

In a typical passive avoidance paradigm, a rat is placed on a brightly illuminated platform facing a dark chamber, the floor of which can be electrified. The natural behavior of the rat is to escape the platform and enter the dark cage. After a few pretraining trials, a mild electric foot shock is delivered in the dark chamber. When placed again on the platform (retention trial), the rat is slower to enter the dark chamber again. A single injection of ACTH$_{4-10}$ markedly increases avoidance latencies. This and other findings (such as the delay of extinction of active avoidance behavior) have been interpreted as a temporary increase in the motivational significance of environmental cues by ACTH (De Wied, 1977).

In fact, peripheral administration of small amounts of peptide increases the excitability of the reticular formation, as shown by the facilitation of driving hippocampal rhythmic slow activity (or theta activity, 6 to 10 Hz) by septal stimulation. These effects are usually interpreted as reflecting an activation along the midbrain limbic pathways and an improvement of attentional processes. Posttrial administration of ACTH modifies passive avoidance learning with a bell-shape dose-response curve. Low doses increase passive avoidance behavior during retention tests, and high doses disrupt learning (Gold and van Buskirk, 1976). This is reminiscent of the shape of the curve relating arousal and performance and suggests that endocrine and/or nervous signals involving ACTH and related peptides may participate in the arousal state of the brain in stress situations, and therefore influence the formation of stimulus-response associations or their behavioral expression.

The same interpretation can be put forward to explain the "anti-amnesic" effects of ACTH. Immediately upon termination of the acquisition trial in a passive avoidance experiment, the rat is placed in a box filled with carbon dioxide until respiratory arrest occurs; it is then revived and returned to its home cage. In these conditions, when a retention test is given 24 hr later, the avoidance latency is shortened ("amnesia"). ACTH treatment reinstates the

Table 5
Selected Effects of Adrenocorticotropic Hormone-Related Peptides

---

Endocrine
  1. Stimulate the synthesis and release of adrenocortical steroids (corticotropic)
  2. Darken frog skin (melanotropic)
Neuroendocrine
  3. Activate the autonomic nervous system with an increase in blood pressure and heart rate
Behavioral
  4. Restore acquisition of active avoidance behavior in hypophysectomized animals
  5. Delay extinction of active avoidance behavior in intact animals
  6. Increase passive avoidance behavior
  7. Reverse amnesia induced by postlearning treatment with carbon dioxide, electroconvulsive shock, or protein synthesis inhibition
  8. Induce excessive grooming behavior and a yawning/stretching syndrome (after intracerebroventricular administration only)

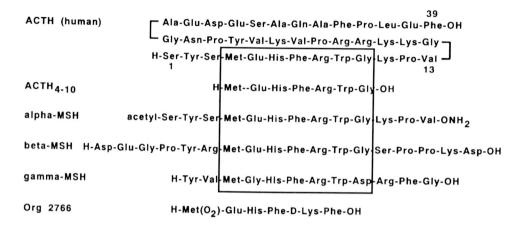

Figure 11. Amino acid sequence of ACTH and melanotropins, showing the common core heptapeptide ACTH4–10 from which derives the synthetic analog Org 2766.

weakened passive avoidance behavior, when given 1 hr before the retention test, but is inactive when given before the amnesic treatment. This is in contrast to vasopressin, which is active in both treatment situations. These results indicate that the peptide does not interfere with information processing but strengthens the significance of environmental cues, which has been reduced by the amnesic treatment (Rigter and van Riezen, 1978).

D. Structure-Activity Studies

Within the numerous peptides derived from POMC emerges a seven-amino acid sequence (-Met-Glu-His-Phe-Arg-Trp-Gly-) common to ACTH (and therefore α-MSH, which is derived from it), β-MSH, and γ-MSH (Figure 11). This common core heptapeptide (referred to as $ACTH_{4-10}$) appears to play a critical role in most of the biological activities of all these related peptides, such as the corticotropic action of ACTH (Schwyzer et al., 1971), the melanotropic properties of the MSHs (Eberle and Schwyzer, 1976), the pressor activity of γ-MSH (Gruber and Callahan, 1989), as well as their effects on avoidance behaviors (van Nispen and Greven, 1982). This necessary "message sequence" is given its specific target information by other parts of the peptides, which can be referred to as "address sequences". Finally, "potentiating sequences" are usually necessary for the active core to express its full potency, by increasing either the intrinsic activity of the peptide on its receptor, or its metabolic stability.

Chemists have produced a large number of analogs to study these structure-activity relationships and have obtained superagonists (up to 4×10^6-fold more potent than $ACTH_{4-10}$ to delay extinction of active avoidance behavior) like $[Met(O_2)^4, D\text{-}Lys^8, Phe^9]ACTH_{4-9}$, known as Org 2766, and a 1000-fold more potent than $ACTH_{4-10}$. This peptide has been developed for clinical use, and can be administered by the oral route. They have also obtained antagonists like $[D\text{-}Phe^7]ACTH_{4-10}$, which accelerates the extinction of active avoidance behavior, an effect similar to that of the naturally occurring peptide γ-MSH (van Nispen and Greven, 1982). On other targets however, these same peptides can behave as agonists. For instance, the cardiovascular actions of $ACTH_{4-10}$ are not present in α- or β-MSH but the D-Phe[7] analog is fully active and γ-MSH is 100-fold more active than the parent heptapeptide. A few examples of structure-activity studies are shown in Table 6.

These experimental data clearly show that the processing of the POMC precursor gives a very large panel of peptides containing the $ACTH_{4-10}$ active core with very different possible

Table 6

Structure-Activity Relationships of Adrenocorticotropic Hormone-
Like Peptides[a]

Peptide	Avoidance extinction (subcutaneous)[b]	Pressor activity (intravenous)[c]	Grooming behavior (i.c.v.)[d]
ACTH	+ (delay)	+	+
ACTH$_{4-10}$	+	+	0
α-MSH	+	0	+
α-MSH	− (acceleration)	+++	ND
[D-Phe^7]ACTH$_{4-10}$	−	+	+

[a]i.c.v., Intracerebroventricular; ND, not determined; +, agonist; −, antagonist; 0, no activity.
[b]Data from van Nispen and Greven, 1982.
[c]Data from Gruber and Callahan, 1989.
[d]Data from Gispen et al., 1975.

biological activities. The net result will depend on the combination of the end-products, and thus possibly on the activity of the processing enzymes in a given projection field.

E. Mechanisms of Action

Although most of the neurotropic effects of ACTH-like peptides are obtained after peripheral administration of microgram amounts, a central site of action has been demonstrated by injecting the peptides in the carotid artery or directly in the brain, and showing that in these conditions they are 10- to 100-fold more potent, respectively. However, the initial target and the route of entry are still under investigation. Other effects, like excessive grooming, are obtained only after intracerebroventricular administration.

Numerous neurochemical effects of ACTH-like peptides have been described. For instance, they interact with opiate receptors and interfere with various effects of opiates, like the narcotic cue or analgesia. They behave *in vitro* like weak partial agonists. These experimental data introduce another level of complexity in the study of POMC-derived peptides since opiate-like peptides, the endorphins, are also generated by the processing of the precursor protein. Excessive grooming, as induced by the intracerebroventricular administration of ACTH-like peptides, can also be elicited by mild stressors, like novel environment exposure, and low doses of amphetamine or morphine, suggesting that it involves opiate and dopamine neuronal circuits. In fact, ACTH-induced excessive grooming can be blocked by dopamine or opiate antagonists. Most interesting, intraventricular administration of ACTH antiserum to neutralize the endogenous peptide reduces excessive grooming induced by novel environment exposure. These results indicate that ACTH neurons can be involved in normal activation of the brain by stressful events. In addition, the expression of the stretching and yawning syndrome after administration of ACTH-like peptides in the cerebral ventricles is dependent on the activation of acetylcholine turnover in the hippocampus.

Several biochemical effects of ACTH-like peptides have been described. These include the stimulation of adenylate and guanylate cyclase, an increased phosphorylation of synaptic membrane proteins, a trophic effect on neurons *in vitro* and *in vivo*, with a stimulation of glucose uptake and protein synthesis. Their respective importance in the aforementioned neurotropic actions remains to be investigated.

F. Conclusions

ACTH is a 39-amino acid polypeptide synthesized in the anterior lobe of the pituitary and characteristically is released under conditions of arousal and stress. It activates the synthesis of glucocorticoid hormones from the adrenal gland that in turn act on carbohydrate and protein metabolism to help the organism meet the metabolite requirements of the behavioral adaptive response to stress. ACTH is derived from a large precursor molecule, POMC, from which comes a succession of biologically active peptides. In addition to its neuroendocrine effect, ACTH also appears to alter behavior independent from adrenal actions. It delays extinction of motivated behavior, an effect generally described as an enhancement of attentional processing, and the hormonally inert analog $ACTH_{4-10}$ is fully active. Other analogs are reportedly even more potent in producing these effects and yet others may act as antagonists. Future studies are needed to evaluate the clinical potential of these analogs and their mechanism of action in the central nervous system.

III. The Behavioral Neuroendocrinology of Opioids

A. Introduction

In 1969, Reynolds (1969) showed that electrical stimulation of the periaqueductal gray (PAG) of rats produced an intense analgesia. It was then demonstrated that like morphine-induced analgesia, electrical stimulation-induced analgesia was reduced by naloxone (Akil et al., 1976). These crucial observations were followed by two main discoveries made in the first half of the 1970s, which started the enormous research activity that has characterized the opiate field in the last 2 decades. Historically the discovery of opioid receptors preceded the isolation and sequencing of endogenous opioid peptides. In 1971, Goldstein et al. established the characteristics of specific opiate binding in brain tissue. Then three groups independently reported stereospecific binding sites in brain tissue in 1973: Simon et al. (1973), Pert and Snyder (1973), and Terenius (1973). The second important discovery was the demonstration by Terenius and Whalström (1975), Hughes et al. (1975), Pasternak et al. (1975), Goldstein (1976), Simantov and Snyder (1976), and Guillemin et al. (1976) that the brain synthesized endogenous opioid peptides that had morphine-like properties and were the putative endogenous ligands of the opiate receptors. Different opioid peptides have been characterized, known as enkephalins (pentapeptides), endorphins, and dynorphins. These opioid peptides are localized in specific neurons. As we will see, the large distribution of opioid neuron innervations within the CNS and the multiplicity of opioid receptors explain the wide range of physiological effects of opioid peptides: cardiovascular, respiratory, and neuroendocrine regulation; thermoregulation; analgesia; consummatory, sexual, aggressive, and defensive behaviors; locomotor activity; learning and memory; and, finally, mediation of endogenous reward, tolerance, and dependence, which could explain opiate addiction.

B. Neuroanatomy

All opioid peptides are derived from three endogenous peptide precursors, which contain also nonopioid peptides cosynthesized from a single precursor: the Pro-opiomelanocortin (POMC), the Pro-enkephalin (or Pre-Proenkephalin A), and the Pro-dynorphin (or Pre-Proenkephalin B). Peptides derived from POMC include the opioid β-endorphin and the nonopioid hormones ACTH and α-MSH (Hollt, 1983).

1. Pro-Opiomelanocortin

The POMC precursor is synthesized both in the pituitary gland as well as in the brain. Hypophysectomy reduces plasma β-endorphin, but brain concentrations are not altered by hypophysectomy. The brain contains a limited amount of β-endorphin neurons located in discrete areas. These neurons have long axons and a widespread diffuse innervation throughout the brain. The major site of immunoreactive β-endorphin/α-MSH/ACTH perikarya in the CNS is the arcuate nucleus of the medial basal hypothalamus in mainly its rostrocaudal extent. Recently, a second less extensive group of POMC neurons has been described in the nucleus tractus solitarius. These neurons are distinct from enkephalin-containing neurons. Rostral projections of arcuate POMC neurons can be traced through periventricular regions of the hypothalamus and preoptic area innervating olfactory-associated areas, septum, diagonal band, amygdala, and throughout the hypothalamus (limbic structures) and thalamus. Caudal projections of these POMC neurons are rather complex and diffuse: posterior hypothalamus mammillary area, periventricular and mesencephalic periaqueductal gray, collicular areas, ventral mesencephalon, raphe nucleus, and dorsal and lateral regions of pons and medulla.

POMC perikarya of the caudal nucleus tractus solitarius innervate caudal medullary reticular formation. POMC fibers detected in the spinal cord arise from either of the two POMC neuronal groups. It is interesting to notice that cortical and hippocampal areas are devoid of POMC innervation (Figure 11 and Table 7).

2. Pro-Enkephalin

Unlike the POMA precursor, which contains only one opioid peptide (β-endorphin), several opioid peptides are derived from Pro-enkephalin, essentially Met- and Leu-enkephalin. The distribution of these two opioid pentapeptides is not parallel, suggesting different neuronal enkephalinergic networks. Enkephalins are synthesized in many neuronal systems throughout the CNS, from the cerebral cortex to the spinal cord, some forming local circuits and others with long-tract projections.

Neurons containing Pro-enkephalin peptides are found at virtually all levels of the neuraxis, in most regions of the telencephalon, including cerebral cortex, olfactory tubercule, amygdala, hippocampus, striatum, accumbens, septum, bed nucleus of stria terminalis, and preoptic area. In the diencephalon perikarya are seen in most hypothalamic nuclei and some thalamic areas. In the midbrain, enkephalinergic cells are localized in the colliculi, periaqueductal gray, and interpeduncular nuclei, and in numerous structures of the pons and medulla. Because of the extensive enkephalinergic innervation, it should be apparent that enkephalin neurons have the potential to influence a wide variety of CNS functions.

3. Pro-Dynorphin

Like Pro-enkephalin, Pro-dynorphin contains several opiate-active peptides, including dynorphin A and B and α- and β-neoendorphin. This precursor is also synthesized throughout the CNS in a wide variety of neuronal systems distributed in cortical areas, striatum, amygdala, hippocampus, several hypothalamic nuclei, midbrain periaqueductal gray, and in numerous brainstem areas and spinal cord dorsal horn.

4. Neurotransmitters or Neuromodulators

Opioid peptides have been shown to meet many of the criteria for neurotransmitters. They appear to be inhibitory transmitters on most if not all brain neurons, and particularly on inhibitory neurons, suggesting that disinhibition may be an important general mechanism of opioid action in the CNS. The coexistence of Met-enkephalin and other putative neurotransmitters such as noradrenaline and serotonin has been reported. This has led to the suggestion

Table 7

Regional Distribution of Opioid Receptors and Opioid Peptides in the Rat Brain[a]

CNS region	Receptors			Peptides		
	μ	δ	κ	POMC	Pro-Enk	Pro-Dyn
I. Telencephalon						
Frontal cortex (laminar)	+++	++	+	0	++	+
Piriform cortex (laminar)	++	++	++	0	++	+
Entorhinal cortex (laminar)	++	++	++	0	+++	+
Amygdala						
Central nucleus	0	0	++	++++	++++	++
Medial nucleus	+++	++	++	+++	+++	+
Lateral nucleus	++++	+++	+++	++	+++	+
Hippocampal formation						
Hippocampus (laminar)	+++	++	+	0	++	+++
Dentate gyrus (laminar)	+++	+	+	0	++	+++
Olfactory tubercle	+	+++	+++	0	++	++
Nucleus accumbens	++++ (patchy)	++++	+++ (ventral)	+	+++	++
Caudate-putamen	++++ (patchy)	++++ (vent-lat)	+++ (vent-med)	0	+++ (patchy)	++
Globus pallidus	+	+	+	0	++++	+++
Medial septum	+++	+	+	+++	+++	0
Bed nucleus stria terminalis	++	++	+++	++++	+++	++
Preoptic area	+	+	++++	+++	+++	++
II. Diencephalon						
Hypothalamus						
Supraoptic nucleus	0	0	++	0	+	+++
Paraventricular nucleus	0	0	++	++++	++++	++++
Arcuate nucleus	0	0	++	++++	+++	++
Ventromedial nucleus	0	+	+++	+	+++	++
Dorsomedial nucleus	+	0	+++	++++	++	++
Lateral hypothalamic area	+	0	++	+++	++	+++
Thalamus						
Periventricular nucleus	0	0	+++	++++	+++	+
Central-medial nucleus	++++	+	++	0	+++	0
Reuniens nucleus	++++	+	++	0	++	0
Medial habenula	+++	+	+++	0	+++	0
III. Mesencephalon						
Interpeduncular nucleus (central)	++++	+++	+++	0	+++	0
Substantia nigra						
Pars compacta	+++	0	0	+	++	+
Pars reticulata	++	+	+	0	+	++++
Ventral tegmental area	++	0	+	++	++	+
Periaqueductal gray (rostral-ventral)	+	0	++	++++	+++	++
Superior/inferior colliculi	++++	+	++	++	+++	+
Dorsal raphe nucleus	++	0	++	+++	++	+
IV. Pons/medulla						
Parabrachial nucleus	+++	0	++	+++	+++	++
Nucleus raphe magnus	++	0	+	+	+++	++
Nucleus reticular gigantocellularis	+	0	+	++	+++	+
Nucleus tractus solitarius (caudal part)	++++	+	+++	+++	+++	+++
Lateral reticular nucleus	+	0	+	+++	+++	+
Spinal trigeminal nucleus	+++	0	++	++	++++	+++
V. Spinal cord						
Substantia gelatinosa	+++	+	++	++	++++	+++

[a]++++, Very dense; +++, dense; ++, moderate; +, low; 0, undetectable.

From Mansour, A., Khachaturian, H., Lewis, M. E., Akil, H., and Watson, S. J., *TINS,* 11, 308, 1988. With permission.

that one of these coexisting substances may function as a neurotransmitter and the other as a neuromodulator, with the general presumption being that the peptide is likely to be the neuromodulator.

C. Multiple Opiate Receptors

1. Distribution Within the CNS

In 1976, Martin and colleagues suggested the existence of multiple opioid receptors. They observed that different opiate drugs induced distinct physiological or behavioral symptoms, and that tolerance developed toward one of these drugs did not result in cross-tolerance to another class of opiate drugs. Further support for this position came from studies using peripheral organ bioassays, in which the relative potencies of different opioids and opiate agonists and antagonists varied according to the tissue bioassay system. On the basis of these results, three classes of opioid receptors were defined: mu (μ) for morphine-like drugs, kappa (κ) for ketocyclazocine-like compounds, and delta (δ) for the vas deferent bioassay, in which enkephalin peptides were found to be particularly potent. This classification subsequently was confirmed by homogenate binding and autoradiographic studies. Opioid receptors are widely distributed throughout the CNS, with particularly dense binding observed in cortical and limbic structures, thalamus nuclei, mesencephalon, pons, medulla, and spinal cord. The distribution of μ, δ, and κ opioid receptors is remarkably different in both their relative abundance across the brain areas and their specific locations (Table 7). While the three of them are present in the telencephalon, only the κ type is present in the hypothalamus. The δ type is particularly absent from the diencephalon, mesencephalon, and the pons medulla. In other cases, some overlap exists in the localization of each of these receptor types. However, their precise anatomical distributions vary markedly and generally appear complementary, as in the neocortex and limbic structures such as hippocampus and olfactory bulbs. In contrast, all receptor types are densely distributed within the caudate putamen and the accumbens; however, while δ and κ receptors have a diffuse distribution, μ receptors are concentrated in clusters or patches (Mansour et al., 1988).

2. Relationship between the Different Opioid Peptide Systems and Multiple Opioid Receptors

The enkephalins, which are the proposed end products in the processing of Pro-enkephalin but not of POMC, have been shown to bind preferentially to δ receptors. On the other hand, all intermediate peptides in the processing of Pro-dynorphin show a selective affinity for the κ receptors. β-Endorphin, the opioid-active end product of POMC precursor, has high affinity for all three sites, μ, κ, and δ. No endogenous peptides with selectivity for the μ receptors have been previously described. However, recent discoveries indicate that a single precursor generates peptides with different receptor selectivity and the selectivity changes as the processing continues. For example, Pro-dynorphin generates first a set of κ-selective opioid peptides (dynorphin$_{1-17}$, α-neo-endorphin) that might be further processed into the δ-specific Leu-enkephalin. This differential processing of the opioid precursor may indicate a biological strategy for yielding peptide products that act at different opioid receptors.

Given the complexity of the distribution of both the opioid receptors and peptide systems in the CNS, it may be premature to attempt to correlate a particular opioid peptidergic system with a receptor type. The complexity is magnified when species differences are considered, since species vary dramatically in the relative abundance of each opioid binding sites. While the distribution of opioid receptor types is well conserved between species in brainstem and spinal cord areas, it varies most markedly in forebrain and midbrain structures (Table 7).

D. Behavioral Neuroendocrinology

In spite of a considerable amount of data on the physiological and behavioral effects induced by intracerebral application of opioid peptides and opiate agonists and antagonists (Table 8), it is still difficult to draw firm conclusions regarding the functional role of different opioid receptor types in any neuronal system. The main reasons are because the physiological effects of opioids are influenced not only by pharmacological variables such as the dose, stability, site of administration, and receptor specificity of the compounds but also by organismic variables such as whether the animal is resting, stressed, injured, or anesthetized. However, it is clear that endogenous opiates are involved in at least three domains: (1) the modulation of the response to pain stimuli and stressors both at the sensory and affective level, (2) reward function, and (3) adaptive functions such as food and water intake and temperature regulation.

1. Antinociception and Stress-Induced Analgesia

One of the most striking properties of opiates and opioid peptides when injected intracerebrally is their antinociceptive nature. They relieve the pain associated with the nociceptive stimuli without significantly altering basic sensations (touch, temperature, and proprioception). After synapsing in the spinal cord, nociceptive fibers ascend at the spinothalamic tract, which consists of two divisions. First, the neospinothalamic tract projects to the ventroposterolateral nucleus of the thalamus and then to the somatosensory cortex with a somatotopic organization

Table 8

Specific Agonists and Antagonists of the Opioid
Receptors

Receptor	Agonists	Antagonists
μ	Morphine	Naloxone
	Dihydromorphine	Naltrexone
	DAGO	Naloxonazine
	Morphiceptine	CTOP
	Casomorphine	CTP
	Metorphamide	Cypromide
	Sufentanil	
δ	Met-Enkephalin	ICI 154.129
	Leu-Enkephalin	ICI 174,864
	DSLET	NTI (naltrindole)
	DTLET	
	DSTBULET	
	BUBU	
	BUBUC	
	DPDPE	
	DPLPE	
	[Tyr-D-Cys-Phe-D-Pen]	
	Dermenkephalin	
κ	U 50.488H	MR 2266
	U 69.593	MR 2034
	Dynorphin$_{1-17}$	WIN 44.441-3
	[D-Pro^{10}]dynorphin$_{1-11}$	
μ, δ, κ	Ethylketocyclazocine	Diprenorphin
	Bremazocine	
	Etorphine	
ε	β-Endorphin	
σ	SKF 10.047	Rimcazole
	DTG	Cinuperone
		BMY 14802-1

(primary pain: quality, intensity, and location of the noxious stimuli). Second, the paleospinothalamic tract projects polysynaptically to the reticular formation, including the periaqueductal gray, to the thalamus and then diffusely to limbic and subcortical areas. This system carries the pain (secondary or subjective pain) associated with noxious stimuli, which explains why pain is highly subjective and depends on the individual characteristics and the situation (Besson and Chaouch, 1987).

Endogenous opioid pain modulatory systems control at different levels nociceptive inputs carried through the paleospinothalamic tract to limbic and subcortical structures, including the periaqueductal gray, nucleus raphe magnus, and medial thalamus. These structures are rich in μ receptors and intracerebral injection of opiates at these sites induce intense analgesia that is preferentially inhibited by naloxone, a μ receptor antagonists, while δ or κ antagonists are ineffective.

Recently, a new subclass of μ receptors has been characterized (μ_1) with very high affinity for morphine and enkephalins. Their presence correlates with the sensitivity to opiate analgesia that is specifically blocked by naloxonazine and naloxonazone, two μ_1-selective antagonists (Pasternak, 1988).

Several lines of evidence suggest that the endogenous opioid systems may play a role in the defensive response of the organism to stressors (Amit and Galina, 1986). They influence motivation, arousal, pain sensation, and other central processes that contribute to adaptive behaviors. Stress induces a naloxone-reversible analgesia (SIA) by releasing endogenous opioid peptides. Moreover, the intensity of SIA depends on the control that an animal can exert over the stressor since the amplitude of SIA is reduced if the animals are exposed to escapable foot shock (Hemingway and Reigle, 1987).

2. Consummatory Behavior

Several lines of evidence suggest direct or indirect control of food and water intake by endogenous opiates. Food intake can be induced by peripheral administration of low doses of morphine or intracerebroventricular infusion of β-endorphin, both effects being reduced by peripheral or central administration of naloxone. Genetically obese mice or rats stop overeating in response to opiate antagonists (Margules et al., 1978) and higher doses of opiate antagonists can reduce feeding in normal rats. Similarly, a role of endogenous opiates in stress-induced eating has been proposed on the basis of reversibility by opiate antagonists (μ). Opiate agonists usually stimulate fluid intake, while naloxone reduces water intake in water-deprived and undeprived animals, effects that are not reduced by ablation of pituitary β-endorphin (hypophysectomy). However, drinking stimulated by cellular dehydration, hypovolemia, angiotensin II, or eating is generally reduced by central application of β-endorphin, which suggests a complex interaction between endogenous opiates and fluid intake.

3. Other Adaptive Processes

A physiological role of endogenous opioids in regulating sexual behavior has been proposed since naloxone was found to stimulate copulatory response in male rats and lordosis behavior in female rats, both of them being potently inhibited by intracerebral application of β-endorphin.

The role of β-endorphin in thermoregulation is complex and varies with ambient temperature. This opioid peptide induces hyperthermia when rats are exposed to cold and hypothermia when exposed to heat stress.

4. Brain Opiates and Reward Function

It is striking that opioid peptides in high concentration in a number of CNS sites are implicated directly in the evaluation of sensory stimuli. As seen above, they also are found in limbic structures such as the amygdala, where highly integrated sensory information is processed, and in the ventral tegmental area source of the ascending mesolimbic dopaminergic (DA) neurons and the nucleus accumbens (ventral striatum). This mesolimbic dopamin system serves an enabling function for sensorimotor integration. In spite of conflicting hypotheses, the rewarding effects of opiates appear to be due to the activation of opiate receptors at least at two brain sites, first in the ventral tegmental area (Bozarth and Wise, 1983), which produces the activation of mesolimbic DA neurons (psychostimulant effect) (Kelley et al., 1980), and second, in the nucleus accumbens (Stinus et al., 1986). The abuse liability of psychostimulants (cocaine, amphetamine) and opiates (heroin, morphine) may be directly related to their ability to sensitize the neural substrate involved in natural reward. A complex balance exists in the involvement of DA and endogenous opiate in the control of the reward system (Figures 12 and 13) since the chronic inhibition of DA activity (specific lesion or chronic neuroleptic treatment) induces a dramatic increase of the appetitive effects of opiates (Stinus et al., 1989).

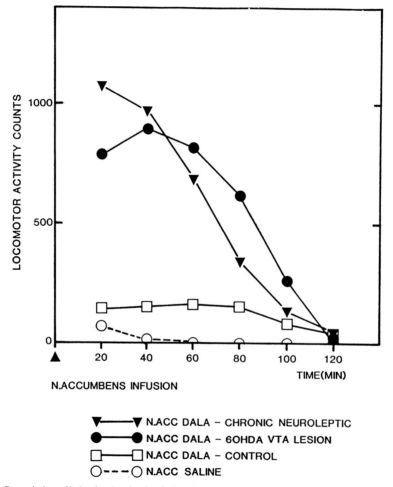

Figure 12. Potentiation of behavioral activation induced by injection of D-Ala-Met-enkephalin (DALA) into the nucleus accumbens (N.ACC) after either (●) lesion of DA-A10 neurons (6-OHDA VTA lesion) or (▼) chronic neuroleptic treatment. □, Control; ○, saline. (From Stinus, L., Nadaud, D., Jauregui, J., and Kelley, A. E., *Biol. Psychiatry*, 21, 34, 1986. With permission.)

EFFECT OF CHRONIC NEUROLEPTIC TREATMENT

ON HEROIN INTRAVEINOUS SELF-ADMINISTRATION

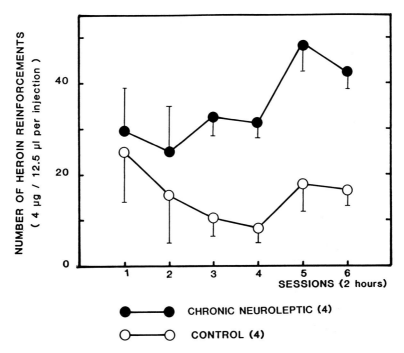

Figure 13. The intravenous self-administration of a very low dose of heroin (subthreshold dose for control rats) is considerably increased after a chronic neuroleptic treatment (long-acting neuroleptic flupentixol decanoate for 1 month). •, Chronic neuroleptic (4); °, control (4). (From Stinus, L., Nadaud, D., Deminiere, J. M., Jauregui, J., Hand, T. T., and Le Moal, M., *Biol. Psychiatry,* 26, 363, 1989. With permission.)

E. Tolerance to Dependence on Opioids

The rapid development of tolerance and dependence is one of the best known properties of exogenous opiates (heroin, morphine), which is also produced by repeated administrations of opioid peptides. Tolerance is defined as the loss in responsiveness to a drug, or the increase in the dose of the drug required to elicit a given response. Dependence is defined according to the abnormalities that appeared after the drug was withdrawn. Tolerance and dependence can be considered as adaptive biological processes that develop in order to reduce the drug action. This adaptive process persists after the drug has been cleared from the brain, leaving an opposing reaction unopposed (abstinence syndrome) (Koob et al., 1989). Several biological mechanisms have been hypothesized to be involved in tolerance and dependence observed after repeated application of opiates. These include suppression of production or release of endogenous opioid peptides, down regulation of opiate receptors, or uncoupling of the receptor from its second messenger system. However, these adaptive mechanisms have yet to be directly linked to opiate tolerance and dependence. Repeated administration of morphine induces reduction of its analgesic effect. This tolerance is augmented if the drug is injected in the presence of environmental cues previously associated to the drug injection (Siegel, 1975). If, after establishment of tolerance to morphine-induced analgesia, rats received a test injection of the drug in the presence of a novel environment, a normal analgesic effect is recorded, indicating that tolerance is a learned response. A particularly attractive hypothesis to explain these results is the opponent process theory developed by Solomon (1989). It supposes that many reinforcers, including addictive drugs, arouse positive and hedonic processes (a) that are opposed by negative affective and hedonic processes (b). The a-processes are hypothesized to be simple, stable, and to follow the reinforcer (drug) closely. In contrast, the b-processes are of longer latency, slow to build up in strength, and slow to decay. The intense pleasure induced by opiates would reflect the a-process and the withdrawal syndrome the opponent b-process. In normal conditions, the b-processes are latent, and could be triggered by environmental or social cues associated in the past to the drug effects. The retrieval of this conditioned b-process may explain the withdrawal (craving) and relapse in former heroin addicts. One of the important neural substrates for the acute reinforcing effects of opiate drugs (the a-process) in nondependent rats is in the region of the nucleus accumbens (Koob et al., 1989). This same region may become sensitized during the development of dependence, and thus may be responsible for the aversive stimulus properties associated with opiate withdrawal (b-process). Unknown at this time is the exact role for opioid peptides or opiate receptors in these phenomena or the role of neurochemical (even neuropeptidergic) systems that modulate the action of opiates (Yang et al., 1985).

F. Conclusions

Opioid peptides are derived from three endogenous precursors, Pro-opiomelanocortin (POMC), Pro-enkephalin, and Pro-dynorphin. β-Endorphin is derived from POMC and is located in the pituitary, with a limited distribution in the central nervous system (CNS). In contrast, the enkephalins are derived from Pro-enkephalin and have a widespread CNS distribution; dynorphins are derived from Pro-dynorphin and also have a widespread CNS distribution. There are also multiple opioid receptors that correspond somewhat to different opioid peptides. β-Endorphin has a high affinity for all three receptor subtypes, whereas some dynorphins are selective for κ sites and Leu-enkephalin is selective for δ sites. This diversity of peptides and receptor subtypes provides a rich neurobiological substrate for the behavioral and functional effects of opioid peptides, including antinociception, consummatory behavior, sexual behavior, and reward. New work suggests that opioid peptides in the mesolimbic system may be involved in reinforcement, and future studies may define how these systems act to influence the motivational aspects of opiate dependence.

Acknowledgments

We thank MEM word processing of the Scripps Research Institute for their excellent help in preparation of the manuscript.

References

Akil, H., Mayer, D. J., and Liebeskind, J. C., Antagonism of stimulation-produced analgesia by naloxone, a narcotic antagonist, *Science,* 191, 961, 1976.

Albers, H. E., Pollock, J., Simmons, W. H., and Ferris, C. F., A V1-like receptor mediates vasopressin-induced flank marking behavior in hamster hypothalamus, *J. Neurosci.,* 6, 2085, 1986.

Amit, Z. and Galina, Z. H., Stress-induced analgesia: adaptive pain suppression, *Physiol. Rev.,* 66, 1091, 1986.

Benjamini, E., Shimizu, M., Young, J. D., and Leung, C. Y., Immunochemical studies on the tobacco mosaic virus protein. VII. The binding of octanoylated peptides of the tobacco mosaic virus protein with antibodies to the protein, *Biochemistry*, 7, 1261, 1968.

Besson, J. M. and Chaouch, A., Peripheral and spinal mechanism of nociception, *Physiol. Rev.*, 67, 67, 1987.

Bluthé, R. M., Dantzer, R., Mormède, P., and Le Moal, M., Specificity of aversive stimulus properties of vasopressin, *Psychopharmacology*, 87, 238, 1985a.

Bluthé, R. M., Dantzer, R., and Le Moal, M., Peripheral injections of vasopressin control behavior by way of interoceptive signals for hypertension, *Behav. Brain Res.*, 18, 31, 1985b.

Bluthé, R. M., Schoenen, J., and Dantzer, R., Androgen-dependent vasopressinergic neurons are involved in social recognition in rats, *Brain Res.*, 519, 150, 1990.

Bozarth, M. A. and Wise, R. A., Neural substrate of opiate reinforcement, *Prog. Neuropsychopharmacol.*, 7, 569, 1983.

Buijs, R. M., Vasopressin and oxytocin. Their role in neurotransmission, *Pharmacol. Ther.*, 22, 127, 1983.

Chrétien, M., Genjannet, S., Gossard, F., Gianoulakis, C., Crine, P., Lis, M., and Seidah, N. G., From beta-lipotropin to beta-endorphin and "pro-opio-melanocortin", *Can. J. Biochem.*, 57, 1111, 1979.

Dantzer, R., Bluthé, R. M., Koob, G. F., and Le Moal, M., Modulation of social memory in male rats by neurohypophyseal peptides, *Psychopharmacology*, 91, 363, 1987.

Dantzer, R., Koob, G. F., Bluthé, R. M., and Le Moal, M., Septal vasopressin modulates social memory in male rats, *Brain Res.*, 457, 143, 1988.

De Kloet, E. R. and Ruel, J. M. H. M., Feedback action and tonic influence of corticosteroids on brain function: a concept arising from the heterogeneity of brain receptor systems, *Psychoneuroendocrinology*, 12, 83, 1987.

De Vries, G. J. and Al-Shamma, H. A., Sex differences in hormonal responses of vasopressin pathways in the rat brain, *J. Neurobiol.*, 21, 686, 1990.

De Vries, G. J., Buijs, R. M., and Sluiter, A. A., Gonadal hormone actions on the morphology of the vasopressinergic innervation of the adult rat brain, *Brain Res.*, 298, 141, 1984.

De Vries, G. J., Buijs, R. M., Van Leeuwen, F. W., Caffé, A. R., and Swaab, D. F., The vasopressinergic innervation of the brain in normal and castrated rats, *J. Comp. Neurol.*, 233, 236, 1985.

De Wied, D., The influence of the posterior and intermediate lobe of the pituitary and pituitary peptides on the maintenance of a conditioned avoidance response in rats, *Int. J. Neuropharmacol.*, 4, 157, 1965.

De Wied, D., Long term effect of vasopressin on the maintenance of a conditioned avoidance response in rats, *Nature (London)*, 232, 58, 1971.

De Wied, D., Behavioral effects of intraventricularly administered vasopressin and vasopressin fragments, *Life Sci.*, 19, 685, 1976.

De Wied, D., Pituitary adrenal system hormones and behavior, *Acta Endocrinol.*, 85 (Suppl. 214), 9, 1977.

De Wied, D., Peptides and behavior, *Life Sci.*, 20, 195, 1977.

De Wied, D., The importance of vasopressin in memory, *Trends Neurosci.*, 7, 62, 1984a.

De Wied, D., The importance of vasopressin in memory, *Trends Neurosci.*, 7, 109, 1984b.

De Wied, D. and Bohus, B., Long term and short term effects on retention of a conditioned avoidance response in rats by treatment with long acting pitressin and α-MSH, *Nature (London)*, 212, 1484, 1966.

Deyo, S. N., Shoemaker, W. J., Ettenberg, A., Bloom, F. E., and Koob, G. F., Subcutaneous administration of behaviorally effective doses of arginine vasopressin change brain AVP content only in median eminence, *Neuroendocrinology*, 42, 260, 1986.

Doris, P. A., Vasopressin and central integrative processes, *Neuroendocrinology*, 38, 75, 1984.

Eberle, A. and Schwyzer, R., Hormone-receptor interactions. The message sequence of alpha-melanotropin: demonstration of two active sites, *Clin. Endocrinol.*, 5 (Suppl.), S41, 1976.

Ermisch, A., Landgraf, R., and Möbius, P., Vasopressin and oxytocin in brain areas of rats with high or low behavioral performance, *Brain Res.*, 379, 24, 1986.

Ettenberg, A., Intracerebroventricular application of a vasopressin antagonist peptide prevents the behavioral action of vasopressin, *Behav. Brain Res.*, 14, 201, 1984.

Ettenberg, A., Le Moal, M., Koob, G. F., and Bloom, F. E., Vasopressin potentiation in the performance of a learned appetitive task: reversal by a pressor antagonist analog of vasopressin, *Pharmacol. Biochem. Behav.*, 18, 645, 1983a.

Ettenberg, A., Van der Kooy, D., Le Moal, M., Koob, G. F., and Bloom, F. E., Can aversive properties of (peripherally-injected) vasopressin account for its putative role in memory?, *Behav. Brain Res.*, 7, 331, 1983b.

Ferris, C. F., Albers, H. E., Wesolowski, S. M., Goldman, B. D., and Leeman, S. E., Vasopressin injected into the hypothalamus triggers a stereotypic behavior in golden hamsters, *Science*, 224, 521, 1984.

Gash, D. M. and Thomas, G. J., What is the importance of vasopressin in memory processes, *TINS*, 6, 197, 1983.

Gash, D. M. and Thomas, G. J., Reply from D. M. Gash and G. J. Thomas, *TINS*, 7, 64, 1984.

Gillies, G. and Lowry, P., Corticotrophin releasing factor may be modulated vasopressin, *Nature (London)*, 278, 463, 1979.

Gillies, G. E., Linton, E. A., and Lowry, P. J., Corticotropin releasing activity of the new CRF is potentiated several times by vasopressin, *Science*, 299, 355, 1982.

Gold, P. E. and van Buskirk, R., Enhancement and impairment of memory processes with post-trial injections of adrenocorticotropic hormone, *Behav. Biol.*, 16, 387, 1976.

Goldstein, A., Opioid peptides (endorphins) in pituitary and brain, *Science*, 193, 1081, 1976.

Goldstein, A., Lowney, L. I., and Pal, B. K., Stereospecific and nonspecific interactions of the morphine congener levorphanol in subcellular fractions of mouse brain, *Proc. Natl. Acad. Sci. U.S.A.*, 68, 1742, 1971.

Goudsmit, E., Fliers, E., and Swaab, D. F., Testosterone supplementation restores vasopressin innervation in the senescent rat brain, *Brain Peptides*, 173, 306, 1988.

Gruber, K. A. and Callahan, M. F., ACTH-(4–10) through alpha-MSH: Evidence for a new class of central autonomic nervous system-regulating peptides, *Am. J. Physiol.*, 257, R681, 1989.

Guillemin, R., Ling, N., and Burgus, R., Endorphines, peptides, d'origine hypothalamique et neurohypophysaire à activité morphinomimétique. Isolement et structure moléculaire de l'α-endorphine, *C.R. Acad. Sci. Paris*, 282, 783, 1976.

Hays, R. M., Agents affecting the renal conservation of water, in *The Pharmacological Basis of Therapeutics*, 6th ed., Gilman, A. G., Goodman, L. S., and Gilman, A., Eds., Macmillan, New York, 1980, 916.

Hemingway, R. B. and Reigle, T. G., The involvement of endogenous opiate systems in learned helplessness and stress-induced analgesia, *Psychopharmacology*, 93, 353, 1987.

Hermes, M. L. H. J., Buijs, R. M., Masson-Pévet, M., Van Der Woude, T. P., Pévet, P., Brenklé, R., and Kirsch, R., Central vasopressin infusion prevents hibernation in the European hamster (*Cricetus cricetus*), *Proc. Natl. Acad. Sci. U.S.A.*, 86, 6408, 1989.

Hollt, V., Multiple endogenous opioid peptides, *TINS*, 6, 24, 1983.

Hughes, J., Smith, T. W., Kosterlitz, H. W., Fothergill, L. A., Morgan, B. A., and Morris, H. R., Identification of two related pentapeptides from the brain with potent opiate agonist activity, *Nature (London)* 258, 577, 1975.

Kelley, A. E., Stinus, L., and Iversen, S. D., Interactions between D-Ala-Met-enkephalin, A10 dopaminergic neurones, and spontaneous behavior in the rat, *Behav. Brain Res.*, 1, 3, 1980.

Khachaturian, H., Lewis, M. E., Schafer, M. K.-H., and Watson, S. J., The anatomy of CNS opioid systems, *Trends Neurosci.*, 8, 111, 1985.

Koob, G. F., Le Moal, M., Gaffori, O., Manning, M., Sawyer, W. H., Rivier, J., and Bloom, F. E., Arginine vasopressin and a vasopressin antagonist peptide: opposite effects on extinction of active avoidance in rats, *Regul. Peptides*, 2, 153, 1981.

Koob, G. F., Dantzer, R., Bluthé, R. M., Lebrun, C., Bloom, F. E., and Le Moal, M., Central injections of arginine vasopressin prolong extinction of active avoidance, *Peptides*, 7, 213, 1985a.

Koob, G. F., Dantzer, R., Rodriguez, F., Bloom, F. E., and Le Moal, M., Osmotic stress mimics effects of vasopressin on learned behavior, *Nature (London)*, 315, 750, 1985b.

Koob, G. F., Lebrun, C., Dantzer, R., and Le Moal, M., Role of neuropeptides in learning versus performance: focus on vasopressin, unpublished, 1989a.

Koob, G. F., Stinus, L., Le Moal, M., and Bloom, F. E., Opponent process theory of motivation: neurobiological evidence from studies of opiate dependence, *Neurosci. Behav. Rev.*, 13, 135, 1989b.

Le Moal, M., Koob, G. F., Koda, L. Y., Bloom, F. E., Manning, M., Sawyer, W. H., and Rivier, J., Vasopressin antagonist peptide: blockade of pressor receptor prevents behavioral action of vasopressin, *Nature (London)*, 291, 491, 1981.

Le Moal, M., Dantzer, R., Mormede, P., Baduel, A., Lebrun, C., Ettenberg, A., Van der Kooy, D., Wenger, J., Deyo, S., Koob, G. F., and Bloom, F. E., Behavioral effects of peripheral administration of arginine vasopressin: a review of our search for a mode of action and a hypothesis, *Psychoneuroendocrinology*, 9, 319, 1984.

Le Moal, M., Bluthé, R. M., Dantzer, R., Bloom, F. E., and Koob, G. F., The role of arginine vasopressin and other neuropeptides in brain-body integration, in *Cognitive Neurochemistry*, Stahl, S. M., Iversen, S. D., and Goodman, E. C., Eds., Oxford University Press, New York, 1987a, 203.

Le Moal, M., Dantzer, R., Michaud, B., and Koob, G. F., Centrally injected arginine vasopressin (AVP) facilitates social memory in rats, *Neurosci. Lett.*, 77, 353, 1987b.

Lebrun, C., Le Moal, M., Koob, G. F., and Bloom, F. E., Vasopressin pressor antagonist injected centrally reverses peripheral behavioral effects of vasopressin but only at doses that reverse increases in blood pressure, *Regul. Peptides*, 11, 173, 1985.

Lebrun, C., Le Moal, M., Dantzer, R., Bloom, F. E., and Koob, G. F., Hypertonic saline mimics the effects of vasopressin on inhibitory avoidance, *Behav. Neural Biol.*, 47, 130, 1987.

Manning, M. and Sawyer, W. H., Design and uses of selective agonistic and antagonistic analogs of the neuropeptides oxytocin and vasopressin, *TINS*, 7, 6, 1984.

Mansour, A., Khachaturian, H., Lewis, M. E., Akil, H., and Watson, S. J., Anatomy of CNS opioid receptors, *TINS*, 11, 308, 1988.

Margules, D. L., Moisset, B., Lewis, M. J., Shibuya, H., and Pert, C., Beta-endorphin is associated with overeating in genetically obese mice (*ob/ob*) and rats (*fa/fa*), *Science*, 202, 988, 1978.

Martin, W. R., Eades, C. G., Thompson, J. A., Huppler, R. E., and Gilbert, P. E., Effects of morphine and morphine-like drugs in the nondependent and morphine-dependent chronic spinal dog, *J. Pharmacol. Exp. Ther.*, 197, 517, 1976.

Matshuguchi, H., Sharabi, F. M., Gordon, F. J., Johnson, A. K., and Schmid, P. G., Blood pressure and heart rate responses to microinjection of vasopressin into the nucleus tractus solitarius region of the rat, *Neuropharmacology*, 21, 687, 1982.

Mirsky, I. A., Miller, R., and Stein, M., Relation of adrenocortical activity and adaptive behavior, *Psychosom. Med.*, 15, 574, 1953.

Mormède, P., Le Moal, M., and Dantzer, R., Analysis of the dual mechanism of ACTH release by arginine vasopressin and it analogs in conscious rats, *Regul. Peptides*, 12, 175, 1985.

Nakanishi, S., Inoue, A., Kita, T., Nakamura, M., Chang, A. C. Y., Cohen, S. N., and Numa, S., Nucleotide sequence of cloned c-DNA for bovine corticotropin-beta-lipotropin precursor, *Nature (London)*, 278, 423, 1979.

Naylor, A. M., Gubitz, G. J., Dinarello, C. A., and Veale, W. L., Central effects of vasopressin and 1-desamino-8-D-arginine vasopressin (DDAVP) on interleukin-1 fever in the rat, *Brain Res.*, 401, 173, 1987.

Packard, M. G. and Ettenberg, A., Effects of peripherally injected vasopressin on the extinction of a spatial learning task in rats, *Regul. Peptides*, 11, 51, 1985.

Pardridge, W. M., Neuropeptides and the blood-brain barrier, *Ann. Rev. Physiol.*, 45, 73, 1983.

Pasternak, G. W., Multiple morphine and enkephalin receptors and the relief of pain, *JAMA*, 269, 1362, 1988.

Pasternak, G. W., Goodman, R., and Snyder, S. H., An endogenous morphine-like factor in mammalian brain, *Life Sci.*, 16, 1765, 1975.

Perlow, M. J., Reppert, S. M., Artman, H. A., Fisher, D. A., Seif, S. M., and Robinson, A. G., Oxytocin, vasopressin and estrogen-stimulated neurophysin: daily patterns of concentration in cerebrospinal fluid, *Science*, 216, 1416, 1982.

Pert, C. B. and Snyder, S. H., Opiate receptor: demonstration in nervous tissue, *Science*, 179, 1011, 1973.

Reppert, S. M., Artman, H. G., Swaminanthan, S., and Fisher, D. A., Vasopressin exhibits a rhythmic pattern in cerebrospinal fluid but not in blood, *Science*, 231, 1256, 1981.

Reppert, S. M., Schwartz, W. J., and Uhl, G. R., Arginine vasopressin: a novel peptide rhythm in cerebrospinal fluid, *TINS*, 10, 76, 1987.

Reynolds, D. V., Surgery in the rat during electrical analgesia induced by focal stimulation, *Science*, 164, 444, 1969.

Rigter, H. and van Riezen, H., Hormones and memory, in *Psychopharmacology: A Generation of Progress*, Lipton, M. A., DiMascio, A., and Killam, K. F., Eds., Raven Press, New York, 1978, 677.

Saghal, A., A critique of the vasopressin memory hypothesis, *Psychopharmacology*, 83, 215, 1984.

Sawyer, W. H., Vertebrate neurohypophysial principles, *Endocrinology*, 75, 981, 1964.

Sawyer, W. J. and Manning, M., The development of vasopressin antagonists, *Fed. Proc.*, 43, 87, 1984.

Schwyzer, R., Schiller, P., Seeling, S., and Sayers, G., Isolated adrenal cells: log dose response curves for steroidogenesis induced by ACTH1–24, ACTH1–10, ACTA4–10 and ACTH5–10, *Fed. Eur. Biochem. Soc. Lett.*, 19, 229, 1971.

Siegel, S., Evidence from rats that morphine tolerance is a learned response, *J. Comp. Physiol. Psychol.*, 89, 489, 1975.

Simantov, R. and Snyder, S. H., Morphine-like peptides in mammalian brain: isolation, structure elucidation, and interactions with the opiate receptor, *Proc. Natl. Acad. Sci. U.S.A.*, 73, 2515, 1976.

Simon, E. J., Hiller, J. M., Edelman, I., Stereospecific binding of the potent narcotic analgesic ^{3}H-etorphine to rat-brain homogenate, *Proc. Natl. Acad. Sci. U.S.A.*, 70, 1947, 1973.

Smith, I. and Funder, J. W., Proopiomelanocortin processing in the pituitary, central nervous system, and peripheral tissues, *Endocrine Rev.*, 9, 159, 1988.

Södersten, P., Henning, M., Melin, P., and Ludin, S., Vasopressin alters female sexual behavior by acting on the brain independently of alterations in blood pressure, *Nature (London)*, 301, 608, 1983.

Sofroniew, M. V. and Weindl, A., Projections from the parvocellular vasopressin and neurophysin-containing neurons of the suprachiasmatic nucleus, *Am. J. Anat.*, 153, 391, 1978.

Solomon, R. L., The opponent process theory of acquired motivation, *Am. Psychol.*, 35, 691, 1989.

Stinus, L., Nadaud, D., Jauregui, J., and Kelley, A. E., Chronic treatment with five different neuroleptics elicits behavioral sensitivity to opiate infusion into the nucleus accumbens, *Biol. Psychiatry*, 21, 34, 1986.

Stinus, L., Nadaud, D., Deminiere, J. M., Jauregui, J., Hand, T. T., and Le Moal, M., Chronic flupentixol treatment potentiates the reinforcing properties of systemic heroin administration, *Biol. Psychiatry*, 26, 363, 1989.

Terenius, L., Stereospecific interaction between narcotic analgesics and a synaptic plasma membrane fraction of rat cerebral cortex, *Acta Pharmacol. Toxicol.*, 32, 317, 1973.

Terenius, L. and Wahlström, A., Search for an endogenous ligand for the opiate receptor, *Acta Physiol. Scand.*, 94, 74, 1975.

Van Nispen, J. W. and Greven, H. M., Structure-activity relationships of peptides derived from ACTH, beta-LPH and MSH with regard to avoidance behavior in rats, *Pharmacol. Ther.*, 16, 67, 1982.

Van Ree, J. M., Bohus, B., Versteeg, D. H., De Wied, D., Neurohypophyseal principles and memory processes, *Biochem. Pharmacol.*, 27, 1793, 1978.

Yang, H. Y. T., Fratta, W., Majane, E. A., and Costa, E., Isolation sequencing, synthesis and pharmacological characterization of two brain neuropeptides that modulate the action of morphine, *Proc. Natl. Acad. Sci. U.S.A.*, 82, 7757, 1985.

Zerbe, R. L., Bayorth, M. A., and Feuerstein, G., Vasopressin: an essential pressor factor for blood recovery following hemorrhage, *Peptides*, 3, 509, 1982.

14

Psychiatric Abnormalities in Endocrine Disorders

ROGER G. KATHOL
Department of Psychiatry and Internal Medicine
University of Iowa
Iowa City, Iowa

I. Introduction

The number of endocrine disorders in which psychiatric disturbances has been described is extremely large, particularly when considering that case reports comprise a significant part of the literature. To improve our current understanding of psychiatric factors in endocrine disease, this chapter will examine, in detail, data about the presence of psychiatric comorbidity in endocrine conditions that are seen either with some frequency (diabetes mellitus, hyperthyroidism, hypothyroidism) or which, although uncommon, are reported to have a high frequency of psychiatric symptoms [hyperthyroidism, hypothyroidism, Cushing's syndrome (hypercortisolemia), and hyperparathyroidism].

The majority of this chapter will deal with a review of research studies of patients presenting with the disease in question rather than a summary of case reports. This, in part, is done to obviate the potential for suggesting that a relationship between the endocrine disease and psychiatric symptoms is present when, in fact, it is not, as can occur in multiple case reports. It has the added advantage of providing the reader with an understanding of what can and should be expected psychiatrically in the *typical patient* with one of the endocrine disorders listed above. If the psychiatric presentation is typical for the endocrine disorder, then treatment of the endocrine disorder itself along with psychological support may be all that is necessary to return the patient to emotional stability. If, on the other hand, the presentation is atypical, then it could mean that the psychiatric symptoms may be related to an alternative cause, such as an underlying psychiatric disturbance, which would require more thorough independent evaluation in addition to primary psychiatric intervention. Of course, the disadvantage of the approach taken in this chapter is that it necessarily excludes information related to rare psychiatric presentations of these endocrine diseases. For each disease unusual presentations will be briefly discussed, if warranted, but not emphasized.

In addition to limiting the number of endocrine conditions reviewed in this chapter to those listed above, special attention will be given to the frequency of occurrence and to the treatment of depression, anxiety, dilirium/organic psychosis, and dementia. Although other psychiatric conditions (anorexia, alcoholism, schizophrenia, etc.) may occur in patients with endocrine disease, they are more likely to be co-existent with rather than related to the endocrine disease in question. Personality change is also frequently cited as one of the early manifestations of endocrine disorders. Reference to this fact will be made in the text when appropriate; however, it should be noted that any chronic change in a person's physical condition can result in a change in the way a person reacts to certain situations (thus an apparent "personality change"). The personality change may also be a reflection of the development of a clinical syndrome (depression, anxiety, etc.) rather than a true change in personality. The fact remains that the majority of patients demonstrating this adaptive behavior do not have a personality *disorder*. Furthermore, specific changes in personality are not characteristic of specific endocrine states and, therefore, would not help in leading to a diagnosis of the underlying endocrine disease in isolation. For this reason personality changes will not be emphasized unless patterns of consistent personality alterations emerge that would be of clinical assistance.

A final note should be made about how psychiatric "disorders" have been identified in patients with endocrine disease. Many of the studies that will be cited were performed before the publication of DSM III (APA, 1980) or DSM-III-R (APA, 1987) and, therefore, rely on psychiatric evaluations that use a diagnostic classification discordant with current nomenclature. Alternatively, studies rely on the use of symptom scales to identify those with psychiatric disturbance. The criterion cutpoints on these symptom scales, however, uniformly have not been validated in patients with medical illness. Utilization of "clinical" diagnoses in the old classification systems (and even in the new classification system when nonstructured interviews are performed) and symptoms scale cutpoints is part of the reason for massive discrepancies among studies in the frequency of psychiatric comorbidity with the endocrine diseases. An example of this is illustrated by Abed et al. (1987), who found in a study of 51 acromegalic patients that the incidence of depression is no greater than that found in the general population. A literature of case reports, however, emphasizes depression as a potential complication of acromegaly (Fava et al., 1987). For this reason, diagnoses made by standardized criteria as a result of structured interviews in studies of patient populations will be given greater weight than those provided from questionnaires, retrospective reviews, or case reports.

II. Diabetes Mellitus

Unlike the other endocrine diseases reviewed in this chapter, diabetes mellitus is a chronic condition, characterized by exacerbations and remissions, which requires close monitoring in many cases. One could argue that the same could be said for hypothyroidism, hyperthyroidism, and Cushing's disease since long-term observation and therapy are often required. Diabetes, however, is different because it often requires daily blood glucose monitoring, modification of the diet, and controlled exercise to prevent long-term complications. For this reason much has been written about the stresses associated with the life changes involved, but until recently few studies had investigated the prevalence of psychiatric illness.

During the past 3 years, several well-formulated studies of the psychiatric manifestations seen in patients with diabetes mellitus have been published (Table 1). From these, it is suggested that clinical depression and/or generalized anxiety are frequently seen in patients with diabetes. The works of Lustman et al. (1986) and Wilkinson et al. (1988) show that at any one time 10% of patients will manifest symptoms of major depression while the study of Lustman et al. (1986) reports that 22% will demonstrate generalized anxiety. Both of these conditions are seen with greater frequency than in the general population. Interestingly, panic disorder is not included in the conditions noted to have an increased frequency.

The work of Lustman et al. (1986) compared the presence of psychiatric symptoms to the degree of control of the diabetes as manifest by hemoglobin A_1 levels. They found that those with more poorly controlled diabetes were much more likely to have a history of psychiatric symptoms and, perhaps more importantly, psychiatric symptoms at the time of interview.

Table 1
Psychiatric Manifestations in Patients with Diabetes Mellitus[a]

Study	Diagnostic technique	Illnesses identified	Frequency	Comments
Lustman, 1986	DIS	Generalized anxiety disorder	36/93	Six to seven times general population prevalence
			20/93	Current GAD
		Major depression	37/114	Same as above
			116/114	Current MD
		Dysthymic disorder	20/114	
		Agoraphobia	18/114	
Wilkinson, 1987	CIS	Depressive neurosis	16/92	All indicate current depression
		Major depression	5/92	No anxiety reported
Popkin et al., 1988	DIS	Generalized anxiety disorder	13/41	Prevalence
		Major depression	18/75	Prevalence
		Sexual dysfunction	18/75	
		agoraphobia	8/75	

[a]Abbreviations: DIS, Diagnostic Interview Schedule; CIS, Clinical Interview Schedule; GAD, generalized anxiety disorder; MD, major depression.

Although it is known that acute psychological stress does not cause changes in circulating levels of glucose, ketones, free fatty acids, or glucagon (Kemmer et al., 1986), Lustman et al. suggest that chronic stress experienced during depression and/or anxiety (or other less common psychiatric conditions) may influence metabolic stability. An alternative could be that uncontrolled diabetes leads to a greater number of psychiatric symptoms and thus the diagnosis of major depression and anxiety.

Eighteen of 75 patients in the study of Popkin et al. (1988) reported sexual dysfunction. This finding is in accordance with studies that specifically address problems of sexual function in diabetics (Jensen, 1981; Newman and Bertelson, 1986). Although one might expect that the dysfunction is related to diabetic control, in fact, studies have not consistently been able to document this fact. A relationship, however, has been found between impotence in males and vascular complications (Karalan et al., 1977) and between dyspareunia and urinary tract infections in females (Newman and Bertelson, 1986).

In addition to the psychiatric disorders described above, which occur with increased frequency in patients with diabetes, Bale (1973) suggests that impairment of anterograde memory (new word learning) may also occur in diabetics, and particularly in those exposed to episodes of hypoglycemia. This report that 17 of 100 diabetics and none of 100 controls were considered to have brain damage has not been replicated. All 15 with damage on the Walton-Black scale (new word learning) who were tested with the Wechsler Adult Intelligence Scale had full-scale IQs in the normal range while 14 of the 15 had no discrepancy between the verbal and performance sections. When this is coupled with the fact that an organic brain syndrome is not identified in the cohorts of patients reported by Lustman et al. (1986), Wilkinson et al. (1988), and Popkin et al. (1988), it suggests that memory impairment, if it occurs, is not a significant psychiatric problem in diabetics. Thus when it is seen, alternative causes should be explored until further data supporting a relationship with diabetes becomes available.

In summary, diabetes mellitus has a high prevalence of generalized anxiety disorder, major depression, and sexual dysfunction. To date there have been no studies that address whether and what type of intervention may be helpful in preventing or alleviating these symptoms. Certainly the association of these with diabetic control suggests that optimizing blood sugar regulation should be one of the measures included in the therapeutic plan. Since diabetes is a chronic condition in which only palliative care (diet, weight loss, insulin, etc.) can be given in most cases (some can now receive a pancreas transplantation), other measures besides optimizing medical management should be considered in the psychiatric intervention plan. These may include education, support, and psychopharmacology.

III. Hyperthyroidism

It is helpful to have an appreciation for the history of the diagnosis and treatment of hyperthyroidism (Table 2) in order to understand the significant changes that have occurred not only in the way that psychiatric symptoms present but also in how they are conceptualized and treated. About the time that Lugol solution (iodine) was introduced as a preoperative medication in the treatment of hyperthyroidism, there was a shift in psychiatric symptoms from manic-depression and exhaustion psychosis (delirium) with a high associated mortality (Table 3) to anxiety and depression with little associated mortality (Table 4). Psychiatric symptoms associated with hyperthyroidism became more limited in scope and less frequently required the special attention of psychiatrists. Psychiatric hospitalization was usually unnecessary and effective treatment for both medical and psychiatric manifestations of the thyrotoxicosis could be administered by the primary physician. This switch in the psychiatric presentation, however, led to a need for greater awareness of psychiatrists to exclude hyperthyroidism (and hypothyroidism) as a cause for primary symptoms of depression and anxiety since the physical symptoms of hyperthyroidism may be subtle or nonexistent.

In addition to a shift in psychiatric symptom presentation, when effective treatment for thyrotoxicosis became available, there is also a greater appreciation for the probable role of

Table 2
History of Advances in Diagnosing and Treating Hyperthyroidism

1656	Wharton first described thyroid gland
1820	Rush said larger size of the thyroid gland in women was "necessary to guard the female system from the influence of the more numerous causes of irritation and vexation of the mind to which they are exposed than the male sex"
1820	Hofrichter rebuked Rush theory: "If it were indeed true that the thyroid contains more blood at some times than others, this effect would be visible to the naked eye; in this case women would certainly have long ceased to go about with bare necks, for husbands would have learned to recognize the swelling of this gland as a danger signal of threatening trouble from their better halves"
1825	Hyperthyroidism described by Parry
1835	Characterization of disease by Graves and Basedow
1800s–1920s	Surgical treatment had high mortality — 50–70% when associated with psychiatric symptoms
1930s	Preoperative use of iodine
1940s	Introduction of antithyroid medications (thioureas)
1950	PBI first used
1950s	Use of steroids preoperatively
1950s	Use of ^{131}I
1964	Assay for T_4 developed

Table 3

Symptoms (Operative Era — 1830–1940)

Study	N	Male:female	Age	Severity	Comments
Packard, 1909	82	20:62	34	Mild to severe	High incidence of depression and excitement 30% mortality rate Some new cases but most from reports in literature of time
Johnson, 1928	2286		53	None to severe	1% of thyrotoxics develop delirium (24/2286); series from Cleveland Clinic
Dunlap and Moersch, 1935	143	35:108	50	Moderate to severe	73% Graves; 21% toxic multinodular; 6% nontoxic goiter 60% mortality rate Mayo Clinic files 72% either toxic "exhaustion psychosis" or "acute delirium" (78% mortality) 19% manic-depressive (depression most frequent)

Table 4

Symptoms (Antithyroid Drug Era — after 1940s)[a]

Study	N	Male:female	Age	Severity	Comments
Lidz, 1949	15	3:12	30s	Not stated	9/14 depressed; no description of criteria given
Robbins and Vinson, 1960	10	3:7	42	Not stated	1/10 psychosis, 1/10 anxious; no criteria
Wilson et al., 1962	26	1:25	37	Not stated	15/26 dysphoric; 2/26 elated; 6/25 anxious; no criteria
Hermann and Quarton, 1965	24	NS	NS	Not stated	Anxiety a sensory phenomenon
Artunkal and Togrol, 1964	20	0:20	36	Not stated	Increase in depression and anxiety score on MMPI; not changed with treatment
Whybrow et al., 1969	10	3:7	43	Mean PBI, 14.6 ($N = 3.5$–8.8)	2/10 depression; 2/10 anxiety; 2/10 paranoia on MMPI; 4/10 confusion; "subjective mental disturbance"
MacCrimmon et al., 1979	19	0:19	39	All T_4 11.5 All ^{131}I uptake 60%	High depression scores on MMPI and Present State Schedule
Rockey and Griep, 1980	14	3:11	40	T_4 — all elevated	1/14 depressed; psychiatric diagnoses not specifically looked for

[a]Abbreviations: N, number; NS, not stated; MMPI, Minnesota Multiphasic Personality Inventory.

this altered hormone state in the production of symptoms. Initially, it was thought that hyperthyroidism was caused by psychic trauma (Bram, 1927); however, this theory was discarded when Hermann and Quarton (1965) demonstrated that patients with hyperthyroidism were no more likely to have antecedent stresses than a matched control population of patients with euthymic goiter. Now emotional changes are considered manifestations of cerebral changes from the altered hormonal environment, but they could also be extensions of the physical symptoms themselves. One of the problems in diagnosing psychiatric disease in patients with hyperthyroidism is that the symptoms of hyperthyroidism overlap to such a great extent with those of the principal psychiatric conditions (anxiety and depression) that occur in these patients (Table 5). In a study of 33 patients with hyperthyroidism presenting to an outpatient endocrinology practice (Kathol and Delahunt, 1986), 80% met DSM-III criteria for generalized anxiety disorder and 31% met DSM-III criteria for depression when symptoms were taken at face value. As might be expected by the overlap of thyroid and anxiety symptoms, the severity of the hyperthyroidism, as assessed both by symptoms and thyroxine blood levels, correlated closely with the number of anxiety symptoms (Kathol et al., 1986).

Depression occurred much less frequently than anxiety and did not correlate with the severity of hyperthyroidism. There was no increase in the number with a personal or family history of depression between depressed and nondepressed patients. There was, however, a low incidence of suicidal ideation (20%) when compared to patients with primary affective disorder (80%). These findings suggest that depression associated with hyperthyroidism is qualitatively different than that seen in patients with primary affective disorder.

A number of studies suggests that effective treatment of the hyperthyroidism with antithyroid drugs, radioactive iodine, or surgery will result in a resolution of psychiatric symptoms (Dunlap and Moersch, 1935; Wilson et al., 1962; Whybrow et al., 1969; MacCrimmon et al., 1979; and Kathol et al., 1986). In most cases, the improvement occurs within the first month of treatment. Occasional patients have, however, been described who did not show resolution in depressive symptoms even though their thyroid condition normalized (Whybrow et al., 1969; Rockey and Griep, 1980). Because the vast majority show resolution with treatment of the hyperthyroidism itself, it is possible that these exceptional cases represent those with underlying primary affective disorder that happened to occur concurrently with the onset of their hyperthyroidism.

In summary, hyperthyroidism is often accompanied by symptoms that suggest generalized anxiety and major depression. Since there is such an overlap of symptoms between the endocrine disease itself and anxiety and depression, one can successfully argue that psychiatric comorbidity in hyperthyroidism does not exist at all but is artifactual, especially in the case of anxiety. The fact that depression resolves with treatment of the thyrotoxicosis supports this

Table 5
Comparison of Hyperthyroid to Depressive Symptoms

Hyperthyroid	Anxiety/panic	Depressive
Shakiness	Shakiness	
Palpitations	Palpitations	
Insomnia	Insomnia	Insomnia
Fatigue/weakness	Fatigue	Fatigue/weakness
Shortness of breath	Dyspnea	
Weight loss		Weight loss/anorexia
Nervousness	Anxiety	
Irritability	Irritability	Irritability
Impaired concentration	Poor concentration	Impaired concentration
Other symptoms		
Heat intolerance	Sweating	Agitation/retardation
Impaired memory	Chest pain	Loss in interest
Menstrual change	Faintness	Worthlessness/guilt
Change in face	Choking	Thoughts of death/suicide
Change in hair	Fear of dying	
Change in skin	Dizziness	
	Unreality	
	Paresthesias	
	Hot/cold flashes	

notion as well, although the lack of correlation with thyrotoxic symptoms does not. Psychotic and delirious symptoms can occur in patients with hyperthyroidism, as is exemplified by studies performed prior to 1935. These symptoms are much less common nowadays because the disease can be identified easily much earlier in its course. When psychosis and delirium are the presenting psychiatric problems, they suggest that the patient likely has more advanced disease or that an alternative cause for the psychiatric symptoms may coexist.

IV. Hypothyroidism

The treatment for hypothyroidism first became available in 1890. Prior to that time, many of the patients with this condition spent their final days in mental hospitals. The description of one of the first patients to be treated with thyroid extract was reported by Drs. Shaw and Stansfield in 1892 and provides an informative picture of the problems that could occur for these patients:

Mrs. H, married in 1879 at the age of 20, had her first child in 1880, second in 1882, and third in 1887. My recollection of the case was that following the birth of the second child she had an attack of lactational melancholia and inflicted a wound on her throat. She was aphonic for three months, but recovered everything except full voice tone after treatment with electricity and massage. It was assumed that the thyroid had suffered injury during this suicide attempt.

Symptoms of myxedema were first noticed when she was pregnant with her third child. The principal mental symptoms were mental confusion and inability to concentrate or employ herself. She had considerable insight into her mental state and became languid and disinterested in her occupation and her children. She was under the treatment of Sir William Broadbent for about a year in 1890–1891, phosphorus being given exclusively. The prognosis at that time was very bad and the patient was given only months to live. The mental condition became worse and she was certified and sent to the Banstead Asylum in April, 1891.

To the ordinary symptoms of myxedema were added occasional stupor, aphonia, rigidity, and erotomania. She would periodically get into other patients' beds and when being bathed, unless the nurses were careful, would seize and almost strangle them in the excess of her sexual desire. All sorts of remedies were tried without avail: hot baths, massage, injections of pilocarpine (until, indeed, profuse salivation resulted), tonics, and electricity.

Finally, it was decided to treat the patient with glycerine extract of the thyroid of the sheep. The Committee purchased the sheep, killed them, and dissected out the thyroid. A 20 percent glycerine extract was made by pounding and macerating the gland for forty-eight hours and then straining it through several layers of very fine muslin. The patient was given an injection every second day. The reaction was most remarkable. In ten weeks' time Mrs. H was out on trial and at the expiration of her trial she was discharged recovered.

Dr. Stansfield followed the patient for some time thereafter. He recollected that about four months after discharge, and five months after the last injection, the symptoms began to recur. The patient was then instructed to obtain the gland from the butcher and take it in daily small doses in the raw state, either in port wine or in a mouthful of soup. This method of treatment was carried out until the advent of the thyroid tabloid.

Within three years of her discharge from the asylum she made two tours of the United States. Despite the occurrence of mental changes before the myxedema developed, there appeared little doubt that the former depended on the latter.

Shaw, 1892 and Barham, 1912

Like hyperthyroidism, the psychiatric comorbidity associated with hypothyroidism is largely related to the duration of symptoms and degree of hypothyroidism prior to clinical diagnosis. Many case reports document that depression and dementia are the two cardinal psychiatric manifestations of hypothyroidism. The first unselected prospective study of psychiatric comorbidity in patients with hypothyroidism was performed by Whybrow et al. (1969). In this landmark study, they showed that five of seven patients were subjectively depressed at the time of evaluation while six of seven showed impairment of cognitive function. One additional patient was "bad tempered" while another was described as anxious. Of interest, the symptoms of depression improved in all of the four who were followed, including one who had a psychotic depression, with treatment of the thyroid condition alone. On the other hand, two of the three patients with cognitive impairment of the Trailmaking Test failed to improve when the protein-bound iodine returned to the normal range.

Jain (1972) used a semistructured clinical evaluation to assess the presence of psychiatric disease in consecutive patients entering the nuclear medicine department with the diagnosis of hypothyroidism. No criteria defining why patients were identified as emotionally disturbed were given. Jain found that 13 of 30 (43%) patients had a clinical depression, 10 (30%) had symptoms of anxiety, and 8 (27%) were confused. There was no relationship of the depressive symptoms to the severity of thyroid dysfunction while those with symptoms of anxiety were more likely to have less severe disease and those with cognitive dysfunction more severe disease. Psychotic symptoms did occur in two patients but in one they were related to long-standing schizophrenia and in the other the relationship to depressive symptoms was not stated. The latter patient had severe hypothyroidism.

Two important additional facts emerge from the work of Jain (1972). First, there is no increased family history of depression in depressed patients with hypothyroidism. This suggests that the depression associated with hypothyroidism does not carry a genetic predisposition as does primary depressive disease. Second, treatment of the thyroid condition alone is sufficient to cause a decrease or resolution in the depressive and anxiety symptoms even in severely affected patients.

Cognitive dysfunction in patients with hypothyroidism has been recognized for many years (Jain, 1972) and accounts for approximately 3% of patients with dementia (Larson et al., 1986). When one thinks of hypothyroidism, one thinks of "reversible" dementia. That this premise is probably incorrect was suggested by the work of Whybrow et al. (1969) and substantiated by Clarfield (1988). In the review by Clarfield (1988), only one of seven patients followed up with dementia associated with hypothyroidism had a complete recovery. This points out the importance of early detection of hypothyroidism in patients showing signs of early thyroid dysfunction (including psychiatric).

Psychiatric comorbidity does not occur only during the onset and progression of hypothyroidism, it also can occur during the initiation of its treatment. Josephson and MacKenzie (1980) reviewed the reports of 18 patients who developed mania when hypothyroid patients were started on thyroid replacement. This reaction typically occurred during the first week of therapy and spontaneously resolved within 3 to 5 weeks while continuing thyroid replacement. Patients who experienced this reaction had a greater personal and family history of psychiatric illness and therefore could have been genetically predisposed to the development of the symptoms. Antimanic therapy was not necessary to control symptoms in most cases.

In summary, depression is more frequently encountered in patients with hypothyroidism than anxiety but both resolve when thyroid replacement is given. Psychosis and delirium were more common presentations in this disease before early detection was possible. Memory disturbance is probably related to the severity and duration of hypothyroidism and in most cases is only partially reversible with thyroid replacement. Treatment of hypothyroidism can cause a short episode of mania that resolves spontaneously.

V. Cushing's Syndrome

A review by Ettigi and Brown (1978) suggested that depression, psychosis, and organic brain syndrome are the principle psychiatric manifestations in patients with Cushing's syndrome. A number of research studies (Table 6) have been published since that review that allow us to refine this general conclusion. First, depression is seen in approximately 70% of

Table 6
Psychiatric Manifestations in Patients with Cushing's Syndrome[a]

Study	Diagnostic technique	Illnesses identified	Frequency	Comments
Jeffcoate et al., 1979	Clinical	Depression	21/38	Four severe
		Mania	2/38	
		Delirium	1/38	
Cohen, 1980	Clinical	Depression	25/29	Five severe; one dilusional
		Mania	1/29	
Kelly et al., 1980	PSE	Depression	8/12	One severe
Haskett, 1985	SADS-L	Depression	25/30	Retrospective; two delusional
		Mania	4/30	Five more had mania

[a]Abbreviations: PSE, Present State Examination; SADS-L, Schedule for Schizophrenia and Affective Disorder — Lifetime Version.

patients with Cushing's syndrome (perhaps the highest percentage of any medical illness) (Kathol, 1985). Twenty percent of these patients are considered to have incapacitating depression and suicide attempts are frequently seen. Second, psychosis, when it occurs (4 to 8% of those with depression), is usually related to the depression (psychotic depression). Nonaffective psychotic symptoms are uncommon. And third, delirium (acute organic brain syndrome) does not occur often, but can, as with any other serious medical illness. On the other hand, memory impairment (chronic organic brain syndrome), particularly nonverbal memory, occurs in up to two thirds of patients with Cushing's syndrome (Whelan et al., 1980). Although a change in memory capabilities can be elicited on clinical examination with serial 7's and remembering three things at 15 min, the memory difficulties are generally subclinical. Perhaps as important as the frequency of reportings of these psychiatric syndromes is the fact that the studies in Table 6 and those by others (Starr, 1952; Starkman et al., 1981) do not report an increased incidence of other psychiatric illnesses.

Several lines of evidence suggest that the mood changes associated with Cushing's syndrome are qualitatively similar to those seen in patients with primary affective disorder. First, the frequency of suicidal ideation is approximately 80%, a figure similar to that found with primary depression (Haskett, 1985). Suicidal ideation in patients with depression associated with other medical illnesses, on the other hand, is around 20% (Cavanaugh et al., 1983). Second, psychotic depression is rarely seen in patients with depression associated with other medical illness, while in patients with Cushing's syndrome it is present in up to 8% (Haskett, 1985). This figure is less than the 18% found in inpatients with primary depression (Winokur, 1989), but would likely be close to the frequency found in a mixture of inpatients and outpatients. And third, there appears to be a relationship of depression to the presence of hypercortisolemia in patients with intermittent Cushing's syndrome (Kathol, 1985). Such a relationship is similar to that recorded for patients with primary depression (Kathol, 1985c).

Despite these similarities, depression in patients with Cushing's syndrome and primary affective disorder differ in other ways. Both Haskett (1985) and Hudson et al. (1987) demonstrated that there was no increased family history for affective disorder in first degree relatives of patients with Cushing's syndrome. Such is not the case in patients with primary affective disorder (Weissman et al., 1984). Another difference between primary depression and depression secondary to Cushing's syndrome is that treatment of the Cushing's syndrome alone is sufficient to resolve the depressive symptoms, albeit sometimes there may be a 2- to 6-month delay between correction of serum cortisol and euthymia (Jeffcoate et al., 1979; Haskett, 1985).

It is worth commenting further on the important common bond, elevated cortisol levels, between Cushing's syndrome with a high frequency and severity of depression and primary major depression. There are multiple causes of hypercortisolemia in patients with Cushing's syndrome. It can occur as a result of hypersecretion of corticotropin-releasing hormone (CRH) (Belsky et al., 1985; Schteingart et al., 1986). It can occur as a result of hypersecretion of adrenocorticotropic hormone (ACTH), both ectopically produced and as a result of pituitary adenoma (Crapo, 1979; Besser and Edwards, 1972), and it can occur as a result of direct cortisol production as in patients with adrenal adenomas (Crapo, 1979; Besser and Edwards, 1972). Now, if there is a relationship between hypercortisolemia and depression, is it most closely related to CRH, ACTH, or cortisol? At this time, the evidence suggests that cortisol or by-products in the production of cortisol are more likely related to the development of symptoms than ACTH or CRH, as is reviewed in Table 7.

One of the principal arguments against this is that depression sometimes does not improve rapidly after correction of cortisol elevation. The reason that psychiatric symptoms in patients with Cushing's disease do not rapidly resolve when serum cortisol returns to the normal range is not well understood. It could have to do with the time it takes for intra- and extracellular metabolic processes to return to normal even in the face of physiologic circulating cortisol levels. At the current time, delayed clinical improvement is important not so much in the need to understand the temporal relationship between the two, but to be aware that even patients effectively treated for their Cushing's syndrome can continue to manifest severe depressive symptoms with the attendant risks of suicide. For this reason close psychiatric follow-up is as important as medical.

In summary, affective disorder, primarily depression but also mania, is seen frequently in patients with Cushing's syndrome. The depressions in these patients are often severe as manifest by psychotic symptoms and suicidal ideation. Identifiable, but usually clinically insignificant, memory disturbance also occurs with some frequency. These symptoms typically resolve with treatment of the hypercortisolemia, which could play an etiologic role in their development.

VI. Hyperparathyroidism

The best prospective studies (Petersen, 1968; Joborn et al., 1988a) investigating psychiatric comorbidity in patients with hyperparathyroidism did not use the syndrome approach to diagnosis. Petersen (1968) identified "personality changes," divided into moderate, severe,

Table 7
Evidence Suggesting that Cortisol and not ACTH or CRH Are Related to the Development of Depression[a]

Finding	Cortisol	ACTH	CRH	Ref.
Depression is commonly associated with Cushing's syndrome of adrenal origin	+	−	−	Kathol, 1985
Significant correlation of ACTH and cortisol levels to depression symptoms present	+	+		Starkman et al., 1981
Paucity of depression in patients with Nelson's syndrome and congenital adrenal hyperplasia	+	−	−	Feldman et al., 1987; Jeffcoate et al., 1979; Buckler et al., 1988
Elevated CSF CRH in depression; low CSF CRH in Cushing's disease	+		−	Nemeroff et al., 1984; Tomori et al., 1983
Correction of depression with one but not ACTH in patients with Cushing's syndrome	+	−	−	Jeffcoate et al., 1979; Kathol, 1985

[a]+, Suggestive; −, not suggestive.

and psychotic, in 36 of 54 patients. Although Petersen indicated that the majority of these represented affective disturbances, in fact, this was suggested by individual symptoms such as loss of initiative and spontaneity, dejection, listlessness, moroseness, irascibility, explosiveness, and suicidal tendencies rather than a syndrome complex. None of the patients required hospitalization and no description was given about what constituted moderate, severe, and psychotic difficulties. Despite these limitations Petersen was able to show that when psychiatric symptoms occurred they were likely to be related to the level of hypercalcemia rather than parathyroid hormone levels and that the symptoms resolved after hypercalcemia was corrected.

Joborn et al. (1988) were unable to reproduce the findings of Petersen (1968), which suggest that the degree of psychiatric symptoms is related to the level of hypercalcemia; since their patients were less severely ill. They used the Comprehensive Psychopathological Rating Scale (CPRS; Asberg et al., 1978) to identify psychiatric changes and documented that treatment of the hypercalcemia alone caused significant improvement in psychiatric symptoms. During their evaluations spinal fluid examinations revealed that cerebrospinal fluid (CSF) 5-hydroxyindole-acetic acid (5-HIAA) levels were lower in those with more severe psychiatric disturbance and returned toward normal levels with treatment of the disease. This suggests that serotoninergic neurotransmitters may be involved in the development of psychiatric symptoms (Joborn et al., 1988b). Unfortunately, the CPRS does not allow an assessment of which complex of symptoms (depression, anxiety, dementia, etc.) is most closely correlated with the CSF 5-HIAA levels.

Alarcon and Franceschini (1984) have reviewed other, mostly retrospective, studies of psychiatric symptoms in patients with hyperparathyroidism. These studies also suggest that depression is the major psychiatric presentation in patients with hyperparathyroidism. Unlike the other disorders discussed in this chapter, however, it is impossible from these studies to determine whether there are similarities between the depression in these patients and those with primary psychiatric disease. It is still possible that the symptoms scales that are used in most of these studies are identifying overlapping symptoms between hyperparathyroidism and depression (fatigue, weakness, listlessness, etc.) rather than symptoms of a depressive syndrome (dysphoria, loss of interest, guilt, hopelessness, pessimism, suicidal ideation, etc.). Therefore, the symptoms could represent artifactual depression.

In addition to reviewing the studies that had been performed up to 1984, Alarcon and Franceschini (1984) also summarize the case reports in a table. This does not help to understand what should "typically" be expected in patients with hyperparathyroidism but it does illustrate that a wide variety of psychiatric symptoms that can be seen in patients with hyperparathyroidism (delusions and hallucinations, delirium, depression, memory disturbance, coma, catatonia, and lethargy) and can occur even at relatively low serum calcium concentrations. Interestingly, mania is not mentioned in either these case reports or in the studies cited.

In addition to depression (or personality changes), several investigators suggest that memory impairment occurs in patients with hyperparathyroidism. Relatively few studies actually document this hypothesis. Cogan et al. (1978) performed memory testing on 13 patients with hyperparathyroidism and found that performance on the Raven Progressive Matrices and the Trailmaking Tests improved after parathyroidectomy. A surgical control group also showed significant postoperative change on the Trailmaking Test but not the Raven in this study. Petersen (1968) also suggests that up to 7 of 54 patients exhibited memory impairment in the absence of an acute confusional state (delirium). The means by which they were assessed, however, was not described. Petersen indicated that cognitive deficits improved when the hypercalcemia was corrected.

Joborn et al. (1986) retrospectively assessed the charts of 552 patients who had undergone an operation for primary hyperparathyroidism. They found that 13 (2.3%) with an average age of 73 were demented. It is impossible to tell from this study whether this number represents an increase from that which would be expected in the general population. Interestingly, none of those identified with memory difficulties were younger than 61 years.

In summary, symptoms resembling depression but occasionally accompanied by psychotic features occur in 20 to 60% of patients with hyperparathyroidism. These tend to be related to the level of serum calcium (Petersen, 1968), particularly when calcium levels rise above a threshold of 12 mg%, and possibly to the presence of a low CSF 5-HIAA (Joborn et al., 1988). Psychiatric symptoms can also occur at only slightly elevated calcium levels if case reports do not merely represent patients with coexistent primary psychiatric disease. The psychiatric symptoms tend to resolve with treatment of the hypercalcemia. Memory dysfunction has been suggested in a number of studies but has not been adequately substantiated through clinical investigation.

VII. Conclusions

In 1978, Ettigi and Brown wrote an excellent review of psychiatric manifestations of endocrine disorders. In it they included a summary table that suggested the frequency with which psychiatric symptoms occurred in several of the more common endocrine disorders. The information reviewed in this chapter updates that summary table for four of the conditions listed in their review and adds one that they did not address (Table 8).

Depression and anxiety are the most common psychiatric symptoms that occur in hyperthyroidism, hypothyroidism, and diabetes mellitus. Depression (and mania) are almost exclusively the psychiatric symptoms seen in patients with Cushing's disease. Psychiatric syndromes in patients with hyperparathyroidism have not been established but the studies that have been performed suggest that affective symptoms are the most common at low calcium levels while cognitive disturbances also occur when calcium levels rise.

Memory disturbances are reported in patients with hyperparathyroidism, hypothyroidism, diabetes, and Cushing's syndrome. The only condition in which this has been studied in some detail is in those with hypothyroidism. With the other three endocrine disorders, memory difficulties are usually subclinical. It is incorrect to assume that memory dysfunction in patients with hypothyroidism is reversible.

Table 8

Common Psychiatric Manifestations of Endocrine Disturbances

Psychiatric symptoms	Diabetes mellitus	Hyperthyroidism	Hypothyroidism	Cushing's syndrome	Hyperpara-thyroidism
Depression	+[a]	+++[b]	+++[c]	++++[d]	+++[e]
Mania	0	0	0	++	0
Anxiety	++[f]	+++[g]	++[c]	0	0
Memory impairment	+	0	++	+	+
Delirium/psychosis	0	0	0	0	0
Sexual dysfunction	+++				

[a]0, 65%; +, 5–10%; ++, 11–30%; +++, 31–50%; ++++, >50%.
[b]Qualitatively different than primary major depression — no psychotic depression, 20% rather than 80% suicidal ideation, no increased family history.
[c]Based on semistructured medical clinical interview without defined criteria.
[d]Similar in quality to primary major depression but with no increased family history.
[e]Suggested from clinical evaluations but no diagnostic criteria.
[f]Primarily generalized anxiety disorder.
[g]Probably related to overlap of symptoms.

In all of the endocrine disorders discussed above with the exception of diabetes, the psychiatric symptoms have been shown to resolve with treatment of the endocrine condition alone. Since there is morbidity associated with the use of psychiatric medications, this is important to understand. There is, however, occasionally a delay between the correction of the endocrine condition and the resolution of the psychiatric symptoms by one or more months, just as is seen with tricyclic antidepressants. For this reason, patients require follow-up for their psychiatric symptoms, especially in the case of patients with Cushing's syndrome, while correcting the hormone imbalance.

Since diabetes is a chronic condition with a high psychiatric morbidity, intervention with primary psychiatric therapies may be of benefit although this has not been proven to date. Optimizing medical management is an important first step in improving psychiatric morbidity.

References

Abed, R. T., Clark, J., Elbadawy, H. F., and Cliffe, M. J., Psychiatric morbidity in acromegaly, *Acta Psychiatr. Scand.*, 75, 635, 1987.

Alarcon, R. D., and Franceschini, S. A., Hyperparathyroidism and paranoid psychosis case report and review of the literature, *Br. J. Psychiatry*, 145, 477, 1984.

American Psychiatric Association, *Diagnostic and Statistical Manual of Mental Disorders*, 3rd ed., APA Press, Washington, D.C., 1980.

American Psychiatric Association, *Diagnostic and Statistical Manual of Mental Disorders*, 3rd ed. (revised), APA Press, Washington, D.C., 1987.

Artunkal, S. and Togrol, B., Psychological studies in hyperthyroidism, in *Brain Thyroid Relationships*, No. 18, Ciba Foundation Series, London, 1964.

Asberg, M., Perris, C., Schalling, D., and Sedvall, G., The CPRS — development and applications of a psychiatric rating scale, *Acta Psychiatr. Scand.*, (Suppl. 271), 1978.

Bale, R. N., Brain damage in diabetes mellitus, *Br. J. Psychiatry*, 122, 337, 1973.

Barham, G. F., Insanity with myxedema, *J. Ment. Sci.*, 58, 226, 1912.

Belsky, J. L., Cuello, B., Swanson, L. W., Simmons, D. M., Jarrett, R. M., and Braza, F., Cushing's syndrome due to ectopic production of corticotropin-releasing factor, *J. Clin. Endocrinol. Metab.*, 60, 496, 1985.

Besser, G. M. and Edwards, C. R. W., Cushing's syndrome, in *Clinics of Endocrinology and Metabolism*, Vol. 1, Mason, A. S., Ed., W. B. Saunders, London, 1972, 451.

Bram, I., Psychic trauma in pathogenesis of exophthalmic goiter, *Endocrinology*, 11, 106, 1927.

Buckler, H. M., Freeman, H., Chetty, M. C. P., and Anderson, D. C., Nelson's syndrome and behavioral changes reversed by selective adenomectomy, *Br. J. Psychiatry*, 152, 412, 1988.

Cavanaugh, S., Clark, D. C., and Gibbons, R. D., Diagnosing depression in the hospitalized medically ill, *Psychosomatics*, 24, 809, 1983.

Clarfield, A. M., The reversible dementias: do they reverse?, *Ann. Int. Med.*, 476, 1988.

Cogan, M. G., Covey, C. M., Arieff, A. I., Wisniewski, A., and Clark, O. H., Central nervous system manifestations of hyperparathyroidism, *Am. J. Med.*, 65, 963, 1978.

Cohen, S. I., Cushing's syndrome: a psychiatric study of 29 patients, *Br. J. Psychiatry*, 136, 120, 1980.

Crapo, L., Cushing's syndrome: a review of diagnostic tests, *Metabolism*, 28, 955, 1979.

Dunlap, H. F. and Moersch, F. P., Psychic manifestations associated with hyperthyroidism, *Am. J. Psychiatr.*, 91, 1215, 1935.

Ettigi, P. G. and Brown, G. M., Brain disorders associated with endocrine dysfunction, *Psychiatr. Clin. N. Am.*, 1, 117, 1978.

Fava, G. A., Sonino, N., and Morphy, M. A., Major depression associated with endocrine disease, *Psychiatr. Dev.*, 4, 321, 1987.

Feldman, S. R., Krishnan, F. E. R., McPherson, H., and Meglin, D. E., Organic affective disorder in a patient with congenital adrenal hyperplasia, *Biol. Psychiatry*, 22, 767, 1987.

Haskett, R. F., Diagnostic categorization of psychiatric disturbance in Cushing's syndrome, *Am. J. Psychiatry,* 142, 911, 1985.

Hermann, H. T. and Quarton, G. C., Psychological changes and psychogenesis in thyroid hormone disorders, *J. Clin. Endocrinol.,* 25, 327, 1965.

Hudson, J. I., Hudson, M. S., Griffing, G. T., Melby, J. C., and Pope, H. G., Jr., Phenomenology and family history of affective disorder in Cushing's disease, *Am. J. Psychiatry,* 144, 951, 1987.

Jain, V. K., A psychiatric study of hypothyroidism, *Psychiatr. Clin.,* 5, 121, 1972.

Jeffcoate, W. H., Silverstone, J. T., Edwards, C. R. W., and Besser, G. M., Psychiatric manifestations of Cushing's syndrome: response to lowering of plasma cortisol, *Q. J. Med.,* 191, 465, 1979.

Jensen, S. B., Diabetic sexual dysfunction: a comparative study of 160 insulin treated diabetic men and women and an age-matched control group, *Arch. Sex. Behav.,* 10, 493, 1981.

Joborn, C., Jetta, J., Frisk, P., Palmer, M., Akerstrom, G., and Ljunghall, S., Primary hyperparathyroidism in patients with organic brain syndrome, *Acta Med. Scand.,* 219, 91, 1986.

Joborn, C., Hetta, J., Johansson, H., Rastad, J., Agren, H., Akerstrom, G., and Ljunghall, S., Psychiatric morbidity in primary hyperparathyroidism, *World J. Surg.,* 12, 476, 1988a.

Joborn, C., Hetta, J., Rastad, J., Agren, H., Akerstrom, G., and Ljunghall, S., Psychiatric symptoms and cerebrospinal fluid monoamine metabolites in primary hyperparathyroidism, *Biol. Psychiatry,* 23, 149, 1988b.

Johnson, W. O., Psychosis and hyperthyroidism, *J. Nerv. Ment. Dis.,* 67, 558, 1928.

Josephson, A. M. and Mackenzie, T. B., Thyroid-induced mania in hypothyroid patients, *Br. J. Psychiatry,* 137, 222, 1980.

Karalan, I., Scott, F., Salis, P., Attia, S., Ware, J., Altinei, A., and Williams, R., Nocturnal erections, differential diagnosis of impotence, *Am. J. Surg.,* 138, 278, 1977.

Kathol, R. G., Etiologic implications of corticosteroid changes in affective disorder, *Psychiatry Med.,* 3, 135, 1985a.

Kathol, R. G., Circannual rhythm and peak frequency of corticosteroid excretion: relationship to affective disorder, *Psychiatry Med.,* 3, 53, 1985b.

Kathol, R. G., Persistent evaluation of urinary free cortisol and loss of circannual periodicity in recovered depressed patients. A trait finding, *J. Aff. Dis.,* 8, 137, 1985c.

Kathol, R. G. and Delahunt, J. W., The relationship of anxiety and depression of symptoms of hyperthyroidism using operational criteria, *Gen. Hosp. Psychiatry,* 8, 23, 1986.

Kathol, R. G., Turner, R., and Delahunt, J., Depression and anxiety associated with hyperthyroidism: response to antithyroid therapy, *Psychosomatics* 27, No. 7, 1986.

Kathol, R. G., Jaeckle, R. S., Lopez, J. F., and Meller, W. H., Pathophysiology of HPA axis abnormalities in patients with major depression: an update, *Am. J. Psychiatry,* 146, 3, 1989.

Kelly, W. F., Checkley, S. A., and Bender, D. A., Cushing's syndrome, tryptophan and depression, *Br. J. Psychiatry,* 136, 125, 1980.

Kemmer, F. W., Bisping, R., Steingruber, H. J., Baar, H., Hardtmann, F., Schlaghecke, R., and Berger, M., Psychological stress and metabolic control in patients with type I diabetes mellitus, *N. Engl. J. Med.,* 314, 1078, 1986.

Larson, E. B., Reifler, B. V., Sumi, S. M., Canfield, C. G., and Chinn, N. M., Diagnostic tests in the evaluation of dementia: a prospective study of 200 elderly outpatients, *Arch. Intern. Med.,* 146, p.1917, 1986.

Lidz, T., Emotional factors in the etiology of hyperthyroidism: the report of a preliminary survey, Paper presented at the meeting of the Society for Research in Psychosomatic Problems, May, 1949.

Lustman, P. J., Griffith, L. S., Clouse, R. E., and Cryer, P. E., Psychiatric illness in diabetes mellitus: relationship to symptoms and glucose control, *J. Nerv. Ment. Disease,* 174, 736, 1986.

MacCrimmon, D. J., Wallace, J. E., Goldbert, W. M., and Streiner, D. L., Emotional disturbance and cognitive deficits in hyperthyroidism, *Psychosom. Med.,* 41, 331, 1979.

Nemeroff, C. B., Widerlov, E., and Bissette, G., Elevated concentrations of CSF corticotropin releasing factor-like immunoreactivity in depressed patients, *Science,* 226, 1342, 1984.

Newman, A. S. and Bertelson, A. D., Sexual dysfunction in diabetic women, *J. Behav. Med.,* 9, 261, 1986.

Packard, F. H., American journal of insanity: an analysis of psychoses associated with Graves' disease, Paper presented at the meeting of the American Medico-Psychological Association, Atlantic City, NJ, June 1–4, 1909.

Petersen, P., Psychiatric disorders in primary hyperparathyroidism, *J. Clin. Endocrinol. Metab.,* 28, 1491, 1968.

Popkin, M. E., Callies, A. L., Lentz, R. D., Colon, E. A., and Sutherland, D. E., Prevalence of major depression, simple phobia, and other psychiatric disorders in patients with long-standing type I diabetes mellitus, *Arch. Gen. Psychiatry,* 45, 64, 1988.

Robbins, L. R. and Vinson, D. B., Objective psychologic assessment of the thyrotoxic patient and the response to treatment: preliminary report, *J. Clin. Endocrinol.,* 20, 120, 1960.

Rockey, P. H. and Griep, R. J., Behavioral dysfunction in hyperthyroidism: improvement with treatment, *Arch. Intern. Med.,* 140, 1194, 1980.

Schteingart, D. E., Lloyd, R. V., Akil, H., Chandler, W. F., Ibarra-Perez, G., Rosen, S. G., and Ogletree, R., Cushing's syndrome secondary to ectopic corticotropin-releasing hormone-adrenocorticotropin secretion, *J. Clin. Endocrinol. Metab.,* 63, 770, 1986.

Shaw, C., Case of myxedema with restless melancholia treated by injections of thyroid juice: recovery, *Br. Med. J.,* 451, 1892.

Starkman, M. N., Schteingart, D. E., and Schork, M. A., Depressed mood and other psychiatric manifestations of Cushing's syndrome: relationship to hormone levels, *Psychosom. Med.,* 43, 3, 1981.

Starr, A. M., Personality changes in Cushing's syndrome, *J. Clin. Endocrinol.,* 12, 502, 1952.

Tomori, N., Suda, T., and Tozawa, F., Immunoreactive corticotropine releasing factor concentration in cerebrospinal fluid from patients with hypothalamic-pituitary-adrenal disorders, *J. Clin. Endocrinol. Med.,* 57, 1305, 1983.

Weissman, M. M., Gershon, E. S., Kidd, K. K., Prusoff, B. A., Leckman, J. F., Dibble, E., Hamovit, J., Thompson, W. D., Pauls, D. L., and Guroff, J. J., Psychiatric disorders in the relatives of probands with affective disorder, *Arch. Gen. Psychiatry,* 41, 13, 1984.

Whelan, T. B., Schteingart, D. E., Startman, N. M., et al., Neuropsychological deficits in Cushing's syndrome, *J. Nerv. Ment. Dis.,* 168, 753, 1980.

Whybrow, P. C., Prange, A. J., Treadway, C. R., and Treadway, C. R., Mental changes accompanying thyroid gland dysfunction, *Arch. Gen. Psychiatry,* 20, 48, 1969.

Wilkinson, G., Borsey, D. Q., Leslie, P., Newton, R. W., Lind, C., and Ballinger, C. B., Psychiatry morbidity and social problems in patients with insulin-dependent diabetes mellitus, *Br. J. Psychiatry,* 153, 38, 1988.

Wilson, W. P., Johnson, J. E., and Smith, R. B., Affective change in thyrotoxicosis and experimental hypermetabolism, *Recent Adv. Biol. Psychiatry,* 4, 234, 1962.

Winokur, G., The schizoaffective continuum: Euclid's second axiom, *Ann. Clin. Psychiatry,* 1, 19, 1989.

15

Neuroendocrine Alterations in Psychiatric Disorders

CHARLES B. NEMEROFF
Department of Psychiatry
Emory University School of Medicine
Atlanta, Georgia

and

K. RANGA R. KRISHNAN
Department of Psychiatry
Duke University Medical Center
Durham, North Carolina

I. Introduction

In the past 25 years multidisciplinary approaches to the study of the major mental disorders have provided incontrovertible evidence that disorders such as major depression with melancholia, schizophrenia, and panic disorder are, in fact, disorders of the central nervous system (CNS), and not, as previously thought, "functional" disorders secondary to poor child rearing, poor parenting, or mild psychosocial stressors. This conclusion is supported by data obtained from (1) genetic/family studies, (2) brain-imaging methods, including magnetic resonance imaging (MRI), positron-emission tomography (PET), and single proton emission computed tomography (SPECT), (3) neurochemical studies, including measurement of neurotransmitters, their metabolites and receptors in brain tissue or body fluids (urine, cerebrospinal fluid, or plasma), (4) studies of the mechanisms of action of antidepressant, anxiolytic, and antipsychotic drugs, (5) electrophysiological studies, including electroencephalogram (EEG), evoked potentials, and brain electroactivity mapping (BEAM), and (6) neuroendocrine studies. It is this last category that is the subject of this chapter.

Although it has long been appreciated that patients with endocrine disorders commonly exhibit psychiatric symptoms (see Kathol, this volume), the notion that particular psychiatric disorders are associated with relatively specific neuroendocrine alterations, perhaps related to the pathophysiology of the disorder, is a relatively new concept. We discuss below each of the major endocrine axes and their alterations in the major psychiatric disorders. Space constraints preclude an encyclopedic review of this area and the interested reader may refer to Copolov and Rubin (1988), Brown et al. (1988), Halbreich (1987), and Brown (1988).

II. Growth Hormone

The secretion of growth hormone (GH) is regulated by the complex interaction of neural and endocrine influences, both stimulatory and inhibitory (Martin, 1976). This control is achieved by at least two hypothalamic hormones, growth hormone-releasing hormone (GRF) and somatostatin. These hormones are synthesized and released from neurons in the hypothalamus. In addition, there is evidence that monoamines, primarily dopamine, norepinephrine, and serotonin, act to modulate the release of these hypothalamic hypophysiotropic hormones.

Almost 10 years ago, GRF$_{1-40}$ and GRF$_{1-44}$ were isolated and sequenced from pancreatic tumors causing acromegaly (Thorner et al., 1983; Guillemin et al., 1982). The biological activity of GRF resides in the 29 amino acids at the amino-terminal end of the molecule. GRF stimulates both the release and synthesis of GH in the somatotroph cells of the anterior pituitary (Lamberts and Oosterom, 1985). Somatostatin inhibits the release of GH from the somatotroph cells. Its effect on the synthesis of GH has been less carefully investigated. GRF is found predominantly in the arcuate nucleus of the hypothalamus, SRIF in the periventricular nucleus. Both peptides are released from nerve terminals in the median eminence and transported in the hypothalamo-hypophysial portal system to the anterior pituitary, where they act on somatotrophs.

There is considerable evidence to suggest that norepinephrine, dopamine, and serotonin have a stimulatory role in the central regulation of GH secretion (Martin, 1976). L-Dopa causes release of GH in humans (Boyd et al., 1970). Apomorphine, a centrally active dopamine agonist, also stimulates the release of GH (Lal et al., 1973). L-Tryptophan and 5-hydroxytryptophan serotonin precursors cause GH release, although the effect is much smaller than that observed with L-dopa (Muller et al., 1974; Imura et al., 1973). Methysergide and cyproheptadine, serotonin receptor antagonists, block the GH response to hypoglycemia. Norepinephrine can release GH and this effect is blocked by phentolamine, indicating a role for α-adrenergic receptors in GH secretion (Toivola et al., 1972). The central α$_2$ antagonist, clonidine, also stimulates GH release (Lal et al., 1975a). In view of the role of catecholamines and indoleamines in regulating GH secretion, and their putative role in the pathophysiology of affective disorders and schizophrenia, several studies that have examined GH regulation in patients with these psychiatric disorders have been conducted. This field has recently been comprehensively reviewed by Risch (1991).

A. Growth Hormone Regulation in Affective Disorders: Circadian Pattern

Growth hormone under basal conditions is secreted in pulses that are highest in the first few hours of the night. Age is a major determinant of GH secretion; GH secretion decreases with increasing age (Finkelstein et al., 1972). Mendlewicz et al. (1985) studied the 24-hr secretion of plasma GH in 16 patients with major depression (8 unipolar and 8 bipolar) compared with 8 age- and sex-matched controls. Both unipolar and bipolar depressed patients secreted more GH than normal subjects, and this hypersecretion occurred during waking hours rather than during sleep. The increase was about sixfold in unipolar depression and about fourfold in bipolar depression. In this study, a relationship between nocturnal GH secretion and depression was not found. An earlier study by Schilkrut et al. (1975) suggested that GH secretion was disturbed during the night in depressed patients, and that depressed patients had a diminished nocturnal GH release. They hypothesized that GH abnormalities in depressed patients were secondary to disrupted sleep architecture, and also reported a diminished association between nocturnal GH spikes and slow wave sleep. Mendlewicz et al. (1985) also found a diminished association between nocturnal GH spikes and slow wave sleep stages, and suggested that this finding may be related to the inhibitory effect of diurnal hypersecretion of GH.

B. Growth Hormone Response to Dopamine Agonists

An early study suggested that the GH response to L-dopa was decreased in patients with unipolar depression, as well as in patients with bipolar depression (Sachar et al., 1973). Sachar et al. (1975) subsequently demonstrated that after controlling for age and sex, there were no differences in GH response to L-dopa between depressed patients and control subjects. Gold et al. (1976) reported that bipolar, but not unipolar, patients had an increased GH response, although Maany et al. (1979) were unable to confirm these findings. Several studies examining GH responses to apomorphine found no differences between depressed patients and normal controls (Casper et al., 1977; Frazer, 1975; Maany et al., 1979). Taken together, these reports suggest that the dopaminergic regulation of GH secretion is not altered in depression (Risch et al., 1990).

C. Noradrenergic Agonists

Clonidine, an α_2-adrenergic agonist, stimulates GH secretion. GH response to intravenous clonidine has been reported to be significantly reduced in patients with endogenous depression in comparison to subjects with neurotic depression (Matussek et al., 1980; reviewed by Matussek, 1988) or normal controls. Siever et al. (1982) reported that in a group of 19 depressed patients and 20 controls, the blunted GH response to clonidine in the depressed group was not related to age or sex. They also demonstrated a negative correlation between plasma MHPG values and the magnitude of the GH response to clonidine, and suggested on the basis of this study that the diminished GH response to clonidine in depression may be secondary to decreased α_2-adrenergic receptor responsiveness. The blunted GH response to clonidine was also observed in depressed patients by Charney et al. (1982) and Checkley et al. (1981). Indeed, the blunted GH response to clonidine is considered by some to be the most reproducible and specific finding in the biology of affective disorders. Langer et al. (1975) reported that the GH response to D-amphetamine was blunted in patients with endogenous depression. This was confirmed by Arato et al. (1983), who showed that this blunting was not related to dexamethasone suppression test results. Halbreich et al. (1982), using dextroamphetamine, which also releases GH through an adrenergic mechanism, reported that the blunted GH response was seen only in endogenously depressed postmenopausal females. They did not observe a diminished GH response in males, although it must be noted that their sample size was quite small.

Recent studies that used parenteral desmethylimipramine (DMI) have also demonstrated that GH responses to DMI are reduced in endogenous depressives (Laakman et al., 1977), and that this blunting was blocked by the α_2-adrenergic antagonists, phentolamine and yohimbine (Laakman, 1986). Recently Dinan and Barry (1990) reported that the GH response to orally administered DMI (1 mg/kg) is blunted in depressed patients, both endogenous and nonendogenous subtypes, when compared to controls. This concatenation of results indicates that there appears to be diminished α_2-adrenergic responsiveness in depression.

D. Growth Hormone Response to TRH

Brambilla et al. (1978) reported an aberrant GH response to thyrotropin-releasing hormone (TRH) in depressed subjects. Similar findings have been reported by Maeda et al. (1975), Winokur et al. (1983), and Brown et al. (1988), but not by Gregiore et al. (1977). An aberrant GH response to TRH has also been observed in patients with acromegaly or hypothyroidism, and although not consistently demonstrable in depression, it is possible that this may be an indication of subclinical hypothyroidism in some patients with depression.

E. Hypoglycemia-Induced Growth Hormone Response

Early studies (Carroll, 1972; Sachar et al., 1973b) suggested that depressed patients have a diminished GH response to insulin-induced hypoglycemia. They also suggested that the hypoglycemic response to insulin was less diminished during the depressed period. Gregiore et al. (1977), Endo and Endo (1974), and other authors have also reported a blunted GH response to insulin tolerance testing in subjects with depression. Endo and Endo (1974) and Gregiore et al. (1977) have reported that this abnormality returns to normal after recovery from the depression. Casper and Davis (1977) demonstrated a blunted GH response to hypoglycemia in both depressed and hypomanic patients and Grof et al. (1982), Gruen et al. (1975), and Kathol et al. (1983) confirmed this finding. These results were not confirmed by Koslow et al. (1982) and Berger et al. (1982). Garver et al. (1975) implicated a role for norepinephrine in the blunted GH response to insulin, and demonstrated a positive correlation between GH response and urinary catecholamine and MHPG excretion. Another factor responsible for the blunted GH response to insulin might be the hypercortisolemia commonly observed in depressed patients (Nathan et al., 1981).

F. Growth Hormone-Releasing Factor

With the availability of synthetic GRF, it became possible to study the GH response to GRF in subjects with depression. The results from these studies have been discordant. Our group (Krishnan et al., 1988) as well as others (Phillip Gold, National Institute of Mental Health, personal communication) have demonstrated minimal differences between depressed patients and control subjects. In our study of 19 depressed patients and 19 age- and sex-matched controls (Krishnan et al., 1988), a few of the depressed subjects had an increased GRF-induced response when compared to control subjects, but certainly no attenuated response. This contrasts with the studies of Lesch et al. (1987a, b), who reported that depressed patients exhibit a blunted GH response to GRF. Moreover, Lesch et al. (1988) correlated the GH response to GRF to the blunted GH response to clonidine, indicating that these two findings may be related. Risch et al. (1991) also observed a blunted GH response to GRF in depressed patients.

The differences between the aforementioned studies and those of Lesch may be due to the length of the drug-free interval, age of the subjects, and possibly to the fact that GRF_{1-44} was used by Lesch and Risch and GRF_{1-40} was used by our group. Another confound is that the GH response to GRF is extremely variable and is influenced by sex, age, menstrual cycle, and body weight. In fact, Krishnan et al. (1988) reported that in normal weight subjects, body weight is correlated to the GH response to GRF. Because this has not been standardized in most studies, it is possible that such nonspecific factors may account for the variance in results obtained by different groups. Further studies using GRF are required to clarify these issues.

G. Alzheimer's Disease

GH regulation has also been studied in Alzheimer's disease, primarily because patients with Alzheimer's disease have a significant reduction in central nervous system concentrations of somatostatin (Nemeroff et al., 1989a). If patients with Alzheimer's disease have a long-standing reduction in the availability of hypothalamic somatostatin, then alterations in pituitary GH secretion may result. We did not, however, find a difference between Alzheimer's patients and control subjects in the GH response to GRF (Nemeroff et al., 1989b). This finding is in accordance with the results of Steardo et al. (1984), who observed a normal GH response to GRF in Alzheimer's disease. Cacabelos et al. (1988) reported that patients with early onset

Alzheimer's disease show an exaggeraged GH response to GRF, unlike those with late onset disease. Nemeroff et al. (1989b) primarily studied individuals with late onset disease. These findings are concordant with the neurochemical studies of Rosser et al. (1984), who reported that patients with early onset Alzheimer's disease show the most marked reductions in cortical somatostatin immunoreactivity. Based on these studies, it would appear that the GH response to GRF may be altered primarily in individuals with the early onset form of the disease and its use as a diagnostic adjunct in Alzheimer's disease, if any, would be limited to those subjects.

H. Schizophrenia

GH concentrations are of interest to investigators in schizophrenia research because GH secretion is, to some extent, under the influence of dopamine, the catecholamine neurotransmitter thought to play a preeminent role in the pathophysiology of schizophrenia. Brambilla et al. (1975) observed normal GH secretion in male schizophrenic patients. Most investigators have reported that drug-free schizophrenic subjects have normal basal GH concentrations (Pandey et al., 1977). The apomorphine-induced GH response has been studied in patients with schizophrenia in some detail. In general, GH responses to apomorphine in chronic schizophrenia tend to be blunted (Ettigi et al., 1976). In acute schizophrenic subjects, an increased GH response has been noted (Pandey et al., 1977). Meltzer et al. (1984) measured the apomorphine-induced GH response in schizophrenia and in other psychoses and observed no differences between the different diagnostic groups and the controls. They did, however, note a significant correlation between GH response to apomorphine and psychosis ratings. Some authors have suggested that an increased hormone response in acute schizophrenic subjects may predict good therapeutic response (Hollister et al., 1980), whereas an increased hormonal response in chronic patients may predict relapse (Cleghorn et al., 1980). One of the problems in studying GH regulation by dopamine in schizophrenia is the fact that psychotropic medications affect the response. In fact, Ettigi et al. (1976) reported diminished GH responses to apomorphine in patients who were withdrawn from chronic drug treatment, especially in individuals with tardive dyskinesia. The GH response to amphetamine does not differ significantly between patients with schizophrenia and normal subjects, although one study reported a blunted GH response to methylphenidate in patients with schizophrenia (Janowsky et al., 1978). Tamminga et al. (1977) suggested that schizophrenic patients may exhibit a blunted GH response to apomorphine, but there was no significant difference in GH response between subjects with and without tardive dyskinesia.

As noted above, the rationale for all of these studies is the hypothesis that there is pathophysiological involvement of the tuberoinfundibular dopaminergic system in schizophrenia. Although there is considerable evidence for a pathophysiological role for the mesocorticolimbic dopamine (DA) system in schizophrenia, there is little evidence for a role of this major hypothalamic DA system in this disorder. It is possible that the GH response may be greater in subjects with acute schizophrenia and less in subjects with chronic schizophrenia, but at this time the evidence must be taken to be equivocal. Matussek et al. (1980) demonstrated an elevated GH response to clonidine in schizophrenia, and suggested that this represents increased α_2-adrenergic receptor sensitivity in schizophrenic patients. However, this clearly requires further confirmation. The major methodological problems in all these studies is the effect of neuroleptic treatment, and possible confounds related to nonspecific factors such as body weight, weight change, etc. Well-designed studies, controlling for all these factors and involving a large number of subjects, need to be undertaken to clarify the issue of whether the tuberoinfundular dopaminergic system and its control of GH secretion is pathologically involved in schizophrenia.

I. Anorexia Nervosa

Basal plasma GH concentrations are elevated in more than half of anorectic patients (Landen et al., 1966; Marks et al., 1965). GH concentrations in these patients are related to body weight and weight loss (Marks et al., 1965) and return to normal after the patients start eating a normal calorie diet (Casper et al., 1977). GH changes are probably related to the low-calorie diet and are similar to those seen in individuals with malnutrition (Garfinkel et al., 1975; Alvarez et al., 1972). The GH response to insulin is blunted in anorexia nervosa (Marks et al., 1965; Vigensky and Loriaux, 1977). A blunted GH response to L-dopa and apomorphine (Casper et al., 1977; Sherman and Halmi, 1977) has also been reported in these patients. These abnormalities are also corrected by refeeding on a balanced diet. Similar to patients with affective disorder, an aberrant GH response to TRH is observed in these patients (Maeda et al., 1976). Casper et al. (1977) also reported an elevated GH response to a glucose load in subjects with anorexia nervosa. This is paradoxical because hyperglycemia characteristically suppresses GH secretion in normal controls. GH alterations in anorexia nervosa are probably related to changes in food intake and thus may be secondary to the illness rather than being primarily involved in the etiopathogenesis of the disorder.

III. Hypothalamic-Pituitary-Adrenal Axis

Because the hypothalamic-pituitary-adrenal (HPA) axis plays an integral role in the pathophysiology of stress, and stress has long been thought to precipitate episodes of affective disorder in genetically vulnerable individuals, it has been the best studied of all the endocrine axes in psychiatric disorders. An understanding of the physiological regulation of the HPA axis is important to evaluate HPA axis disturbances reported in certain psychiatric disorders.

For several years, adrenocorticotropic hormone (ACTH) was considered to be the sole agent regulating cortisol release from the adrenal cortex. Recent evidence suggests that this view may be incomplete. Krieger and Allen (1975) showed that there were periods when there was a dissociation between plasma ACTH and plasma cortisol concentrations. Fehm reported a number of such instances, e.g., after the noon meal (Fehm et al., 1984), after the administration of methamphetamine (Fehm et al., 1983), and in the early morning (Fehm et al., 1984b), when plasma cortisol concentrations could rise without a preceding or concomitant change in plasma ACTH concentration. Recently we noted that about half the time there is no relationship between the occurrence of cortisol peaks and ACTH peaks in normal subjects (Krishnan et al., 1990a). These studies suggest that a number of non-ACTH-dependent mechanisms may be involved, including direct sympathetic activation of the adrenal cortex, activation by a paracrine mechanism involving chemical messengers produced in the adrenal medulla, and other peptides that directly stimulate the adrenal cortex, such as γ-melanocyte-stimulating hormone (γ-MSH), GH, interferons, etc. (for a detailed discussion of these mechanisms, see Krishnan et al., 1988). At the level of the anterior pituitary corticotroph, a number of factors regulate the secretion of ACTH. These include corticotropin-releasing factor (CRF), vasopressin, somatostatin, vasoactive intestinal polypeptide, catecholamines (both α- and β-adrenergic mechanisms), angiotensin, and glucocorticoids.

Corticotropin-releasing factor, a 41 amino acid-containing peptide, was finally characterized, sequenced, and synthesized approximately 10 years ago (Vale et al., 1981). It stimulates the synthesis of the ACTH and the β-endorphin precursor pro-opiomelanocortin (POMC), as well as the release of ACTH and other adenohypophysial products of POMC. Vasopressin also releases ACTH from corticotrophs, although its effect is minimal compared to the effect of

CRF. However, vasopressin potentiates the action of CRF on the corticotroph, amplifying the effect threefold. Catecholamines act directly on the pituitary primarily through a β-adrenergic mechanism in humans, although this has not been well substantiated. In addition, there is a negative feedback effect of glucocorticoids on the adenohypophysial corticotroph. Glucocorticoid feedback also occurs at extrahypothalamic sites, primarily the hippocampus. CRF and vasopressin regulate the ACTH response to various stressors. CRF is the major modulator of the ACTH response to stress, with vasopressin playing an adjunctive role. In contrast, the stress response to hemodynamic (hemorrhage) stimuli seems to be primarily mediated by vasopressin. Norepinephrine, via a central α_1-adrenergic mechanism, plays an important role in regulating HPA axis activity in humans. Dopamine has little effect on HPA axis activity, serotonin exerts a stimulatory influence, whereas γ-aminobutyric acid (GABA) and opioid peptides inhibit HPA axis activity. The fact that the HPA axis is regulated by a number of neurotransmitters implicated in the pathogenesis of psychiatric disorders has led to considerable study of HPA axis hormone secretion in psychiatric disorders. For a detailed discussion of this area, see Krishnan et al. (1991a).

A. Affective Disorders

The HPA axis has been most extensively studied in patients with affective disorders (Stokes and Sikes, 1988). The vast majority of studies have indicated that patients with affective disorders during the depressed phase exhibit increased secretion of cortisol as measured by 24-hr urinary free cortisol. Early studies indicated that depressed patients show elevated plasma corticosteroid concentrations, which were highest in the most severely depressed subjects (Gibbons, 1962). These studies also suggested that plasma glucocorticoid levels return to normal following successful ECT or antidepressant treatment. Sachar et al. (1970) investigated the cortisol production rate in depressed subjects by measuring isotopically labeled cortisol metabolites in urine before treatment and after recovery. The cortisol production rate was elevated during the illness and returned to normal in most subjects after recovery. They also reported a significant positive correlation between cortisol production rate and certain symptoms of depression and anxiety. Carpenter and Bunney (1971) also found an increased cortisol production rate in depressed patients. Carroll and Mendels (1976) reported

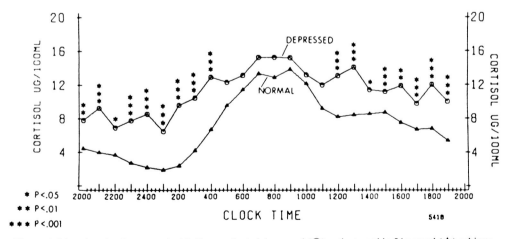

Figure 1. Mean hourly plasma cortisol in 7 unmedicated depressed (○) patients and in 54 normal (▲) subjects. Differences between depressed patients and normals: *, $p < 0.05$; **, $p < 0.01$; ***, $p < 0.001$. (From Sachar, E. J., *Prog. Brain Res.*, 42, 81, 1975. With permission.)

that hospitalized depressed patients had elevated 24-hr urinary free cortisol concentrations and, moreover, this was greater than what was found in other psychiatric patients. In a significant number of these subjects, cortisol concentrations were similar to that seen in Cushing's disease.

Sachar et al. (1970) reported that the 24-hr mean serum cortisol concentrations are elevated in drug-free depressed patients (Figure 1). They suggested that there was an increase in both the number and the magnitude of the cortisol secretory episodes. In addition, this group found that cortisol was inordinately secreted during the late evening and early part of the morning in depressed patients (Sachar et al., 1973a). They also reported a phase advance for the nadir and quiescent period of cortisol and ACTH secretion in depressed subjects when compared to normal controls (Sachar, 1975). Similar findings were reported by other groups (Carroll et al., 1976; Fullerton et al., 1968). We have also noted that patients with depression have high cortisol concentrations in the early morning and night compared to normal controls (Krishnan et al., 1988). Our findings were similar to other authors in that the degree and extent of ACTH rise did not parallel that observed with cortisol (Linkowski et al., 1985). These findings suggest that there is an increase in the sensitivity of the adrenal cortex to ACTH in depressed subjects. In a pioneering study, Amsterdam et al. (1983) reported that depressed patients exhibited an increased cortisol response to $ACTH_{1-24}$ (250 µg), when compared to normal controls, concordant with an increase in adrenocortical responsiveness to ACTH in depression. Kalin et al. (1987) reported that depressed DST (dexamethasone suppression test) nonsuppressors had markedly increased cortisol responses to $ACTH_{1-24}$ (250 µg intravenously) compared to depressed DST suppressors. Jaeckle et al. (1987) conducted a similar study in which $ACTH_{1-24}$ was administered to 38 patients with major depression and to 34 normal control subjects. Patients with major depression were noted to have higher basal plasma cortisol concentrations and a greater increase in plasma cortisol concentration 60 min after $ACTH_{1-24}$ than normal control subjects. Depressed DST nonsuppressors had significantly higher 60-min cortisol concentrations and cortisol increases after ACTH than did normal subjects and depressed DST suppressors. A positive correlation between cortisol response to ACTH and postdexamethasone cortisol concentrations was also found. These findings, taken together, indicate that there is increased adrenocortical responsiveness to ACTH in depression.

Because these studies indicated that depressed patients exhibit an increased cortisol response to high pharmacological doses of ACTH, we conducted a study to assess whether the response was due to increased sensitivity of the adrenal cortex to ACTH (Krishnan et al., 1990b). A threshold dose of $ACTH_{1-24}$ was therefore administered to 11 depressed patients and 12 controls to determine if there is an increased adrenocortical response in depression. Subjects were pretreated with 4 mg of dexamethasone at 11 p.m. the night before the administration of ACTH to eliminate the confounding influence of baseline ACTH fluctuations. $ACTH_{1-24}$ (50 ng) was administered at 8:00 a.m. There was no difference in the rise of plasma cortisol concentrations after this low dose of $ACTH_{1-24}$ administration between depressed patients and control subjects, suggesting that there is no significant change in adrenocortical sensitivity between depressed patients and controls. The study suggests that the enhanced cortisol response observed after high doses of ACTH may reflect adrenocortical hypertrophy, rather than an increased sensitivity to the ACTH receptors.

Using computed tomography, a pilot study by Amsterdam et al. (1987) and a recent study by our group (Nemeroff et al., 1991a) demonstrated increased adrenal gland size in patients with depression. In addition, Zis and Zis (1987) reported that individuals who committed suicide have increased postmortem adrenal gland weights compared to controls. Although the enlargement of the adrenal gland could reflect either hypertrophy of the adrenal cortex or an enlargement of the adrenal medulla, it is most likely due to adrenocortical enlargement. The reasons for this are threefold: (1) the adrenal medulla constitutes less than 10% of the adrenal gland and to account for the increase in size noted in depressed subjects the medulla would have to increase severalfold in size (Neville and O'Hare, 1982); (2) adrenal medullary cells, which are derived from the neural crest, are not known to increase in size or multiply except when neoplastic; and (3) adrenocortical cells are capable of both hypertrophy and hyperplasia. Enlargement of the adrenal gland in patients with depression is thus likely to reflect chronic and persistent HPA axis activation.

A number of studies have measured the ACTH response to exogenously administered CRF. CRF, when administered at a dose of 1 μg/kg, produces a robust ACTH and cortisol response in humans (Schuemeyer et al., 1984). Doses higher than 1 μg/kg are associated with significant side effects and do not produce a greater ACTH or cortisol response. Ovine CRF (oCRF) has a longer half-life in humans than human CRF and has been used in most studies of psychiatric patients. The oCRF-induced ACTH response is blunted in drug-free depressed patients compared to normal subjects (Gold et al., 1984). Gold et al. (1984) suggested that this finding of an attenuated response to CRF in depression was due to the negative feedback effects of elevated cortisol concentrations. This was supported by their finding of a significant inverse correlation between basal plasma cortisol concentrations and ACTH response to CRF. Of additional interest is the fact that the plasma cortisol response to CRF is not different between depressed patients and controls, and that the ACTH:cortisol ratio is higher in depressed patients compared to control subjects, indicating that the adrenocortical response to ACTH is elevated in patients with depression (Gold et al., 1984). The blunted ACTH response to CRF has been confirmed by other authors (Kathol et al., 1989), and a similar finding has been reported using human CRF (Holsboer et al., 1984). The blunted ACTH response is seen only in the evening (Holsboer et al., 1984), during the quiescent phase of HPA axis activity. This response is state dependent and returns to normal after successful treatment of depression (Amsterdam et al., 1988). A recent study by Holsboer et al. (1987) and a similar study by our group indicate that after dexamethasone pretreatment, depressed patients have higher ACTH and cortisol responses after exogenous CRF than normal subjects. Lisansky et al. (1989) and Von Bardeleben et al. (1987) have also shown the ACTH response to CRF after metyrapone administration (metyrapone is used to inhibit cortisol synthesis and therefore eliminate feedback) is increased in depressed patients compared to controls. These data, taken together, indicate that the blunted ACTH response to CRF in depression is not merely due to the hypercortisolemia and resultant negative feedback. The corticotroph may be sensitized to CRF, possibly by increased secretion of vasopressin, which when administered concomitantly with CRF can convert normal controls to DST nonsuppressors (Von Bardeleben et al., 1985), or there is hypersensitivity of the corticotroph. Animal studies indicate that chronic CRF administration can lead to an increase in the number and volume of corticotrophs (Westlund et al., 1987; Gertz et al., 1987). It is therefore possible that there is an increase in pituitary gland size in depression. Indeed, utilizing magnetic resonance imaging, we have recently shown in a study of 19 depressed patients and 19 age- and sex-matched controls that the pituitary gland is enlarged in depressed patients (Krishnan et al., 1991b).

B. Dexamethasone Suppression Test

The DST is undoubtedly the most intensively studied single test of HPA axis activity in patients with depression and it has generated considerable controversy in the literature (Arana and Mossman, 1988). Carroll et al. (1968) reported a failure of suppression of plasma hydroxycorticosteroid levels after the administration of the synthetic glucocorticoid dexamethasone in patients with severe depression, which normalized after recovery from the depression. Stokes et al. (1975), in a seminal study, also demonstrated dexamethasone nonsuppression in drug-free depressed patients. Carroll et al. (1976) reported that many patients with depression

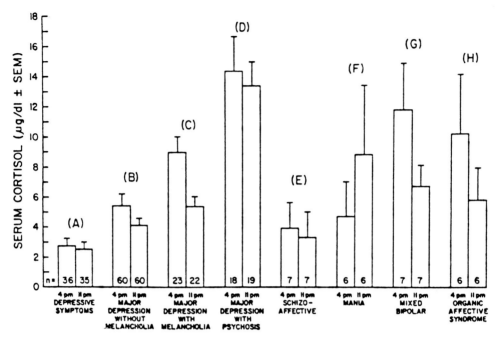

Figure 2. Cortisol levels at 4 p.m. and 11 p.m. of depressed patients with DSM-III diagnoses after oral administration of 1 mg of dexamethasone. (From Evans et al., 1983.)

have an abnormal escape of suppression rather than absolute resistance; thus after the administration of dexamethasone there is in normal volunteers a 24-hr suppression of cortisol, but patients with depression tend to escape from this suppression well before 24 hr. They suggested that this abnormality could be used as a diagnostic marker for depression (Carroll, 1982).

In a landmark publication, Carroll and associates (1981) reported that DST nonsuppression had a 67% sensitivity and a 96% specificity for the diagnosis of melancholia in psychiatric patients hospitalized on a research unit. Since the publication of this report, numerous investigators studied this phenomenon with both concordant and discordant results. Evans and Nemeroff (1984) studied this question in a clinical setting, and showed that the prevalence rate of an abnormal DST increases from the low rate of 14% in patients with depressive symptoms, to 48% in major depression without melancholia, 78% in major depression with melancholia, and finally to the highest rate of 95% in major depression with psychosis (Figure 2). Interestingly, these findings are similar to the results of a recent review of DST results in over 5000 patients (Arana et al., 1985). Remarkably, these findings are also similar to that reported for a clinical setting in a state psychiatric hospital (Krishnan et al., 1987).

Summarizing a vast literature, these data indicate that the DST is unlikely to be useful as a screening test for melancholia or major depression. However, the DST does appear to be useful in distinguishing between subjects with melancholia from those with schizophrenia, and patients with psychotic depression from patients with schizophrenia. A high incidence of DST nonsuppression has been reported in psychiatric disorders other than depression, including mania and dementia, suggesting that the DST is not specific for distinguishing these conditions from depression. The DST may also be useful in identifying adolescent patients with atypical signs and symptoms of depression (Extein et al., 1982; Evans et al., 1987). Evans et al. (1986) demonstrated that the DST is useful in identifying cancer patients with concurrent depression.

When chronic pain patients with and without major depression were compared using items from a modified version of the Hamilton Depression Scale and the Montgomery-Asberg Depression Scale in relation to the DST, depression-related items were useful discriminators between DST suppressors and nonsuppressors (Krishnan et al., 1985). The symptoms that were particularly useful were sleep disturbance, weight change, and reduced appetite, and these symptoms were particularly indicative of the occurrence of DST nonsuppression (Krishnan et al., 1985).

A potential confound in the diagnostic utility of the DST is the finding that plasma dexamethasone concentrations are highly variable and appear to be lower in patients who are DST nonsuppressors than in those who are DST suppressors (Arana et al., 1984; Holsboer et al., 1984, 1986). There have been several reports of significant negative correlations between postdexamethasone plasma cortisol concentrations and plasma dexamethasone concentrations (Johnson et al., 1984). In contrast, a number of investigators have been unable to find such an association between plasma dexamethasone concentration and DST response (Carroll et al., 1980). Discrepancies in the literature may be due to methodological factors, subject selection, sampling times, differences in assay sensitivity and specificity, artifacts associated with uncharacterized dexamethasone metabolites, and the use of unextracted plasma in the radioimmunoassay for plasma dexamethasone. In a recent study Ritchie et al. (1990) have demonstrated that there is a significant inverse relationship between dexamethasone levels and plasma cortisol concentrations, but they found no significant difference in plasma dexamethasone concentration between suppressors and nonsuppressors when patients with a diagnosis of major depression were considered. Most investigators believe that depressed patients do exhibit lower plasma dexamethasone concentrations than controls but that this does not account for DST nonsuppression.

An early report suggested that the DST might be useful for predicting the response to antidepressant treatment (Brown and Shuey, 1980). The studies that have attempted to control for placebo response found that DST suppressors have a high response rate to placebo, with the implication being that DST nonsuppressors may require somatic antidepressant treatment (Shrivastawa et al., 1985). However, this requires further study. Rush et al. (1984) reported that depressed patients with shortened rapid eye movement (REM) latency who also exhibited DST nonsuppression failed to respond to cognitive therapy, whereas depressed DST suppressors responded to cognitive therapy. The presence or absence of an abnormal DST does not predict response to either noradrenergic or serotonergic antidepressants (Simon et al., 1986). An abnormal DST in patients who have previously normalized on clinical improvement is a harbinger for early relapse (Nemeroff and Evans, 1984). Carroll (1985) pooled data on 102 patients who had an abnormal DST on admission and noted that 34% of these patients at time of discharge had an abnormal DST. Of these, 83% had a poor clinical outcome. Arana et al. (1985) also noted that a majority of the patients who remained DST positive on discharge had a poor outcome. An association between DST nonsuppression and suicide has been suggested by Carroll et al. (1981) and Coryell and Schlesser (1981).

C. Neuroanatomical and Cognitive Changes in Relation to HPA Axis Hyperactivity in Depression

Ventricular enlargement and cerebral atrophy are commonly observed in patients with major depression (Pearlson and Veroff, 1981). The ventricular-brain ratio (VBR) has been correlated with 24-hr urinary-free cortisol concentrations (Kellner et al., 1983), although Targum et al. (1983) did not find any significant relationship between DST results and VBR. In contrast, Rothschild et al. (1988) reported a positive correlation between VBR and maximal postdexamethasone plasma cortisol concentration. We recently studied 46 patients with major depression in whom both magnetic resonance imaging (MRI) and a standard 1-mg DST was obtained (Rao et al., 1989). The VBR was measured as described by Synek and Rubin (1976). There were 22 DST suppressors and 24 DST nonsuppressors. There was a strong positive correlation between the maximal postdexamethasone plasma cortisol concentration and VBR ($r = 0.51$, $p = 0.0003$); DST nonsuppressors had a higher VBR than DST suppressors. Recent studies have also suggested that there is a relationship between the cognitive impairment observed in depression and hypercortisolemia (Rubinow et al., 1983). Currently several researchers are investigating the relationship between specific types of cognitive impairment and hypercortisolemia. Such a relationship is suggested by studies of patients with Cushing's disease, in which elevated plasma cortisol concentrations are often associated with specific types of cognitive impairment (Starkman and Schteingart, 1981). One particular impairment that is related to high cortisol concentrations is the Halstead Category Test (Rubinow et al., 1983). The Halstead Category Test is a measure of abstracting ability and it is of interest to note that this test is more poorly performed by patients who have elevated 24-hr urinary free cortisol concentrations. This study provides a physiological basis for the poor outcome of patients with hypercortisolemia in cognitive therapy.

D. Insulin Tolerance Test

When insulin is administered to normal subjects, a rise in plasma ACTH and cortisol concentrations results. A number of studies have indicated that this increase in HPA axis activity in response to insulin is blunted in depressed patients (Carroll, 1972; Gregiore, 1977). However, recent studies have indicated that the insulin tolerance test (ITT) does not differentiate depressed subjects from normal controls. Further studies are required to assess this finding. Another HPA axis stimulation test that has been evaluated in depression is the D-amphetamine cortisol test or the methamphetamine cortisol test (Checkley, 1979). D-Amphetamine or methamphetamine produces a rise in plasma cortisol concentrations. This cortisol rise has been reported to be blunted in depressed patients compared to controls (Checkley et al., 1979; Sachar et al., 1980). This response is similar to that observed with GH and suggests changes in β-adrenoreceptor regulation in depression. Another pharmacological challenge test that has been studied is the desipramine cortisol test; desipramine stimulates cortisol release via a noradrenergic mechanism (Stewart et al., 1984). Depressed patients compared to controls were reported to have a blunted cortisol response to desipramine (Asnis et al., 1986). These studies provide further evidence of subsensitivity of the noradrenergic system in depressed patients.

E. The Role of Corticotropin-Releasing Factor in the Pathogenesis of Depression

Once the chemical identity of CRF was elucidated (*vide supra*), immunohistochemical and radioimmunoassay methods were utilized to determine the distribution of the peptide in the mammalian central nervous system (see Petrusz, this volume). In brief, CRF is found not only within the so-called endocrine hypothalamus (paraventricular nucleus, which projects to the median eminence) but in extrahypothalamic brain areas that subserve affective, cognitive, and autonomic functions. These areas include the locus coeruleus, dorsal motor nucleus of the vagus, hippocampus, cerebral cortex, amygdala, and certain parts of the basal ganglia. There is little doubt that CRF functions as a neurotransmitter substance in the CNS. Not only is the peptide distributed heterogeneously throughout the CNS, but the high-affinity CRF-binding sites are as well. In addition, CRF is preferentially localized in the synaptosomal fraction after density gradient centrifugation and is released from brain slices by depolarizing concentrations of potassium, in a calcium-dependent manner. Furthermore, CRF is degraded by peptidases, and after iontophoretic application CRF alters the firing rate of certain CNS neurons. The gene coding for the CRF precursor has been elucidated and CRF mRNA levels can be measured as an index of CRF biosynthesis rates. These data have been recently reviewed (Nemeroff, 1991).

Because CRF is the major physiological regulator of the HPA axis, by virtue of its potent action on ACTH secretion, it was plausible to determine whether CRF hypersecretion contributes to the hypercortisolemia observed in patients with major depression. In addition, a further impetus to assess the role for CRF in depression comes from studies in laboratory animals that have demonstrated that direct central administration of CRF produces behavioral effects remarkably similar to the cardinal signs and symptoms of major depression, including decreased libido, decreased appetite, psychomotor alterations, and disturbed sleep (Table 1). These findings led to the measurement of CRF in cerebrospinal fluid (CSF) of drug-free patients with major depression, and patients with other psychiatric diagnoses. Our group has conducted six studies. In our first study, we measured the CSF concentration of CRF in 10 normal controls, 23 depressed patients, 11 schizophrenics, and 29 demented patients. The CSF concentration of CRF was elevated in the depressed patients compared to all of the other groups; 11 of the 23 depressed patients had CSF CRF concentrations higher than the highest normal controls (Nemeroff et al., 1984). In our second study we measured the CSF concentration of CRF in 54 depressed women, 138 neurological controls, 23 schizophrenic patients, and 6 manic patients (Figure 3). The depressed patients exhibited a marked two-fold elevation in CSF CRF concentrations (Banki et al., 1987). In a third study we reported that patients with major depression had higher CSF CRF levels than patients with chronic pain (France et al., 1988). Our fourth study, conducted in Budapest, also found increased CSF CRF concentrations

Table 1

Similarities between Signs and Symptoms of Major Depression (DSM III-R Criteria) and the Behavioral Effects of Centrally Administered CRF in Laboratory Animals

DSM III-R major depression	Effect of centrally administered CRF
1. Depressed mood (irritable mood in children and adolescents) most of day, nearly every day, as indicated either by subjective account or observations by others	1. Mimics the behavioral despair syndrome observed after maternal separation in rhesus monkey infants
2. Markedly diminished interest or pleasures in all or almost all activities most of day, nearly every day	2. Diminishes sexual behavior in male and female rats
3. Significant weight loss or weight gain when not dieting or decrease or increase in appetite nearly every day	3. Decreases food consumption in rats
4. Insomnia or hypersomnia nearly every day	4. Disrupts normal sleep patterns with concomitant EEG changes
5. Psychomotor agitation or retardation nearly every day	5. Increases locomotor activity in a familiar environment and produces "stresslike" alterations in locomotion in a novel environment
6. Fatigue or loss of energy nearly every day	6. No data
7. Feelings of worthlessness or excessive or inappropriate guilt nearly every day	7. No data
8. Diminished ability to think or concentrate or indecisiveness nearly every day	8. No data
9. Recurrent thoughts of death, recurrent suicidal ideation or a suicide attempt	9. No data

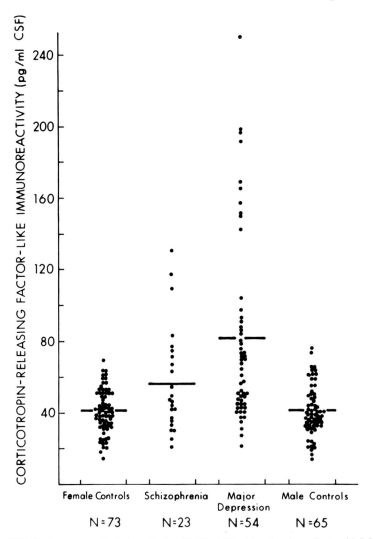

Figure 3. CSF CRF-like immunoreactivity in patients with DSM-III schizophrenia, patients with DSM-III major depression, and control subjects with various peripheral neurological diseases. (From Banki, C. M., Bissette, G., Arato, M., O'Connor, L., and Nemeroff, C. B., *Am. J. Psychiatry,* 144, 873, 1987. With permission.)

in depressed patients (Arato et al., 1986). A fifth study was conducted in which we measured CSF CRF concentrations collected postmortem from the intracisternal space in depressed suicide victims and sudden death controls. Again CSF CRF concentrations were elevated in the depressed group (Arato et al., 1989). Finally, we have recently shown (Nemeroff et al., 1991) that the increase in CSF CRF concentrations that occurs in depression, like the concomitant hypercortisolemia, normalizes on recovery. Nine drug-free psychotically depressed patients had elevated CSF CRF concentrations that were significantly reduced after electroconvulsive therapy and clinical improvement. The increases in CSF CRF concentrations have been confirmed by Risch et al. (1991), by Pitts et al. (1990), and by Roy et al. (1987) in DST nonsuppressors.

In order to determine whether chronic CRF hypersecretion results in CRF receptor down regulation, we measured the number and affinity of CRF receptors in the frontal cortex of 26

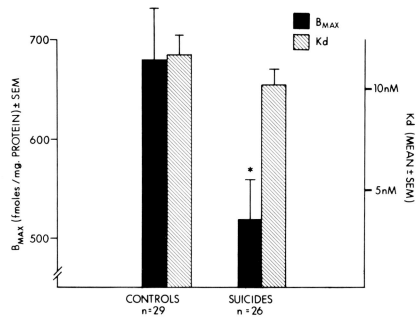

Figure 4. Maximum binding (B_{max}) and dissociation affinity constant (K_d of ^{125}I-labeled Tyr^0-ovine CRF-binding sites in frontal cortex in suicide victims and control subjects. Values are mean ± SEM. There was a 23% decrease in the B_{max} in suicide victims compared with control subject ($P = 0.020$ by Student's t test). Analysis of individual B_{max} values showed normal distributions in both suicide and control populations. (Adapted from Nemeroff et al., 1988.)

suicide victims and 29 controls (Nemeroff et al., 1988). The suicide victims exhibited a marked decrease in CRF receptor number (Figure 4), consistent with the hypothesis that chronic hypersecretion of the peptide produced a long-lasting reduction in CRF receptor density.

This concatenation of findings supports the hypothesis that CRF is hypersecreted in depressed patients, resulting in both behavioral signs and symptoms, and increased HPA axis activity. In subsequent studies, measurement of CRF mRNA levels in discrete postmortem brain areas will provide information as to which CRF neuronal systems are hyperactive in depression (Nemeroff, 1988).

F. Schizophrenia

Early studies indicated that patients with schizophrenia do not have increased plasma cortisol concentrations (Carroll, 1976). However, some studies have indicated that patients with schizophrenia are hypercortisolemic (Dewan et al., 1982). The DST nonsuppression rate in schizophrenia varies from 0 to 70%, with a mean rate of approximately 20%. The range appears to reflect the type of patients, activity of the patients, presence of associated symptoms of depression, and the effects of hospitalization (Evans and Golden, 1987). Patients with schizoaffective disorder, especially the schizoaffective depressed subtype, have very high rates of DST nonsuppression (Krishnan et al., 1988). When the DST is performed within 1 to 2 days of hospitalization, the stress of admission can result in high rates of nonsuppression, regardless of diagnosis (Herz et al., 1985).

The CRF stimulation test has also been conducted in patients with schizophrenia. Cortisol and ACTH responses to CRF in patients with schizophrenia appear to be normal (Roy et al.,

1986). In most studies in which CSF CRF concentrations have been measured, schizophrenic patients exhibit normal values.

G. Alzheimer's Disease

Although early studies indicated that demented patients do not have significant abnormalities in the HPA axis (Carroll et al., 1981), recent findings indicate that patients with Alzheimer's disease do not suppress plasma cortisol when administered dexamethasone (Spar and Gerner, 1982; Krishnan et al., 1988). The DST nonsuppression observed in patients with Alzheimer's disease has been related to the severity of the dementia (Jenike and Albert, 1984). However, in contrast, in a recent study we did not find any relationship between severity of dementia and maximal postdexamethasone cortisol concentration (Krishnan et al., 1988). We also did not find any relationship between severity of depression in these patients and the occurrence of DST nonsuppression (Krishnan et al., 1988). Occurrence of DST abnormalities in patients with Alzheimer's disease has been attributed to hippocampal pathology. Sapolsky et al. (1987) have shown that the hippocampus is of major importance in regulating HPA axis activity. Glucocorticoid feedback at the level of the hippocampus is responsible for turning off the HPA axis response to stress. Thus, in Alzheimer's disease, destruction of hippocampal neurons and loss of the feedback system may account for increased rates of DST nonsuppression.

IV. The Hypothalamo-Pituitary-Thyroid Axis

Although it has long been appreciated that patients with primary hypothyroidism exhibit many of the signs and symptoms of major depression, considerable evidence has accumulated over the past decade that supports the hypothesis that a sizeable proportion of drug-free depressed patients exhibit abnormalities in the hypothalamic-pituitary-thyroid (HPT) axis, and these alterations have been hypothesized to contribute to depressive symptoms.

Like the other neuroendocrine axes, the HPT axis is organized hierarchically. Thyrotropin-releasing hormone (TRH), a tripeptide (pGlu-His-Pro-NH_2) discovered in 1970 (see Lechen, this volume), is a hypothalamic hypophysiotropic hormone that is synthesized within the hypothalamus, and released from nerve endings in the median eminence. Once released from the median eminence, TRH is transported from the hypothalamus to the anterior pituitary gland within the vessels of the hypothalamo-hypophysial portal system. Within the adenohypophysis, TRH binds to TRH receptors on the thyrotrophs, resulting in release of thyrotropin, also known as thyroid-stimulating hormone (TSH), into the systemic circulation. At the thyroid, TSH causes the release of the two major thyroid hormones, triiodothyronine (T_3) and thyroxine (T_4). Thyroid hormones feed back at the adenohypophysis to inhibit TSH release and at the hypothalamus to inhibit TRH release and synthesis.

In primary or grade I hypothyroidism, plasma concentrations of thyroid hormones are decreased, plasma TSH concentrations are increased due to loss of negative feedback, and the TRH-induced TSH response is markedly exaggerated. In grade II hypothyroidism, plasma concentrations of T_3 and T_4 are still within the normal range but basal plasma TSH concentrations are elevated, and the TRH-induced TSH response is exaggerated. In grade III (subclinical) hypothyroidism, plasma concentrations of both TSH and thyroid hormones are normal but the TRH response to TSH is exaggerated.

In primary hyperthyroidism, plasma concentrations of T_3 and T_4 are elevated, basal TSH concentrations are reduced, especially if an ultrasensitive TSH assay is utilized, and the TSH response to TRH is blunted or absent.

In depressed patients, the normal nocturnal rise in plasma TSH concentrations is diminished (Goldstein et al., 1980; Weeke and Weeke, 1980; Bartalena et al., 1990), and this finding is a more sensitive indicator of depression than the TRH stimulation test (vide infra).

A. The Thyrotropin Release to TRH in Depression

Shortly after the discovery of the chemical identity of TRH, a TRH stimulation test was standardized. TRH (500 µg) is administered intravenously over 1 min and blood samples are collected at 30-min intervals for 2 to 3 hr. Several investigators, beginning with the pioneering observations of Prange et al. (1972) and Kastin et al. (1972), have observed that approximately 25% of depressed patients, although euthyroid by any of the usual endocrinological criteria, exhibit a blunted TSH response to TRH (Loosen and Prange, 1982; Mendlewicz et al., 1979). Although the best documented cause of an attenuated TSH response to TRH is hyperthyroidism, no evidence of excessive thyroid hormone secretion in depression has been found. Another potential physiological cause of a blunted TSH response to TRH is somatostatin (SRIF) hypersecretion, but depressed patients exhibit reduced CSF concentrations of SRIF compared to normal controls (vide supra).

Recently Duval et al. (1990) performed TRH stimulation tests using 200 µg at both 8 a.m. and 11 p.m. in normal controls. The difference between the 11 p.m. ΔTSH and 8 a.m. ΔTSH, which they termed $\Delta\Delta$TSH, was markedly lower in the depressed patients. The diagnostic sensitivity was 89%, specificity was 95%.

One putative mechanism to explain the blunted TSH response to TRH in drug-free depressed patients would be chronic hypersecretion of TRH, which theoretically could result in a reduced number of TRH receptors on the adenohypophysial thyrotrophs, so-called "down regulation". More than 10 years ago, our group demonstrated that chronic (2 to 3 week) administration of TRH in rats results in down regulation of TRH receptors in the anterior pituitary gland, as assessed by decreased plasma concentrations of TSH, T_3, and T_4, and a blunted TSH response to TRH (Nemeroff et al., 1980). At approximately the same time, Kirkegaard et al. (1979) reported that depressed patients had elevated CSF concentrations of TRH when compared to controls. This finding was concordant with the hypothesis that TRH is hypersecreted in depressed patients, but there were problems with the TRH radioimmunoassay used, including poor sensitivity and cross-reactivity with urea and SRIF. Our group recently measured the concentration of CSF TRH using a sensitive and specific antiserum generously provided by Dr. A. Winokur (University of Pennsylvania) in 14 drug-free patients with major depression, 12 controls with peripheral neurological disease, 4 patients with somatization disorder, and 2 manic patients. The depressed patients exhibited markedly higher CSF TRH concentrations (Banki et al., 1988). These findings confirm and extend the previous report of Kirkegaard et al. (1979), who, as noted above, demonstrated elevated CSF TRH concentrations in patients with DSM-III major depression. All of the depressed patients in our study were severely depressed, and 13 of 14 were either melancholic or psychotic. No differences in age, sex, body weight, and body height appeared to influence the results. Eleven of the 14 depressed patients had higher CSF TRH concentrations than the highest concentration found in the control subjects. This separation between depressed patients and control subjects was much greater than that achieved by a standard TRH stimulation test. Moreover, no elevation in TRH concentrations could be found in four patients with somatization disorder and in two patients with florid, psychotic mania. The latter observation suggests that elevated CSF TRH is neither related to psychosis *per se* nor associated with motor hyperactivity. However, the small number of manic patients studied renders it impossible to determine the specificity of the increased CSF TRH concentrations for depression. Other potentially confounding influences on CSF TRH concentrations, such as circadian rhythm differences and rostral-caudal gradients, remain unexplored.

The specificity of the elevated CSF concentrations of TRH in depressed patients has been studied in a few small studies. In drug-free patients with anorexia nervosa, CSF TRH is not increased (Lesem et al., 1990), nor do patients with Alzheimer's disease, anxiety disorders, or alcoholism show any alterations in CSF TRH (Fossey et al., 1990; Roy et al., 1990). Recently Adinoff et al. (1991) found a significant inverse relationship between the integrated TSH response to TRH and CSF TRH concentrations in 13 drug-free male alcoholics, a group that also exhibits TSH blunting to TRH. Taken together, these data indicate that TRH hypersecretion may underlie the attenuated TSH response to TRH.

B. Symptomless Autoimmune Thyroiditis and Depression

Although the blunted TSH response to TRH in depressed patients has received considerable attention, approximately 15% of depressed patients exhibit an exaggerated TSH response to TRH. This finding was studied most intensively by Gold et al. (1982) and has led to the realization that a sizeable number of depressed patients with exaggerated TSH responses to TRH and normal baseline plasma TSH and thyroid hormone concentrations have, by definition, grade III hypothyroidism. In their initial study, Gold et al. (1982) reported that of 15 patients with clearly elevated TSH responses to TRH, 9 had detectable circulating anti-microsomal thyroid and/or anti-thyroglobulin antibodies. This was the first report that depressed patients suffer from a greater than expected incidence of symptomless autoimmune thyroiditis (SAT), which is postulated to underlie the high incidence of subclinical (grade III) hypothyroidism.

The prevalence of anti-thyroid antibodies in depressed patients has been studied. In our first study (Nemeroff et al., 1985), we measured the presence of anti-microsomal and anti-thyroglobulin thyroid antibodies in 45 psychiatric inpatients with prominent depressive symptoms (28 with DSM-III major depression). Nine of the patients (20%) had detectable titers of anti-thyroid antibodies, a rate considerably higher than the 5 to 10% observed in the normal population. In a follow-up study (Haggarty et al., 1987), the relationship between the presence of anti-thyroid antibodies and the presence of cortisol nonsuppression to dexamethasone (DST) in depressed patients was determined. DST nonsuppression has been well studied in depressed inpatients (vide supra) and is thought to represent a measure of disease severity by some investigators. A standard 1-mg DST was performed. A single blood sample was obtained prior to dexamethasone administration for the measurement of anti-thyroid antibodies. A total of 124 adolescent and adult inpatients were studied. Our results in this second study confirmed and extended those obtained in our first study. Of the 102 patients who fulfilled criteria for major affective disorder (major depression, mixed bipolar disorder, etc.), 20% exhibited detectable thyroid antibodies. In addition, approximately 50% of these depressed patients exhibited DST nonsuppression. DST nonsuppressors were more likely than DST suppressors to exhibit thyroid abnormalities.

A third study (Haggarty et al., 1990) sought to determine the prevalence rate of autoimmune thyroiditis in subtypes of affective disorder, and the relationship of prior lithium exposure to the presence of anti-thyroid antibodies in 173 consecutively admitted psychiatric inpatients. Patients with bipolar illness had a higher rate of symptomless autoimmune thyroiditis when compared to patients with unipolar depression. In spite of the prevailing notion that lithium exposure increases the prevalence of autoimmune thyroiditis, presumably because of its well-documented direct anti-thyroid effect, there was no relationship in this study between prior lithium exposure and the presence of anti-thyroglobulin or anti-microsomal thyroid antibodies. Interestingly, Bauer et al. (1990) found a very high rate of grade I (23%), grade II (27%), and grade III (10%) hypothyroidism in rapid cycling bipolar patients.

In spite of years of concerted study, it is almost remarkable how little we know of the role of the HPT axis in the pathophysiology of affective disorders. Nevertheless, considerable progress has been made in recent years. First, it is evident that a sizeable proportion of depressed patients, in particular those with bipolar illness, exhibit relatively high rates of autoimmune thyroiditis, as evidenced by the presence of anti-thyroid antibodies. Once thought to be merely secondary to prior lithium exposure, this is clearly not the case (Calebrese et al., 1985; Haggarty et al., 1990; Bauer et al., 1990). Early in the course of autoimmune thyroid disease, plasma TSH concentrations are increased in order to maintain normal plasma T_3 and T_4 concentrations as the negative feedback effect of thyroid hormones is decreased. Perhaps this results in TRH hypersecretion, necessary to increase TSH secretion and secondary to lack of T_3 and T_4 feedback on TRH neurons in the hypothalamus. Clearly CSF TRH concentrations should be measured in depressed patients with autoimmune thyroiditis to test this hypothesis.

The issue of treatment of depressed patients with symptomless autoimmune thyroiditis remains an issue of paramount importance. Is treatment with exogenous thyroid hormone alone sufficient to normalize their mood state? There are anecdotal accounts of treating such patients successfully with T_4 alone, and there is a large literature reviewed by Prange et al. (1976) demonstrating reduced effectiveness of tricyclic antidepressants in patients with frank hypothyroidism. Targum et al. (1984) reported that depressed patients refractory to tricyclic antidepressants who responded to T_3 supplementation had an increased prevalence rate of subclinical hypothyroidism. In addition Russ and Ackerman (1989) recent confirmed the lack of efficacy of antidepressants in depressed hypothyroid patients.

The high rate of autoimmune thyroiditis, and subclinical hypothyroidism, in bipolar patients is of interest in view of the recent studies of Bauer and Whybrow (1990), who reported therapeutic responses of rapid-cycling bipolar patients to high doses of thyroid hormones.

The blunted TSH response to TRH observed in approximately 25% of depressed patients, as well as in abstinent alcoholics, remains mechanistically enigmatic. The recent report that lymphocytes from depressed patients secrete less TSH in response to TRH *in vitro* than that observed in normal controls highlights the apparent cellular universality of this finding (Wassel et al., 1990). However, our studies would suggest that chronic TRH hypersecretion, as evidenced by increased CSF TRH concentrations, results in adenohypophysial TRH receptor down regulation. The finding of an inverse relationship between CSF TRH concentrations and the TSH response to TRH in our pilot study of alcoholic patients supports this view. Direct evidence of TRH receptor down regulation would, however, be more desirable. Such a study could be conducted in post-mortem pituitary and brain tissue obtained from depressed suicide victims and age- and sex-matched controls or alternately one could develop a radioligand for the TRH receptor and to measure TRH binding sites using positron-emission tomography (PET).

Finally there is a large literature on the use of thyroid hormone, usually T_3, to potentiate the therapeutic effects of tricyclic antidepressants and to convert antidepressant nonresponders to responders. This phenomenon was first observed by Prange and co-workers (1969) in depressed patients, has recently been reviewed (Prange et al., 1980), and has also recently been observed in patients with panic disorder (Stein and Uhde, 1990).

V. Conclusion

We have focused on alterations in three of the major neuroendocrine axes in psychiatric disorders: the HPA, HPT, and growth hormone systems. There is unequivocal evidence that each of these are altered in patients with affective disorders. It seems clear that these alterations are due to pathophysiological changes in the CNS of these patients. This neuroendocrine window strategy has been particularly fruitful in research in affective disorders and, to a lesser extent, anorexia nervosa, but not very helpful in schizophrenia. Moreover, alterations in secretion of the hormones of the hypothalamic-pituitary-gonadal axis and in prolactin secretion in the major psychiatric disorders have been less closely scrutinized, and the extant findings remain less robust and more discordant. As more multidisciplinary tools become available, the specific brain areas mediating these abnormal neuroendocrine responses in patients with psychiatric disorders will be elucidated. Whether these neuroendocrine changes are responsible for the behavioral signs and symptoms of these diseases remains unclear.

Acknowledgments

We are grateful to Nancy Winter for preparation of this manuscript. The authors are supported by NIMH MH-42088, MH-39415, MH-40524, MH-40159, MH-45975, MH-46791, and MH-44716.

References

Adinoff, B., Nemeroff, C. B., Bissette, G., Martin, P. R., and Linnoila, M., Inverse relationship between CSF TRH concentrations and the TSH response to TRH in abstinent alcoholics, *Am. J. Psychiatry*, 148, 1586—1588, 1991.

Alvarez, L. C., Dimas, C. O., Castro, A., Rossman, L. G., Vanderlaan, E., and Vanderlaan, W., Growth hormone in malnutrition, *J. Clin. Endocrinol. Metab.*, 34, 400, 1972.

Amsterdam, J. D., Winokur, A., Abelman, E., Irwin, L., Rickels, K., Cosyntropin (ACTH) stimulation test in depressed patients and healthy volunteers, *Am. J. Psychiatry*, 140, 907, 1983.

Amsterdam, J. D., Marinelli, D. L., Arger, P., and Winokur, A., Assessment of adrenal gland volume by C.T. in depressed patients and healthy volunteers. A pilot study, *Psychiatry Res.*, 21, 189, 1987.

Amsterdam, J. D., Maislin, G., Winokur, A., Berwish, N., Kling, M., and Gold, P., The O CRH test before and after clinical recovery from depression, *J. Affective Disorders*, 14, 213, 1988.

Arana, G. W. and Mossman, D., The DST and depression: approaches to the use of a laboratory test in psychiatry, *Neurol. Clin.*, 6, 21, 1988.

Arana, G. W., Workman, B. J., and Baldesarrini, R. J., Association between low plasma levels of dexamethasone and elevated levels of cortisol in psychiatric patients given dexamethasone, *Am. J. Psychiatry*, 141, 1619, 1984.

Arana, G. W., Baldesarrini, R. J., and Ornsteen, M., The dexamethasone suppression test for diagnosis and prognosis in psychiatry, *Arch. Gen. Psychiatry*, 42, 1193, 1985.

Arato, M., Rihmer, Z., Banki, C. M., and Grof, P., The relationships of neuroendocrine tests in endogenous depression, *Biol. Psychiatry*, 7, 715, 1983.

Arato, M., Banki, C. M., Nemeroff, C. B., and Bissette, G., Hypothalamic-pituitary-adrenal axis and suicide, *Ann. N.Y. Acad. Sci.*, 487, 263, 1986.

Arato, M., Banki, C. M., Bissette, G., and Nemeroff, C. B., Elevated CSF CRF in suicide victims, *Biol. Psychiatry*, 25, 355, 1989.

Asnis, G. M. and Lemus, C. Z., Cortisol secretion in psychiatric disorders, in *Handbook of Clinical Psychoneuroendocrinology*, Nemeroff, C. B. and Loosen, P. I., Eds., Guilford Press, New York, 1987.

Asnis, G. M., Lemus, C. Z., and Halbreich, U., The desipramine cortisol test: a selective noradrenergic challenge, *Psychopharmacol. Bull.*, 22, 577, 1986.

Banki, C. M., Bissette, G., Arato, M., O'Connor, L., and Nemeroff, C. B., Cerebrospinal fluid corticotropin-releasing factor-like immunoreactivity in depression and schizophrenia, *Am. J. Psychiatry,* 144, 873, 1987.

Banki, C. M., Bissette, G., Arato, M., and Nemeroff, C. B., Elevation of immunoreactive CSF TRH in depressed patients, *Am. J. Psychiatry,* 145, 1526, 1988.

Bartalena, L., Placidi, G. F., Martino, E., Falcone, M., Pellegrini, L., Dell'osso, L., Pacchiarotti, A., and Pinchera, A., Nocturnal serum thyrotropin (TSH) surge and the TSH response to TSH-releasing hormone: dissociated behavior in untreated depressives, *J. Clin. Endocrinol. Metab.,* 71, 650, 1990.

Bauer, M. S. and Whybrow, P. C., Rapid cycling bipolar affective disorder. II. Treatment of refractory rapid cycling with high-dose levothyroxine: a preliminary study, *Arch. Gen. Psychiatry,* 47, 435, 1990.

Bauer, M. S., Whybrow, P. C., and Winokur, A., Rapid cycling bipolar affective disorder. I. Association with grade I hypothyroidism, *Arch. Gen. Psychiatry,* 47, 427, 1990.

Berger, M., Doew, P., Lund, R., Bronisch, P., and Zerssen, V. D., Neuroendocrinological and neurophysiological studies in major depressive disorders, *Biol. Psychiatry,* 17, 1217, 1982.

Boyd, A. E., Lebovitz, H. E., and Pfeiffer, J. B., Stimulation of growth hormone secretion by L-DOPA, *N. Engl. J. Med.,* 283, 1425, 1970.

Brambilla, F., Guerrin, A., Guastalla, A., Rovere, C., and Riggi, F., Neuroendocrine effects of haldol in chronic schizophrenia, *Psychopharmacología,* 44, 17, 1975.

Brambilla, F., Smeraldi, E., Sacchetti, E., Negri, F., Cocchi, D., and Muller, E., Deranged anterior pituitary responsiveness to hypothalamic hormones in depressed patients, *Arch. Gen. Psychiatr,* 35, 1231, 1978.

Brown, W. A., Predictors of placebo response in depression, *Psychopharmacol. Bull.,* 24, 14, 1988.

Brown, W. A. and Shuey, I., Response to dexamethasone and subtype of depression, *Arch. Gen. Psychiatry,* 41, 1090, 1980.

Brown, G. M., Steiner, M., and Grof, P., Neuroendocrinology of affective disorder, in *Clinical Neuroendocrinology,* Cohn, R., Brown, G. M., and Van Loon, G. R., Eds., Blackwell Scientific, Boston, 1988, 461.

Cacabelos, R., Niigawa, H., Ikemura, Y., Yanagi, Y., Panaka, S., Rodriguez-Arano, M. D., Gomez-Pan, A., and Nishimura, T., GHRH induced GH response in patients with senile dementia of the Alzheimer type, *Acta Endocrinol.,* 117, 295, 1988.

Calabrese, J. R., Gulledge, A. D., Hahn, K., Skwerer, R., Kotz, M., Schumaker, O. P., Gupta, M. K., Krupp, N., and Gold, P. W., The development of thyroiditis in patients receiving long-term lithium therapy, *Am. J. Psychiatry,* 142, 1318, 1985.

Carpenter, W. and Bunney, W., Adrenal cortical activity in depressive illness, *Am. J. Psychiatry,* 128, 31, 1971.

Carroll, B. J., Plasma cortisol levels in depression, in *Depressive Illness, Research Studies,* Davies, B., Carroll, B., and Moubray, R., Eds., Charles C Thomas, Springfield, IL, 1963, 69.

Carroll, B. J., The hypothalamo-pituitary-adrenal axis, in *Depressive Illness: Some Research Studies,* Davis, B., Carroll, B. J., and Mowbray, R., Eds., Charles C Thomas, Springfield, IL, 1972, 23.

Carroll, B. J., The dexamethasone suppression test for melancholia, *Br. J. Psychiatry,* 140, 292, 1982.

Carroll, B. J., Dexamethasone suppression test. A review of contemporary confusion, *J. Clin. Psychiatry,* 46, 13, 1985.

Carroll, B. J. and Mendels, J., Neuroendocrine regulation in affective disorder, in *Hormones, Behavior and Psychopathology,* Sachar, E., Ed., Raven Press, New York, 1976, 197.

Carroll, B. J., Martin, F. I. R., and Davies, B., Resistance to suppression by dexamethasone of plasma 11 OHCS levels in severe depressive illness, *Br. Med. J.,* 3, 285, 1968.

Carroll, B. J., Curtis, G. C., and Mendels, J., Neuroendocrine regulation in depression. I. Limbic system-adrenocortical dysfunction, *Arch. Gen. Psychiatry,* 33, 1039, 1976a.

Carroll, B. J., Curtis, G., and Mendels, J., Neuroendocrine regulation in depression: discrimination of depressed from nondepressed patients, *Arch. Gen. Psychiatry,* 33, 1051, 1976b.

Carroll, B. J., Schroeder, K., Mukhopadhyay, S., Greden, J. F., Feinberg, M., Ritchie, J., and Tarika, J., Plasma dexamethasone concentrations and cortisol suppression responses in patients with endogenous depression, *J. Clin. Endocrinol. Metab.,* 51, 433, 1980.

Carroll, B. J., Feinberg, M., Greden, J. F., Tarika, J., Albala, A. A., Hasket, R. F., James, N. M., Krantol, Z., Lohr, N., Steiner, M., De Vigne, J. P., and Young, E., A specific laboratory test for the diagnosis of melancholia, *Arch. Gen. Psychiatry,* 38, 15, 1981a.

Carroll, B. J., Greden, J. F., and Feinberg, M., Suicide neuroendocrine dysfunction and CSF 5-HIAA concentrations in depression, in *Recent Advances in Neuropsychopharmacology,* Angrist, B., Ed., Pergamon Press, Oxford, 1981b, 307.

Casper, R. and Davis, J., Neuroendocrine and amine studies in affective illness, *Psychoneuroendocrinology,* 2, 105, 1977.

Casper, R. C., Davis, J. M., and Pandey, G. N., The effect of nutritional status and weight changes on hypothalamic function tests in anorexia nervosa, in *Anorexia Nervosa,* Vigersky, R. A., Ed., Raven Press, New York, 1977a, 137.

Casper, R. C., Davis, J. M., Pandey, G. N., Garver, D. L., and Dekirmenjian, H., Neuroendocrine and amine studies in affective illness, *Psychoneuroendocrinology,* 2, 103, 1977b.

Charney, D. S., Henninger, G. R., Steinberg, D. E., Hafstad, K. M., Gildeings, S., and Landis, D. H., Adrenergic receptor sensitivity in depression: effects of clonidine in depressed patients and health controls, *Arch. Gen. Psychiatry,* 39, 290, 1982.

Checkley, S. A., Corticosteroid and growth hormone response to methylamphetamine in depressive illness, *Psychiatr. Med.,* 9, 107, 1979.

Checkley, S. A., Slade, A. P., and Shur, P., Growth hormone and other responses to clonidine in patients with endogenous depression, *Br. J. Psychiatry,* 138, 51, 1988.

Cleghorn, J. M., Brown, G. M., and Brown, P. J., Apomorphine in schizophrenia, *Comm. Psychopharmacol.,* 4, 277, 1980.

Copolov, D. L. and Rubin, R. T., Endocrine disturbances in affective disorders and schizophrenia, in *Handbook of Clinical Psychoneuroendocrinology,* Nemeroff, C. B. and Loosen, P. T., Eds., Guilford Press, New York, 1988, 160.

Coryell, W. and Schlesser, M. A., Suicide and the DST in unipolar depression, *Am. J. Psychiatry,* 138, 1120, 1981.

Dewan, M. J., Pandurangi, A. K., Boucher, M. L., Levy, B. F., and Major, L. F., Abnormal dexamethasone suppression test results in chronic schizophrenic patients, *Am. J. Psychiatry,* 139, 1501, 1982.

Dinan, T. G. and Barry, S., Responses of growth hormone to desipramine in endogenous and non-endogenous depression, *Br. J. Psychiatry,* 156, 680, 1990.

Duval, F., Macher, J.-P., and Mokrani, M.-C., Difference between evening and morning thyrotropin responses to protirelin in major depressive episode, *Arch. Gen. Psychiatry,* 47, 443, 1990.

Endo, M. and Endo, J., Endocrine studies in depression, in *Psychoneuroendocrinologie,* Hatotani, N., Ed., S. Karger, Basel, 1974, 22.

Ettigi, P., Nair, N. P. V., Lal, S., Cervantes, P., and Guyda, H., Effects of apomorphine on growth hormone and prolactin secretion in schizophrenic patients with or without oral dyskinesia, *J. Neurol. Neurosci. Psychiatry,* 39, 870, 1976.

Evans, D. L. and Golden, R. J., The dexamethasone suppression test. A review, in *Handbook of Clinical Psychoneuroendocrinology,* Loosen, P. T. and Nemeroff, C. B., Eds., Guilford Press, New York, 1987, 313.

Evans, D. L. and Nemeroff, C. B., Use of dexamethasone suppression test using DSM III criteria on an inpatient psychiatric unit, *Am. J. Psychiatry,* 141, 1465, 1984.

Evans, D. L., McCartney, C. F., Nemeroff, C. B., Raft, D., Quade, D., Golden, R. N., Haggerty, J. J., Holmes, V., Simon, J. S., Droba, M., Mason, G. A., and Fowler, W. C., Depression in women treated for gynecological cancer: clinical and neuroendocrine assessment, *Am. J. Psychiatry,* 143, 447, 1986.

Evans, D. L., Nemeroff, C. B., Haggerty, J. J., Jr., and Pederson, C. A., Use of the dexamethasone-suppression test within DSMIII criteria in psychiatrically hospitalized adolescents, *Psychoneuroendocrinology,* 12, 203, 1987.

Extein, I., Rosenberg, G., Pottash, A. L. C., and Gold, M., The dexamethasone suppression test in depressed adolescents, *Am. J. Psychiatry.,* 139, 1617, 1982.

Fehm, H. L., Holl, R., Klein, E., and Voigt, K. H., The meal related peak in plasma cortisol is not mediated by radioimmunoassayable ACTH, *Clin. Physiol. Biochem.,* 1, 329, 1983.

Fehm, H. L., Holl, R., and Klein, E., Evidence for ACTH unrelated mechanisms in the regulation of cortisol secretion in man, *Klin. Wochenschr.,* 62, 19, 1984a.

Fehm, H. L., Klein, E., Holl, R., and Voigt, K. H., Evidence for extra pituitary mechanisms mediating the morning peak of plasma cortisol in man, *J. Clin. Endocrinol. Metab.,* 58, 410, 1984b.

Finkelstein, J. W., Roffwarg, H. P., Boyar, R. M., Kream, J., and Hellman, L., Age-related changes in the twenty-four-hour spontaneous secretion of growth hormone, *J. Clin. Endocrinol. Metab.,* 35, 665, 1972.

Fossey, M. D., Lydiarel, R. B., Larara, M. T., Bissette, G., Nemeroff, C. B., and Balleyer, J. C., CSF thyrotropin-releasing hormone in patients with anxiety disorders, *Biol. Psychiat.,* 27, Suppl. 167A, 1990.

France, R. D., Urban, B., Krishnan, K. R. R., Bissette, G., Banki, C. M., Nemeroff, C. B., and Spielman, F. J., CSF corticotropin-releasing factor-like immunoreactivity in chronic pain patients with and without major depression, *Biol. Psychiatry,* 23, 86, 1988.

Frazer, J., Adrenergic responses to depression: implications for a receptor defect, in *Psychobiology of Depression,* Mendels, J., Ed., Spectrum, New York, 1975.

Fullerton, D. J., Wenzel, F. J., Laenz, F., and Fahs, H., Circadian rhythm of adrenal cortical activity in depression. II. A comparison of depressed patients with normal subjects, *Arch. Gen. Psychiatry,* 19, 674, 1968.

Garfinkel, P. E., Brown, G. H., Stancer, H. C., and Moldofsky, H., Hypothalamic pituitary function in anorexia nervosa, *Arch. Gen. Psychiatry,* 32, 739, 1975.

Garver, D., Pandey, G., Derkmenjian, H., and Jones, F. D., Growth hormone and catecholamines in affective disease, *Am. J. Psychiatry,* 132, 1149, 1975.

Gertz, B. J., Cantreras, L. N., McComb, D. J., Kovacs, K., Tyrrell, J. B., and Dallman, M. F., Chronic administration of corticotropin-releasing factor increases pituitary corticotroph number, *Endocrinology,* 120, 381, 1987.

Gibbons, J. L., Plasma cortisol in depressive illness, *J. Psychiatr. Res.,* 1, 162, 1962.

Gold, M. S., Pottash, A. L. C., and Extein, I., Hypothyroidism and Depression, *J. Am. Med. Assoc.,* 245, 1919, 1981.

Gold, M. S., Pottash, A. C., and Extein, I., Symptomless autoimmune thyroiditis in depression, *Psychiatry Res.,* 6, 261, 1982.

Gold, P. W., Goodwin, F. K., Wehr, T., Robar, R., and Sack, R., Growth hormone and prolactin response to levodopa in affective illness, *Lancet,* 2, 1308, 1976.

Gold, P. W., Chrousos, G. P., Kellner, C. H., Post, R. M., Roy, A., Augerinas, P., Schulte, H., Oldfield, E. H., and Loriaux, D. L., Psychiatric implications of basic and clinical studies with corticotropin-releasing factor, *Am. J. Psychiatry,* 141, 619, 1984.

Goldstein, J., Van Cauter, E., Linkowski, P., Vanhaelst, L., and Mendlewicz, J., Thyrotropin nyctohemeral pattern in primary depression. Difference between unipolar and bipolar women, *Life Sci.,* 27, 1695, 1980.

Gregiore, F., Braumann, H., Buck, R., and Corvitain, J., Hormone release in depressed patients before and after recovery, *Psychoneuroendocrinology,* 2, 303, 1977.

Grof, E., Brown, G. M., and Grof, P., Neuroendocrine responses as an indicator of recurrence liability in primary affective illness, *Br. J. Psychiat.,* 140, 320, 1982.

Gruen, P. H., Sacher, E. J., Altman, N., Sassin, J., Growth hormone responses to hypoglycemia in postmenopausal depressed women, *Arch. Gen. Psychiatry,* 32, 31, 1975.

Guillemin, R., Brazeau, P., Bohlen, P., Esch, F., Ling, N., and Wehrenburg, W., Growth-hormone releasing factor from a minor pancreatic tumor that caused acromegaly, *Science,* 218, 585, 1982.

Haggarty, J. J., Simon, J. S., Evans, D. L., and Nemeroff, C. B., Relationship of serum TSH concentration and antithyroid antibodies to diagnosis and DST response in psychiatric inpatients, *Am. J. Psychiat.,* 144, 1491, 1987.

Haggarty, J. J., Evans, D. L., Golden, R. N., Pedersen, C. A., Simon, J. S., and Nemeroff, C. B., The presence of anti-thyroid antibodies in patients with affective and non-affective psychiatric disorders, *Biol. Psychiatry,* 27, 51, 1990.

Halbreich, U., Ed., *Hormones and Depression,* Raven Press, New York, 1987.

Halbreich, U., Sachar, E. J., Asnis, G. M., Quitkin, F., Nathan, R. S., Halpern, F. S., and Klein, D. F., Growth hormone response to D-amphetamine in depressed patients and normal subjects, *Arch. Gen. Psychiatry,* 39, 189, 1982.

Herz, M. I., Fara, G. A., Molnar, G., and Edwards, L., The DST in newly hospitalized schizophrenic patients, *Am. J. Psychiatry,* 142, 127, 1985.

Hollister, L. E., Davis, K. L., and Berger, P., Apomorphine in schizophrenia, *Commun. Psychopharmacol.,* 4, 277, 1980.

Holsboer, F., Von Bardeleben, U., Gerken, A., and Muller, D., Blunted corticotropin and normal cortisol response to human corticotropin-releasing factor in depression, *N. Engl. J. Med.,* 311, 1137, 1984a.

Holsboer, F., Haack, D., Gerken, A., and Vecoci, P., Plasma dexamethasone concentrations and different suppression response of cortisol and corticosterone in depressives and controls, *Biol. Psychiatry,* 19, 281, 1984b.

Holsboer, F., Wiedemann, K., and Boll, E., Shortened dexamethasone half life in depressed dexamethasone nonsuppressors, *Arch. Gen. Psychiatry,* 43, 813, 1986.

Holsboer, F., Von Bardeleben, U., Wiedemann, K., Muller, O. A., and Stalla, G. K., Serial assessment of corticotropin-releasing hormone after dexamethasone in depression. Application for pathophysiology of DST nonsuppression, *Biol. Psychiatry,* 22, 228, 1987.

Holsboer, F., Stalla, G. K., Von Bardeleben, U., Hamman, K., Muller, H., and Muller, O. A., Acute adrenocortical stimulation by recombinant gamma interferon in human controls, *Life Sci.,* 42, 1, 1988.

Imura, H., Nakai, Y., and Hoshimi, T., Effect of 5-hydroxytryptophan (5-HTP) on growth hormone and ACTH release in man, *J. Clin. Endocrinol. Metab.,* 36, 204, 1973.

Jaeckle, R. S., Kathol, R. G., Lopez, J. F., Meller, W. H., and Krummel, S. J., Enhanced adrenal sensitivity to exogenous ACTH stimulation in major depression, *Arch. Gen. Psychiatry,* 44, 233, 1987.

Janowsky, D. S., Leichner, P., Parker, D., Judd, L. L., Huey, L., and Clopton, P., The effect of methylphenidate on serum growth hormone, *Arch. Gen. Psychiatry,* 15, 1384, 1978.

Jenike, M. A. and Albert, M. S., The dexamethasone suppression test in patients with presenile and senile dementia of the Alzheimer type, *J. Am. Geriatric Soc.,* 32, 441, 1984.

Johnson, G. F., Hunt, G., Kerr, K., and Caterson, I., Dexamethasone suppression test and plasma dexamethasone levels in depressed patients, *Psychiatry Res.,* 13, 305, 1984.

Kalin, N. H., Dawson, G., Tariot, P., Shelton, S., Barksdale, C., Weiler, S., and Thieneman, M., Function of the adrenal cortex in patients with major depression, *Psychiatry Res.,* 22, 117, 1987.

Kastin, A. J., Schalch, D. S., Ehrensing, R. H., and Anderson, M. S., Improvement in mental depression with decreased thyrotropin response after administration of thyrotropin-releasing hormone, *Lancet,* 2, 740, 1972.

Kathol, R. G., Sherman, B. M., Winokur, G., Lewis, D., and Schlesser, M., Dexamethasone suppression, protirelin stimulation, and insulin infusion in subtypes of recovered depressive patients, *Psychiatric Res.,* 9, 99, 1983.

Kathol, R. G., Haeckle, R. S., Lopez, J. F., and Muller, W. H., Consistent reduction of ACTH responses to stimulation with CRH, vasopressin and hypoglycaemia in patients with depression, *Br. J. Psychiatry,* 155, 468, 1989.

Kellner, C. H., Rubinow, D. R., Gold, P. W., and Post, R. M., Relationship of cortisol hypersecretion to brain CT scan alterations in depressed patients, *Psychiatry Res.,* 8, 191, 1983.

Kirkegaard, C. J., Faber, J., Hummer, L., and Rogowski, P., Increased levels of TRH in cerebrospinal fluid from patients with endogenous depression, *Psychoneuroendocrinology,* 4, 227, 1979.

Koslow, S. H., Stokes, P. E., Mendels, J., Ramsey, A., and Casper, R., Insulin tolerance test, human growth hormone response and insulin resistance in primary unipolar depressed, bipolar depressed and control subjects, *Psychol. Med.,* 12, 45, 1982.

Krieger, D. T., Serotonin regulation of ACTH secretion, in *ACTH and Related Peptides,* Vol. 297, Krieger, D. T. and Ganong, W. F., Eds., New York Academy of Sciences, New York, 1977, 527.

Krieger, D. T. and Allen, W., Relationship of bioassayable and immunoassayable plasma ACTH and cortisol concentration in normal subjects and patients with Cushing's syndrome, *J. Clin. Endocrinol. Metab.*, 10, 675, 1975.

Krishnan, K. R. R., France, R. D., Pelton, S., McCann, U. D., Manepalli, A. N., and Davidson, J. R. T., What does the dexamethasone suppression test identify?, *Biol. Psychiatry*, 20, 957, 1985.

Krishnan, K. R. R., Davidson, J. R. T., Rayasam, R., Tanas, K. S., Shope, F. S. and Pelton, S., Diagnostic utility of the dexamethasone suppression test, *Biol. Psychiatry*, 22, 618, 1987.

Krishnan, K. R. R., Heyman, A., Ritchie, J. C., Utley, C. M., Dawson, D. V., and Rogers, H., Depression in early onset Alzheimer's disease. Clinical and neuroendocrine correlates, *Biol. Psychiatry*, 24, 937, 1988a.

Krishnan, K. R. R., Ritchie, J. C., Manepalli, A. N., Venkataraman, S., France, R. D., Nemeroff, C. B., and Carroll, B. J., What is the relationship between plasma ACTH and cortisol in normal human and depressed patients, in *HPA Axis, Physiology, Pathophysiology and Psychiatric Implications*, Schatzberg, A. F. and Nemeroff, C. B., Eds., Raven Press, New York, 1988b, 115.

Krishnan, K. R. R., Manepalli, A. N., Ritchie, J. C., Daughtry, G., Pelton, S., Nemeroff, C. B., and Carroll, B. J., Nocturnal and early morning secretion of ACTH and cortisol in humans, *Biol. Psychiatry*, 28, 47, 1990a.

Krishnan, K. R. R., Ritchie, J. C., Saunders, W. B., Nemeroff, C. B., and Carroll, B. J., Adrenocortical sensitivity to low dose ACTH administration in depressed patients, *Biol. Psychiatry*, 27, 930, 1990b.

Krishnan, K. R. R., Doraiswamy, P. M., Venkataraman, S., Reed, D., and Ritchie, J. C., Current concepts in HPA axis regulation, in *The Role of Neuropeptides in Stress Pathogenesis and Disease*, McCubbin, J., Kaufman, P., and Nemeroff, C. B., Eds., Academic Press, New York, 1991a, 19.

Krishnan, K. R. R., Doraiswamy, P. M., Lurie, S. N., Figiel, G. S., Husain, M. M., Boyko, O. H., Ellinwood, E. H., Jr., and Nemeroff, C. B., Pituitary size in depression, *J. Clin. Endocrinol. Metab.*, 72, 256, 1991b.

Laakman, G. F., Schumacher, G., Benkert, O., and Werder, K., Stimulation of growth hormone secretion by desipramines and chlorimipramine in man, *J. Clin. Endocrinol. Metab.*, 44, 101, 1977.

Laakman, G., Zygan, K., Schoen, H. W., and Weiss, A., Wittmann, M., Meissner, R., and Blaschke, D., Effects of receptor blockers (methysergide, propranolol, phentolamine, yohimbine, prazosin) on desipramine induced pituitary hormone stimulation. I. Growth hormone, *Psychoneuroendocrinology*, 11, 447, 1986.

Lal, S., de la Vega, C., Sourkes, T. L., and Friesen, H. G., Effects of apomorphine on growth hormone, prolactin, luteinizing hormone and follicle-stimulating hormone levels in human serum, *J. Clin. Endocrinol. Metab.*, 37, 719, 1973.

Lal, S., Martin, J. B., de la Vega, C., and Friesen, H. G., Comparison of the effect of apomorphine and L-DOPA on serum growth hormone levels in man, *Clin. Endocrinol.*, 4, 277, 1975.

Lamberts, S. W. J. and Oosterom, R., Regulation of growth hormone secretion, *Frontiers Horm. Res.*, 14, 137, 1985.

Landen, J., Howarth, N., and Greenwood, F. C., Plasma sugar free fatty acid, growth hormone response to insulin II in patients with hypothalamic or pituitary dysfunction or anorexia nervosa, *J. Clin. Invest.*, 45, 437, 1966.

Langer, G., Heinze, G., Reim, B., and Matussek, N., Reduced growth hormone response to amphetamine in endogenous depression, *Arch. Gen. Psychiatry*, 33, 1471, 1975.

Lesch, K. P., Laux, G., Erb, A., Pfuller, H., and Beckmann, H., Attenuated growth hormone response to growth hormone RH in major depressive disorder, *Biol. Psychiatry*, 22, 1495, 1987a.

Lesch, K. P., Laux, G., Pfuller, H., Erb, A., and Beckmann, H., Growth hormone response to GH-releasing hormone in depression, *J. Clin. Endocrinol. Metab.*, 65, 1278, 1987b.

Lesch, K. P., Laux, G., Erb, A., Pfuller, H., and Beckmann, H., Growth hormone response to growth hormone RH in depression. Correlates with growth hormone release following clonidine, *Psychiatry Res.*, 25, 301, 1988.

Lesem, M. D., Kaye, W. H., Bissette, G., Jimerson, D. C., and Nemeroff, C. B., Low CSF immunoreactive-TRH levels in anorexia, in Proc. American Psychiatric Association, 143rd Annual Meeting, New Research Abstracts, 1990, 240.

Linkowski, P., Mendelewig, J., LeClerq, R., Brasseur, M., Hubain, P., Goldstein, J., Copinschi, G., and Lauter, E. V., The 24 hour profile of ACTH and cortisol in major depressive illness, *J. Clin. Endocrinol. Metab.*, 61, 429, 1985.

Lisansky, J., Peake, G. T., Strassman, R., Qualls, C., Meikle, A. W., Risch, S. C., Fava, G. A., Zownir-Brazis, M., Hochla, P., and Britton, D., Augmented pituitary corticotropin response to a threshold dosage of human corticotropin-releasing hormone in depressives pretreated with metyrapone, *Arch. Gen. Psychiatry*, 46, 641, 1989.

Loosen, P. T. and Prange, A. J., Serum thyrotropin response to thyrotropin-releasing hormone in psychiatric patients: A review, *Am. J. Psychiatry*, 139, 405, 1982.

Maany, I., Mendels, J., Frazer, A., and Brunswick, D., Growth hormone release in depression, *Neuropsychobiology*, 5, 282, 1979.

Maeda, K., Kato, Y., Ohgo, S., Chihara, K., Yoshimoto, Y., Yamaguchi, N., Kuromaro, S., and Imura, H., Growth hormone and prolactin release after injection of thyrotropin releasing hormone in patients with depression, *J. Clin. Endocrinol. Metab.*, 40, 501, 1975.

Marks, V. and Bannister, R. G., Pituitary and adrenal function in undernutrition with mental illness (including anorexia nervosa), *Br. J. Psychiatry*, 109, 480, 1963.

Marks, V., Howarth, N., and Greenwood, F. C., Plasma growth hormone levels in chronic starvation in man, *Nature (London)*, 208, 686, 1965.

Martin, J. B., Brain regulation of growth hormone secretion, in *Frontiers in Neuroendocrinology*, Vol. 4, Martini, L. and Ganong, W. F., Eds., Raven Press, New York, 1976, 129.

Matussek, N., Catecholamines and mood neuroendocrine aspects, in *Current Topics in Neuroendocrinology*, Vol. 8, Gantt, D. and Pfaff, D., Eds., Springer-Verlag, Berlin, 1988, 141.

Matussek, N., Ackenheil, M., Hippius, H., Muller, F., Schroeder, H., Schultes, H., and Wasilewski, B., Effects of clonidine on growth hormone release in psychiatric patients and controls, *Psychiatry Res.*, 2, 25, 1980.

Meltzer, H. Y., Kolakowska, T., Fang, V. S., Fogg, L., Robertson, A., Lewine, R., Stratulevitz, M., and Bosch, D., Growth hormone and PRL response to apomorphine in schizophrenia and the major affective disorders, *Arch. Gen. Psychiatry*, 41, 512, 1984.

Mendlewicz, J., Linowski, P., and Brauman, H., TSH responses to TRH in women with unipolar and bipolar depression, *Lancet*, 2, 1079, 1979.

Mendlewicz, J., Linkowski, P., Kerkhofs, M., Desmedt, D., Golstein, J., Copinschi, G., and Van Cauter, E., Diurnal hypersecretion of growth hormone in depression, *J. Clin. Endo. Metab.*, 60, 505, 1985.

Mortola, J. F., Liv, J. H., Gillin, J. C., Rasmussen, D. D., and Yen, S. S., Pulsatile rhythms of ACTH and cortisol in women with endogenous depression: evidence for increased ACTH pulse freqeuency, *J. Clin. Endocrinol. Metab.*, 65, 962, 1987.

Muller, E. E., Brambilla, F., Cavagnini, F., and Peracchi, M., and Panerai, A., Slight effect of L-tryptophan on growth hormone release in normal human subjects, *J. Clin. Endocrinol. Metab.*, 39, 1, 1974.

Nathan, R. S., Sachar, E. J., Asmis, G. M., Halbreich, U., and Halpern, F. S., Relative insulin insensitivity and cortisol secretion in depressed patients, *Psychiatry Res.*, 4, 291, 1981.

Nemeroff, C. B., The role of corticotropin-releasing factor in the pathogenesis of major depression, *Pharmacopsychiatry*, 21, 76, 1988.

Nemeroff, C. B., Corticotropin-releasing factor, in *Neuropeptides and Psychiatric Disorders*, Nemeroff, C. B., Ed., APA Press, Washington, D.C., 1991, 75.

Nemeroff, C. B. and Evans, D. L., Correlation between the dexamethasone suppression test in depressed patients and clinical response, *Am. J. Psychiatry*, 141, 247, 1984.

Nemeroff, C. B., Bissette, G., Martin, J. B., Brazeau, P., Vale, W., Kizer, J. S., and Prange, A. J., Jr., Effect of chronic treatment with thyrotropin-releasing hormone (TRH) or an analog of TRH (linear-β-alanine TRH) on the hypothalamic-pituitary-thyroid axis, *Neuroendocrinology*, 30, 193, 1980.

Nemeroff, C. B., Widerlov, E., Bissette, G., Walleus, H., Karlsson, I., Eklund, K., Kilts, C. D., Loosen, P. T., and Vale, W., Elevated concentrations of CSF corticotropin-releasing factor-like immunore-activity in depressed patients, *Science*, 226, 1342, 1984.

Nemeroff, C. B., Simon, J. S., Haggerty, J. J., and Evans, D. L., Antithyroid antibodies in depressed patients, *Am. J. Psychiatry*, 142, 840, 1985.

Nemeroff, C. B., Owens, M. J., Bissette, G., Andorn, A. C., and Stanley, M., Reduced corticotropin-releasing factor (CRF) binding sites in the frontal cortex of suicides, *Arch. Gen. Psychiatry*, 45, 577, 1988.

Nemeroff, C. B., Kizer, J. S., Reynolds, G. P. and Bissette, G., Neuropeptides in Alzheimer's disease: a post-mortem study, *Regul. Peptides,* 25, 123, 1989a.

Nemeroff, C. B., Krishnan, K. R. R., Belkin, B. M., Ritchie, J. C., Clark, C., Vale, W., Rivier, J., and Thorner, M. O., Growth hormone response to GHRF in Alzheimer's disease, *Neuroendocrinology,* 50, 663, 1989b.

Nemeroff, C. B., Bissette, G., Akil, H., and Fink, M., Cerebrospinal fluid neuropeptides in depressed patients treated with ECT: corticotropin-releasing factor β-endorphin and somatostatin, *Br. J. Psychiatry,* 158, 59, 1991.

Nemeroff, C. B., Krishnan, K. R. R., Reed, D., Leder, R., Beam, C., and Dunnick, N. R., Adrenal gland enlargement in major depression: a computed tomography study, *Arch. Gen. Psychiatry,* in press.

Neville, A. M. and O'Hare, M. J., *The Human Adrenal Cortex. An Integrated Approach*, Springer Verlag, Berlin, 1982.

Pandey, G. N., Garver, D. L., Tamminga, C., Eriksen, S., Ali, L., and Davis, J. M., Post synaptic supersensitivity in schizophrenia, *Am. J. Psychiatry,* 134, 518, 1977.

Pearlson, G. D. and Veroff, A. E., Computerized tomographic changes in manic depressive illness, *Lancet,* 1, 470, 1981.

Pitts, A. F., Kathol, R. G., Gehris, T. L., Samuelson, S. D., Carroll, B. T., Mehter, W. H., Carter, J., Nemeroff, C. B., and Bissette, G., Elevated cerebrospinal fluid corticotropin-releasing hormone and arginine vasopressin in depressed patients with dexamethanone non-suppression, *Soc. Neurosci. Abstr.,* 16, 454, 1990.

Prange, A. J., Wilson, I. C., Rabon, A. M., and Lipton, M. A., Enhancement of imipramine antidepressant activity by thyroid hormone, *Am. J. Psychiatry,* 126, 457, 1969.

Prange, A. J., Wilson, I. C., Lara, P. P., Alltop, L. B., and Breese, G. R., Effects of thyrotropin-releasing hormone in depression, *Lancet,* 1, 999, 1972.

Prange, A. J., Wilson, I. C., Breese, G. R., and Lipton, M. A., Hormonal alteration of imipramine response: a review, in *Hormones, Behavior and Psychopathology,* Sachar, E. J., Ed., Raven Press, New York, 1976, 41.

Prange, A. J., Loosen, P. T., Wilson, I., and Lipton, M. A., The therapeutic use of hormones of the thyroid axis in depression, in *Neurobiology of Mood Disorders,* Post, C. R. and Ballenger, J., Eds., Williams & Wilkins, Baltimore, 1980, 311.

Rao, V. P., Krishnan, K. R., Goli, V., Saunder, W. B., Ellinwood, E. H., Blazer, D. G., and Nemeroff, C. B., Neuroanatomic changes and hypothalamo-pituitary-adrenal axis abnormalities, *Biol. Psychiatry,* 26, 729, 1989.

Risch, S. C., Growth hormone-releasing factor and growth hormone, in *Neuropeptides in Psychiatric Disorders,* Nemeroff, C. B., Ed., APA Press, Washington, D.C., 1991, 93.

Risch, S. C., Lewine, R. J., Kalin, N. H., Jewart, R. D., Risby, E. D., Caudle, J. M., Stipetic, M., Turner, J., Eccard, M. B., and Pollard, W. E., Limbic-hypothalamic-pituitary-adrenal axis activity and ventricular-to-brain ratio studies in affective illness and schizophrenia, *Neuropsychopharmacology,* in press, 1992.

Ritchie, J., Belkin, B. M., Krishnan, K. R. R., Nemeroff, C. B., and Carroll, B. J., Plasma dexamethasone concentration and the dexamethasone suppresstion test, *Biol. Psychiatry,* 27, 159, 1990.

Rosser, M. N., Iversen, L. L., Reynolds, G. P., Mountjoy, C., and Roth, M., Neurochemical characteristics of early and late onset of Alzheimer's disease, *Br. Med. J.,* 288, 961, 1984.

Rothschild, A. J., Benes, F., Woods, B., Bakanas, E., and Schatzberg, A. F., Cortisol and brain CT relationships in depression, in *Proc. 141st Ann. Meeting of the Am. Psychiat. Association,* 1988.

Roy, A., Pickar, D., Doran, A., Wolkowitz, O., Gallucci, W., Chrousos, G., and Gold, P., The corticotropin releasing hormone stimulation test in chronic schizophrenia, *Am. J. Psychiatry,* 143, 1393, 1986.

Roy, A., Pickar, D., Paul, S., Doran, A., Chrousos, G. P., and Gold, P. W., CSF corticotropin-releasing hormone in depressed patients and normal control subjects, *Am. J. Psychiatry,* 144, 641, 1987.

Roy, A., Bissette, G., Nemeroff, C. B., DeJong, J., Ravitz, B., Adinoff, B., and Linnoila, M., Cerebrospinal fluid thyrotropin-releasing hormone concentrations in alcoholics and normal controls, *Biol. Psychiatry,* 28, 767, 1990.

Rubinow, D. R., Post, R. N., Savard, R., and Gold, P. W., Cortisol hypersecretion and cognitive impairment in depression, *Arch. Gen. Psychiatry,* 40, 409, 1983.

Rush, J. A., A phase II study of cognitive therapy of depression, in *Psychotherapy Research: Where Are We and Where Should We Be?,* Williams, J. B. and Spitzer, R. L., Eds., Guilford Press, New York, 1984.

Russ, M. J. and Ackerman, S. H., Antidepressant treatment response in depressed hypothyroid patients, *Hosp. Community Psychiatry,* 40, 954, 1989.

Sachar, E. J., Twenty-four hour cortisol secretion patterns in depressed and manic patients, *Prog. Brain Res.,* 42, 81, 1975.

Sachar, E., Hellman, L., Fukushima, D., and Gallagher, T., Cortisol production in depressive illness, *Arch. Gen. Psychiatry,* 23, 289, 1970.

Sachar, E., Hellman, L., Roffwarg, H., Halpern, F., Fukushima, D., and Gallagher, T., Disrupted 24 hour patterns of cortisol secretion in psychotic depression, *Arch. Gen. Psychiatry,* 28, 19, 1973a.

Sachar, E., Frantz, A., Altman, N., and Sassin, J., Growth hormone and prolactin in unipolar and bipolar depression patient response to hypoglycemia and L-DOPA, *Am. J. Psychiatry,* 130, 1362, 1973b.

Sachar, E. J., Altman, N., Gruen, P. H., Glassman, A., and Halpern, F. S., Growth hormone response to L-DOPA in relation to menopause depression and plasma level of L-DOPA, *Arch. Gen. Psychiatry,* 32, 502, 1975.

Sachar, E. J., Asnis, G. M., Nathan, R. S., Halbreich, U., Tabriji, M. N., and Halpern, F. S., Dextroamphetamine and cortisol in depression, *Arch. Gen. Psychiatry,* 37, 755, 1980.

Sapolsky, R., Armine, M., and Packar, M. A., Stress and glucocorticoids in aging, *Endocrinol. Metab. Clin.,* 16, 965, 1987.

Schilkrut, R., Chandra, O., Osswald, M., Ruther, E., Baarfusser, B., and Mattussek, N., Growth hormone during sleep and with thermal stimulation in depressed patients, *Neuropsychobiology,* 1, 70, 1975.

Schimmelbusch, W. H., Mueller, P. S., and Schelps, J., Posture correlation between insulin resistance and duration of hospitalization in untreated schizophrenia, *Br. J. Psychiatry,* 118, 429, 1971.

Schuemeyer, H., Avgerinos, P. C., Gold, P. W., Gallucci, W. T., Tomai, T. P., Cutler, G. P., Loriaux, D. L., and Chrousos, G. P., Human corticotropin releasing factor dose response and time course of ACTH and cortisol secretion in man, *J. Clin. Endocrinol. Metab.,* 59, 1103, 1984.

Sherman, B. and Halmi, K. A., Effect of nutritional rehabilitation on hypothalamic pituitary function in anorexia nervosa, in *Anorexia Nervosa,* Vigensky, R. A., Ed., Raven Press, New York, 1977, 211.

Shrivastara, S., Schimmer, R., Brown, W. A., and Arato, M., DST predicts poor placebo response in depression, #94, in Abstracts of the APA Annual Meeting, Dallas, TX, 1985.

Siever, L. J., Uhde, T. W., Silberman, E. K., Jimerson, D. C., Aloi, J. A., Post, R. M., and Murphy, D. L., Growth hormone response to clonidine as a probe of noradrenergic receptor responsiveness in affective disorder patients and controls, *Psychiatry Res.,* 6, 171, 1982.

Simon, J. S., Evans, D. L., and Nemeroff, C. B., The dexamethasone suppression test and antidepressant response in major depression, *J. Psychiatr. Res.,* 21, 313, 1987.

Spar, J. E. and Gerner, R., Dose dexamethasone suppression test distinguish dementia from depression, *Am. J. Psychiatry,* 139, 238, 1982.

Starkman, M. N. and Schteingart, D. E., Neuropsychiatric manifestations of patients with Cushing syndrome, *Arch. Gen. Psychiatry,* 141, 215, 1981.

Steardo, L., Tamminga, C. A., and Barone, P., CSF somatostatin immunoreactivity and growth hormone plasma levels in Alzheimer's disease, *Neuroendocrinol. Lett.,* 6, 291, 1984.

Stein, M. B. and Uhde, T. W., Triiodothyronine potentiation of tricyclic antidepressant treatment in patients with panic disorder, *Biol. Psychiatry,* 28, 1061, 1990.

Stewart, J. W., Quitkin, F., McGrath, P. J., Liebowitz, M. R., Harrison, W., Rabkin, J. G., Novacenko, H., Antich, J. P., and Asnis, G. N., Cortisol response to dextroamphetamine stimulation in depressed outpatients, *Psychiatry Res.,* 12, 195, 1984.

Stokes, P. and Sikes, C. R., The hypothalamic-pituitary-adrenocortical axis in major depression, *Endocrinol. Metab. Clin. N. Am.,* 17, 1, 1988.

Stokes, P. E., Pick, G. R., Stoll, P. M., and Nunn, W. D., Pituitary-adrenal function in depressed patients: resistance to dexamethasone suppression, *J. Psychiatr. Res.,* 12, 271, 1975.

Synek, V. and Rubin, J. R., Ventricular brain ratio using plain metric measurements of EMI scan, *Br. J. Radiol.,* 49, 233, 1976.

Tamminga, C. A., Smith, R. C., Pandey, G. N., Frohman, L. A., and Davis, J. M., A neuroendocrine study of supersensitivity in T.D., *Arch. Gen. Psychiatry,* 34, 1199, 1977.

Targum, S. D., Rosen, L. N., Delisi, L. E., and Weinberger, D. R., Cerebral ventricular size in major depressive disorder, *Biol. Psychiatry,* 18, 329, 1983.

Targum, S. D., Greenberg, R. D., and Harmon, R. L., Thyroid hormone and the TRH stimulation test in refractory depression, *J. Clin. Psychiat.,* 45, 345, 1984.

Thorner, M. O., Rivier, J., Spiess, J., Borges, J. L., Vance, M. L., Bloom, S. R., Rogol, A. D., Cronin, M. J., Kaiser, S., Evans, W. S., Webster, J. D., Machod, R. M., and Vale, W., Human pancreatic GHRF selectively stimulates GH secretion in man, *Lancet,* 1, 24, 1983.

Toivola, P. T. K., Gale, C. C., Goodner, C. J., and Werrbach, J. H., Central α-adrenergic regulation of growth hormone and insulin, *Hormones,* 3, 193, 1972.

Vale, W., Spiess, J., Rivier, C., and Rivier, J., Characterization of a 41 residue ovine hypothalamic peptide that stimulates secretion of corticotropin of β-endorphin, *Science,* 213, 1394, 1981.

Vigensky, R. A. and Loriaux, D., Anorexia nervosa as a model of hypothalamic dysfunction, in *Anorexia Nervosa,* Vigensky, R. A., Ed., Raven Press, New York, 1977, 109.

Von Bardeleben, U., Holsboer, F., Stalla, G. K., and Muller, O. A., Combined administration of human corticotropin-releasing factor and lysine vasopressin induces cortisol escape from dexamethasone suppression in healthy subjects, *Life Sci.,* 37, 1613, 1985.

Von Bardeleben, U., Benker, O., and Holsboer, F., Clinical and neuroendocrine effects of Zotepine — a new neuroleptic drug, *Pharmacopsychiatry,* 20(1), 28, 1987.

Von Bardeleben, U., Stalla, G. K., Muller, O. A., and Holsboer, F., Blunting of ACTH response to human CRF in depressed patients is avoided by metyrapone treatment, *Biol. Psychiatry,* 24, 782, 1988.

Weeke, A. and Weeke, J., The 24-hour pattern of serum TSH in patients with endogenous depression, *Acta Psychiatr. Scand.,* 62, 69, 1980.

Westlund, K. N., Aguilera, G., and Childs, G. V., Quantification of morphological changes in pituitary corticotrophs by *in vivo* CRF stimulation and adrenalectomy, *Endocrinology,* 120, 381, 1987.

Winokur, A., Amsterdam, J. D., Oper, J., Mendels, J., Snyder, P. J., Caroff, S. N., and Brunswick, D. J., Multiple hormonal responses to protirelin (TRH) in depressed patients, *Arch. Gen. Psychiatry,* 40, 525, 1983.

Zis, K. D. and Zis, A., Increased adrenal weight in victims of violent suicide, *Am. J. Psychiatry,* 144, 1214, 1987.

Section IV
Clinical Neuroendocrinology

John E. Morley, Section Editor

16
Clinical Neuroendocrinology

PIERRE BOULOUX
Royal Free Hospital
London, England

and

ASHLEY GROSSMAN
The Medical College of St. Bartholomew's Hospital
London, England

I. Disorders of the Hypothalamus and Anterior Pituitary

A. The Hypothalamus

1. Introduction

The hypothalamus regulates the hormone-secreting cells of the anterior pituitary through production and hypothalamo-pituitary portal venous delivery of stimulatory and inhibitory hormones. The hypothalamus and pituitary act as a single functional unit that can be affected by many pathological processes, but because of their close interrelationship it is frequently difficult on clinical grounds alone to determine whether defective pituitary function results from primary pituitary disease, or secondary to hypothalamic dysfunction.

Lesions of the hypothalamus may present with abnormal cerebral function, behavioral disturbance, or by hypophysial dysfunction. In general, hypothalamic disease leads to deficiency of anterior pituitary hormone production; however, withdrawal of inhibitory dopaminergic tone to pituitary lactotrophs will result in hyperprolactinemia with its diverse manifestations. Some hypothalamic neurons are under similar restraint; thus, loss of inhibitory regulation of gonadotropin-releasing hormone (GnRH)-secreting cells in the hypothalamic arcuate and supraoptic nuclei in the prepubertal child may trigger precocious puberty: this situation occasionally follows disease of the posterior hypothalamus (e.g., pinealomas). Pituitary disease usually presents with symptoms and signs of hormone excess or insufficiency, or because of the space-occupying effect of a tumor.

2. Clinical Presentation of Hypothalamic Disease

Hypothalamic disease (see classification in Table 1) may present with evidence of hypogonadism, menstrual disturbance, precocious puberty, cranial diabetes insipidus (DI), or feeding disorders (obesity and hyperphagia). Disorders of thirst perception, somnolence, emaciation, anorexia and disturbance of thermoregulation may also occur, reflecting the large number of physiological functions regulated by hypothalamic nuclei. The anatomical localization of the optic chiasm makes it particularly vulnerable to pathological processes in the anterior hypothalamus.

445

Table 1
Classification of Hypothalamic Disorders

Tumors	Trauma
Craniopharyngioma	Subarachnoid hemorrhage
Glioma	AV malformations
Hamartomas	Aneurysms
Dysgerminoma	Surgical or traumatic stalk section
Histiocytosis X	Inflammatory disease
Leukemia	Meningitis
Neuroblastoma	Encephalitis
Meningioma	Sarcoidosis
Colloid cyst of third ventricle	Hydatid disease
Ependymoma	AIDS
Angioma	Miscellaneous
Lymphoma	Chronic hydrocephalus
Teratoma	Raised intracranial pressure
Secondary deposits	Radiotherapy damage
Pineal tumors	Anorexia nervosa
Germ cell tumors	Exercise-induced amenorrhea
Pineal parenchymal tumors	Poor growth due to psychosocial deprivation
	Depression

DI is almost invariable in hypothalamic disease, and often a presenting feature. Full expression of DI requires the presence of adequate amounts of circulating cortisol, and may thus be masked in the presence of coincidental adrenocorticotropin (ACTH) deficiency. Trauma, granulomas [tuberculous (TB) and sarcoid], and tumors (primary and secondary) are the usual causes of acquired DI, but in a significant number of cases no structural lesion is revealed; in such cases, autoimmune processes may be operative, or possibly vascular events within the hypothalamus. Rarely, demyelinating processes may have affected hypothalamic function.

3. Other Hormone Deficiency States

Deficiency of one or more hypothalamic-pituitary-releasing hormones can lead to selective pituitary insufficiency. Selective deficiency of thyrotropin-releasing hormone (TRH) is rare, and leads to "tertiary hypothyroidism". In such cases, an intravenous TRH test (200 to 500 µg) will give a characteristic pattern of response, with the 60-min thyroid-stimulating hormone (TSH) response exceeding the 20-min value. Gonadotropin-releasing hormone deficiency may occur either singly or in combination with other releasing hormone deficiencies. In Kallmann's syndrome, hypogonadotropic hypogonadism (due to GnRH deficiency) is associated with anosmia.

Growth hormone-releasing hormone (GHRH) deficiency appears to be responsible for many cases of idiopathic growth hormone (GH) deficiency in childhood, since these children often have a GH response to the exogenous administration of GHRH (Ross et al., 1987). There have been a number of authenticated reports of corticotropin-releasing hormone (CRH) deficiency associated with hypoadrenalism. Defective dopamine synthesis and delivery to the lactotroph is associated with hyperprolactinemia.

4. Diagnostic Evaluation of Hypothalamo-Pituitary Disorders

The diagnostic evaluation of hypothalamo-pituitary disease has several objectives, the most important of which are to (1) identify the presence of any space-occupying lesion in the area, and (2) characterize the extent of resulting hypothalamo-pituitary dysfunction. This diagnostic approach relies first and foremost on history taking and physical examination.

Thereafter, biochemical and hormonal assessment is required, as well as neuroradiological and neuroophthalmological assessment.

5. Hormonal Evaluation

a. Basal

The measurement of basal hormone levels, both pituitary and target hormones, is essential. In practice, this means an 0900-hr sample for ACTH, cortisol, TSH, T_4 and T_3, luteinizing hormone (LH), follicle-stimulating hormone (FSH), estradiol and testosterone (where appropriate), prolactin, GH, and plasma and urine osmolality.

b. Dynamic

In addition to measurements of basal hormonal status, dynamic testing of the hypothalamo-pituitary axis is usually required. Three tests, the insulin tolerance test, the clomiphene test and the water deprivation test, are used clinically to test the integrity of the hypothalamo-pituitary axis.

In the insulin tolerance test, soluble insulin, in a dose of 0.15 U/kg, is given intravenously to a fasting individual; the ensuing neuroglycopenia will stimulate ACTH and GH release (via CRH, vasopressin, and GHRH, respectively). The test is of particular value in the assessment of the hypothalamo-pituitary-adrenal axis. Diseases of the hypothalamus lead to defective release of these hypothalamo-hypophysiotropic hormones with inadequate ACTH (and thus cortisol) and GH in response to hypoglycemia (glucose nadir < 2.2 mmol/l) . Diseases of the pituitary lead to similar defective responses.

In the clomiphene test, the LH and FSH responses to the anti-estrogen clomiphene test the integrity of the hypothalamo-pituitary axis; clomiphene may act as an agonist in patients with low or undetectable estrogen levels, and in such cases the LH and FSH responses may actually be depressed following its administration. The normal response to clomiphene is an elevation of LH and FSH, the result of increased GnRH secretion following antagonism of the normal feedback processes, operating in part at the level of the hypothalamus. Failure of LH and FSH response to clomiphene can result from both hypothalamic and pituitary disorders.

Water deprivation tests are discussed fully in Chapter 19 on posterior pituitary disorders.

6. Pituitary Releasing Hormone Tests

Synthetic TRH, GnRH, GHRH, and CRH are available for clinical testing of TSH, LH and FSH, GH, and ACTH reserves, respectively. These releasing hormones will stimulate only the readily releasable pools of pituitary hormones. Their diagnostic applications have been reviewed elsewhere (Besser and Ross, 1989), and only a brief outline is given here.

7. TRH Test

TRH (200 to 500 μg) is administered intravenously, and the TSH response measured at 0, 20, and 60 min. Patients with destructive pituitary lesions show an attenuated or absent TSH response to TRH (although not invariably), whereas those with hypothalamic disease show a delayed peak response, with the 60-min TSH value exceeding the 20-min value. A flat TSH response to TRH also occurs in patients with thyrotoxicosis and ophthalmic Graves' disease. In primary hypothyroidism, the basal TSH is elevated, and the TSH response to TRH exaggerated. The TSH response to TRH is characteristically flat in situations of prolonged inappropriate cortisol excess (Cushing's syndrome).

8. GnRH Test

The response of LH and FSH to 100 μg of intravenous GnRH depends on age, sex, degree of sexual maturation, and in women, the phase of the menstrual cycle. In the prepubertal child, the FSH response exceeds the LH response, whereas the opposite is observed in sexual maturity. In situations of prolonged GnRH deficiency (e.g., Kallmann's syndrome), there may be no LH or FSH response to intravenous GnRH initially, but after a suitable period of priming with GnRH, the pituitary responsiveness is restored. An absent LH/FSH response to clomiphene accompanied by LH/FSH responsiveness to GnRH is suggestive of a hypothalamic disturbance.

9. GHRH Test

The GH response to GHRH is reasonably constant during life. Failure of GH release with the insulin-hypoglycemia test, yet a GH response to GHRH, suggests the presence of hypothalamic GHRH deficiency. This appears to underlie many cases of idiopathic GH deficiency in childhood. A flat GH response to GHRH occurs in destructive pituitary lesions, and in patients with Cushing's syndrome of any cause. Some patients with acromegaly have an exaggerated GH response to GHRH despite having an elevated basal GH level (Wood et al., 1983).

10. CRF Test

Failure of the ACTH/cortisol response to hypoglycemia in the presence of responsiveness to exogenous CRF suggests a hypothalamic disturbance with CRF deficiency. An exaggerated ACTH/cortisol response to CRF is seen in most cases of Cushing's disease (Muller et al., 1983). In normal individuals, the ACTH/cortisol response depends on the initial basal cortisol level, the largest incremental rises occurring in subjects with the lowest basal cortisol levels (Lytras et al., 1984).

11. Neuroradiological Investigation
a. Plain Radiography

Posteroanterior (PA) and right lateral films of the skull with correct positioning of the patient have been essential in the past, but are usually now only used as a screening test. Pituitary tumors generally increase sellar size. Small intrasellar tumors may be associated with small blisters in the contour of the sella. Larger tumors may cause a double floor, due to unequal expansion of the sellar floor between the two sides. In such cases, the PA projection may indicate a slope to the sellar floor. However, recent evidence suggests that many minor changes in sellar anatomy may not be related to pathology. Some pituitary tumors spontaneously infarct and undergo calcification, resulting in the rare appearance of a pituitary stone. Calcification in the pituitary area may be caused by craniopharyngioma, meningiomas, calcification in the walls of aneurysms, chordomas, and extremely rarely hydatid disease. Sellar tomography is now rarely undertaken.

b. Computed Tomography Scanning

Computed axial tomography (CT), with high dose intravenous contrast, is the present imaging technique of choice in the radiological assessment of hypothalamo-pituitary disease in most centers. Using a thin slice technique (1- to 2-mm cuts), the technique allows high resolution with precise visualization of the pituitary gland, stalk, and surrounding structures. Multiple adjacent sagittal sections may be taken through the pituitary gland, and then reformatted in a coronal plane. Although direct coronal sections may be scanned, in practice the patient has to hyperextend his neck, making the procedure uncomfortable. The normal pituitary gland has a reasonably homogeneous density, the upper border being flat or concave, and not extending rostral to the interclinoid line. Microadenomas appear as hypodense lesions, and less commonly as isodense or even hyperdense. Larger lesions cause bulging of the sellar contents, causing an upward convexity. The stalk may be displaced to the contralateral side by the tumor, this effect being best seen on the coronal reformatted images. The resolution of present generation CT scanners is on the order of 3 to 4 mm. Meso- or macroadenomas (greater than 1 cm) are readily visualized, and cystic lesions are easily recognized. Large tumors with temporal lobe, retroclival, cerebellopontine, and cavernous sinus extensions are easily delineated.

Knowledge of the range of appearances of the normal pituitary contour remains incomplete. It has become evident that the gland may swell physiologically during the menstrual cycle (generating a convex upper border; Henshaw et al., 1984), during pregnancy, and in the immediate post-partum period. Furthermore, small innocuous hypodense areas may also occur. Primary target gland failure (hypothyroidism, Addison's disease, menopause) may also cause isodense swelling of the pituitary, and this may cause diagnostic confusion. Contrast enhancement may help identify aneurysmal dilatation of the carotid, and will also show early delineation of the "tuft" of portal vessels.

c. MRI

Greater definition of the hypothalamus, median eminence , pituitary stalk, and pituitary gland may be achieved with the latest generation magnetic resonance imaging (MRI) scanners (Kaufman, 1984). The introduction of the contrast medium gadolinium has further enhanced the resolution of MRI. Small tumors appear as low-density focal lesions on the T1-weighted scans, and high intensity on the T2-weighted scans (see Figure 1). A disadvantage of the method is that calcification is not readily identified unless it is gross. In contrast, it is the imaging technique of choice in identifying pituitary apoplexy (see Figure 2).

12. Neuroophthalmological Evaluation of Hypothalamo-Pituitary Disorders

Bedside visual field testing using a small red target and a confrontation technique is exceedingly valuable in determining the presence and extent of a visual field defect. Typical pituitary lesions expanding upward compress the optic chiasm from below, and cause an initial superior quadrantinopia and then a bitemporal hemianopia. Lesions expanding from above downward (e.g., anterior communicating artery aneurysms) may also produce a similar visual field defect, early lesions causing an inferior bitemporal quadrantinopia, progressing eventually to a bitemporal hemianopia.

Formal perimetry should be carried out using a Goldmann perimeter, and visual evoked responses (VERs) should be used in cases where there is equivocal evidence of optic pathway compression. The major advantage of using VERs is the capacity to evaluate individual portions of the visual field.

13. General Principles of Management of Hypothalamo-Pituitary Disease

When hypopituitarism is present, pituitary hormone replacement should be given (see Table 2). The dose of hydrocortisone will need to be increased under conditions of stress. For example, a patient undergoing major surgery will require intramuscular hydrocortisone, 100 mg with the premedication and 100 mg intramuscularly (i.m.) every 6 hr for 48 to 72 hr postoperatively, prior to resuming his usual replacement dose.

B. Disorders of the Hypothalamus

1. Craniopharyngioma

Craniopharyngioma accounts for up to 10% of brain tumors in childhood, although 27% of tumors first present after the age of 40 (Ross-Russell and Pennybacker, 1961). They arise from embryonal squamous cell rests that represent residual epithelium from the stomadeum, which migrated upward to form the anterior pituitary gland. Over half the lesions arise from within the anterior pituitary, the remainder being found above the sella (Carmel, 1985). Lesions are usually partly cystic, and calcification may occur within the wall.

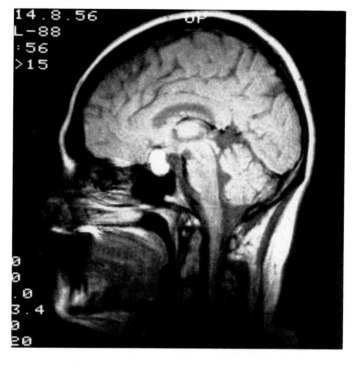

A

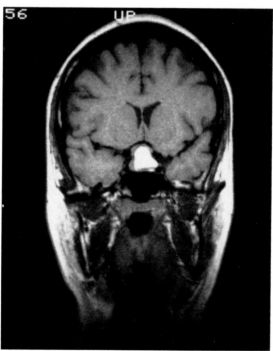

B

Figure 1. (A) Sagittal; (B) coronal. MR scan of patient with pituitary apoplexy in a preexisting tumor. There is hyperintensity within an enlarged gland that shows suprasellar extension, causing optic chiasma compression and elevation of the anterior cerebral arteries. The hematoma is bulging into the left cavernous sinus between the limbs of the carotid siphon on the left.

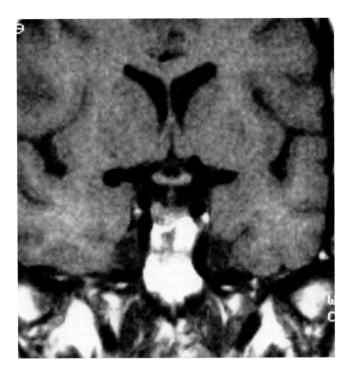

Figure 2. MR coronal scan showing a right-sided pituitary microadenoma. The floor of the pituitary fossa is depressed on the right and the optic chiasm and pituitary stalk visualized.

Table 2
Hormone Replacement in the Hypopituitary Patient

Hormone	Usual replacement dose
Hydrocortisone	20 mg on waking
	10 mg evening
Thyroxine	0.1–0.2 mg/day
Ethinyl estradiol	30 mg/day continuously
Medroxyprogesterone acetate	5–10mg/day for last 14 days of cycle
Testosterone undecanoate	40 mg t.d.s.
Desmopressin	10 µg intranasally 1–2 times daily

The clinical presentation depends on the size and location of the tumor as well as any degree of coincidental hypopituitarism. Some lesions therefore mimic pituitary tumors. In children, raised intracranial pressure due to compression and interruption of the normal pathway for cerebrospinal fluid (CSF) flow may occur, with headache, vomiting, papilloedema and visual field defect (Bartlett, 1971). The position of the optic chiasma (pre- or post-fixed) determines the nature and severity of the visual field defect. Bitemporal visual field defects may be seen, and there may be damage to the 3rd, 4th and 6th cranial nerves. Focal cerebral deficits may be present in patients with largely extrasellar lesions. Endocrine impairment may be associated with short stature, retarded bone age, and delayed pubertal development in children, variable degrees of hypogonadism in adults, and with menstrual irregularity, decreased libido, and impotence in males (Baskin and Wilson, 1986). Diabetes insipidus is a frequent presenting complaint and other hypothalamic disturbances, such as eating disorders with obesity and thermoregulatory defects, may be present. In adults, variable degrees of intellectual impairment and in extreme cases dementia are occasionally seen (Bartlett, 1971).

Investigation usually reveals an abnormal pituitary fossa (50 to 70% cases), and intracranial calcification presents in up to 90% of childhood cases. This may be patchy rather than curvilinear. Calcification of a lesion in childhood is highly suggestive of a craniopharyngioma but may occur in pituitary adenomas, chordomas, meningiomas, aneurysms, secondary carcinomas, and teratomas in adults. The cystic lesions are generally filled with an oily, cholesterol-rich liquid. Recently, it has been shown that cyst fluid contains human chorionic gonadotrophin (β-hCG) and indeed this may act as a tumor marker for such lesions (Harris et al., 1988). Computed tomography (CT) scanning and MRI are the imaging modalities of choice. CT scans will usually reveal a predominantly (although not invariably) cystic lesion enclosing one or multiple cysts. Low attenuation on CT scanning is related to the cholesterol content. Arteriography may be helpful in defining the anatomy further prior to attempted excision.

In terms of treatment, surgery is usually required, and if the lesion has a predominantly suprasellar component transfrontal craniotomy is indicated. Total excision is rarely achieved, and after surgical debulking radiotherapy is indicated to reduce the chances of recurrence. Complete removal should rarely be attempted, as this greatly increases the possibility of severe neurological defect. Pituitary hormone replacement treatment may be required prior to any surgical intervention and to correct any post-operative hypopituitarism.

2. Other Lesions in the Suprasellar Region
a. Rathke's Pouch Cyst

Rathke's pouch cysts are derived from the area between the pars intermedia and the infundibular process, and are usually intrasellar. Occasionally they are suprasellar and may present with a visual field defect or hypothalamic dysfunction (Ringer and Barley, 1972). Variable degrees of hypopituitarism may be present. Often the diagnosis of a Rathke's pouch cyst is made only at surgery, when a pituitary adenoma had previously been suspected.

b. Chordoma

Chordomas arise from the notochordal remnants in the clivus, which usually produce destruction of the basisphenoid (Dahlin and MacCarty, 1952). The most common clinical presentation is with headaches, visual disturbance, neck pain, and nasopharyngeal obstruction. The 3rd, 4th and 6th cranial nerves may be affected. Endocrine disturbances are uncommon, but when they occur cause variable pituitary insufficiency (de Cremoux et al., 1980). A "pseudoprolactinoma" syndrome with hyperprolactinemia secondary to stalk compression may occur. Radiologically, there is bone destruction and calcification. Surgical extirpation is rarely complete. The lesions are not usually radioresponsive.

c. Arachnoid Cyst

Arachnoid cysts produce their clinical manifestations by a mass effect, visual symptoms being consequent upon compression of optic nerves, chiasm, or tracts. Hydrocephalus secondary to compression of the foramen of Munro may occur. The etiology of these lesions is currently speculative (Kasdon et al., 1977): trauma, adhesive arachnoiditis secondary to infection, and a congenital developmental defect of the subarachnoid space have all been suggested. In addition to the mass effects produced, lesions may cause variable degrees of hypopituitarism. Treatment is surgical, with either internal or external drainage, or marsupialization.

d. Germinomas of the Hypothalamus (Atypical Teratoma, Ectopic Pinealoma)

Hypothalamic germinomas occur in one of three sites (Kagevama and Belsky, 1961). Ventral hypothalamic lesions are usually associated with germinomas in the pineal region, and are probably metastatic lesions from the pineal. When they arise in the anterior third of the hypothalamus, compression of the foramina of Munro may lead to hydrocephalus. Inferior extension may then lead to compression of the optic nerves and chiasm. Extension into the sella is rare, but when it occurs may mimic a pituitary adenoma. Clinically, patients present with diabetes insipidus, visual disturbance (visual field defects with optic atrophy), headache, and other features of raised intracranial pressure. Young patients may present with stunted growth, and obesity and variable degrees of hypogonadism and hypopituitarism may be present (Takenchi et al., 1978). The typical CT finding is that of an isodense lesion in the suprasellar region that enhances markedly with contrast (Naidich et al., 1976). Lesions metastasize within the CNS in about 10% of cases, and in such instances tumor cells may be found on examination of the cerebrospinal fluid.

β-hCG is usually present in the CSF and occasionally in the circulation, as may be α-fetoprotein (Nenwelt et al., 1980). These are important diagnostic markers of the disorder. Circulating hCG levels may cause stimulation of gonadal steroid secretion, causing premature pubertal development and gynecomastia in males. Lesions in the posterior hypothalamus can also induce true precocious puberty by disinhibiting the restraining influence of the pineal on GnRH-secreting cells. Lesions arising from the pineal region can cause abnormalities of pupillary and eye movement, as in Parinaud's syndrome. The tumor tends to be exquisitely radiosensitive, but chemotherapy plays an increasing part in the management of these tumors.

e. Optic Nerve Gliomas

Optic nerve gliomas are rare, occurring both in childhood and in adults. In childhood, lesions tend to be anterior and behave in a benign manner (Oxenhandler and Sayers, 1978), whereas in adulthood a more malignant pattern is seen (Manor et al., 1976). The childhood form is associated with neurofibromatosis. Patients present with visual failure, headache, and proptosis (Oxenhandler and Sayers, 1978). Larger lesions may present with hydrocephalus and signs of raised intracranial pressure, and occasionally precocious puberty in childhood. In adults, retroocular pain and visual loss may occur, usually affecting the optic chiasm. Skull X-rays may show enlargement of the optic foramen. However, CT scanning is the imaging technique of choice and there is usually contrast enhancement of the lesion. Magnetic resonance imaging (MRI) scanning can also provide excellent resolution of the optic chiasm. Treatment is by radiotherapy.

f. Hypothalamic Glioma

The classical presentation of hypothalamic glioma is the diencephalic syndrome, patients presenting with cachexia, weight loss, diabetes insipidus, and visual impairment. Chiasmatic involvement is common, and may lead to optic atrophy. The tumor usually arises in the anterior third of the hypothalamus, and infiltrates the floor of the third ventricle. Skull X-rays may show erosion of the tuberculum sellae and undercutting of the anterior clinoids. CT scanning will usually reveal an enhancing suprasellar mass. Treatment is usually palliative, the lesions rarely being radioresponsive.

g. Parasellar Meningioma

Parasellar meningioma can arise from the tuberculum sellae, the planum, and occasionally the diaphragma sellae. They may also grow from the sphenoid ridge and the cavernous sinus (Trobe et al., 1978). Lesions are usually small. Occasionally they arise from the arachnoid tissue of a herniated diaphragma and may then mimic a pituitary tumor. Visual failure, optic atrophy, and mild hyperprolactinemia are not uncommon, panhypopituitarism much less so. Radiologically, hyperostosis of the tuberculum sellae, planum, or sphenoid ridge may be seen. CT scanning is the imaging technique of choice, and usually shows a uniform, well-enhancing lesion. When the lesions are inoperable, radiotherapy is the only treatment.

h. Aneurysms Mimicking Pituitary Adenomas

Aneurysms of the carotid are occasionally intrasellar, thus leading to hypopituitarism

(White and Ballantine, 1961). Suprasellar aneurysms usually cause visual field defects. The presence of supraorbital pain, episodes of sudden severe headache, or cranial nerve palsies are suggestive of the presence of an aneurysm. Endocrine disorders related to the presence of an aneurysm include disorders of menstruation, diabetes insipidus, short stature, and ACTH and TSH deficiency. Plain radiography usually discloses an asymmetrical pituitary fossa, with erosion of the ipsilateral anterior clinoid. A thin rim of calcification in the wall is not specific as it may also be found in cases of craniopharyngioma. Arteriography is the imaging technique of choice, although CT scanning immediately after injection of intravenous contrast may show a homogeneous intense blush.

3. Granulomatous Disorders Affecting the Hypothalamus
a. Histiocytosis X

Histiocytosis X is the term now applied to the three disorders eosinophilic granuloma, Hand-Schüller-Christian disease, and Letterer-Siwe disease. The endocrinopathy that results from this disorder is variable (Tibbs et al., 1978), but there is a predilection for hypothalamic involvement. Almost one half of patients have diabetes insipidus, which is usually the presenting complaint (Pressman et al., 1975). Punched-out lesions of the skull or of the mandible are common. Long bones may be similarly affected. CT scanning usually shows an enhancing mass in the region of the hypothalamus.The lesions respond to small doses of radiotherapy (1000 to 1500 cGy over 2 to 3 weeks), as do lesions elsewhere in the skeleton. The presence of extracranial lesions greatly facilitates the diagnosis, but where these are absent, biopsy may be required. The prognosis is good for older children and adults with patchy bone lesions, but the disease may be relentlessly progressive in some cases. Spontaneous healing occasionally occurs. The therapeutic role of high-dose corticosteroids is controversial.

b. Neurosarcoid

Although sarcoidosis is a systemic disorder, involvement of the CNS is a relatively rare event, occurring in 15 to 20% of cases. The hypothalamus is a preferred site of CNS involvement (Selenkow et al., 1959). At this site, the disease usually causes a granulomatous or adhesive arachnoiditis, and invasion of the floor of the third ventricle. Diabetes insipidus is common, as is hyperprolactinemia, due to interruption of delivery of dopamine to the lactotrophs. The diagnosis is made by establishing the presence of sarcoid elsewhere in the body, although occasionally a biopsy is required with isolated neurosarcoidosis. Serum acetylcholinesterase (ACE) levels are often raised in this condition and oligoclonal bands may be present within the CSF. The CT scanning appearances are not specific. Treatment is by corticosteroids combined with immunosuppression.

c. Tuberculosis

In tuberculous meningitis, a dense, plaquelike exudate at the base of the brain can involve the sellar and parasellar region. Occasionally, a tuberculoma may compress the pituitary or the hypothalamus directly, thereby causing dysfunction secondary to dilatation of the third ventricle. A number of hypothalamic syndromes have been described in this context, including sleep disturbances, precocious sexual development, hyperphagia and obesity, and diabetes insipidus. Virtually all patients have evidence of active tuberculosis elsewhere. Treatment is with antituberculous chemotherapy.

4. Miscellaneous Hypothalamic Disorders
a. Radiation Damage to the Hypothalamus

Patients who have undergone cranial irradiation may develop selective deficiency of releasing hormone production. For example, children having undergone cranial irradiation for medulloblastoma can develop GHRH deficiency and short stature.

b. Anorexia Nervosa

Anorexia nervosa affects young women, usually below 25 years of age, and is characterized by an obsessive fear of obesity that is not diminished by weight loss. There is a distortion of body image such that patients imagine themselves to be overweight even when they are grossly cachectic. Weight loss usually exceeds 25% of the ideal body weight. There is absence of any medical illness to account for the weight loss. Patients are invariably amenorrheic due to a reversion to a prepubertal state. Other clinical features include the presence of lanugo hair, bradycardia, constipation, periods of overactivity, cold intolerance, and occasionally parotid enlargement secondary to malnutrition. Peripheral edema may be present. The prognosis is frequently poor, and patients are susceptible to relapses. Behavior therapy and admission to hospital to supervise a high-calorie diet are the usual treatments. Menses usually but not invariably resume after a period of adequate weight gain. Similar menstrual disturbance may also be seen in women who exercise to excess.

c. Depressive Illness

Loss of cirdadian variation in cortisol levels and lack of dexamethasone suppressibility are the characteristic hallmarks of endogenous depressive illness. The TSH response to TRH is also attenuated. However, although cortisol production rates are elevated, patients do not usually appear cushingoid.

C. Pituitary Disorders

1. Tumors

For the most part pituitary tumors are benign lesions that make up between 10 and 15% of intracranial tumors in surgical material, and up to 23% of unselected adult autopsies. Rarely, the pituitary may be the site of a metastatic deposit from a primary tumor outside the central nervous system. Most primary lesions originate within the sella turcica, and are usually slow growing. Extension of such tumors to the suprasellar region may cause visual field defects and headache resulting from stretching of the diaphragma sella. Cranial nerve palsies, involving the oculomotor, supratrochlear, and abducens nerve, may occur with cavernous sinus involvement. Rarely, inferior extension into the sphenoid sinus and nasopharynx and forward extension into the ethmoidal air spaces occur. CSF rhinorrhea may ensue. Occasionally tumors are truly massive, extending into the hypothalamus, the temporal lobe, or in the retroclival space with compression of the pons. In these cases, severe neurological deficits may be seen. Pituitary carcinomas are rare, and are diagnosed in the presence of unequivocal extracranial metastases.

Pituitary adenomas may be functionless or lead to oversecretion of hormones. GH hypersecretion is associated with gigantism in childhood (prior to epiphyseal fusion of long bones) and acromegaly in adulthood. ACTH hypersecretion is associated with Cushing's disease, while hyperprolactinemia is associated with the amenorrhea-galactorrhea syndrome and infertility. TSH hypersecretion is a rare cause of thyrotoxicosis. LH-FSHomas are usually large tumors and may be associated with either normal or abnormal gonadal function.

2. Classification

Attempts at classification have caused a great deal of confusion. Historically, tumors were classified on the basis of cytoplasmic staining characteristics, size (microadenomas, < 1-cm diameter; macroadenomas > 1-cm diameter), growth patterns (diffuse, invasive, intrasellar, extrasellar), or endocrine activity [GH, ACTH, prolactin (PRL), TSH, FSH/LH, α subunit, plurihormonal, and nonsecreting]. There is little now to commend the use of classification by staining characteristics. Thus chromophobe adenomas are capable of secreting GH, PRL, ACTH, TSH, and LH and FSH.

3. Pathogenesis

The etiology is unknown in most cases. There is little evidence that hypersecretion of a hypothalamic releasing peptide leads to tumor production, although it may lead to hyperplasia. In theory, adenoma could supervene on a background of hyperplasia, but there is little evidence for this sequence of events in most cases, with the exception of true "feedback" tumors (some cases of TSHomas in primary hypothyroidism and Nelson's syndrome occurring in Addison's disease). Ectopic GHRH secretion leads to somatotroph hyperplasia, and similar hyperplasia may be seen in association with the very rare hypothalamic gangliocytomas. With pituitary prolactinomas, a popular if unproven theory suggests that infarction/interruption of blood flow to a portion of the pituitary leads to disinhibition of the normal inhibitory dopaminergic tone to a population of lactotrophs. Alternatively, these cells could receive an anomalous arterial supply from the pituitary capsule devoid of the usual dopamine content.

4. Prolactin-Secreting Tumors

Hyperprolactinemia is a common endocrine problem, and has several causes. It may be defined as persistent elevation of prolactin above 20 ng/ml in the absence of pregnancy or postpartum lactation. Prolactin secretion from the pituitary is under predominantly inhibitory control from hypothalamic dopamine, which is transported to the lactotrophs via the hypothalamo-hypophysial portal circulation. Thus, lesions destroying the dopamine-synthesizing neurons, lesions that impair the normal delivery of dopamine to the lactotroph, or inhibit the action of dopamine on its lactotroph receptor (e.g., dopamine antagonists), will cause pathological hyperprolactinemia. The causes of hyperprolactinaemia are diverse and shown in Table 3.

5. Clinical Features

Gonadal dysfunction is the most common manifestation of hyperprolactinemia in the female, with disruption of menstrual cyclicity (amenorrhea, oligomenorrhea, luteal insufficiency), loss of libido, and galactorrhea (Nabarro, 1982). The lesions are usually slow growing, and in our experience it is not unknown to see patients whose duration of secondary amenorrhea exceeds 20 years. Infertility is a common presentation. For the most part, tumors are small at presentation (prolactin-secreting microadenomas), the remainder of anterior pituitary function being preserved. In a proportion of patients, a suprasellar extension is present at the time of presentation, with visual field defect. In addition to the hormonal changes, patients appear to have a relatively high incidence of psychological disturbance (hostility, anxiety, depression), which may relate to central actions of prolactin.

Men with hyperprolactinemia tend to present later in the course of their disease. Gonadal dysfunction is gradual, and patients may not readily admit to problems of impotence and loss of libido. Seminal emissions tend to be of low volume, but sperm count is maintained until significant gonadotropin deficiency occurs. Impotence is frequent in patients with hyperprolactinemia (Carter et al., 1978), although hyperprolactinemia is a rare cause of impotence. Because of the late presentation, tumors are frequently large (macroadenomas) at the time of presentation and visual field defects due to chiasmatic compression are common. Rarely, tumors can be truly massive, extending into the temporal lobes and prepontine regions, or invading the sphenoid and ethmoidal sinuses. In both sexes, prolactinomas may be a cause of delayed sexual maturation; the larger tumors may also impair growth by impaired growth hormone secretion.

Table 3
Causes of Hyperprolactinemia

Hypothalamic disorders	Drugs
Tumors	Neuroleptics
Craniopharyngioma	Perphenazine
Germinoma	Fluphenazine
Glioma	Chlorpromazine
Colloid cyst of the third ventricle	Haloperidol
Hamartoma	Metoclopramide
Metastatic tumor	Sulpiride
Infiltrative disorders	Domperidone
Sarcoidosis	Other drugs
Tuberculosis	Methyl dopa
Histiocytosis X	Reserpine
Infection	Estrogens
Hydatid disease	Opiates
Encephalitis	Intravenous cimetidine
Radiotherapy	
	Miscellaneous
Pituitary Disorders	
	Hypothyroidism
Prolactinoma	Chronic renal failure
Acromegaly	Cirrhosis
Pituitary stalk section	Chest wall lesions, spinal cord lesions, breast
Empty sella syndrome	stimulation
Functional stalk section ("pseudoprolactinoma")	Idiopathic

6. Biochemical Features

Several prolactin levels should be determined to confirm the diagnosis of hyperprolactinemia, particularly when levels are only marginally raised. This is to avoid spurious elevations consequent on the occurrence of a spontaneous peak, or the effect of a stressful venepuncture. The finding of hyperprolactinemia should prompt a search for underlying causes such as hypothyroidism, pregnancy, renal failure, and drug ingestion. When these causes have been ruled out, the diagnosis is most commonly found to be due to a prolactin-secreting tumor. However, a larger number of intracranial lesions may cause hyperprolactinemia (see Table 3), and CT scanning is mandatory. High-resolution CT with contrast enhancement and reformatted pictures in the coronal and sagittal planes and the use of 1.5-mm collimations will usually reveal the presence of a pituitary tumor. In general, space-occupying lesions that cause effective stalk section do not cause hyperprolactinemia exceeding 2000 mU/l (100 ng/ml). Patients with macroadenomas usually have prolactin levels exceeding 4000 mU/l (200 ng/ml). A number of dynamic tests have been advocated to differentiate between the hyperprolactinemia caused by a prolactin-secreting adenoma and that due to hypothalamic causes or effective stalk section, including TRH, metoclopramide, and domperidone (Ferrari et al., 1982). In our opinion, none is clinically useful.

7. Causes of Hypogonadism in Prolactinoma

Several mechanisms may contribute to the hypogonadism associated with hyperprolactinemia (Bouloux and Grossman, 1987). Persistent hyperprolactinemia is thought to increase dopamine synthesis and turnover in the median eminence. This may in turn be responsible for suppressing the activity of GnRH-secreting neurons, which disrupts the normal pattern of GnRH and thus LH and FSH pulsatility. There is some evidence that this effect is mediated by increased opioidergic tone, since administration of naloxone by infusion will restore the normal frequency and amplitude of LH and FSH pulses. In addition, tumor may compress and destroy gonadotropin-secreting cells directly, leading to pituitary hypogonadism. There is evidence that prolactin may also interfere with the actions of the gonadotropins on their target organs.

8. Tests of Anterior Pituitary Function.

As with all pituitary tumors, both basal and dynamic testing of anterior pituitary function should be undertaken, and 9 a.m. cortisol, T_4, TSH, LH, FSH, estradiol, and testosterone should be measured. An insulin tolerance test should be carried out to evaluate the GH and cortisol responses to hypoglycemia with large tumors, and paired plasma and urinary osmolality carried out to exclude diabetes insipidus.

9. Treatment of Prolactinoma

Because of risks of pituitary dysfunction, enlargement of tumor with visual field defects and cranial nerve palsies, and the long-term consequences of hypogonadism (particularly osteoporosis), prolactinomas should be treated under most circumstances. The three treatment modalities to be considered are medical (using dopamine agonists), surgical (transsphenoidal hypophysectomy), and external beam irradiation.

10.   Medical Treatment

Dopamine agonists such as bromocriptine, lisuride, and terguride lower prolactin levels by mimicking the action of endogenous dopamine on the lactotroph membrane. Tumorous cells stop synthesizing prolactin, and lose cytoplasmic volume. Mitotic activity is attenuated or stopped and the lesions shrink, often dramatically. Pressure effects may be relieved within days of starting treatment (Thorner et al., 1980), and normal hypothalamo-pituitary relationships resumed. Thus, not infrequently, previously abnormal GH and cortisol responses to ITT are normalized, and normal pulsatile gonadotropin secretion resumed. Menses are regularized, and fertility is often rapidly demonstrated (Thorner et al., 1974). Some tumors, albeit a minority, do not exhibit the usual exquisite sensitivity to dopamine agonists, and larger doses than the conventional ones [i.e., 15 to 30 mg in divided doses rather than the usual 2.5 mg t.d.s. (three times a day)] are required to control the hyperprolactinemia. While tumor shrinkage is rapid, there is evidence for a more prolonged effect, with further shrinkage occurring over a matter of months to years. However, discontinuation of treatment is almost invariably associated with recurrence of hyperprolactinemia, and therefore this treatment cannot be considered definitive. For small lesions it is customary to treat with bromocriptine alone for a minimum of 2 years. If fertility is desired, patients are requested to discontinue treatment as soon as pregnancy is suspected. The risks of tumor expansion in cases of microadenomas are small; however, should pregnancy occur, careful regular monitoring of visual fields is required. In terms of side effects, nausea, vomiting, and postural hypotension can be obviated if the starting dose is small and taken in the middle of a meal. The drug should be taken with food at all times to slow absorption, and only gradually built up over a period of weeks to the final dose.

11.   Radiotherapy

In our experience meso- and macroadenomas should be shrunk by a dopamine agonist, and then irradiated before pregnancy is attempted. It is then customary to administer 4500 cGy in 25 fractions over 35 days to the original tumor volume as assessed by CT scanning. Follow-up of such patients show that after 10 years approximately 50% will become normoprolactinemic, while a proportion will show evidence of partial hypopituitarism requiring replacement therapy (Grossman et al., 1984). However, gonadotropin therapy takes many years to develop and patients are therefore capable of completing their family without recourse to exogenous gonadotropin administration. Radiotherapy is indicated particularly to obviate the tendency to potential catastrophic tumor enlargement during pregnancy. During treatment, skin erythema and epilation at the portals of entry of the rays are inevitable. Longer term complications include hypopituitarism, optic nerve or chiasmatic damage, carcinogenesis, and brain necrosis. These are rare when a three-field approach with dose fractionation is employed.

12. Surgery

There is considerable controversy concerning the use of transsphenoidal surgery in the management of prolactinomas. Patients with the best responses to medical treatment are the very group likely to have a good result following surgery (i.e., those with microadenomas), with normalization of prolactin in 60 to 88% of cases. However, recurrence of hyperprolactinemia occurs in 12 to 40% of patients after 5 years (Serri et al., 1983). Surgery is indicated where the tumors appear refractory to bromocriptine, although this is unusual. These are usually macroadenomas, and radiotherapy should be given post-operatively, as surgical extirpation is rarely complete. Thus, only 37% of women and 12% of men with significant suprasellar extension achieve a satisfactory remission following surgery. Pretreatment with prolactin above 4000 mU/l (200 ng/ml) does not significantly improve the chances for a cure by surgery alone (Hardy, 1984). The likelihood of hypopituitarism is greater in such instances. Intolerance to bromocriptine or major psychosis with treatment may also constitute an indication for surgery.

D. Acromegaly

Acromegaly is the clinical syndrome produced by prolonged inappropriate excessive secretion of growth hormone. It is most usually associated with a pituitary tumor, and more rarely associated with GHRH secretion from an ectopic source with consequent somatotroph hyperplasia. The prevalence is estimated to be 4 to 6 per 100,000 population (Alexander et al., 1980). It is a disease of middle age with female preponderance. Gigantism is the term given to describe the sequelae of GH excess before skeletal maturation is complete. The tumor is usually an eosinophilic adenoma, but may be a chromophobe adenoma. Tumors are capable of cosecreting prolactin and more rarely TSH. Because of the insidious onset of acromegaly, tumors have tended to be fairly large at presentation, although in recent years we have seen an increasing proportion of microadenomas.

1. Clinical Features of Acromegaly

The systemic manifestations of acromegaly result from the bone and soft tissue enlargement caused by GH excess (see Figure 3). A typical patient presents with thickening of the skin, coarse facial features, large nose, thick lips, and deep facial folds, particularly frontal furrows. There is progressive enlargement of the hands and feet; patients have to keep changing shoe and glove size. Hyperhydrosis is invariably present, and the skin is oily. Cutaneous fibromas, fleshy tags, sebaceous cysts, and acanthosis nigricans and hirsuties in females may occur. The voice is deep and resonant. An enlarged tongue (rarely to the point of causing obstruction) and overgrowth of buccal soft tissue can impair mastication. The jaw protrudes (prognathism) and there is widening of interdental separation, food tending to stick between the teeth. Kyphosis is frequent. Sinuses are enlarged, particularly the frontal sinuses. The supraorbital ridges are prominent, and may limit the upper visual fields. There is a tendency to premature osteoarthritis, affecting not only the weight-bearing joints, but also the glenohumeral joint. The width of cartilage is increased. Soft tissue overgrowth is thought to be

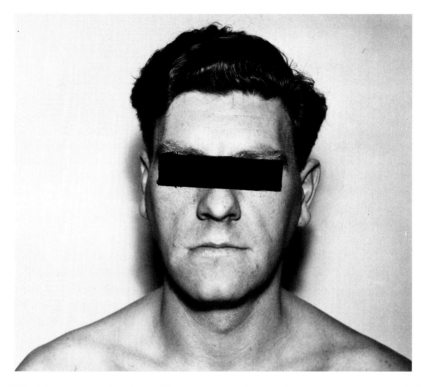

Figure 3. Facial appearance of patient with early acromegaly. The features are coarsened, and the bony protuberances prominent. Prognathism is present.

responsible for the tendency to peripheral nerve compression syndromes, particularly the median nerve at the wrist. Hypertension occurs in up to 30% of acromegalic patients, but does not necessarily resolve with treatment. Left ventricular hypertrophy is common, but dilated "acromegalic cardiomyopathy," associated with congestive cardiac failure and arrhythmias, is more rare. Glucose intolerance is common (up to 70%). Rarely, acromegaly may represent one component of the MEN 1 syndrome, with hyperparathyroism and pancreatic islet cell tumors.

Untreated, cardiovascular morbidity and mortality is the dominant consequence of acromegaly (Nabarro, 1987). Patients have a 10-fold increase in cardiovascular mortality. Earlier series showed that up to 90% of acromegalic patients die before the age of 60 years (Wright et al., 1970). Treatment has been shown to significantly improve the prognosis.

2. Biochemical Findings in Acromegaly

The pulsatile nature of normal GH secretion is maintained in acromegaly, but the GH spikes are higher, and GH levels fail to return to normal (i.e., undetectable) levels between bursts. Although the total amount of GH secreted over 24 hr is increased in acromegaly, there appears to be no direct relationship between the clinical severity of the disease and the circulating levels of GH. GH dynamics are also abnormal in acromegaly, and in 50% of cases there is a paradoxical rise in GH secretion following oral glucose administration (GH is normally suppressed following glucose administration). Further, both TRH and GnRH may occasionally be provocative stimuli for GH release in acromegaly, whereas these are normally inert in normal individuals.

GH exerts its biological actions partly by induction of insulin-like growth factor (IGF)-I (somatomedin C), produced predominantly but not exclusively by the liver, and partly by a direct action. Direct actions of GH are the diabetic actions, lipolysis, amino acid transport, and phosphate retention. IGF-I levels are better correlated with the severity of acromegaly than GH levels (Clemmons et al., 1979).

3. Treatment of Acromegaly

Medical, surgical, and radiotherapy (alone or in combination) treatments are used in the management of acromegaly. Treatment has three principal goals: normalization of GH hypersecretion, elimination of the mass effects of the tumor, and restoration of normal pituitary function. Treatment is tailored to the individual. In young patients, an aggressive approach is warranted, and usually involves transsphenoidal hypophysectomy followed by radiotherapy (usually three-field external beam irradiation) if GH levels remain outside the normal (i.e., undetectable) range. In elderly patients a less aggressive approach may be warranted, but surgery may have to be performed if visual field impairment is present. Reduction of tumor mass in general, and consequent reduction of GH output, will increase the effectiveness of subsequent radiation therapy.

4. Results of Medical Treatment for Acromegaly

Apart from the use of bromocriptine in the treatment of acromegaly, several pharmacological modalities have been used in an attempt to suppress GH hypersecretion. These include high doses of glucocorticoids, medroxyprogesterone acetate, chlorpromazine, phentolamine, fenfluramine, sulpiride, sodium valproate, pirenzepine, and cyproheptadine. None is therapeutically useful, although estradiol (McCullagh et al., 1955) has been shown to induce some biochemical and clinical improvement in acromegaly without an alteration in GH levels, probably by suppressing IGF-I levels (Clemmons et al., 1980).

The use of dopamine agonists in the treatment of acromegaly has its origins in the observation that L-dopa caused transient reduction in plasma GH levels in some 50% of acromegalic patients (Liuzzi, 1972). Bromocriptine (2-bromo-α-ergocryptine) is currently the most widely used dopamine agonist in the treatment of acromegaly. In general, bromocriptine lowers GH levels to a variable degree, but in a dose-dependent fashion in most patients, with improvement in biochemical indices (Wass et al., 1977). Tumor shrinkage has been documented in some studies, although this is rarely dramatic (Oppizzi et al., 1984). Other dopamine agonists in clinical use include lergotrile mesylate, pergolide, mesulergine, and cabergoline. In general, their side effects resemble those of bromocriptine. While these agents were formally used in conjunction with radiotherapy, to a large extent they have been replaced by octreotide (see below).

Although the infusion of native somatostatin was originally shown to cause dramatic falls in GH levels in acromegalics (Besser et al., 1974), this compound was found to be unsuitable for clinical use because of its short half-life (2 to 3 min), and the need for continuous intravenous administration. Furthermore it was unselective, and the suppression of insulin secretion lead to glucose intolerance. The recently developed somatostatin analog octreotide is a cyclic octapeptide retaining the essential tetrapeptide sequence that confers biological activity, but being relatively resistant to enzymatic degradation. The compound has 40 to 2000 times greater activity in suppressing GH levels, and is only one third as potent as somatostatin in suppressing insulin secretion (Marbech et al., 1988). Its half-life in the human is approximately 120 min, with GH hormone levels suppressed approximately 8 hr after a single subcutaneous (s.c.) dose. Significant GH suppression in acromegalics may be accomplished by 100 μg s.c., every 8 hr. Most series have shown dramatic reductions in GH secretion and clinical improvement following treatment of acromegaly with octreotide. Normal GH levels are achieved in 50 to 60% of patients, with similar normalization of IGF-I levels. The clinical response to treatment is rapid, with significant diminution of sweating and weight loss, and alleviation of acral paresthesiae. Only about 10% of patients fail to show an improvement with treatment. Steatorrhea with flatulence and abdominal pain occasionally occurs at the beginning of treatment, and is thought to result from the suppression of pancreatic exocrine secretion. The drug may accelerate the formation of gallstones, and ultrasonic examination of the gall bladder is advisable on prolonged treatment.

5. Surgery

Transsphenoidal adenomectomy is used in most patients with acromegaly. In one series of 214 patients, 56% had a GH level less than 10 mU/l after surgery (Ross and Wilson, 1988). New hypopituitarism occurred in 5.2% of patients. However, 28 to 56% of patients with detectable GH levels after surgery fail to respond normally to dynamic testing, suggesting the presence of residual tumor. Small tumors give the best chance of cure following transsphenoidal adenomectomy (up to 88%); on the other hand, patients with suprasellar extensions are rarely cured by surgery alone. It is likely that the definition of "cure" following treatment has not been sufficiently rigorous, and that many patients said to be cured are destined to have recurrences with time.

6. Radiation Therapy

Radiation therapy has been used singly or as an adjunct to surgery. The three types of radiotherapy are external beam (EBI), proton beam, and interstitial radiation. With our form of EBI, a total dose of 4500 cGy is delivered in 180-cGy fractions over 25 treatment days using a linear accelerator. Three portals of entry are used, two temporal and one frontal route. About 80% of patients respond to EBI by a fall in GH levels, with a 50% fall in GH levels occurring within 2 years and an approximately 15% fall annually thereafter (Eastman et al., 1979). The lower the starting GH levels the higher the chance of cure with this method of treatment. It has been estimated that there is a 60% chance of achieving a GH level below 10 mU/l 10 to 15 years after radiotherapy, 40% below 5 mU/l, and 20% below 2 mU/l. However, the incidence of hypopituitarism undoubtedly rises with time. In one series (Eastman et al., 1979), the incidence rose from 17% pretreatment to 29% at 2 years, 42% at 5 years, and 50% at 10 years. Patients therefore require regular review to detect hypopituitarism early so the adequate pituitary replacement may be given.

Proton beam and interstitial irradiation may produce a more rapid fall in GH levels, but the incidence of hypopituitarism is similar to EBI and the techniques are less readily available.

E. ACTH-Secreting Pituitary Tumors

Cushing's syndrome is the name given to the clinical manifestations of persistent and inappropriate secretion of cortisol. Cushing's disease is the name given to ACTH hypersecretion from the pituitary gland. In the majority of cases this results from a basophil microadenoma, and only in a minority from diffuse hyperplasia of the corticotrophs.

1. Clinical Features of Cushing's Disease

The clinical manifestations of Cushing's disease are diverse and affect most organs of the body. Patients are typically plethoric with a "moon face" and have a redistribution of body fat with truncal obesity, abdominal striae, thin skin with easy bruising, hirsuties, and marked myopathy, particularly proximally (Figure 4). Hypertension and psychiatric manifestations are common. Other features are listed in Table 4. The symptoms are usually insidious in onset, evolving over a period of years. Inspection of a series of photographs may help establish the onset of the disease.

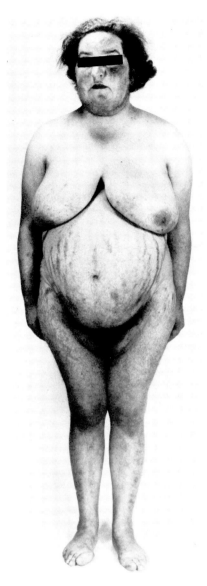

Figure 4. Appearance of a patient with florid Cushing's disease. There is truncal obesity, facial plethora, a moon face, thin arms and legs, proximal myopathy, and abdominal striae.

2. Diagnostic Evaluation of Cushing's Syndrome

The characteristics of abnormal ACTH secretion in Cushing's disease include loss of the circadian rhythm of cortisol secretion, and abnormal negative feedback threshold for cortisol release. The disorder is capable of cycling with normal cortisol dynamics on occasion with pathological secretion at other times. This rhythmicity can occur at intervals of days, weeks, or months, and can pose problems during diagnostic evaluation.

When the condition is suspected on clinical grounds, preliminary testing should include measurement of urinary free cortisol (corrected for creatinine clearance), or the use of a low-dose dexamethasone suppression test. This involves the administration of 0.5 mg dexamethasone every 6 hr for 48 hr, with the measurement of cortisol before and 6 hr after the last dose of the

Table 4
Clinical Features of Cushing's Disease

General	Psychiatric
Obesity (truncal)	Depression
Hypertension	Psychosis
Heaviness	Gonadal
Chemosis	Menstrual irregularity
Cutaneous	Impotence
Facial plethora	Loss of libido
"Moon face"	Muscle and skeletal
Thin skin	Weakness
Ecchymosis	Osteoporosis
Striae (especially abdominal)	Collapsed vertebrae
Supraclavicular fat pads	Fractured ribs
"Buffalo hump"	Metabolic
Hyperpigmentation	Glucose intolerance (diabetes)
Acne	Hypokalemia
Hirsuties	Alkalosis (especially ectopic ACTH)
Thinning hair	Polyuria

drug. Normal subjects have undetectable circulating cortisols after 48 hr of dexamethasone. The test may be carried out on an out-patient basis, provided the drug is taken at the appropriate times. Some centers use an overnight dexamethasone suppression test (1 mg last thing at night orally), with a plasma cortisol estimation the following morning. Normal subjects have undetectable cortisol levels whereas patients with Cushing's fail to suppress their cortisol levels completely. However, each laboratory may need to develop its own normal range. In addition, patients with Cushing's syndrome of any cause fail to demonstrate the usual rise in cortisol in response to an insulin tolerance test (see below). A low-dose dexamethasone test, followed immediately by a high-dose dexamethasone suppression test (2 mg dexamethasone orally every 6 hr for 48 hr) may then be carried out. Characteristically, patients with Cushing's disease suppress their circulating cortisols to less than 50% of their starting baseline value on high-dose dexamethasone, although a minority (about 20%) do not (Howlett et al., 1986).

A detectable ACTH level signifies that the disorder is caused either by pituitary disease or ectopic ACTH secretion. The intravenous CRF test (100 μg i.v.) is helpful in distinguishing between these two possibilities (Chrousos et al., 1984; Nieman et al., 1986; Grossman et al., 1988). Patients with basophil adenomas characteristically have an exuberant cortical response to CRF, whereas there is no response in the ectopic ACTH syndrome. This is because the high circulating cortisol in the latter will have switched off the normal corticotrophs, such that they become unresponsive to the action of exogenous CRF. Because of its lack of sensitivity and specificity, we no longer perform the metyrapone test.

Because of the frequently inconclusive nature of the aforementioned tests, it is sometimes necessary to proceed to a venous ACTH catheter study before finally establishing the diagnosis. High ACTH levels within the internal jugular veins are suggestive of a pituitary-dependent cause (Findling et al., 1981). The use of bilateral simultaneous inferior petrosal sinus catheters for ACTH before and after intravenous CRF has further increased diagnostic accuracy (vide infra).

Shortened versions of the high-dose dexamethasone test (e.g., 8 mg as a single dose at 22:00, followed by a 9 a.m. cortisol estimation) have been advocated (Bruno et al., 1985). The diagnostic efficacy or predictive power (defined by the ratio of the number of cases in which the diagnosis is correctly predicted and the total number of cases) of the overnight high-dose test is reported as 82.5% vs. 84.6% for the classic Liddle test.

All tests have a certain degree of false positive and false negative results. In particular, the low-dose overnight dexamethasone suppression test gives a false positive result in up to 30% of patients. This lack of sensitivity and specificity means that in practice the clinician must use a battery of tests before being certain of the diagnosis. Cyclical Cushing's syndrome, as previously mentioned, can also lead to inconclusive results.

3. Diagnostic Imaging in Cushing's Syndrome

CT scanning of the pituitary is mandatory when a basophil adenoma is suspected, plain radiography of the sella turcica being abnormal in very few cases. The lesion responsible is usually small, and lesions are visualized only in 20 to 30% of cases using CT scanning. The lesion is usually hypodense or enhancing. The appearances are not specific, however, and may be found incidentally due to nonsecreting tumors or small intrapituitary cysts. More recently, MR scanning has been used in the diagnosis of microadenomas; this diagnostic modality has a higher resolution than CT scanning. Petrosal sinus venous sampling for ACTH following CRF administration, with simultaneous peripheral venous sampling, has greatly assisted both the diagnosis and lateralization of the lesion. A plasma ACTH gradient (petrosal/peripheral gradient exceeding 2.0) verifies the pituitary source of the tumor (Findling et al., 1981), this difference being accentuated following CRF administration. So as to correct for unequal dilution by nonpituitary venous blood, other pituitary hormones such as prolactin, TSH, and α subunit are measured in some centers. However, most studies have shown that the uncorrected ACTH value gives the highest descriminating value.

Despite all these investigations, the diagnosis of pituitary-dependent Cushing's disease may not be made with certainty in some cases. CT scanning of the chest and upper abdomen using 1-cm cuts is advisable in all cases to exclude a possible ectopic source. In ACTH-dependent Cushing's syndrome the adrenals are usually bulky and hyperplastic. Adrenal adenomas and carcinomas are easily identifiable on CT scanning. The overactive gland invariably causes suppression of the contralateral healthy adrenal gland (because of negative feedback switching off ACTH secretion). The high resolution obtained by CT scanning has dispensed with the need for adrenal scintigraphy, except that this investigative tool may be useful in the diagnosis of primary nodular hyperplasia of the adrenals, where uptake of the radionuclide is bilateral. Bilateral adrenalectomy is the treatment of choice in such cases.

A not infrequent diagnostic pitfall occurs in alcoholic pseudo-Cushing's. Alcohol in some but not all individuals can lead to the biochemical and many of the clinical features of Cushing's disease (truncal obesity, proximal myopathy, facial plethora). Urinary free cortisol may be elevated. The elevated cortisol levels may not suppress with low- or high-dose dexamethasone, and there is frequently a failure of response to insulin-induced hypoglycemia. These abnormal cortisol dynamics rapidly normalize with abstinence from alcohol. The presence of abnormal liver enzymes and unexplained macrocytosis are useful pointers to the presence of this etiology. Similarly, endogenous depression is characterized by the absence of of a normal circadian rhythm for cortisol and dexamethasone nonsuppressibility. However, the cortisol response to insulin-induced hypoglycemia is usually intact in such patients. Although often having high cortisol levels, depressed patients rarely show the physical manifestations of Cushing's syndrome.

4. Nelson's Syndrome

Nelson's syndrome is the term given to describe the occurrence of an aggressive invasive ACTH-secreting pituitary tumor that classically arises a number of years after the treatment of pituitary-dependent Cushing's disease by bilateral adrenalectomy alone. It is thought to represent the clinical progression of a preexisting adenoma. The condition occurs less frequently if prophylactic pituitary irradiation has been given shortly after the adrenalectomy. Patients have extremely high ACTH levels that do not suppress completely following glucocorticoid administration; hyperpigmentation is invariable, and pressure symptoms secondary to suprasellar and cavernous sinus extension may be present. There is a high incidence of concomitant hypopituitarism. Treatment is by surgical debulking followed by radiotherapy, but even this combination may not be curative.

5. Treatment of Cushing's Disease

The four treatment modalities currently available in the treatment of Cushing's disease are transsphenoidal surgery, pituitary irradiation, adrenalectomy, and medical treatment. These have been used singly or in combination.

6. Transsphenoidal Surgery

Transsphenoidal surgery (TSS) This is the current first-line treatment and when successful is truly curative (Boggan et al., 1983). Thus, if the lesion can be located at the time of surgery and resected with preservation of residual pituitary tissue, patients can enjoy long-term remission without loss of pituitary function. The recognition of the causative lesion tends to be operator dependent. Preoperative CT scanning and inferior petrosal sinus sampling usually assist localization of the lesion. In cases where the tumor is not detected by imaging techniques, provided the biochemical abnormalities strongly suggest the presence of a pituitary tumor, a transsphenoidal exploration is indicated. In such cases a lesion will be identified in up to 90% of cases. In our experience, an undetectable cortisol level within 24 to 48 hr following TSS is a strong prognostic indicator of cure. It may take several months (even years) before normal corticotroph function is resumed in such cases, the patient requiring glucocorticoid replacement in the interim. Detectable cortisol levels post-TSS usually signify residual tumor. In such cases it is customary to reexplore the pituitary within a week of the first operation and attempt a pituitary clearance. If cortisol levels remain detectable, radiotherapy is indicated: the price is invariably some degree of hypopituitarism.

TSS can be used successfully in childhood Cushing's disease. Following successful resection, growth retardation is followed by catch-up growth, and hypogonadism followed by pubertal maturation.

7. Pituitary Irradiation

External beam irradiation has been shown to be most effective in childhood Cushing's disease and in patients under the age of 40. Remission is particularly rapid in childhood cases (Jennings et al., 1977), but in adults the remission is slower, occurring over several years. In the interim patients require control of their disease with medical treatment (vide infra). However, normal residual pituitary function is usually preserved, and hypopituitarism is rare. Heavy particle beam irradiation and Bragg peak proton irradiation appear to be more effective than conventional external beam irradiation, although the incidence of hypopituitarism is increased. A similar high incidence of hypopituitarism occurs in patients in whom yttrium or gold have been implanted into the pituitary.

8. Adrenalectomy

In patients in whom TSS has failed and in whom medical treatment is not effective, bilateral adrenalectomy is the treatment of choice. Although the beneficial effects are immediate, this treatment fails to treat the underlying cause, and unless radiotherapy is administered there is a risk of Nelson's syndrome supervening in later years.

9. Medical Treatment

Drug management of Cushing's disease has attempted to control hypercortisolism by two main mechanisms: either by manipulating the neurotransmitter control of CRF secretion, or by directly inhibiting the cortisol synthesis from the adrenal gland. The former has been attempted with cyproheptadine and bromocriptine; cyproheptadine works by an unknown mechanism and is limited by side effects, while bromocriptine is very rarely effective. There is some evidence that sodium valproate may ocasionally be useful.

10. Metyrapone

Metyrapone is an 11β-hydroxysteroid inhibitor. In a dose range of 250 mg t.d.s. to 4 g/day, cortisol secretion can usually be reduced to within the normal range in patients with Cushing's disease (Jeffcoate et al., 1977); this is associated with an elevation of deoxycortisol and androgen precursors. The rise in ACTH following treatment in Cushing's disease is usually modest, and insufficient to overcome the block. Hypertension and hirsuties are common side effects. The drug can also cause nausea and vomiting. It remains a useful compound in the medical control of Cushing's disease. Drugs such as aminoglutethimide, trilostane, and ketoconazole are rarely useful, the latter in particular being hepatototoxic. The adrenolytic drug o'p'DDD (mitotane), is highly effective but causes unacceptable hypercholesterolemia.

F. Glycoprotein Hormone-Secreting Tumors

1. Gonadotroph Cell Adenomas

Gonadotroph cell adenomas secrete gonadotropins and/or their subunits. The normal gonadotroph secretes both LH and FSH, glycoproteins composed of two subunits, α and β. The α subunit is common to all glycoprotein hormones (TSH, hCG), whereas the β subunit is unique to each hormone. It has been shown that under normal circumstances, the α subunit is synthesized in excess of the β subunit, so that the latter is the rate-limiting step in the synthesis of the intact glycoprotein hormone. Up to 17% of a series of 139 men with previously untreated pituitary macroadenomas were found to have a gonadotropin-secreting tumor (Snyder, 1985). Although this represents an overestimate of the proportion of gonadotropin-secreting tumors in all pituitary tumors (i.e., microadenomas and macroadenomas), gonadotropinomas are certainly not rare. Tumors may secrete intact LH, FSH, and α subunit, alone or in combination. Hypersecretion of intact FSH is most commonly seen. Clinically, these patients present as nonfunctioning tumors (see below), although occasionally macrotestes may be present. Treatment is as for nonfunctioning tumors, as medical therapy is rarely effective.

2. Thyrotropin-Secreting Pituitary Tumors

Thyrotropin-secreting pituitary tumors may occur as "feedback" tumors in cases of primary hypothyroidism, or *de novo,* causing thyrotoxicosis. Both are extremely rare. In the former, regression may sometimes occur with thyroid replacement therapy, suggesting the presence of thyrotroph hyperplasia rather than as autonomous tumor. TSH secreting tumors may also cause thyrotoxicosis. Unlike with Graves' disease there is not the usual female-to-male preponderance. The disorder has been described with an age range of 17 to 76 years. In all cases there is thyroid enlargement (Afrasiabi et al., 1979), but in addition to the usual features of thyrotoxicosis, there is an absence of pretibial myxedema and ophthalmopathy. Biochemically, circulating TSH is elevated in the presence of raised total and free T_4 and T_3. The condition must be distinguished from TSH elevation resulting from central resistance to thyroid hormone. Patients with thyrotropinomas usually have an excess of circulating α subunit. Further, the elevation of TSH levels may be inversely related to the biological potency. These paradoxical characteristics are thought to be related to abnormal glycosylation of TSH. Cosecretion of GH and prolactin is common in these tumors, and even more rare is gonadotropin secretion.

The major differential diagnosis is with patients with the syndrome of inappropriate TSH secretion. In such patients there may be a generalized resistance to the actions of T_4. In cases where the pituitary is most affected, there may be clinical hyperthyroidism, whereas patients with generalized tissue resistance are euthyroid or frankly hypothyroid. Surgery with or without external beam irradiation is the current treatment of choice. Medical therapy with antithyroid medication is appropriate prior to surgery. There is no evidence of long-term remission resulting from treatment with dopamine agonists or somatostatin.

G. Functionless or Nonsecreting Pituitary Tumors

Functionless or nonsecreting pituitary tumors account for up to 30% of pituitary tumors. Because they do not produce the characteristic clinical syndrome associated with hormone excess, these tumors tend to present because of mass effects — headache, visual loss, and symptoms of hypopituitarism. Although previously thought to be functionless, it is now recognized that these tumors do in fact synthesize and occasionally secrete glycoprotein subunits. Such tumors tend to be macroadenomas, and thus present with symptoms of suprasellar or extrasellar extension. Thus, visual field defects and cranial nerve palsies are not uncommon. Occasionally such patients present with pituitary apoplexy, with sudden severe headache and visual embarrassment.

Patients may present with partial or total hypopituitarism; GH and gonadotropin deficiency are most frequently seen. Modest hyperprolactinemia (up to 2000 to 3000 mU/l) is caused by effective stalk compression, and impairment of the delivery of dopamine to the lactotrophs. Impaired pituitary adrenal function may be demonstrable on dynamic testing.

Management

In most cases the mass effects of the tumor warrant surgery as the first-line treatment. An attempt at radical clearance is usually made by transsphenoidal hypophysectomy, even in the presence of suprasellar extensions. This usually achieves adequate decompression of the optic pathways. It is rare for pituitary function to recover fully after such procedures. However, in cases where pituitary function was intact prior to surgery, it is usual for such function to be preserved in the aftermath of surgery (Harris et al., 1989). In this center it is customary to irradiate all patients with nonfunctioning tumors after surgery to prevent recurrence.

H. Miscellaneous Disorders

1. Pituitary Infarction and Apoplexy

Pituitary tumors occasionally infarct spontaneously or bleeding may occur within them. Hypopituitarism, partial or complete, may ensue. In Sheehan's syndrome (post-partum hypopituitarism), patients become hypopituitary and fail to lactate. This is secondary to severe post-partum hemorrhage with hypotension, with subsequent infarction of the pituitary. Patients with pituitary apoplexy present with sudden severe headache, often with some features of meningism. Rapid expansion of the tumor may cause rapid onset of visual field defect. MRI is the best imaging modality for demonstrating this condition.

2. Empty Sella Syndrome

Empty sella syndrome is the term used to describe the radiological appearance of an abnormal pituitary fossa but with only a small rim of pituitary tissue at its base. Two mechanisms are thought to contribute to this appearance: a defect in the diaphragma sella may allow herniation of the suprasellar cistern into the pituitary fossa, thereby compressing pituitary tissue; alternatively, a pituitary tumor may have been present originally, but following spontaneous infarction only the normal pituitary remains. This condition is usually diagnosed incidentally as part of the investigation for an abnormal pituitary fossa. There are no endocrine abnormalities in cases arising from cisternal herniation, although following infarction of a tumor there may be a degree of hypopituitarism.

3. Lymphocytic Hypophysitis

Lymphocytic hypophysitis is thought to be an autoimmune disorder of the hypophysis and is a rare cause of hypopituitarism.

4. Pituitary Fibrosis

Pituitary fibrosis is rare and is associated with fibrosis elsewhere (e.g., mediatinal fibrosis, testicular fibrosis). It is associated with hypopituitarism. CT scan appearances are not specific and the lesion may be confused radiologically with a pituitary tumor.

5. Hemochromatosis

Iron deposition may occur in the pituitary associated with partial hypopituitarism, usually affecting the gonadotropin-producing cells.

References

Afrasiabi, A., Valents, L., and Gwinup, G., A TSH-producing pituitary tumour causing hyperthyroidism: presentation of a case and review of the literature, *Acta Endocrinol.*, 92, 448, 1979.

Alexander, L., Appleton, D., Hall, R., Ross W. M., and Wilkinson, R., Epidemiology of acromegaly in the Newcastle region, *Clin. Endocrinol.*, 12, 71, 1980.

Bartlett, J. R., Craniopharyngiomas — a summary of 85 cases, *J. Neurol., Neurosurg. Psychiatry*, 34, 37, 1971.

Baskin, D. S. and Wilson, C. B., Surgical management of cranipharyngiomas, *J. Neurosurg.*, 65, 22, 1986.

Bauer, W., Briner, U., Doepfner, W., Haller, R., Huguenin, R., Marbach, P., Petcher, T. J., and Pless, M., SMS 201-995. A very potent and selective octapeptide analog of somatostatin with prolonged action, *Life Sci.*, 31, 1133, 1982.

Besser, G. M. and Ross, R. J. M., Are hypothalamic releasing hormones useful in the diagnosis of endocrine disorders?, *Recent Adv. Endocrinol. Metab.*, 3, 135, 1989.

Besser, G. M., Mortimer, G. H., Carr, D., Schally, A. V., Coy, D. H., Evered, D., Kastin, A. J., Tunbridge, W. M. G., and Thorner, M. O., Growth hormone release inhibiting hormone in acromegaly, *Br. Med. J.*, 1, 352, 1974.

Boggan, J. E., Tyrrell, J. B., and Wilson, C. B., Transphenoidal microsurgical managment of Cushing's disease. Report of 100 cases, *J. Neurosurg.*, 59, 195, 1983.

Bouloux, P. M. and Grossman, A., Hyperprolactinaemia and sexual function in the male, *Br. J. Hosp. Med.*, June, 503, 1987.

Bruno, O. D., Ross, M. A., Contreras, L. N., Gomes, R. M., Galparsola, G., Cazado, E., Krai, M., Leber, B., and Arias, D., Nocturnal high dose dexamethasone suppression test in the etiological diagnosis of Cushing's syndrome, *Br. Acta Endocrinol.*, 109, 158, 1985.

Carmel, P., Craniopharyngioma, in *Neurosurgery*, Vol. 1, McGraw Hill, New York, 1985, 905.

Carter, J. N., Tyson, J. E., Tolis, G., Van Vliet, S., Fairman, C., and Friesen, H. G., Secreting hormones and hypogonadism in 22 men, *N. Engl. J. Med.*, 299, 847, 1978.

Chrousos, G. P., Schulte, H. M., Oldfield, E. H., Gold, P. W., Cutler, A. G., Jr., and Loriaux, D. L., The corticotrophin-releasing factor stimulation test: an aid in the evaluation of patients with Cushing's syndrome, *N. Engl. J. Med.,* 310, 622, 1984.

Clemmons, D. R., Van Wyk, J. J., Ridgeway, E. C., Kliman, B., and Kjellberg, R. W., Evaluation of acromegaly by radioimmunoassay of somatomedin C, *N. Engl. J. Med.,* 301, 1138, 1979.

Clemmons, D. R., Underwood, L. E., Ridgeway, E. C., Kliman, B., Kiellberg, R. N., and Van Wyke, J. J., Oestradiol treatment of acromegaly following treatment with oestrogens, *Diabetes,* 4, 13, 1980.

Dahlin, D. C. and MacCarty, C. S., Chordoma. A study of 9 cases, *Cancer,* 5, 1170, 1952.

de Cremoux, P., Turpin, G., Hamon, P., and de Gennas, J. L., Les chromosomes intrasellaires, *Semin. Hopitaux Paris,* 1169, 1980.

Eastman, R. C., Gorden, P., and Roth, J., Conventional super voltage irradiation is an effective treatment for acromegaly, *J. Clin. Endocrinol. Metab.,* 48, 931, 1979.

Ferrari, C., Rampin, P., Benco, R., Caldara, R., Scardvelli, C., and Crosigniani, P. G., Functional characterisation of hypothalamic hyperprolactinaemia, *J. Clin. Endocrinol. Metab.,* 55, 897, 1982.

Findling, J. W., Aron, D. C., Tyrrel, J. B., Shinsako, J. H., Fitzgerald, P. A., Norman, D., Wilson, C. B., and Forsham, P. H., Selective venous sampling for ACTH in Cushing's syndrome: differentiation between Cushing's disease and the ectopic ACTH syndrome, *Ann. Intern. Med.,* 94, 647, 1981.

Grossman, A., Cohen, B. L., Charlesworth, M., Plowman, N., Rees, L. H., Wass, J. A. H., Jones, A. C., and Besser, G. M., Treatment of prolactinomas with megavoltage radiotherapy, *Br. Med. J.,* 288, 1105, 1984.

Grossman, A., Howlett, T. A., Perry, L., Coy, D. H., Savage, M. O., Lavender, P., Rees, L. H., and Besser, G. M., CRF in the differential diagnosis of Cushing's syndrome: a comparison with the dexamethasone suppression test, *Clin. Endocrinol.,* 29, 167, 1988.

Hardy, J., Transphenoidal microsurgery of prolactinomas, in *Secretory Tumours of the Pituitary Gland,* Black, P. M., Zervas, N. T., Ridgeway, E. C., et al., Eds., Raven Press, New York, 1984.

Harris, P. E., Perry, L., Chard, T., Chandry, L., Cooke, B. A., Touzel, R., Coates, P., Lowe, D. G., Afshar, F., Wass, J. A. H., and Besser, G. M., Immunoreactive human chorionic gonadotrophin from the cyst fluid and CSF of patients with craniopharyngioma, *Clin. Endocrinol.,* 29, 503, 1988.

Harris, P. E., Afshar, F., Coates, P., Doniach, I., Wass, J. A. H., Besser, G. M., and Grossman, A., The effects of transsphenoidal surgery on endocrine function and visual fields in patients with functionless pituitary tumours, *Q. J. Med.,* 265, 417, 1989.

Henshaw, D. B., Jr., Hasso, A. N., Thompson, J. R., and Davidson, B. J., High resolution computer tomography in the postpartum pituitary gland, *Neuroradiology,* 26, 299, 1984.

Howlett, T. A., Drury, P. L., and Perry, L., Diagnosis and management of ACTH-dependent Cushing's syndrome: comparison of the features in ectopic and pituitary ACTH production, *Clin. Endocrinol.,* 24, 699, 1986.

Jeffcoate, W. J., Rees, L. H., Tomlin, S., Jones, A. E., Edwards, C. R. W., and Besser, G. M., Metyrapone in the long term management of Cushing's disease with pituitary irradiation, *N. Engl. J. Med.,* 2, 215, 1977.

Jennings, A. S., Liddle, G. W., and Orth, D. N., Results of treating childhood Cushing's disease with pituitary irradiation, *N. Engl. J. Med.,* 297, 957, 1977.

Kagevama, N. and Belsky, R., Ectopic pincaloma in the chiasmal region, *Neurology,* 11, 318, 1961.

Kasdon, D. L., Dongeas, E. A., and Brougham, M. F., Suprasellar arachnoid cyst diagnosis preoperatively by computerised tomography scanning, *Surg. Neurol.,* 7, 299, 1977.

Kaufman, B., Magnetic resonance imaging of the pituitary gland, *Radiol. Clin. N. Am.,* 22, 975, 1984.

Liuzzi, A., Chiodini, P. G., Botalla, A., Cremascoli, G., and Silvestrini, F., Inhibitiory effect of L-dopa on GH release in acromegalic patients, *J. Clin. Endocrinol. Metab.,* 35, 941, 1972.

Lytras, N., Grossman, A., Perry, L., Tomlin, S., Wass, J. A. H., Coy, D. H., Schall, A. V., Rees. L. H., and Besser, G. M., Corticotrophin releasing factor 6 responses in normal subjects and patients with disorders of the hypothalamus and pituitary, *Clin. Endocrinol.,* 20, 71, 1984.

Manor, R. S., Israeli, J., and Sandbank, U., Malignant optic glioma in a 70-year-old patient, *Arch. Ophthalmol.,* 94, 1142, 1976.

Marbech, P., Andres, H., and Azria, M., Chemical structure, pharmacodynamics profile and pharma-cokinetics of SMS 201-995 (somatostatin) in, *Somatostatin in the Treatment of Acromegaly,* Lambert, S. W. J., Ed., Springer-Verlag, New York, 1988, 53.

McCullagh, E. P., Beck, J. C., and Schlaffenburg, G. A., Control of diabetes and other features of acromegaly following treatment with oestrogens, *Diabetes,* 4, 13, 1955.

Muller, O. A., Stall, G. K., and Werder, V. K., Corticotrophin releasing factor: a new look for the differential diagnosis of Cushing's syndrome, *J. Clin. Endocrinol. Metab.,* 57, 227, 1983.

Nabarro, J. D. N., Pituitary prolactinomas, *Clin. Endocrinol.,* 17, 129, 1982.

Nabarro, J. S. N., Acromegaly, *Clin. Endocrinol.,* 26, 481, 1987.

Naidich, T. P., Pinto, R. S., Kushner, M. J., Evaluation of sellar and parasellar masses by computed tomography, *Radiology,* 120(1), 91, 1976.

Nenwelt, E. A., Frenkel, E. P., and Smith, R. G., Suprasellar germinomas (ectopic pinealomas): aspects of immunological characterization and successful chemotherapeutic responses in recurrent disease, *Neurosurgery,* 7, 352, 1980.

Nieman, L. K., Chrousos, A. P., Oldfield, E. H., Argerinos, P. C., and Cutler, G. B., Jr., Ovine corticotropin-releasing hormone stimlation test and the dexamethasone suppression test in the differential diagnosis of Cushing's syndrome, *Ann. Intern. Med.,* 105, 862, 1986.

Oldfield, E. H., Chrousos, G. P., Schulte, H. M., Schaaf, M., McKeaver, P. E., Krudy, A. G., Cutler, G. B. J., Lorianx, D. L., and Doppman, J. L., Preoperative localisation of ACTH secreting microadenoma by bilateral and simultaneous inferior petronal venous sinus sampling, *N. Engl. J. Med.,* 312, 100, 1988.

Oppizzi, G., Liuzzi, A., Chiodini, P. G., Dallabonzana, D., Spelta, B., Silvestrini, F., Borghi, G., and Toran, C., Dopaminergic treatment of acromegaly: different effects on hormone secretion and tumour size, *J. Clin. Endocrinol. Metab.,* 58, 988, 1984.

Oxenhandler, D. C. and Sayers, M. P., The dilemma of childhood optic gliomas, *J. Neurosurg.,* 48, 34, 1978.

Pressman, D., Waldron, R. L., and Wood, E. H., Hystiocytosis X of the hypothalamus, *Br. J. Radiol.,* 48, 176, 1975.

Ringer, S. P. and Barley, O. T., Rathke's cleft cyst, *J. Neurol., Neurosurg. Psychiatry,* 35, 693, 1972.

Ross, D. A. and Wilson, C. B., Results of transsphenoidal microsurgery for growth hormone-secreting pituitary adenoma in a series of 214 patients, *J. Neurosurg.,* 68, 854, 1988.

Ross, R. J. M., Tsagarakis, S., Grossman, A., Preece, M. A., Davies, P. S. W., Rees, L. H., Savage, M. O., and Besser, G. M., Treatment of growth hormone deficiency with growth hormone releasing hormone, *Lancet,* 1, 5, 1987.

Ross-Russell, R. W. and Pennybacker, J. B., Craniopharyngioma in the elderly, *J. Neurol., Neurosurg. Psychiatry,* 24, 1, 1961.

Rovitt, R. L. and Duane, T. D., Cushing's syndrome and pituitary tumours. Pathophysiology and ovular manifestations of ACTH-secreting pituitary adenomas, *Am. J. Med.,* 46, 416, 1969.

Selenkow, H. A., Tyler, H. R., Matson, D. D., and Nelson, D. H., Hypopituitarism due to hypothalamic sarcoidosis, *Am. J. Med. Sci.,* 238, 456, 1959.

Serri, O., Rasio, E., Beauregard, H., Hardy, J., and Somma, M., Recurrence of hyper prolacinnaemia after selective transphenoidal adenomectomy in women with prolactinoma, *N. Engl. J. Med.,* 309, 280, 1983.

Snyder, P. J., Gonadotropin cell adenomas of the pituitary, *Endocrine Rev.,* 6, 552, 1985.

Swartz, J. D., Russel, K. B., Basili, B. A., O'Donnell, P. C., and Popky, G. L., High resolution computed tomographic appearance of the intrasellar contents in women of childbearing age, *Radiology,* 147, 115, 1983.

Takenchi, J., Handa, H., and Nagata, I., Supresellar germinoma, *J. Neurosurg.,* 49, 41, 1978.

Thorner, M. O., McNeilly, S., Hagen, C., Edwards, C. R. W., Rees, L. H., and Besser, G. M., Long term treatment of galactinoma and hypogonadism with bromocriptine, *Br. Med. J.,* 2, 419, 1974.

Thorner, M. O., Martin, W. H., Rogol, A. D., Morris, P. J., Perryman, R. L., Conway, B. P., Howard, S. S., Wolfman, M. G., and Macleod, R. M., Rapid regression of pituitary prolactinoma during bromocriptine treatment, *J. Clin. Endocrinol. Metab.,* 51, 438, 1980.

Tibbs, P. A., Chaela, V., and Mortaro, R. H., Isolated hystiocytosis of the hypothalamus, *J. Neurosurg.*, 49, 929, 1978.

Trobe, J. D., Glaser, J. S., and Post, J. D., Meningiomas and aneurysms of the cavernous sinus. Neuroophthalmological features, *Arch. Ophthalmol.*, 96, 457, 1978.

Wass, J. A. H., Thorner, M. O., Morris, D. V., Rees, L. H., Stuart Mason, A., Jones, A. E., and Besser, G. M., Long-term treatment of acromegaly with bromocriptine, *Br. Med. J.*, 1, 875, 1977.

White, J. C. and Ballantine, H. T., Jr., Intrasellar aneurysms simulating hypophyseal tumours, *J. Neurosurg.*, 18, 34, 1961.

Wood, A. M., Ch'ng, J. L. C., Adams, F. C., Webster, J. D., Joplin, G. G., Machiter, K., and Bloom, S. R., Abnormalities of growth hormone release in response to human pancreatic growth hormone releasing hormone (GRF (1-44)) in acromegaly and hypopituitarism, *Br. Med. J.*, 286, 1687, 1983.

Wright, A. D., Hill, D. M., Lowy, C., et al., Mortality of acromegaly, *Q. J. Med.*, 39, 1—16, 1970.

17

Pediatric Neuroendocrinology: Growth and Puberty

ORA HIRSCH PESCOVITZ

Departments of Pediatrics, Physiology, and Biophysics
Indiana University Medical Center
James Whitcomb Riley Hospital for Children
Indianapolis, Indiana

I. Introduction

The advances made in neuroendocrinology during the past decade will have their greatest impact in the pediatric population. Although all aspects of neuroendocrinology apply to children, this chapter will focus only on growth and puberty, as they are unique to pediatrics.

II. Growth

Normal childhood growth is dependent on genetic, hormonal, environmental, psychosocial, nutritional, and medical factors. Some of the hormones and neurotransmitters that work alone or in synchrony with each other to regulate growth are listed in Table 1. The relative importance of each is dependent on developmental stage. For example, while thyroid hormone, growth hormone (GH), and insulin-like growth factor I (IGF-I) are most important for childhood growth, they may be less important during prenatal growth. In contrast, insulin-like growth factor II (IGF-II) and placental growth factors may be more important in fetal growth than they are later in life.

Growth disorders account for the bulk of referrals to pediatric endocrinologists. Most commonly, short children are referred to exclude serious organic lesions. Parents may be concerned about peer isolation and ridicule at an age when social acceptance is paramount to an emerging concept of self-image. On the other hand, excessive growth, while more accepted by our society, may indicate organic abnormalities and also necessitates appropriate evaluation and therapy.

A. The Growth Hormone Axis

1. Hypothalamus (Growth Hormone-Releasing Hormone and Somatostatin)

The hypothalamus contains two peptides that act in concert to regulate GH production and secretion. Somatostatin is a tetradecapeptide that inhibits GH release. Growth hormone-releasing hormone (GHRH) is a 44-amino acid polypeptide that stimulates GH release in a dose-dependent, although heterogeneous manner (Gelato et al.). In 1982, GHRH was sequenced from two pancreatic islet cell tumors (Guillemin et al.; Rivier et al.). Pancreatic GHRH has now been shown to be identical to hypothalamic GHRH (Esch et al.).

Table 1
Factors Involved in Growth

Classical hormones	Neuropeptides (continued)
Growth hormone	Substance P
Thyroid hormone	Neurotensin
Gonadal sex steroids	Bombesin
Adrenal sex steroids	Galanin
Glucocorticoids	Vasopressin
Peptide growth factors	MSH
IGF-I	POMC
IGF-II	β-Endorphin
EGF	α-Endorphin
PDGF	Enkephalins
FGF	PHI
TGF-α	Neuropeptide Y
TGF-β	Motilin
Neuropeptides	Catecholamines
GHRH	Neurotransmitters
Somatostatin	Dopamine
TRH	Norepinephrine
CRH	5-Hydroxytryptamine
GnRH	Acetylcholine
ACTH	γ-Aminobutyric acid
VIP	

GHRH has been evaluated as a diagnostic tool in the assessment of children with growth disorders. As a group, children with classical GH deficiency have lower GH responses to GHRH than normal children. However, between 40 and 80% of children with classical GH deficiency have measureable responses to GHRH (Takano et al., Schriock et al., Rogol et al., Gelato et al.). Therefore, it is not likely to be useful as a diagnostic test in the evaluation of GH deficiency. Furthermore, repeated administration of GHRH to children with GH deficiency (even those with minimal responses to an initial GHRH challenge) results in enhanced GH responses and increased IGF-I secretion (Borges et al.). These data suggest that the majority of children with GH deficiency have a hypothalamic defect that results in somatotroph unresponsiveness or atrophy, and that GHRH has the potential to be an effective therapeutic agent in GH deficiency.

2. Pituitary (Growth Hormone)

Growth hormone is produced by acidophilic cells known as somatotrophs that reside in the lateral sections of the adenohypophysis. GH is a 21,500-kDa single-chain polypeptide consisting of 191 amino acids. It circulates bound to a specific high-affinity binding protein that is probably a part of the GH receptor (Baumann, Shaw, and Winter). Growth hormone secretion occurs in a pulsatile fashion with higher amplitude pulses occurring at night during slow-wave sleep, or sleep phases 3 and 4 (Muller). Increased secretion of GH also occurs in response to exercise, physical or emotional stress, hypoglycemia, and increased amino acid secretion. Neurotransmitters are important in regulating both GHRH and somatostatin, and may also directly affect GH secretion at the pituitary level. It is known that α-adrenergic agents, such as clonidine, are potent stimulators of GH while cholinergic muscarinic antagonists, such as atropine and pirenzepine, inhibit GH secretion. These agents are felt to act via stimulation or inhibition of hypothalamic GHRH. Beta blockers like propranolol probably stimulate GH secretion through inhibition of somatostatin. The precise mechanisms by which L-dopa, GABA (γ-aminobutyric acid), opiates, and the serotonin precursor 5-hydroxytryptophan enhance GH secretion are still under study. Thyroid hormone, glucocorticoids, and sex steroids also influence GH secretion, as does IGF-I, which has pituitary and hypothalamic receptors.

Growth hormone promotes growth in almost every tissue and increases nitrogen retention. It stimulates protein synthesis in bone, muscle, liver, and kidneys, leading to decreased blood urea nitrogen and amino acid levels. It also causes a reduction of free fatty acids and an increase in circulating nonesterified fatty acids. The GH-deficient child often has decreased muscle mass and increased fat deposition that will decrease with GH replacement. Growth hormone causes glucose transport into the intracellular compartments of skeletal muscle and adipose tissue that leads to a transient decrease in blood sugar. In GH deficiency, insulin production is usually decreased and there may be extreme sensitivity to the effects of exogenous insulin. GH therapy will result in increased pancreatic production of insulin, but it also appears to antagonize the effects of insulin at the target tissues. Although not common in subjects receiving physiologic GH therapy, glucose intolerance is a relatively common feature of GH excess. Hypoglycemia frequently accompanies GH deficiency and may even be the major symptom, especially in the neonatal period.

3. Periphery (Insulin-Like Growth Factors)

Growth hormone stimulates linear growth of the organism at the level of the tissues, bone, and cartilage. *In vitro,* direct administration of GH to cartilage explants results in minimal metabolic effects while administration of serum from normal animals leads to sulfate and thymidine incorporation into cartilage and cellular proliferation (Salmon and Daughaday). Because of this effect on sulfate incorporation, the name "sulfation factor" was originally given to the serum factor responsible for these effects. Serum from hypophysectomized animals is unable to induce cellular proliferation and growth, while GH replacement of hypophysectomized animals restores the growth-promoting capacity of serum. Because of the ability to mediate the somatogenic effects of GH, this factor was later termed somatomedin C (Van Wyk). More recently insulin-like activity and cross-reactivity with the insulin receptor was demonstrated, leading to the current terminology of *insulin-like growth factors* (IGFs).

The two predominant IGFs in human serum are IGF-I, which is GH dependent, and IGF-II, which does not appear to be regulated by GH to the same degree as IGF-I. IGF-II may have its major role in metabolism and/or fetal growth and development (Adams et al.). The IGFs circulate bound to carrier proteins that are also regulated by GH (Zapf, Waldvogel, and Froesch). At least six IGF-binding proteins have been identified and it is possible that each tissue makes its own IGF-binding protein. The precise role of the binding proteins is unknown. Since they also may be regulated by GH, it is likely that they participate in the physiologic actions of the IGFs. It has been postulated that these binding proteins might stabilize the circulating IGFs, causing them to have prolonged and increased biologic activity. In contrast, they have also been postulated to interfere with the binding of free IGFs to their respective receptors, resulting in an inhibitory effect on the action of the IGFs.

It appears as though both IGF-I and IGF-II act as endocrine, as well as paracrine and autocrine, factors. Receptors have been found in hepatocytes, chondrocytes, adipocytes, and placental monocytes and lymphocytes. The liver makes the greatest contribution to the circulating pool of IGF-I but almost every tissue has been shown to contain both peptide and mRNA. *In vitro,* insulin-like growth factors stimulate DNA, RNA, and protein synthesis in a variety of cell lines, including cartilage. They stimulate glucose uptake and transport of glucose into glycogen. *In vivo,* they result in a prolonged reduction in blood sugar with increased incorporation of glucose into glycogen and lipids. Whether all the growth-promoting effects of GH are due to IGF-I is still unknown. Administration of IGF-I alone stimulates body and organ weight gain in hypophysectomized rats, but may have less of an effect on linear growth than administration of GH. *In vitro,* GH and IGF-I can stimulate unilateral bone growth (Russell and Spencer; Isgaard et al.). The most appealing hypothesis to date suggests that GH and IGF-I interact with bone cells at different stages of differentiation. GH may act on young differentiating chondrocytes or prechondrocytes, while IGF-I may act at the level of proliferative chondrocytes (Isaksson et al.).

B. Growth Hormone Secretory Dynamics

Growth hormone secretion is associated with age and pubertal stage. A single, random GH determination is not characteristic of GH secretory dynamics because of the pulsatile nature of GH secretion. Pharmacologic stimulation tests have been designed to induce the release of GH via stimulation of GHRH, inhibition of somatostatin, or direct pituitary effects. Stimuli that have been used to induce GH secretion include L-dopa, arginine, clonidine, propranolol, insulin, glucagon, sex steroids, and exercise. Classical GH deficiency is currently defined by an inadequate response to two or more of these stimuli (peak GH level <10 ng/ml). Unfortunately, there are a number of pitfalls associated with this type of testing. First, the quantitation of GH in serum is dependent on the assay system used and variable results have been obtained when the same sample has been evaluated in different assays (Reiter et al.). Second, the lower limit for a normal response is arbitrary and has been increasing over the years, as GH has become more available as a therapeutic agent. Third, pharmacologic agents only test responsiveness to an acute stimulus and do not provide information regarding endogenous GH secretion.

In order to gather information regarding spontaneous GH secretion, various techniques including frequent GH sampling and continuous blood withdrawal via indwelling venous catheters have been developed. Some short children who respond normally to provocative testing may have abnormal endogenous GH secretion, when tested by these alternate methods. This type of abnormality has been termed neurosecretory dysfunction (Spiliotis et al.). Unfortunately, tests of integrated endogenous GH secretion are also flawed. Sampling subjects on successive nights results in variable test results even when samples are measured in the same assay (Donaldson et al.). Although endogenous GH secretion, determined by frequent sampling techniques, is correlated with responses to pharmacologic stimuli in some studies (Plotnick et al.), in other studies the correlation is poor (Bercu et al., Chalew et al.). The response to endogenous testing does not predict the response to GH therapy (Lin, et al.). Finally, healthy children of normal height may have low GH secretory profiles (Rose, et al., Costin, et al.). Because of these shortcomings, some investigators are now recommending that a 6-month therapeutic trial of GH be administered to any short child regardless of endogenous, or stimulated, GH levels. The growth response to this therapeutic trial could then be used to identify patients who should receive subsequent GH therapy. Unfortunately, this approach is also flawed because almost every child with open epiphyses will demonstrate a short-term increase in growth velocity when treated with a large enough dose of exogenous GH. In summary, making the diagnosis of GH deficiency is difficult, but evaluation of both classical hormonal and auxological criteria is still valuable.

C. Disorders of Short Stature (Table 2)

1. Genetic Short Stature

The most common cause of short stature is familial or *genetic short stature.* Usually, the offspring of tall parents are tall and the offspring of short parents are short. Children with

Table 2
Etiology of Short Stature

Genetic short stature
Constitutional delay of growth and puberty
Psychosocial dwarfism
Chromosomal abnormalities
Skeletal dysplasias
Intrauterine growth retardation
Syndromes not defined by chromosomal abnormalities
Chronic disease
Hormonal abnormalities

genetic short stature are perfectly healthy, grow at a normal growth velocity, have age-appropriate skeletal maturation, normal pubertal development, and are short adults.

2. Constitutional Delay of Growth and Puberty

The second most likely diagnosis in a child referred for evaluation of short stature is *constitutional delay of growth and puberty*. These children often have a positive family history for pubertal delay but the parents are of normal adult stature. Typically, these children are of normal weight and length at birth. They may have a 1- to 2-year period during which growth velocity is decreased between the ages of 1 and 4 years. Subsequently, growth resumes at an age-appropriate rate. There is usually a modest delay in skeletal maturation; however, height is normal when corrected for the skeletal delay. Occasionally, genetic short stature and constitutional delay of growth and puberty occur in the same individual.

3. Psychosocial Dwarfism

Psychosocial dwarfism was originally described in institutionalized infants who did not have the opportunity to develop a unique relationship with a particular caretaker. The syndrome has now been expanded to include growth failure with anorexia and weight loss in otherwise healthy children who do not thrive, even in their home environment. In some cases, appropriate dietary nutrients are withheld from the child and malnutrition is present. In others, caloric intake is adequate but physical and/or psychological abuse exist in the home. The specific mechanism for the impaired growth is not understood. Older children may exhibit bizarre behaviors characterized by extreme polydipsia and polyphagia. Children may drink from toilet bowls and rummage through garbage cans for food, even when adequate food is available. Hormonal abnormalities, including apparent GH deficiency with delayed skeletal maturation, may be present. However, GH therapy does not usually correct the growth failure. The appropriate intervention is to remove the child from his environment and hospitalize him or, preferably, place him in a foster home. Once the environmental situation has been corrected, the majority of children with psychosocial dwarfism resume a normal growth pattern.

4. Turner's Syndrome

Turner's syndrome is characterized by an abnormality of one of the X chromosomes. The incidence of Turner's syndrome is estimated at 1/2000 live-born phenotypic females (Rosenfeld). The syndrome includes defects such as complete absence of one of the X chromosomes (accounting for approximately 60% of cases), structural X chromosomal abnormalities (20% of cases), and mosaicism, with at least one cell line containing a defective X chromosome (20% of cases). The incidence of Turner's syndrome in spontaneous abortuses is estimated at 6 to 7% and most Turner's karyotype fetuses are aborted prior to 28 weeks gestation.

Short stature is the most consistent and striking clinical finding in Turner's syndrome. Other commonly observed features include a short, webbed neck, with a low posterior hairline and rotated ears. Facial abnormalities include micrognathia, high-arched palate, strabismus, and ptosis. Skeletal abnormalities include cubitus valgus, short fourth metacarpals, abnormal upper-to-lower segment ratio, scoliosis, shieldlike chest appearance, and nail dysplasias. Gonadal failure secondary to "streak gonads" and resulting in defective ovarian function is almost uniform in 45 XO subjects but less common in those with other X chromosomal abnormalities and mosaicism. Cardiovascular anomalies, hypertension and renal anomalies are common. A higher incidence of autoimmune conditions characterized by thyroiditis, alopecia, and vitiligo is also associated with Turner's syndrome.

The mean final adult heights of women with Turner's syndrome ranges between 142.0 and 146.8 cm. Subjects from genetically tall families will achieve a greater final adult height than those with short family members. If all of the growth failure were due to the absence of gonadarche and the pubertal growth spurt, one would expect normal intrauterine and prepubertal growth, a growth pattern analogous to that observed in patients with hypogonadotropic hypogonadism. A comprehensive report of growth patterns in 150 untreated Turner's syndrome patients revealed that intrauterine growth is retarded, postnatal growth is normal until a bone age of 2 years, then linear growth is stunted between bone age 2 to 11 years, with continued slow growth into the adolescent period. Because of the gonadal failure, untreated patients will have delayed epiphyseal fusion and growth may continue until the late teens or early 20s. Despite the prolonged growth period, final stature is compromised.

Whether the short stature is secondary to end-organ resistance to the effects of GH or due to some other factor associated with the karyotype abnormality is still not known. Although the majority of girls with Turner's syndrome have normal GH responses to provocative stimuli, several cases of GH deficiency have been documented (Brook, Duke et al., Laczi et al.). Furthermore, even when the responses to provocative stimuli are normal, GH pulse amplitude and frequency are decreased when compared to normal girls (Ross et al.).

Numerous studies have evaluated the role of hormonal therapy in girls with Turner's syndrome. Although there are reports suggesting that sex steroid therapy does not result in increased linear growth (Brook et al.), evidence is increasing that, with appropriate dosages, sex steroids may increase linear growth in Turner's syndrome. Six months of low-dose (100 ng/kg) estradiol in 16 girls with Turner's syndrome, ages 5 to 15 years, resulting in a 70% increase in linear growth when compared to placebo (Ross et al.). Although linear growth improved during this short course of therapy, the impact on predicted height of +0.35 cm was of insufficient biologic significance to conclude that significant improvement in final stature would occur. These studies are still ongoing at the National Institutes of Health (NIH) and the impact on final adult height will be assessed when longer courses of therapy can be evaluated. Most studies evaluating the efficacy of anabolic steroids in increasing linear growth in Turner's syndrome have reported short-term improvements, but with controversial results when evaluated in terms of final adult height (Lev-Ran, Johanson et al., Rosenbloom et al., Urban et al., Joss and Zuppinger). In the most comprehensive prospective, multicenter trial to date, Rosenfeld et al. documented significantly increased 1-year growth rates in children treated with oxandrolone (7.9 cm/year) compared to controls (3.8 cm/year) and even greater 1-year growth with the combination of oxandrolone and GH (9.8 cm/year) (Rosenfeld et al.). Following the first year, the control group and the oxandrolone-only group were treated with GH. Because the study is still ongoing, the impact of this therapy on final adult height is yet to be determined.

The reader should be aware that skeletal dysplasias, chromosomal abnormalities, intrauterine growth retardation, syndromes not defined by chromosomal abnormalities, and chronic systemic disorders can all be associated with short stature. It is common for short stature to be the most significant clinical feature in many of these conditions, but it is beyond the scope of this chapter to discuss these disorders.

Table 3 outlines the endocrine disturbances that can be associated with short stature. Only thyroid hormone deficiency, glucocorticoid excess, and growth hormone deficiency will be discussed.

5. Hypothyroidism

While fetal thyroid hormone may not be important for normal fetal growth, thyroid hormone is necessary for normal neonatal and childhood growth. Thyroid hormone probably acts to stimulate growth both directly, at the level of bone and cartilage, as well as at the hypothalamic-pituitary axis to permit adequate GH production and secretion. GH secretion is impaired in hypothyroid patients and this abnormality can persist for up to 1 month after initiating thyroid replacement therapy. If hypothyroidism occurs in the newborn period, there will be severe developmental delay in addition to growth delay. Additional neonatal findings may include large anterior and posterior fontanelles, macroglossia, umbilical hernia, distended abdomen, skin mottling, jaundice, hoarse cry, dry skin, hyporeflexia, lethargy, feeding problems, and cold intolerance. Unless appropriate thyroid hormone replacement therapy is initiated, brain development will be abnormal and the child will remain mentally retarded.

In older children, the signs and symptoms of hypothyroidism may be of gradual onset, with growth delay as the major clinical feature. There will often be an increase in the ratio of the upper body segment to the lower body segment, due to the relative slow growth of the limbs. Children with hypothyroidism have a dramatic delay in skeletal maturation. They may have dull, placid facial expressions and deteriorating school performance. Delayed dentition, constipation, lethargy, cold intolerance, hyporeflexia, thick and pale skin, galactorrhea, and either delayed or precocious puberty may be associated features. Because the most common cause of acquired hypothyroidism in childhood is chronic lymphocytic or Hashimoto's thyroiditis, the child may also have a palpable goiter.

It is important to consider hypothyroidism in the diagnosis of any short child since in most circumstances it is a condition that is relatively easy to both diagnose and treat.

6. Hypercortisolism

Hypercortisolism of either endogenous or exogenous origin impedes normal growth. The first clinical manifestation of Cushing's syndrome may be short stature, although obesity affecting the face, trunk, back, and abdomen is usually an accompanying feature. The face may be plethoric and acne may be present over the chin, cheeks, nose, chest, and back. Hyperpigmentation, violaceous striae, and hirsutism, with excessive hair over the face, limbs, and suprapubic region, may be present. Glucose intolerance, hypertension, and osteoporosis of the spine may also occur. In children under the age of 7, an adrenocortical carcinoma or adenoma is the most likely etiology of endogenous glucocorticoid excess. In older children, as in adults, adrenocorticotropic hormone (ACTH)-secreting pituitary tumors are more common.

Table 3
Endocrine Causes of Short Stature

Growth hormone deficiency
Thyroid hormone deficiency
Glucocorticoid excess
Rickets
Pseudohypoparathyroidism
Premature epiphyseal fusion: congenital adrenal hyperplasia, virilizing or feminizing
    adrenal or gonadal tumors, central or peripheral precocious puberty

Endogenous hypercortisolism is rare in children but hypercortisolism secondary to the exogenous administration of glucocorticoids is not. Glucocorticoids are commonly used as routine therapy for many pediatric diseases, including asthma, rheumatoid arthritis, inflammatory bowel disease, the nephrotic syndrome, and as immunosuppressive agents for organ and bone marrow transplantation. The physical features and impaired growth associated with endogenous Cushing's syndrome can also occur with exogenous glucocorticoid administration. Any child receiving glucocorticoids for more than 2 to 3 weeks, at daily doses of greater than 25 mg/m^2 of hydrocortisone (or equivalent), is at risk for compromise of linear growth.

The mechanism of the growth failure in hypercortisolism is unknown but may include local tissue resistance to the effects of GH and peptide growth factors. In addition, the normal GH response to hypoglycemia is blunted in the presence of glucocorticoid excess. Even after only 48 hr of high-dose glucocorticoids, GH secretion will be decreased. Whether GH therapy can overcome the growth failure associated with glucocorticoid excess is still unknown.

It is important to consider endogenous Cushing's syndrome in the differential diagnosis of a short, overweight child. Therapy is directed toward removal of the excess glucocorticoid source. In the case of exogenous Cushing's syndrome, it is desirable to carefully weigh the benefits the child is receiving from the glucocorticoid treatment against the potential disadvantages of hypercortisolism. When possible, alternate-day rather than daily glucocorticoid administration is preferable because less growth suppression has been documented with this form of treatment.

7. Growth Hormone Deficiency

Whether fetal GH, like fetal thyroid hormone, is necessary for normal intrauterine growth is still hotly debated. In congenital GH deficiency, birth weight is usually normal, although some investigators have shown that birth length is compromised. The diagnosis of congenital GH deficiency should be considered in any newborn with hypoglycemia, or in male babies with microphallus. Growth impairment usually becomes apparent within the first 2 to 3 years of life. There may be delayed closure of the anterior fontanelle. Dental development as well as skeletal maturation may be delayed. The child will often have a "cherubic" appearance with a truncal fat distribution. Neurologic development is generally normal, although it may be impaired if there have been frequent hypoglycemic episodes, if a central nervous system lesion is present, or if radiation therapy is the cause of the GH deficiency.

GH deficiency may result from numerous etiologies (Table 4). Most commonly, GH deficiency is of idiopathic origin. The incidence of GH deficiency is estimated at 1 of every 60,000 live births in Britain (Pankin). As already discussed, the results obtained from GHRH testing reveal that most children with idiopathic GH deficiency have hypothalamic, rather than pituitary, abnormalities. The majority of cases of idiopathic GH deficiency are sporadic. In some subjects, it is possible to elicit a history of a complicated birth, marked by prolonged labor and some degree of fetal hypoxia. Although a higher incidence of perinatal problems is reported in children with GH deficiency, it has not been possible to clearly demonstrate that traumatic delivery is the usual cause of idiopathic GH deficiency. Varying degrees of hypopituitarism may accompany GH deficiency. While the majority of idiopathic cases have isolated GH deficiency, thyroid-stimulating hormone (TSH), ACTH, and less commonly gonadotropin deficiencies can occur concomitantly.

The GH gene is located on the long arm of chromosome 17 (Miller and Eberhardt, Phillips). An autosomal recessive form of GH deficiency, type IA, is associated with a complete deletion of this gene. These children do not respond well to GH therapy. The lack of an adequate response to GH is felt to be secondary to the development of neutralizing GH antibodies that develop when the foreign antigen, GH, is administered. Another autosomal

Table 4
Causes of Growth Hormone Deficiency

Idiopathic	Vascular
Hereditary	Aneurysms
Sporadic	Infarctions
Brain malformations	Infection
Septo-optic dysplasia	Bacterial
Midline defects	Viral
Tumors	Fungal
Location and tumor type	Infiltrative
Surgical therapy	Autoimmune
Radiation therapy	Histiocytosis
Trauma	Sarcoidosis
Accidents	Metastases
Surgery	
Abuse	

recessive form of GH deficiency, type IB, is associated with the presence, but presumed malfunction, of the GH gene. These children make small amounts of GH and thus do not develop significant titers of neutralizing antibodies against GH. Autosomal dominant (type II) and X-linked (type III) forms of GH deficiency have also been reported. As in GH deficiency type IB, no abnormalities of the GH gene have yet been documented in these disorders.

Congenital abnormalities of brain formation are the second most common cause of neonatal GH deficiency. Abnormalities in the development of the forebrain may result in hypopituitarism. Holoprosencephaly or less severe malformations with hypertelorism, broad-based nasal bridge, cleft lip or palate, or single central maxillary incisor, have all been described in association with hypopituitarism, manifest by GH deficiency. An ectopically located posterior pituitary gland may be associated with the anterior pituitary dysfunction. Deficiencies of other anterior and posterior pituitary hormones frequently accompany the GH deficiency. In the author's experience, septo-optic dysplasia, characterized by an absence of the septum-pellucidum, optic nerve hypoplasia, and hypopituitarism, is the most common of these congenital abnormalities to result in GH deficiency. Posterior pituitary hypofunction, characterized by diabetes insipidus, is also common.

In older children, brain tumors are the second most common etiology of GH deficiency. Primary pituitary tumors are rare in childhood. Brain tumors that have hypothalamic extension or that impair hypothalamic-pituitary function are more commonly associated with GH deficiency. These tumors include gliomas, astrocytomas, ependymomas, meningiomas, pinealomas, medulloblastomas, germinomas, and sarcomas. Not only can central nervous system (CNS) tumors result in GH deficiency, the surgical or radiological treatment of CNS tumors can cause GH deficiency. GH deficiency and other anterior pituitary abnormalities are more likely when high doses of radiation are used (Richards, et al., Oberfield, et al., Shalett et al., Winter and Green). Radiation doses in excess of 2000 rads directed at the hypothalamic-pituitary region will significantly increase a child's risk for anterior pituitary dysfunction.

The tumor that most commonly results in growth failure as a primary feature is the craniopharyngioma. Delayed skeletal maturation, obesity, headaches, and visual impairment may also occur. This tumor presumably arises from the remnants of Rathke's pouch at the junction of the anterior and posterior pituitary gland. It is a slowly growing tumor that may develop cystic areas and areas of calcification. There may be compression of the optic chiasm and nerves, increased intracranial pressure, and abnormalities of hypothalamic, anterior, or posterior pituitary function. The most effective form of therapy is still controversial, but the combination of surgical excision with subsequent radiotherapy is currently recommended.

Following surgery, extreme weight gain, which may be associated with normal or even excessive linear growth, is common. This phenomenon is intriguing because abnormal, and even absent, GH secretion is usually documented following therapy. The factor that stimulates growth in the absence of GH has not been identified, but investigators have suggested that insulin, prolactin, or possibly other CNS products are responsible.

Trauma to the brain, pituitary, or pituitary stalk may result in anterior and/or posterior hypopituitarism. Similarly, surgical damage may occur to the pituitary stalk. Child abuse, characterized by "shaking" of the child's body, can result in either traumatic or vascular pituitary lesions causing hypopituitarism. Other vascular lesions that can cause abnormalities of pituitary function include aneurysms or infarction.

Bacterial, viral, or fungal causes of hypophysitis can lead to varying degrees of hypopituitarism. Infiltrative processes including histiocytosis, sarcoidosis, or metastic disease from distant malignancies may also impair pituitary function. Autoimmune hypophysitis occurs rarely in children and may be associated with autoimmune polyglandular failure.

D. Therapy of Short Stature

1. Growth Hormone

Growth hormone has been the standard form of therapy for GH deficiency since the 1950s, when the principal source was from extracted human pituitaries. Because the supply was scarce, strict criteria were established by the National Pituitary Agency to restrict its availability to children with severe GH deficiency. In 1985, the Food and Drug Administration (FDA) banned its use because of the transmission of a slow virus that induced Jakob-Creutzfeld disease in several subjects who had received pituitary-derived GH (Beardsley). In most countries, pituitary-derived GH is no longer available for general use. Fortunately, several pharmaceutical companies have succeeded in the development of synthetic GH by recombinant DNA technology. Currently, two companies have FDA approval to market GH preparations in the United States (Genentech, San Francisco, CA; Eli Lilly and Co., Indianapolis, IN). In Europe, several additional products are available from other pharmaceutical firms. The current production methods have resulted in unlimited supplies of GH. Unfortunately, the cost of treatment is high, ranging from $10,000 to $30,000/year of treatment per child.

Biosynthetic and pituitary-derived GH are of comparable potency, efficacy, and pharmacokinetic characteristics. Because of the increased availability of GH, treatment of children with conditions aside from classical GH deficiency has become more common. GH is now acceptable therapy in Turner's syndrome (Rosenfeld, et al.), and is being used experimentally in chronic renal failure (Koch et al.), in the treatment of intrauterine growth retardation (Lanes et al.), and to aid in burn and wound healing. In addition, the use of GH to promote linear growth in non-GH-deficient short children is being tested in numerous centers (Genentech Collaborative Study Group). Although initial results demonstrate increased growth rates, final height data are not yet available.

The recommended dose of GH is between 0.15 and 0.5 mg/kg/week, given in at least three weekly injections. Recent data suggest a growth advantage from daily, rather than triweekly, administration. Equal efficacy has been demonstrated with subcutaneous and intramuscular routes of administration. The growth response is generally greatest in the first year of treatment. This effect may represent a period of catch-up growth. In general, younger children exhibit better growth rates than older children. The magnitude of the growth response appears to be dose dependent, with higher doses resulting in greater growth velocity.

Skeletal maturation occurs during GH therapy and correlates with the degree of linear growth. In some peripubertal children, GH therapy results in activation of the hypothalamic-pituitary-gonadal axis and puberty is induced shortly after therapy is initiated. Because skeletal maturation occurs rapidly in puberty, the rate of bone age advancement may exceed the rate of linear growth. This has led some investigators to propose the use of long-acting GnRH analogs to delay puberty in peripubertal or pubertal GH deficient subjects, so that maximal benefit might be achieved from the GH therapy (Stanhope and Brook). Although not demonstrated to be of short-term benefit, several centers have ongoing research protocols to investigate this combination of treatments. In contrast, other investigators have proposed an opposite approach to adjuvant GH therapy. They recommend using anabolic steroids when the growth response to GH is no longer maximal. This combination has been widely used in the Turner's syndrome population, where the risk of hypothalamic-pituitary-gonadal activation is not a significant problem. However, the effect of this combined therapy on final adult height has not been proven to be more effective than GH alone. Thus, it has yet to be shown whether the use of GH in combination with either GnRH analogs or anabolic steroids will result in greater final height than GH treatment alone.

2. Growth Hormone-Releasing Hormone

Since the characterization of growth hormone-releasing hormone (GHRH) in 1982, it has been tested for its diagnostic usefulness in adults and children (Gelato et al., Grossman et al.). It has been shown to stimulate the release of GH in the majority of children with GH deficiency. Repeated stimulation with GHRH will lead to enhanced GH responses, even in GH-deficient children with minimal initial responses (Takano et al.). When group data are analyzed, children with GH deficiency have lower GH responses to GHRH testing. However, because most children with GH deficiency respond to GHRH testing, and there is an overlap in GH responses with normal children, GHRH is not a good diagnostic test for GH deficiency. However, since it does stimulate GH secretion in most children, GHRH has potential useful-ness as a therapeutic agent in the treatment of GH deficiency. Short-term studies have demonstrated increased growth velocity in most GH-deficient children when treated with GHRH (Gelato et al., Thorner et al.). More recently, increases in growth velocity have been demonstrated with up to 18 months of GHRH therapy in GH-deficient children (Ross et al., Thorner et al.). GHRH may have a physiologic advantage over GH in children who have normal somatotroph function. Whether GHRH becomes an alternative to GH therapy will depend on availability and cost, as well as on efficacy and safety. Furthermore, the optimal dose, route, and frequency of administration are yet to be determined.

3. Other Therapy

Other forms of therapy have been used to treat short children with variable success. Cyproheptadine, an antihistamine sertonin antagonist, has been used as adjuvant therapy in the treatment of GH deficiency (Kaplowitz and Jennings). L-Dopa and bromocriptine have been used to treat GH-deficient children (Huseman and Hassing). Clonidine, an α_2-adrenergic agonist, has also been shown to increase linear growth in both GH-deficient children and in those with constitutional delay of growth and puberty (Pintor et al., Castro-Magana et al.). Unfortunately, the effect in non-GH-deficient short children was not substantiated when tested in a double-blind, placebo-controlled trial (Pescovitz and Tan).

E. Disorders of Tall Stature

1. Genetic Tall Stature

As in short stature, genetic background is the most important determinant of tall stature. In general, tall boys come to medical attention less often than short boys because male tall stature is associated with social advantage. Referrals for evaluation of tall stature in girls are more common. Obtaining a bone age radiograph may be helpful, so that a prediction of final adult stature can be determined. Since the social stigmata associated with tall stature are decreasing, a conservative approach is generally recommended, with the mainstay of therapy being simple reassurance. Based on the predicted height, however, some physicians may advocate therapy to decrease final height potential. Numerous studies have evaluated the efficacy of high-dose sex steroid treatment in children with excessive tall stature (Bierich, Prader and Zachman). The primary principle is that although sex steroids promote growth, in high doses they also promote epiphyseal maturation. When the degree of skeletal advancement exceeds the increase in linear growth, epiphyseal fusion will occur and final stature will be decreased. Most of these studies evaluated the impact of high doses of estrogens in tall girls on final height predictions (Bayley-Pinneau, Roche-Weiner-Thissen, Tanner). Regardless of the precise treatment regimen or the method for comparison, these studies concluded that estrogen treatment results in a decrease of 3.5 to 7.3 cm in final height (Crawford). Similar results have been demonstrated from testosterone treatment of boys with excessive tall stature (Zachman et al.). The potential side effects of this therapy include acceleration of puberty, weight gain, hypertension, nausea, increased risk of thromboembolic disease, cystic breast lesions, and endometrial hyperplasia. Because of the potential for serious side effects, therapy to promote epiphyseal fusion should not be undertaken lightly.

2. Premature Sexual Development

Premature sexual development secondary to elevated sex steroids will lead to increased growth velocity. While childhood growth is excessive, final stature is stunted because of premature epiphyseal fusion. The conditions that cause premature sexual development are discussed in detail in Section III.

3. Klinefelter's Syndrome

Boys with chromosomal abnormalities, in particular XXY or XYY karyotypes, have a high incidence of tall stature. The incidence of Klinefelter's syndrome is estimated at 1 in 600 newborn males. These boys tend to have a slim build with small, firm testes. There is decreased cellularity of the testicular tubules with few, or absent, germ cells. There is an increased risk for impaired intellectual function that is most pronounced in the area of language development. At puberty, gynecomastia is often noted. Hypogonadism, whether from primary gondal failure or secondary to hypogonadotropic hypogonadism, is associated with a greater likelihood of tall final stature because of the delay in epiphyseal fusion and the extended growth period. Because this results in increased leg length, the upper:lower body segment ratio is decreased in these subjects.

4. Marfan's Syndrome

Subjects with Marfan's syndrome have disproportionate tall stature with long limbs and arachnodactyly of fingers and toes. There is a tendency to lens dislocations and cataracts. Muscular hypotonia, increased joint flexibility, and cardiac anomalies are common. In appearance, patients with Marfan syndrome resemble subjects with homocystinuria, which is characterized by excretion of large amounts of homocystine in the urine. Homocystinuria is associated with mental retardation. No effective therapy is currently available for either disorder.

5. Cerebral Gigantism

This syndrome is also known as Sotos' syndrome. These children have a unique pheno-type characterized by a large head and prominent forehead, high-arched palate, antimongoloid slant of the palpebral fissures, and tall stature. The skeletal age is usually advanced, and there may be varying degrees of mental retardation. No known diagnostic test or therapy exists.

6. Beckwith-Wiedemann Syndrome

This syndrome is often suspected at birth in large (for gestational age) babies who have prominent macroglossia. They also have an increased incidence of hypoglycemia, umbilical hernia, and hemihypertrophy. While no therapy for the underlying condition exists, these children have an increased risk for the development of Wilm's tumors and adrenal, renal, or hepatic carcinomas. Therefore, tumor surveillance is the mainstay of future evaluations once the diagnosis is made.

7. Growth Hormone Excess

When GH is secreted in excess in adults, it is defined as acromegaly. Although some of these cases may have developed during childhood, GH-producing tumors are rarely reported in children. If GH excess is present before there is complete epiphyseal fusion, linear growth will be rapid and "gigantism" will occur. In addition, there may be coarse facial features, large hands and feet, acral enlargement, excess soft tissue growth, and macrocephaly (Blumberg et al.). The facial features are characterized by prominence of the supraorbital ridges, prominent mandible, and large nose. In addition, there may be kyphosis and osteoporosis. Abnormal glucose tolerance testing, polyuria, and polydipsia may also be present. Hyperprolactinemia is common in children with GH excess. As in the adult population, the possibility of ectopic GHRH secretion exists in the pediatric population. However, most cases of GH excess in childhood are probably secondary to excessive hypothalamic GHRH, or deficient somatostatin, secretion that results in mammosomatotroph hyperplasia.

III. Puberty

A. Clinical Features

Puberty is a transitional stage from the sexually immature to the sexually mature state. It is accompanied by significant changes in hormonal activity, in secondary sexual characteristics, and in behavior. Most females exhibit the first physical signs of secondary sexual development between 9 and 13 years of age, while most males will develop the first signs of puberty between ages 10 and 14.

In girls, the first physical indication of puberty is usually breast budding, termed thelarche. This is generally followed within a few months by pubic hair development, known as pubarche. Girls may also notice increased oiliness of hair and skin, development of acne, increased perspiration and body odor. Frequently, there is an increased interest in makeup and clothes. Family members and friends may report greater moodiness, flirtatious behavior, and emotional lability. An acceleration in growth velocity with the peak of the growth spurt occurring 1 to 2 years prior to menarche is typical. Menarche, or the first menstrual bleed, is the culminating pubertal event in girls. By the time of menarche, most girls have completed more than 75% of pubertal physical development and have achieved more than 90% of their growth potential.

The first clinical sign of puberty in boys is testicular enlargement, followed by pubarche. Boys also experience increased oiliness of hair and skin, perspiration, and body odor. In addition, they may develop generalized body hair, deepening voice, penile erections, and emissions. The physical features are accompanied by a heightened interest in girls. Boys may also experience breast budding during puberty. A small tender "button" of breast tissue appears beneath the areolae of either one or both breasts. The physician must be aware that this is a normal physiologic change, known as pubertal gynecomastia. Although many do not realize that it is a part of normal development, gynecomastia is seen in most pubertal boys. It is important for the physician to provide reassurance for pubertal gynecomastia. However, if the gynecomastia occurs prior to puberty, a comprehensive medical evaluation is indicated. In boys, the peak of the growth spurt occurs about midpuberty and will continue until there is complete epiphyseal fusion and a cessation of linear growth.

B. Hypothalamic-Pituitary-Gonadal Axis

From a hormonal standpoint, puberty is made up of two distinct, dissociated events: adrenarche and gonadarche. Under most circumstances, gonadarche and adrenarche occur in synchrony with each other. However, because they are differentially regulated, they may be dissociated in pathologic states (Sklar et al., Counts et al.).

Adrenarche is a maturational increase in adrenal 17-ketosteroid production characterized by increased circulating levels of dehydroepiandrosterone (DHEA) and its sulfated form, dehydroepiandrosterone sulfate (DHEAS). These factors begin to increase above prepubertal levels at the age of 6 or 7 years in both boys and girls. The mechanism of increased adrenal androgen secretion is unknown. Two major hypotheses predominate. The first hypothesis states that adrenarche represents increased efficiency of the $C_{17,20}$-lyase enzyme system leading to selective conversion of adrenal precursors to DHEA. The second hypothesis states that a pituitary hormone selectively stimulates adrenal androgen production. This putative adrenal androgen-stimulating hormone has not been isolated to date.

Gonadarche is a developmental process associated with increased amplitude and frequency of hypothalamic pulses of gonadotropin-releasing hormone (GnRH). It is also associated with decreased sensitivity of the hypothalamic rheostat, the gonadostat, to negative feedback inhibition from the gonadal sex steroids.

The pulsatile secretion of GnRH is regulated by a putative *pulse generator* that resides in the hypothalamus. GnRH is secreted into the portal circulation and results in the pulsatile pituitary secretion of the gonadotropins, luteinizing hormone (LH) and follicle-stimulating hormone (FSH). Gonadotropin stimulation of the gonad leads to enlargement and sex steroid production. The predominant circulating sex steroid produced by the ovary during puberty is estradiol, while the testis produces testosterone. The sex steroids act peripherally to induce the physical and behavioral features associated with puberty. Sex steroids also act centrally at the level of the hypothalamic-pituitary axis to regulate further gonadotropin secretion. Although sex steroids generally cause negative feedback regulation of gonadotropins, they may also work through positive feedback mechanisms (i.e., the LH surge that results in ovulation is induced by positive feedback from ovarian estradiol).

Both the fetus and the neonate have highly active hypothalamic-pituitary-gonadal axes that result in circulating sex steroids in the range observed during early puberty. The hypothalamic-pituitary-gonadal axis becomes quiescent in the prepubertal period. This is secondary to a maturational process in the central nervous system characterized by a predominance of inhibitory neural pathways. During the quiescent period, sex steroids exert negative feedback and inhibit GnRH and gonadotropin secretion.

One hypothesis for the onset of puberty is the "gonadostat hypothesis". According to this theory, a gonadostat that regulates the negative feedback effects of sex steroids is present somewhere in the central nervous system. At the time of puberty, and after the child has achieved a minimal body mass and degree of skeletal maturation, the setting of the gonadostat is changed so that it becomes less sensitive to the suppressive effects of sex steroids. Because of this decreased sensitivity, the same sex steroid levels no longer have an inhibitory effect on gonadotropin secretion. Thus, pulsatile GnRH and gonadotropin activity ensues. Initially, puberty is characterized by LH-predominant gonadotropin pulses occurring during sleep. As puberty progresses, daytime gonadotropin pulses occur as well.

C. Pubertal Growth

While it is still unclear whether sex steroids of either adrenal or ovarian origin are necessary for normal prepubertal growth, it seems unlikely that they play a critical role (Campos and MacGillivray). However, pubertal growth differs from prepubertal growth in two significant ways. First, the growth velocity is usually 1.5 to 2 times the prepubertal rate. Second, there is more dramatic maturation of the skeleton during pubertal growth. Children with premature gonadarche demonstrate an increased growth velocity at an early chronologic age and children with delayed gonadarche demonstrate a delayed pubertal growth spurt. Those who never experience gonadarche never experience a pubertal growth spurt.

In the condition of isolated hypogonadotropic hypogonadism, adrenarche occurs normally and gonadarche is delayed until hormonal therapy is initiated. The absence of gonadal sex steroids results in pubertal delay, a delay in the pubertal growth spurt, and perhaps a small increase in final adult stature. In constitutional delay of growth and puberty, children experience short stature and delayed pubertal onset (Styne). When spontaneous hypothalamic-pituitary-gonadal activation ensues (sometimes as late as age 17 or 18 years), the pubertal growth spurt is of normal magnitude and the final height is genetically appropriate. The prepubertal growth velocity of 18 agonadal patients with normal sex chromosomes was normal prior to the institution of sex steroid therapy (Campos and MacGillivray). Thus, it seems that the pubertal growth spurt is not essential for the achievement of normal final adult stature. When the pubertal growth spurt is delayed or does not occur at all, prepubertal growth continues and final height is either normal or greater than normal. An exception to this concept is Turner's syndrome, in which short stature is associated with absent gonadal function. However, the short stature in this syndrome is not primarily related to the absence of a pubertal growth spurt. Rather, it is associated with intrauterine and prepubertal growth retardation that is most likely secondary to a deficiency of X-linked gene functions encoded on missing chromosomal material.

Whether measured by pharmacologic stimulation tests or by assessing endogenous GH secretion, there are now good data to support the concept of increasing GH levels at the time of puberty. Several authors found increased GH release in response to pharmacologic stimuli in pubertal compared to prepubertal children (Frasier et al.). Short-term administration of sex steroids prior to provocative GH testing also increases GH secretion (Martin et al., Moll et al., Merimee and Fineberg) and endogenous GH secretion is higher during puberty than before puberty (Thompson et al., Zadik et al.). In a recent study of spontaneous GH secretion in 21 children with idiopathic short stature, 8 of whom received sex steroids and 13 of whom did not, mean 24-hr GH concentrations were greater in sex steroid-treated children (Rose et al.).

The precise mechanism by which sex steroids increase GH secretion is unknown. In primary gonadal failure, GH levels are lower than after sex steroid replacement. GH levels increase significantly following sex steroid replacement in subjects with anorchia (Illig and Prader). Both GH secretion and IGF-I levels are decreased in girls with Turner's syndrome, and estrogen therapy leads to increases in both (Cuttler et al.).

IGF-I levels rise throughout childhood, with a dramatic increase at the time of puberty (Luna et al., Rosenfield et al.). The pubertal increase in IGF-I levels may be due to a direct effect of sex steroids on IGF-I production or an indirect effect mediated through increased GH secretion. During normal puberty, IGF-I levels correlate closely with plasma levels of sex hormones (Rosenfield et al.). Administration of sex steroids to functionally agonadal, GH-intact children results in increased IGF-I levels (Rosenfield and Furlanetto). Furthermore, IGF-I levels are correlated with growth velocity during the early phases of the pubertal growth spurt (Cara et al.). However, in late puberty, when growth velocity is decelerating, IGF-I levels remain high and do not correlate with growth velocity. There are also data to support either no effect or an inhibitory effect of sex steroids on IGF-I, and estradiol has even been used as adjuvant therapy to suppress GH and IGF-I in acromegaly (Wiedemann et al., Clemmons et al.).

These conflicting effects of sex steroids on IGF-I might be explained on the basis of sex steroid dose. In low doses, sex steroids initially act to stimulate GH secretion directly without significant effect on IGF-I. In modest doses that result in circulating levels comparable to those observed in early puberty, the increase in GH secretion leads to an increase in circulating IGF-I. Finally, in high doses, estradiol suppresses IGF-I. It seems likely that sex steroids induce these changes in IGF-I at the level of GH, or even at higher hypothalamic or cortical levels. Support for this hypothesis can be derived from studies in which administration of testosterone to GH-deficient boys is not associated with an increase in IGF-I, while similar therapy in GH-sufficient children results in increased circulating IGF-I levels (Parker et al.).

Children with precocious puberty of either central or peripheral etiology experience a pubertal growth spurt that is comparable in magnitude to the normal pubertal spurt, but which occurs at an inappropriately early chronologic age. Although delayed or absent puberty does not adversely affect final stature, precocious puberty does. A number of studies have evaluated final adult height in children with congenital adrenal hyperplasia (CAH) and all of them document compromised final adult stature in untreated or poorly treated patients. The most comprehensive review of final height in untreated children with precocious puberty was published in 1968 (Sigurjonsdottir and Hayles). Although a heterogeneous group in terms of etiology, all had premature development of secondary sexual characteristics and an early pubertal growth spurt with premature epiphyseal fusion. The final adult height in 27 girls with idiopathic precocious puberty was below 160 cm in all except 1, who had pubertal onset at age 7 years and reached an adult height of >170 cm.

GH secretory dynamics have also been studied in precocious puberty. IGF-I levels are increased for chronologic age but are appropriate for pubertal stage (Pescovitz et al., Harris et al.). Spontaneous GH secretion in children with precocious puberty is increased when compared to normal age-matched prepubertal children (Ross et al.). However, in children with the combination of GH deficiency and precocious puberty, IGF-I levels do not rise into the range appropriate for pubertal status (Cara et al.).

D. Premature Sexual Development

Disorders of puberty can be divided into two major groups: (1) premature sexual development and (2) delayed pubertal development. The most common cause of pubertal delay is constitutional delay of growth and puberty. This condition has already been discussed in the context of linear growth delay. Pubertal delay can also result from primary or secondary gonadal failure. Both primary gonadal failure (i.e., Klinefelter's syndrome, Turner's syndrome) and secondary or tertiary gonadal failure (hypogonadotropic hypogonadism) have already been discussed briefly. This section will focus on premature sexual development.

When the clinical features of puberty appear before the age of 8 in girls or 9 in boys, it is considered premature. Premature sexual development can take the form of isolated pubic hair or breast development, complete isosexual pubertal development, heterosexual pubertal development, or any intermediate form. There are three major categories of precocious puberty: central precocious puberty, peripheral precocious puberty, and combined peripheral and central precocious puberty. In addition, there are some forms of precocious puberty that are of unknown etiology. Central precocious puberty is gonadotropin dependent and is initiated by hypothalamic-pituitary-gonadal activation. Central precocious puberty, therefore, results in pubertal development by a mechanism similar to that observed in normal puberty. Peripheral precocious puberty is gonadotropin independent and therefore does not involve activation of the hypothalamic-pituitary-gonadal axis. Combined precocious puberty involves secondary activation of the hypothalamic-pituitary-gonadal axis in the presence of a primary peripheral cause of abnormal sex steroid elevation.

1. Central Precocious Puberty

Central precocious puberty occurs when there is an increase in endogenous gonadotropin pulse frequency and/or amplitude. In early precocious puberty, as in normal puberty, there is a striking augmentation of gonadotropin pulses at night. Later in the process, the day-night differences in the pulsatile secretory patterns disappear. Both normal and precocious puberty are also characterized by an exaggerated LH response to GnRH compared to the FSH-predominant response of the normal, prepubertal child. The result of increased gonadotropin secretion is enlargement of the gonads, measured as an increase in either testicular or ovarian volume, and an increase in gonadal sex steroid production. The sex steroid secretion results in the development of secondary sexual characteristics, rapid linear growth and skeletal maturation, and behavioral changes. These clinical features are similar to those described above for normal, pubertal children. Children with precocious puberty are comparable to their chronological peers in intellectual and emotional development and thus they should be treated on an age-appropriate, rather than size-appropriate, level.

Most cases of central precocious puberty, especially in girls, are of idiopathic origin. A complete diagnostic evaluation fails to reveal an organic lesion as the etiology of the premature activation of the hypothalamic-pituitary-gonadal axis. Occasionally, there is a familial tendency for premature sexual development. A positive family history is more common in children with only modestly early puberty, that is, girls older than 6 years or boys older than 7 years of age. It is unusual to obtain a positive family history in very young children with central precocious puberty.

Since the hypothalamic-pituitary axis is predominantly under inhibitory control during the prepubertal period, any insult that might disrupt inhibitory neural paths can cause premature activation of the axis. Central precocious puberty has occurred in association with many central nervous system lesions, including head trauma, astrocytomas, gliomas, medulloblastomas, third ventricular cysts, Arnold-Chiari malformations, pinealomas, prolactinomas, or hydrocephalus. The most commonly detected lesion in a child with precocious puberty and no other symptomatology is a hypothalamic hamartoma. Most hamartomas have a characteristic radiographic appearance on either computed tomography (CT) or magnetic resonance imaging (MRI) scanning. They are generally spherical and do not enhance after intravenous contrast during CT scanning. Most children with hypothalamic hamartomas appear to be neurologically normal. The advent of high-resolution CT and MRI scanning is responsible for our ability to diagnose these lesions in some children who previously carried a diagnosis of idiopathic precocious puberty. In select children with hypothalamic hamartomas, there is an increased incidence of seizure disorders, and delayed speech and motor development. An unusual seizure disorder characterized by gelastic, or laughing, seizures occasionally occurs in children with hypothalamic hamartomas and precocious puberty. These children may also experience a variety of other types of seizures.

2. Peripheral Precocious Puberty

Peripheral precocious puberty is gonadotropin-independent pubertal development. The etiology of the secondary sexual development is circulating sex steroids that have either been ingested, or originated from the gonad or the adrenal gland by a gonadotropin-independent process. In peripheral precocious puberty, the hypothalamic-pituitary axis is not activated, and may actually be suppressed, secondary to negative feedback inhibition of the sex steroids. The gonadotropin response to GnRH stimulation is usually characterized by an FSH-predominant pattern while central precocious puberty is more frequently characterized by an LH-predominant pattern. Often, a thorough history and physical examination will direct the physician toward a particular diagnosis and the appropriate diagnostic evaluation. Table 5 summarizes the differential diagnosis of peripheral precocious puberty.

a. Premature Adrenarche

The most common cause of isolated early pubarche is premature adrenarche. Premature adrenarche is a benign condition secondary to premature elevations in adrenal androgens and characterized by modestly elevated dehydroepiandrosterone sulfate (DHEAS) levels. Children may have isolated pubic hair, or there may be axillary hair, acne, perspiration, and body odor. In general, there is no significant growth spurt or skeletal maturation, and girls do not have clitoromegaly. However, it is not uncommon for height and bone age to be at the upper limits of normal for chronologic age. When the diagnosis of premature adrenarche is made, only observation is indicated because there are no long-term sequelae. Occasionally, children with gonadal or adrenal tumors, or late-onset forms of congenital adrenal hyperplasia, will have isolated pubarche. DHEAS, testosterone levels, and gonadal or adrenal ultrasounds may be necessary to exclude tumors. While still considered controversial, an ACTH stimulation test is often recommended to exclude 21-hydroxylase, 11-hydroxylase, and 3β-hydroxysteroid dehydrogenase deficiencies as causes of late-onset congenital adrenal hyperplasia.

Table 5
Differential Diagnosis of Precocious Puberty

Central precocious puberty
Idiopathic
Hypothalamic hamartoma
Other CNS lesions
Peripheral precocious puberty
Premature adrenarche
Exogenous/factitious ingestion of steroids
Adrenal gland
Enzymatic defects: CAH (21-hydroxylase, 11-hydroxylase, 3β-hydroxysteroid dehydrogenase)
Tumors: virilizing or feminizing
Ovary
Cysts
Tumors: virilizing or feminizing
McCune-Albright syndrome
Testis
Tumors: dysgerminomas, Leydig-Sertoli cell
Familial male precocious puberty, also known as testotoxicosis
hCG-secreting tumors: hepatoblastomas, dysgerminomas, pinealomas
Combined peripheral and central precocious puberty
Mechanism unknown
Hypothyroidism
Premature thelarche
Hyperprolactinemia

b. Exogenous/Factitious Ingestion of Steroids

Accidental or intentional ingestion of sex steroids may result in secondary sexual development. The most common offenders are birth control pills, anabolic steroids, and hair or facial creams that contain estrogens or androgens. A careful history should alert the physician to this diagnosis. Elimination of the responsible agent usually results in a reversal of the findings.

c. Adrenal Abnormalities

Defects of adrenal steroidogenesis, known as congenital adrenal hyperplasia, may result in excessive adrenal androgen production and peripheral precocious puberty. The most common adrenal enzymatic abnormalities to result in peripheral precocious puberty are 21-hydroxylase, 11-hydroxylase, and 3β-hydroxysteroid dehydrogenase deficiencies. In 21-hydroxylase and 11-hydroxylase deficiencies, boys may develop pubic hair, acne, body odor, deepending of the voice, penile enlargement, acceleration of linear growth, and/or skeletal maturation. Boys with 3β-hydroxysteroid dehydrogenase deficiency do not pubesce early. In girls, however, 21-hydroxylase, 11-hydroxylase, and 3β-hydroxysteroid dehydrogenase deficiencies may result in early or late childhood virilization characterized by pubic hair, acne, body odor, deepening of the voice, clitoral enlargement, and acceleration of linear growth and/or skeletal maturation.

Because the defective enzymes are necessary for normal cortisol production, patients may suffer from varying degrees of adrenal insufficiency. They may also have mineralocorticoid deficiency and salt wasting (21-hydroxylase deficiency and 3 β-hydroxysteroid dehydrogenase deficiency), or hypertension (11-hydroxylase deficiency). The diagnosis of congenital adrenal hyperplasia is made by measurement of the adrenal metabolites before and after ACTH stimulation. Adrenal precursors that precede an enzymatic block will be elevated when compared with the metabolites that follow the block in the adrenal steroidogenic pathway. Therapy for congenital adrenal hyperplasia consists of carefully monitored glucocorticoid replacement, and mineralocorticoids, if indicated.

Adrenal tumors may produce excessive androgens or estrogens resulting in either virilizing or feminizing premature sexual development. Virilizing tumors are more common than feminizing tumors. Because these tumors are relatively inefficient in producing sex steroids, they tend to be large by the time a diagnosis is made. The diagnosis is confirmed by radiographic techniques including adrenal ultrasound, CT, or MRI scanning. Surgical removal of the tumor is the treatment of choice.

d. Ovarian Abnormalities

Ovarian abnormalities can lead to premature development of secondary sexual characteristics. These abnormalities range from benign ovarian cysts to malignant ovarian tumors. Most feminizing lesions are derived from theca cells, granulosa cells, or a combination of the two cell types. Estrogen-secreting tumors and cysts may be responsible for isolated premature thelarche, vaginal estrogenization, or even menses. Sufficient hormonal secretion from these lesions may result in accelerated linear growth and/or skeletal maturation. The larger lesions can be palpated on a bimanual abdominal-rectal examination and confirmatory diagnosis is made by pelvic ultrasound. Most of these lesions are benign and many ovarian cysts will resolve spontaneously. The other neoplastic lesions require surgical therapy. Ovarian tumors may also cause virilization that results in pubic hair, acne, body odor, clitoromegaly, accelerated linear growth, and/or skeletal maturation. Surgery is the therapy of choice.

McCune-Albright syndrome is a clinical triad consisting of irregularly shaped, *cafe-au-lait* skin pigmentation (Coast of Maine lesions), long bone and skull polyostotic fibrous dysplasia, and precocious puberty. The syndrome may also be associated with other endocrine abnormalities including hyperthyroidism, excessive adrenal production of glucocorticoids, and pituitary hyperfunction, usually characterized by excessive growth hormone and/or prolactin secretion. While the etiology of the multiple endocrine abnormalities is unknown, there appears to be autonomous hyperfunction of the involved endocrine glands associated with a $G_s\alpha$ protein abnormality. Although not proven to be a primary ovarian abnormality, it has been shown that the premature sexual development in young girls with McCune-Albright syndrome is gonadotropin independent (Comite et al., Foster et al., Wierman et al.). Large, frequently unilateral ovarian cysts, which presumably secrete the estrogen responsible for secondary sexual development, may be seen (Foster et al.). Some girls with McCune-Albright syndrome have been treated successfully with testolactone, a drug that prevents estrogen synthesis by blocking the aromatase enzyme responsible for converting testosterone and androstenedione to estradiol and estrone, respectively (Foster et al., Feuillan et al.). This treatment is still considered investigational.

e. Testis Abnormalities

Testicular tumors such as dysgerminomas, Leydig-Sertoli cell tumors, and gonadoblastomas generally result in unilateral and frequently asymmetrical testicular enlargement. Occasionally the tumors are bilateral. Diagnosis is often suspected following physical examination and may be confirmed by testicular ultrasound. Definitive pathologic diagnosis is essential and surgery is the therapy of choice. Adrenal rest tissue may also reside in the testis and may increase in size during adrenarche or secondary to congenital adrenal hyperplasia.

A familial form of premature sexual development has been described that is characterized by Leydig cell hyperplasia and germ cell maturation. It has been termed as both "testotoxicosis" and "familial male precocious puberty" (Rosenthal et al., Pescovitz et al., Egli et al.). It appears to be an autosomal dominant disorder with variable penetrance and sex-limited expression. The syndrome may be analogous to McCune-Albright syndrome in that testosterone secretion and sexual maturation take place in the absence of pubertal gonadotropin activity. Fertility is well preserved in these individuals. Investigational therapy has involved ketoconazole, which interferes with the steroid metabolic pathway as a cytochrome P-450 inhibitor (Holland et al.) or a combination of testolactone and spironolactone, which is also a cytochrome P-450 inhibitor (Laue et al.).

f. Gonadotropin-Secreting Tumors

Tumors have long been recognized as able to cause ectopic hormone secretion. The hormone most commonly produced ectopically that results in premature sexual development is human chorionic gonadotropin (hCG). Human chorionic gonadotropin may be produced by hepatoblastomas, intracranial lesions such as pinealomas, or retroperitoneal tumors. Because hCG is structurally similar to LH, it binds to LH receptors and may activate sex steroid secretion. The history and physical examination may suggest the presence of such a tumor. Therapy is generally surgical with the addition of chemotherapy or radiotherapy, as indicated by the histopathologic diagnosis.

3. Combined Peripheral and Central Precocious Puberty

Activation of the hypothalamic-pituitary-gonadal axis and central precocious puberty has been observed in association with peripheral precocious puberty. The combination of peripheral and central precocious puberty has been reported in children with congenital adrenal hyperplasia, in children with adrenal and ovarian tumors, and in older girls with McCune-Albright syndrome (Pescovitz et al., Foster et al.). Theoretically, any etiology of peripheral precocious puberty might result in secondary central precocious puberty. The mechanism of this central activation is not well described. Hypothetical considerations include direct effects of elevated circulating sex steroids on the hypothalamic GnRH neuron, advanced skeletal maturation that suggests a degree of somatic maturation to the central nervous system, and a release of negative feedback suppression of the gonadotropins following successful therapy of the underlying cause of the peripheral precocious puberty. Therapy should be directed at the underlying cause of peripheral precocious puberty. The central precocious puberty can be treated with long-acting GnRH analogs (see below).

4. Mechanism Unknown
a. Hypothyroidism

Precocious puberty has been described in association with severe, acquired hypothyroidism in girls. The mechanism by which hypothyroidism results in precocity has not been accurately described. It is an unusual form of sexual precocity for a number of reasons. Because of the hypothyroidism, linear growth and skeletal maturation are frequently delayed, rather than advanced. There may be multiple, large follicular ovarian cysts. Frequently, there are elevations in both prolactin and TSH. It has been hypothesized that the elevated TSH levels cross react with ovarian gonadotropin receptors to stimulate ovarian enlargement and sex steroid production. The diagnosis of hypothyroidism should be elicited by the history and physical examinations. Therapy is directed toward thyroid hormone replacement. If central precocious puberty is documented, GnRH analog therapy may be indicated (see below).

b. Premature Thelarche

Girls who present with isolated breast development and no evidence for progressive secondary sexual development, accelerated growth, and/or skeletal maturation, have a condition known as premature thelarche. Premature thelarche is a benign condition but the physiologic processes involved in its development are still unknown. Girls with premature thelarche generally have an FSH-predominant response to GnRH stimulation while girls with classical central precocious puberty usually have an LH-predominant response. Hypotheses to account for the development of premature thelarche include increased breast sensitivity to estrogen, transient estrogen secretion by follicular cysts of the ovary, increased estrogen production from adrenal precursors, increased dietary estrogen, and transient partial activation of the hypothalamic-pituitary-ovarian axis with excessive FSH secretion. Although it is not known which, if any, of these hypotheses is correct, the transition to an LH-predominant response is probably a relatively insensitive measure of pubertal activation of the hypothalamic-pituitary-gonadal axis (Pescovitz et al.). The presence of an FSH-predominant response in a child with premature sexual development cannot, however, be taken as assurance that a child with premature thelarche will not develop central precocious puberty. Furthermore, if other signs consistent with central precocious puberty are present, one can make this diagnosis despite an FSH-predominant response to GnRH, provided that other causes of peripheral precocious puberty have been excluded. If a diagnosis of premature thelarche is made, no intervention is indicated unless further progression occurs, at which time reassessment is indicated.

E. Therapy of Premature Sexual Development

The appropriate therapy for premature sexual development is dependent on the specific diagnosis. Premature thelarche and premature adrenarche should be treated by observation only, while exogenous ingestion of steroids is treated by removing them from the child's environment. The appropriate therapies for the other causes of peripheral precocious puberty have already been reviewed. Surgery, radiation, or chemotherapy may be appropriate for invasive or malignant lesions. This section will emphasize medical therapy for central precocious puberty.

The untreated child with central precocious puberty may face psychosocial trauma from premature pubertal development, the effects of hormonal influences on age-appropriate behavior, and adult short stature secondary to premature epiphyseal fusion. Until the early 1980s, therapy for central precocious puberty was limited to progestational agents, such as medroxyprogesterone acetate. These agents inhibit gonadotropin secretion at the hypothalamic and pituitary levels. While menses ceased and secondary sexual characteristics regressed in some patients, most children continued to experience rapid linear growth and skeletal maturation.

When it became known that continuous infusions of GnRH inhibited gonadotropin secretion, and when long-acting synthetic analog forms became available, they were tested in children with central, gonadotropin-dependent, precocious puberty (Beopple et al.). A variety of different GnRH analogs have been produced that all appear to cause an uncoupling of GnRH receptor occupation and the pituitary response to native GnRH. They differ in potency and in amino acid substitutions (all have at least a single amino acid substitution for glycine in position 6 of the decapeptide). Most can be administered either subcutaneously or by the intranasal route (Luder et al.). The therapy is effective in decreasing endogenous and GnRH-stimulated gonadotropin secretion, in decreasing sex steroid levels, and in decreasing the rates of linear growth and skeletal maturation (Pescovitz et al., Comite et al., Styne et al., Mansfield et al., Beopple et al.). The effects on secondary sexual characteristics have varied with the different analogs, but most result in a cessation of menses, and at least a slowing of the progression of secondary sexual characteristics. The effects of long-term stature are promising, although final height data are not yet available for large numbers of children who have been treated for extended periods. In an analysis of children treated with GnRH analog for 6 years, the rate of bone age advancement per year of chronologic age ($\Delta BA/\Delta CA$) declined from 2.7 to 0.5 (Manasco et al.). For 10 of these children, there was an 18-cm increase in predicted height.

While the long-term effects of these analogs on future sexual and reproductive function have not been assessed, the hormonal suppression they induce is reversible when therapy is discontinued (Manasco et al.), and no serious short-term side effects have been reported.

References

Adams, S. O., Nissley, S. P., Handwerger, S., and Rechler, M. M., Developmental patterns of insulin-like growth factor-1 and 2 synthesis and regulation in rat fibroblasts, *Nature (London)*, 302, 150, 1983.

Baumann, G., Shaw, M. A., and Winter, R. J., Absence of the plasma growth hormone-binding protein in laron-type dwarfism, *J. Clin. Endocrinol. Metab.*, 65, 814, 1987.

Bayley, N. and Pinneau, S. R., Tables for predicting adult height from skeletal age: revised for use with the Greulich-Pyle hand standards, *J. Pediatr.*, 40, 432, 1952.

Beardsley, T., FDA ban on pituitary product, *Nature (London)*, 315, 358, 1985.

Beopple, P. A., Mansfield, M. J., Wierman, M., Rudlin, C. R., Bode, H. H., Crigler, J. F., Crawford, J. D., and Crowley, W. F., Jr., Use of a potent, long-acting agonist of gonadotropin releasing hormone in the treatment of precocious puberty, *Endocrine Rev.*, 7, 24, 1986.

Beopple, P. A., Mansfield, M. J., Link, K., Crawford, J. D., Crigler, J. F., Jr., Kushner, D. C., Blizzard, R. M., and Crowley, W. F., Jr., Impact of sex steroids and their suppression on skeletal growth and maturation, *Am. J. Physiol.* 255 (*Endocrinol. Metab.*, 18), E559, 1988.

Bercu, B. B., Shulman, D., Root, A. W., and Spiliotis, B. E., Growth hormone (GH) provocative testing frequently does not reflect endogenous GH secretion, *J. Clin. Endocrinol. Metab.*, 63, 709, 1986.

Bierich, J. R., Estrogen treatment of girls with constitutional tall stature, *Pediatrics*, 62, 1196, 1978.

Blumberg, D. L., Sklar, C. A., David, R., Rothenberg, S., and Bell, J., Acromegaly in an infant, *Pediatrics*, 83, 998, 1989.

Borges, J. L., Blizzard, R. M., Evans, W. D., Furlanetto, R., Rogol, A. D., Kaiser, D. L., Rivier, J., Vale, W., and Thorner, M. O., Stimulation of growth hormone (GH) and somatomedin C in idiopathic GH-deficient subjects by intermittent pulsatile administration of synthetic human pancreatic tumor GH-releasing factor, *J. Clin. Endocrinol. Metab.*, 59, 1, 1984.

Brook, C. G. D., Growth hormone deficiency in Turner's syndrome, *N. Engl. J. Med.*, 298, 1203, 1987.

Brook, C. G. D., Murset, G. Zachmann, M., and Prader, A., Growth in children with 45, XO Turner's syndrome, *Arch. Dis. Child.*, 49, 789, 1974.

Campos, S. P. and MacGillivray, M. H., Sex steroids do not influence somatic growth in childhood, *Am. J. Dis. Child.*, 143, 942, 1989.

Cara, J. F., Rosenfeld, R. L., and Furlanetto, R. W., A longitudinal study of the relationship of plasma somatomedin-C concentration to the pubertal growth spurt, *Am. J. Dis. Child.*, 141, 562, 1987.

Cara, J. F., Burstein, S., Cuttler, L., Moll, G. W., and Rosenfield, R. L., Growth hormone deficiency impedes the rise in plasma insulin-like growth factor I levels associated with precocious puberty, *J. Pediatr.*, 115, 64, 1989.

Castro-Magana, M., Angulo, M., Fuentes, B., Castelar, M. E., Canas, A., and Espinoza, B., Effect of prolonged clonidine administration on growth hormone concentrations and rate of linear growth in children with constitutional growth delay, *J. Pediatr.*, 109, 784, 1986.

Chalew, S. A., Raiti, S., Armour, K. M., and Kowarski, A., Therapy in short children with subnormal concentrations of growth hormone, *Am. J. Dis. Child.*, 141, 1195, 1987.

Clemmons, D. R., Underwood, L. E., Ridgway, R. C., Kliman, B., Kjellberg, R. N., and Van Wyk, J. J., Estradiol treatment of acromegaly: reduction in immunoreactive somatomedin-C and improvement in metabolic status, *J. Clin. Endocrinol. Metab.*, 69, 571, 1980.

Comite, F., Shawker, T. H., Pescovitz, O. H., Loriaux, D. L., and Cutler, G. B., Jr., Autonomous ovarian function resistant to luteinizing hormone releasing hormone analog therapy in McCune-Albright syndrome, *N. Engl. J. Med.*, 311, 1032, 1984.

Comite, F., Cassorla, F., Dwyer, A., Hench, K., Skerda, M., Cutler, G. B., Jr., Loriaux, D. L., and Pescovitz, O. H., Luteinizing hormone releasing hormone (LHRH) analogue therapy in central precocious puberty: long-term effect on somatic growth, bone maturation and height prediction, *JAMA*, 255, 2613, 1986.

Costin, G., Kaufman, F. R., and Brasel, J. A., Growth hormone secretory dynamics in subjects with normal stature, *J. Pediatr.*, 115, 537, 1989.

Counts, D. R., Pescovitz, O. H., Barnes, K. M., Chrousos, G. P., Sherins, R. J., Comite, F., and Cutler, G. B., Jr., Dissociation of adrenarche and gonadarche in patients with precocious puberty and hypogonadotrophic hypogonadism, *J. Clin. Endocrinol. Metab.*, 64, 1174, 1987.

Crawford, J. D., Treatment of tall girls with estrogen, *Pediatrics*, 62, 1189, 1978.

Cuttler, L., Van Vliet, G., Conte, F. A., Kaplan, S. L., and Grumbach, M. M., Somatomedin-C levels in children and adolescents with gonadal dysgenesis: differences from age-matched normal females and effect of chronic estrogen replacement therapy, *J. Clin. Endocrinol. Metab.*, 60, 1087, 1985.

Donaldson, D. L., Hollowell, J. G., Pan, F. P., Gifford, R. A., and Moore, W. V., Growth hormone secretory profiles: variation on consecutive nights, *J. Pediatr.*, 115, 51, 1989.

Duke, E. M. C., Hussein, D. M., and Hamilton, W., Turner's syndrome associated with growth hormone deficiency, *Scott. Med. J.*, 26, 240, 1981.

Egli, C. A., Rosenthal, S. M., Grumbach, M. M., Montalvo, J. M., and Gondos, B., Pituitary gonadotropin-independent male-limited autosomal dominant sexual precocity in nine generations: familial testotoxicosis, *J. Pediatr.*, 106, 33, 1985.

Esch, F. S., Bohlen, P., Ling, N. C., Brazeau, P. E., Wehrenberg, W. B., and Guillemin, R., Primary structures of three human pancreas peptides with growth hormone releasing activity, *J. Biol. Chem.*, 258, 1806, 1983.

Feuillan, P., Foster, C., Pescovitz, O. H., Hench, K., Shawker, T., Loriaux, D. L., and Cutler, G. B., Jr., Treatment of precocious puberty in McCune-Albright syndrome with the aromatase inhibitor: testolactone, *N. Engl. J. Med.*, 315, 1115, 1986.

Foster, C. M., Ross, J. L., Shawker, T., Pescovitz, O. H., Loriaux, D. L., Cutler, G. B., Jr., and Comite, F., Absence of pubertal gonadotropin secretion in girls with McCune-Albright syndrome, *J. Clin. Endocrinol. Metab.*, 58, 1161, 1984a.

Foster, C. M., Comite, F., Pescovitz, O. H., Ross, J. L., Loriaux, D. L., and Cutler, G. B., Jr., Variable response to a long-acting analog of LHRH in girls with McCune-Albright syndrome, *J. Clin. Endocrinol. Metab.,* 59, 801, 1984b.

Foster, C., Pescovitz, O. H., Comite, F., Feuillan, P., Shawker, T., Loriaux, D. L., and Cutler, G. B., Jr., Testolactone treatment of precocious puberty in McCune-Albright syndrome, *Acta Endocrinol.,* 109, 254, 1985.

Foster, C. M., Feuillan, P., Padmanabhan, V., Pescovitz, O. H., Beitins, I. Z., Comite, F., Shawker, T. H., Loriaux, D. L., and Cutler, G. B., Jr., Plasma estradiol levels and ovarian volume in girls with McCune-Albright syndrome, *Pediatr. Res.,* 20, 859, 1986.

Frasier, S. D., Hilburn, J. M., and Smith, F. G., Effect of adolescence on the serum growth hormone response to hypoglycemia, *J. Pediatr.,* 77, 465, 1970.

Gelato, M. C., Pescovitz, O., Cassorla, F., Loriaux, D. L., and Merriam, G. R., The effects of a growth hormone releasing factor in man, *J. Clin. Endocrinol. Metab.,* 57, 674, 1983.

Gelato, M. C., Ross, J. L., Malozowski, S., Pescovitz, O. H., Skerda, M., Cassorla, F., Loriaux, D. L., and Merriam, G. R., Effects of pulsatile administration of growth hormone (GH)-releasing hormone on short-term linear growth in children with GH deficiency, *J. Clin. Endocrinol. Metab.,* 61, 44, 1985.

Gelato, M. C., Malozowski, S., Nicoletti, M. C., Ross, J. R., Pescovitz, O. H., Rose, S., Loriaux, D. L., Cassorla, F., and Merriam, G. R., Growth hormone responses to growth hormone-releasing hormone during pubertal development in normal boys and girls: comparison to idiopathic short stature and growth hormone deficiency, *J. Clin. Endocrinol. Metab.,* 63, 174, 1986.

Gelato, M. C., Malozowski, S., Pescovitz, O. H., Cassorla, F., Loriaux, D. L., and Merriam, G. R., Growth hormone-releasing hormone: therapeutic perspectives, *Pediatrician,* 14, 162, 1988.

Genentech Collaborative Study Group, Idiopathic short stature: results of a one-year controlled study of human growth hormone treatment, *J. Pediatr.,* 115, 713, 1989.

Grossman, Z., Wass, J. A. H., Suireas-Diaz, J., Savage, M. O., Lytras, N., Coy, D. H., and Besser, G. M., Growth-hormone-releasing factor in growth hormone deficiency: demonstration of a hypothalamic defect in growth hormone release, *Lancet,* 1, 137, 1983.

Guillemin, R., Brazeau, P., Bohlen, P., Esch, F., Ling, N., and Wehrenberg, W. B., Growth hormone releasing factor from a human pancreatic tumor that caused acromegaly, *Science,* 218, 585, 1982.

Harris, D. A., Van Vliet, G., Egli, C. A., Grumbach, M. M., Kaplan, S. L., and Styne, D. M., Somatomedin-C in normal puberty and in true precocious puberty before and after treatment with a potent luteinizing hormone-releasing hormone agonist, *J. Clin. Endocrinol. Metab.,* 61, 152, 1985.

Holland, F. J., Fishman, L., Bailey, J. D., and Fazekas, A. T. A., Ketoconazole in the management of precocious puberty unresponsive to LHRH-analogue therapy, *N. Engl. J. Med.,* 312, 1023, 1985.

Huseman, C. A. and Hassing, J. M., Evidence of dopaminergic stimulation of growth velocity in some hypopituitary children, *J. Clin. Endocrinol. Metab.,* 58, 419, 1984.

Illig, R. and Prader, A., Effect of testosterone on growth hormone secretion in patients with anorchia and delayed puberty, *J. Clin. Endocrinol.,* 30, 615, 1970.

Isaksson, O. G. P., Lindahl, A., Nilsson, A., and Isgaard, J., Mechanism of the stimulatory effect of growth hormone on longitudinal bone growth, *Endocrine Rev.,* 8, 426, 1987.

Isgaard, J., Nilsson, A., Lindahl, A., Jansson, J.-O., and Isaksson, O. G. P., Effects of local administration of GH and IGF-I on longitudinal bone growth in rats, *Am. J. Physiol.,* 250, E367, 1986.

Johanson, A. J., Brasel, J. A., and Blizzard, R. M., Growth in patients with gonadal dysgenesis receiving fluoxymesterone, *J. Pediatr.,* 75, 1015, 1969.

Joss, E. and Zuppinger, K., Oxandrolone in girls with Turner's syndrome: a pair-matched controlled study up to final height, *Acta Paediatr. Scand.,* 73, 674, 1984.

Kaplowitz, P. B. and Jennings, S., Enhancement of linear growth and weight gain by cyproheptadine in children with hypopituitarism receiving growth hormone therapy, *J. Pediatr.,* 110, 140, 1987.

Koch, B. H., Lippe, B. M., Nelson, P. A., Boechat, M. I., Sherman, B. M., and Fine, R. N., Accelerated growth after recombinant human growth hormone treatment of children with chronic renal failure (CRF), *J. Pediatr.,* 115, 365, 1989.

Laczi, F., Julesz, J., Janaky, T., and Laszlo, F. A., Growth hormone reserve capacity in Turner's syndrome, *Horm. Metab. Res.,* 11, 664, 1979.

Lanes, R., Plotnick, L. P., and Lee, P. A., Sustained effect of human growth hormone therapy on children with intrauterine growth retardation, *Pediatrics,* 63, 731, 1979.

Laue, L., Kenigsberg, D., Pescovitz, O. H., Hench, K. D., Barnes, K. M., Loriaux, D. L., and Cutler, G. B., Jr., The treatment of familial male precocious puberty with spironolactone and testolactone, *N. Engl. J. Med.,* 320, 496, 1989.

Lev-Ran, A., Androgens, estrogens, and the ultimate height in XO gonadal dysgenesis, *Am. J. Dis. Child.,* 131, 648, 1977.

Lin, T. H., Kirkland, R. T., Sherman, B. M., and Kirkland, J. L., Growth hormone testing in short children and their response to growth hormone therapy, *J. Pediatr.,* 115, 57, 1989.

Luder, A. S., Holland, F. J., Costigan, D. C., Jenner, M. R., Wielgosz, G., and Fazekas, A. T. A., Intranasal and subcutaneous treatment of central precocious puberty with a long-acting analogue of luteinizing hormone-releasing hormone, *J. Clin. Endocrinol. Metab.,* 58, 966, 1984.

Luna, A. M., Wilson, D. M. Wibbelsmann, C. J., Brown, R. C., Nagashima, R. J., Hintz, R. L., and Rosenfeld, R. G., Somatomedins in adolescence: a cross-sectional study of the effect of puberty on plasma insulin-like growth factor I and II levels, *J. Clin. Endocrinol. Metab.,* 57, 268, 1983.

Manasco, P. K., Pescovitz, O. H., Feuillan, P. P., Barnes, K. M., Jones, J., Hill, S. C., Loriaux, D. L., and Cutler, G. B., Jr., Resumption of puberty after long-term luteinizing hormone releasing hormone agonist treatment of central precocious puberty, *J. Clin. Endocrinol. Metab.,* 67, 368, 1988.

Manasco, P. K., Pescovitz, O. H., Hill, S. C., Jones, J. M., Barnes, K. M., Hench, K. D., Loriaux, D. L., and Cutler, G. B., Six-year results of luteinizing hormone-releasing hormone (LHRH) agonist treatment in children with LHRH-dependent precocious puberty, *J. Pediatr.,* 115, 105, 1989.

Mansfield, M. J., Beardsworth, D. E., Loughlin, J. S., Crawford, J. D., Bode, H. H., Rivier, J., Vale, W., Kushner, D. C., Crigler, J. F., and Crowley, W. F., Jr., Long-term treatment of central precocious puberty with a long-acting analogue of luteinizing hormone-releasing hormone, *N. Engl. J. Med.,* 309, 1286, 1983.

Martin, L. G., Clark, J. W., and Conner, T. B., Growth hormone secretion enhanced by androgens, *J. Clin. Endocrinol. Metab.,* 28, 425, 1968.

Merimee, T. J. and Fineberg, S. E., Studies of the sex based variation of human growth hormone secretion, *J. Clin. Endocrinol.,* 33, 896, 1971.

Miller, W. L. and Eberhardt, N. L., Structure and evaluation of the growth hormone gene family, *Annu. Rev. Med.,* 34, 519, 1983.

Moll, G. W., Jr., Rosenfield, R. L., and Fang, V. S., Administration of low dose estrogen rapidly and directly stimulates growth hormone production, *Am. J. Dis. Child.,* 140, 124, 1968.

Muller, E. E., Neural control of somatotropic function, *Physiol. Rev.,* 67, 962, 1987.

Oberfield, S. E., Allen, J. C., Pollack, J., New, M. I., and Levine, L. S., Long term endocrine sequelae after treatment of medulloblastoma: prospective study of growth and thyroid function, *J. Pediatr.,* 108, 219, 1986.

Pankin, J. M., Incidence of growth hormone deficiency, *Arch. Dis. Child.,* 49, 905, 1974.

Parker, M. W., Johanson, A. J., Rogol, A. D., Kaiser, D. L., and Blizzard, R. M., Effect of testosterone on somatomedin-C concentrations in prepubertal boys, *J. Clin. Endocrinol. Metab.,* 58, 87, 1984.

Pescovitz, O. H. and Tan, E., Clonidine therapy of non-growth hormone deficient short stature, *Lancet,* 2, 874, 1988.

Pescovitz, O. H., Comite, F., Cassorla, F., Dwyer, A. J., Poth, M. A., Sperling, M., Hench, K., McNemar, A., Skerda, M., Loriaux, D. L., and Cutler, G. B., Jr., True precocious puberty complicating congenital adrenal hyperplasia: treatment with a luteinizing hormone releasing hormone analogue, *J. Clin. Endocrinol. Metab.,* 58, 857, 1984.

Pescovitz, O. H., Comite, F., Hench, K., Green, O., Loriaux, D. L., and Cutler, G. B., Jr., Central precocious puberty complicating a virilizing adrenal tumor: treatment with a long-acting LHRH analog, *J. Pediatr.,* 106, 612, 1985a.

Pescovitz, O. H., Rosenfeld, R. G., Hintz, R. L., Comite, F., Barnes, K., Hench, K., Loriaux, D. L., and Cutler, G. B., Jr., The role of somatomedin C and sex steroids in the accelerated growth of precocious puberty, *J. Pediatr.,* 107, 20, 1985b.

Pescovitz, O. H., Comite, F., Hench, K., Barnes, K., McNemar, A., Foster, C., Kenigsberg, D., Loriaux, D. L., and Cutler, G. B., Jr., The NIH experience in precocious puberty: diagnostic subgroups and the response to short-term LHRH analogue therapy, *J. Pediatr.*, 108, 47, 1986.

Pescovitz, O. H., Hench, K., Barnes, K., Loriaux, D. L., and Cutler, G. B., Jr., Premature thelarche and central precocious puberty: a comparative study, *J. Clin. Endocrinol. Metab.*, 67, 474, 1988.

Phillips, J. A., Genetic diagnosis: differentiating growth disorders, *Hosp. Pract.*, 20, 85, 1985.

Pintor, G., Cella, S. G., Corda, R., Locatelli, V., Loche, S., Puggioni, R., and Muller, E. E., Clonidine accelerates growth in children with impaired growth hormone secretion, *Lancet*, 1, 1482, 1985.

Pintor, G., Loche, S., Corda, R., and Muller, E. E., Clonidine treatment for short stature, *Lancet*, 2, 1191, 1988.

Plotnick, L. P., Thompson, R. G., Beitins, I., and Blizzard, R. M., Integrated concentrations of growth hormone correlated with stage of puberty and estrogen levels in girls, *J. Clin. Endocrinol. Metab.*, 38, 436, 1974.

Prader, A. and Zachmann, M., Treatment of excessively tall girls and boys with sex hormones, *Pediatrics*, 62, 1202, 1978.

Reiter, E. O., Morris, A. H., MacGillivray, M. H., and Weber, D. A., Variable estimates of serum growth hormone concentrations by different radioassay systems, *J. Clin. Endocrinol. Metab.*, 66, 68, 1988.

Richards, G. E., Wara, W. M., Grumbach, M. M., Kaplan, S. L., Sheline, G. E., and Conte, F. A., Delayed onset of hypopituitarism: sequelae of therapeutic irradiation of central nervous system, eye, and middle ear tumors, *J. Pediatr.*, 89, 553, 1976.

Rivier, J., Spiess, J., Thorner, M., and Vale, W., Characterization of a growth hormone releasing factor from a human pancreatic islet tumour, *Nature (London)*, 300, 276, 1982.

Roche, A. F., Wainer, H., and Thissen, D., The RWT method for the prediction of adult stature, *Pediatrics*, 56, 1026, 1975.

Rogol, A. D., Blizzard, R. M., Johanson, A. J., Furlanetto, R., Evans, W. S., Rivier, J., Vale, W., and Thorner, M. O., Growth hormone release in response to human pancreatic tumor growth hormone-releasing hormone-40 in children with short stature, *J. Clin. Endocrinol. Metab.*, 59, 580, 1984.

Rose, S. R., Ross, J. L., Uriarte, M., Barnes, K. M., Cassorla, F. G., and Cutler, G. B., Jr., The advantage of measuring stimulated as compared with spontaneous growth hormone levels in the diagnosis of growth hormone deficiency, *N. Engl. J. Med.*, 319, 201, 1988a.

Rose, S. R., Kibarian, M., Gelato, M., Ross, J. L., Turek, J., Gay, K., Merriam, G. R., Cutler, G. B., Jr., and Cassorla, F., Sex steroids increase spontaneous growth hormone secretion in short children, *J. Pediatr. Endocrinol.*, 3, 1, 1988b.

Rosenbloom, A. L. and Frias, J. L., Oxandrolone for growth promotion in Turner syndrome, *Am. J. Dis. Child.*, 125, 385, 1973.

Rosenfeld, R. G., *Turner Syndrome: A Guide for Physicians*, The Turner's Syndrome Society, 1989.

Rosenfeld, R. G., Hintz, R. L., Johanson, A. J., Sherman, B., Brasel, J. A., Burstein, S., Chernausek, S., Compton, P., Frane, J., Gotlin, R. W., Kuntze, J., Lippe, B. M., Mahoney, P. C., Moore, W. V., New, M. I., Saenger, P., and Sybert, V., Three year results of methionyl growth hormone and oxandrolone in Turner syndrome, *J. Pediatr.*, 113, 393, 1988.

Rosenfield, R. L., Furlanetto, R., and Bock, D., Relationship of somatomedin-C concentrations to pubertal changes, *J. Pediatr.*, 103, 723, 1983.

Rosenfield, R. L. and Furlanetto, R., Physiologic testosterone or estradiol induction of puberty increases plasma somatomedin-C, *J. Pediatr.*, 107, 415, 1985.

Rosenthal, S. M., Grumbach, M. M., and Kaplan, S. L., Gonadotropin-independent familial sexual precocity with premature Leydig and germinal cell maturation (familial testotoxicosis); effects of a potent luteinizing hormone-releasing factor agonist and medroxyprogesterone acetate therapy in four cases, *J. Clin. Endocrinol. Metab.*, 57, 571, 1983.

Ross, J. L., Long, L. M., Loriaux, D. L., and Cutler, G. B., Jr., Growth hormone secretory dynamics in Turner syndrome, *J. Pediatr.*, 106, 202, 1985.

Ross, J. L., Long, L. M., Skerda, M., Cassorla, F., Kurtz, D., Loriaux, D. L. and Cutler, G. B., Jr., Effect of low doses of estradiol on 6-month growth rates and predicted height in patients with Turner syndrome, *J. Pediatr.*, 109, 950, 1986.

Ross, J. L., Pescovitz, O. H., Barnes, K., Loriaux, D. L., and Cutler, G. B., Jr., Growth hormone secretory dynamics in children with precocious puberty, *J. Pediatr.*, 110, 369, 1987.

Ross, R. J. M., Tsgarakis, S., Grossman, A., Preece, M. A., Rodda, C., Davies, P. S. W., Rees, L. H., Savage, M. O., and Besser, G. M., Treatment of growth-hormone deficiency with growth-hormone-releasing hormone, *Lancet*, 7, 5, 1987.

Russell, S. M. and Spencer, E. M., Local injections of human or rat growth hormone or of purified human somatomedin-C stimulate unilateral tibial epiphyseal growth in hypophysectomized rats, *Endocrinology*, 116, 2563, 1985.

Salmon, W. D., Jr. and Daughaday, W. H., A hormonally controlled serum factor which stimulates sulfate incorporation by cartilage in vitro, *J. Lab. Clin. Med.*, 49, 825, 1957.

Schriock E. A., Lustig, R. H., Rosenthal, S. M., Kaplan, S. L., and Grumbach, M., Effect of growth hormone (GH)-releasing hormone (GRH) on plasma GH in relation to magnitude and duration of GH deficiency or multiple pituitary hormone deficiencies: evidence for hypothalamic GRH deficiency, *J. Clin. Endocrinol. Metab.*, 58, 1043, 1984.

Shalett, S. M., Beardwell, C. G., Morris-Jones, P. H., and Pearson, D., Growth hormone deficiency after treatment of acute leukemia in children, *Arch. Dis. Child.*, 51, 489, 1976.

Sigurjonsdottir, T. J. and Hayles, A. B., Precocious puberty. A report of 96 cases, *Am. J. Dis. Child.*, 115, 309, 1968.

Sklar, C. A., Kaplan, S. L., and Grumbach, M. M., Evidence for dissociation between adrenarche and gonadarche: studies in patient with idiopathic precocious puberty, gonadal dysgenesis, isolated gonadotropin deficiency, and constitutionally delayed growth and adolescence, *J. Clin. Endocrinol. Metab.*, 51, 548, 1980.

Spiliotis, B. E., August, G. P., Hung, W., Sonis, W., and Mendelson, W., Growth hormone neurosecretory dysfunction, *JAMA*, 251, 2223, 1984.

Stanhope, R. and Brook, C. G. D., The effect of gonadotrophin releasing hormone analogue on height prognosis in growth hormone deficiency and normal puberty, *Eur. J. Pediatr.*, 148, 200, 1988.

Styne, D. M., Delayed puberty, in *Growth Abnormalities*, Hintz, R. L. and Rosenfled, R. G., Eds., Churchill Livingstone, New York, 1987, 141.

Styne, D. M., Harris, D. A., Egli, C. A., Conte, F. A., Kaplan, S. L., Rivier, J., Vale, W., and Grumbach, M. M., Treatment of true precocious puberty with a potent luteinizing hormone-releasing factor agonist: effect on growth, sexual maturation, pelvic sonography, and the hypothalamic-pituitary-gonadal axis, *J. Clin. Endocrinol. Metab.*, 61, 142, 1986.

Takano, K., Hizuka, N., Shizume, K., Asakawa, K., Miyakawa, M., Hirase, N., Shibasaki, T., and Ling, N. C., Plasma growth hormone (GH) response to GH-releasing factor in normal children with short stature and patients with pituitary dwarfism, *J. Clin. Endocrinol. Metab.*, 58, 236, 1984.

Takano, K., Hizuka, N., Shizume, K., Honda, N., and Ling, N. C., Plasma growth hormone (GH) responses to single and repetitive administration of GH releasing factor (hpGRF-44) in normal and GH deficient children, *Acta Endocrinol.*, 108, 11, 1985.

Tanner, J. M., Whitehouse, R. H., Marshall, W. A., Healy, M. J. R., and Goldstein, H., *Assessment of Skeletal Maturity and Prediction of Adult Height. (TW2 Method)*, Academic Press, London, 1975.

Thompson, R. G., Rodriguez, A., Kowarski, A., Migeon, C. J., and Blizzard, R. M., Integrated concentrations of growth hormone correlated with plasma testosterone and bone age in preadolescent and adolescent males, *J. Clin. Endocrinol. Metab.*, 35, 334, 1972.

Thorner, M. O., Reschke, J., Chitwood, J., Rogol, A. D., Furlanetto, R., Rivier, J., Vale, W., and Blizzard, R. M., Acceleration of growth in two children with human growth hormone-releasing factor, *N. Engl. J. Med.*, 312, 1985.

Thorner, M. O., Rogol, A. D., Blizzard, R. M., Klingensmith, G. J., Najjar, J., Misra, R., Burr, I., Chao, G., Martha, P., McDonald, J., Pezzoli, S., Chitwood, J., Furlanetto, R., Rivier, J., Vale, W., Smith, P., and Brook, C., Acceleration of growth rate in growth-hormone deficient children treated with human growth-hormone-releasing hormone, *Pediatr. Res.*, 24, 145, 1988.

Urban, M. D., Lee, P. A., Dorst, J. P., Plotnick, L. P., and Migeon, C. J., Oxandrolone therapy in patients with Turner syndrome, *J. Pediatr.*, 94, 823, 1979.

Van Wyk, J. J., *Hormonal Proteins and Peptides*, Academic Press, New York, 1984, 81.

Weidemann, E., Schwartz, F., and Frantz, A. G., Acute and chronic estrogen effects upon serum somatomedin activity, growth hormone and prolactin in man, *J. Clin. Endocrinol. Metab.*, 42, 942, 1976.

Wierman, M. E., Beardsworth, D. E., Mansfield, M. J., Badger, T. M., Crawford, J. D., Crigler, J. F., Bode, H. H., Loughlin, J. S., Kushner, D. C., Scully, R. E., Hoffman, W. H., and Crowley, W. F., Puberty without gonadotropins: a unique mechanism of sexual development, *N. Engl. J. Med.*, 312, 65, 1985.

Winter, R. J. and Green, O. C., Irradiation-induced growth hormone deficiency: blunted growth response and accelerated skeletal maturation to growth hormone therapy, *J. Pediatr.*, 106, 609, 1985.

Zachmann, M., Ferrandez, A., Murset, G., Gnehm, H. E., and Prader, A., Testosterone treatment of excessively tall boys, *J. Pediatr.*, 88, 116, 1976.

Zadik, Z., Chalew, S. A., McCarter, R. J., Meitas, M., and Kowarski, A. A., The influence of age on the 24-hour integrated concentration of growth hormone in normal individuals, *J. Clin. Endocrinol. Metab.*, 60, 513, 1985.

Zapf, J., Waldvogel, M., and Froesch, E. R., Binding of nonsuppressible insulin-like activity to human serum: evidence for a carrier protein, *Arch. Biochem. Biophys.*, 168, 638, 1975.

18

Reproductive Hormones and Behavior

FRAN E. KAISER AND JOHN E. MORLEY
Division of Geriatric Medicine
St. Louis University Medical Center, and
Geriatric Research, Education, and Clinical Center
St. Louis Veterans Affairs Medical Center
St. Louis, Missouri

Aretaeus of Cappadocia suggested nearly 2000 years ago that hormones affect behavior:

For it is the semen, when possessed of vitality, which makes us to be men, not well braced in limbs, hairy, well voiced, spirited, strong to think and to act, as the characteristics of men prove. For when the semen is not possessed of its vitality, persons become shrivelled, have a sharp tone of voice, lose their hair and their beard, and become effeminate, as the characteristics of eunuchs prove.

The role of hormones and behavior remains an area of much controversy. Subjective assessments, lack of validated measures, and lack of uniformity in the outcome measures have made this a difficult area to assess at best. Our knowledge is rudimentary and the connections between reproductive hormones and other transmitters or effectors that influence behavior, those known and yet to be discovered, remain to be elucidated.

Data regarding prenatal exposure to hormones and their effects on behavior are compelling, but in humans, the assumption that prenatal hormonal exposure affects gender role and gender identity has fallen into question. The suggestion that "you are what you secrete" may not ring as true in humans as in other species. Prenatal testosterone administration has been shown to increase post-partum aggression in female mice, and aggressive behavior in both male and female mice (Saal, 1979; Mann and Svare, 1983). Even proximity to testosterone has been thought to play a role in behavior, with female mice who are positioned between male siblings *in utero* displaying evidence of masculinization and "male" characteristics as adults, with greater aggressive behavior than other females, and increased urinary territorial marking (Saal and Bronson, 1986). In other species, such as rhesus macaques, prenatally androgenized females (treated with testosterone) are born with male genital structures (penis, scrotum, and lack of a vagina) and have behavior that is considered masculine. This masculine behavior includes (if the animal is ovariectomized and further treated with testosterone) male mounting patterns with receptive females, and even ejaculation (Eaton et al., 1973). Furthermore, if prenatally androgenized female monkeys are later treated with estradiol, and are paired with males, these hermaphroditic females were as receptive to male overtures as female control monkeys, indicating hormonal modulation of behavior (Phoenix et al., 1984). Estrogenic effects or the use of antiandrogens can result in a "female" pattern of behavior, and even early estradiol administration to 4-day-old rats will increase female rat behavior (ear wiggling and lordosis) 44 hr later (Williams, 1986; Gladue and Clemens, 1978).

Sexual dimorphism, or the association of certain behaviors with one sex or the other, has been thought to result from prenatal or perinatal exposure to gonadal to gonadal hormones

(Phoenix et al., 1959; McEwen, 1983; MacLusky and Naftolin, 1981; Toran-Alherand, 1980; Feder, 1981; Gorski et al., 1978; Arnold and Gorski, 1984). Neuroanatomic correlates of sexual dimorphism have been described in rat brains. Areas of the brain that seem to be involved in this process include sites at or near areas of gonadotrophic regulation such as the hypothalamus, amygdala, and preoptic areas, with changes in dendritic growth, and cell nuclei showing gender-related differences (MacLusky and Naftolin, 1981; Toran-Alherand, 1980). In rat brain, for example, there are fewer preoptic nonamygdaloid synapses in male rats than in female rats. Evidence of sexual dimorphism has been found in human brain with a larger posterior corpus collosum in females than in males (deLacoste-Utamsing and Holloway, 1982). Which gonadal hormones are involved in this sexual dimorphism remain to be fully elucidated (McEwen, 1981). Testosterone and estrogen enhance preoptic region neuritic proliferation, whereas the administration of 5α-dihydrotestosterone has no effect. Aromatization of androgens, conversion to estrogen, and/or the ratio of androgens to estrogens appears to play an important role in sexual dimorphism (Toran-Alherand, 1980; Beyer et al., 1976; Morali et al., 1977).

These sexually dimorphic changes may have behavioral correlates, most notably in species other than human. Male songbirds are capable of singing, while females are not. It has been shown that selective androgen uptake in brain areas associated with singing fosters the sexual diversity in this event (Konishi, 1985). In humans, it is difficult to ascertain whether the early (pre- and perinatal) hormonal milieu exerts influence on behavior. With prenatal exposure to androgens, such as one sees in congenital adrenal hyperplasia (the most common cause of female pseudohermaphroditism) or with early progesterone exposure, there have been reports of increased "masculine" (tomboyish) behavior (Ehrhardt et al., 1968a, b). Dalton (1968) reported attainment of developmental milestones, such as standing and walking, in 1-year-old children whose mothers had been treated with progestational agents for toxemia of pregnancy.

Measures of timidity in children (using response to novel toys) followed longitudinally and assessed in 6- to 18-month old children also appeared to be related to hormones. In male children, an inverse correlation was found to exist between cord concentrations of testosterone and progesterone vs. expression of timidity, whereas cord estradiol concentrations were positively related to timidity. No such correlation could be found in female children (Jacklin et al., 1983).

A role for testosterone in self-reported aggressive behavior in adolescent males has been noted (Olweus et al., 1988). In this study, items that involved a response to provocation and lower frustration levels appeared to correlate to testosterone concentrations among Swedish male teenagers (Olweus et al., 1988). Unfortunately, this was not examined in a group of comparable Swedish female teenagers.

As society alters its views of specific "male and female" behaviors, and greater fluidity and shifting of roles for both genders occurs in various societies, this area of "gender-specific behaviors" is bound to undergo even further change.

I. Gender Identity (Karyotypes and Gonadal Sex)

The first aspect of gender identity begins with the genetic sex of an individual, which is determined at the time of conception (see Table 1). Gonadal sex begins when the undifferentiated (unisex) gonad — either through the effect of the H-Y antigen or other Y-linked or autosomal genes (or their absence), causes the gonad to develop into either a testis or ovary (Wachtel et al., 1975; Simpson, 1982). Expression of the H-Y antigen may result in testicular organogen-

Table 1
Components of Sexual Differentiation

Genetic sex
    Chromosomal determination
Gonadal sex
    Y chromosome and/or H-Y antigen
Ductular sex
    Male: regression of paramesonephric ducts due to anti-Müllerian hormone; development of epididymis,
        vas deferens, seminal vesicles due to testosterone
    Female: nonsuppression of Müllerian structures, resulting in uteran, fallopian tube, and upper vaginal
        development. Regression of Wolffian ducts
External sex
    Male
    Female
    Sexually ambiguous
Social (rearing) sexual orientation
Hormonal sex
Gender preference
Gender behavior

esis. However, it is likely that the H-Y antigen lacks some specificity in this role, as some female to male transsexuals, as well as some phenotypic females with gonadal dysgenesis, have been shown to possess an H-Y antigen (Wachtel et al., 1980; Eicher et al., 1979; Engel et al., 1980). In any event, external genital development in females results from an intrinsic tendency to feminize in the absence of androgenic stimulation, and masculinization occurs with the presence of androgenic stimulation by testosterone and 5-dihydrotestosterone (5-DHT) by the 12th fetal week. Similar levels of plasma estradiol are found in the male and female fetus. Internal ductular sex results from stimulation of Wolffian duct development in the male by testosterone, and regression of Müllerian duct development by Sertoli cell secretion of anti-Müllerian hormone.

It is beyond the scope of this chapter to fully cover all causes and manifestations of abnormal sexual development, and Table 2 lists an abbreviated classification of problems with sexual development.

Chromosomal abnormalities occur in 1 of 200 newborns. Klinefelter's syndrome with an XXY or variant pattern can range from nearly normal gonadal function in individuals with mosaicism to levels of testosterone that are exceedingly low, while serum and urinary gonadotropins are elevated. A higher prevalence of mental retardation has been found with Klinefelter's syndrome (Ferguson-Smith, 1959). Walzer et al. (1978) noted that boys under the age of 3 years with the XXY pattern were more passive, and showed less activity than boys with normal karyotypes; while Bancroft and colleagues found XXY boys to rate themselves as more insecure, and with less self-esteem than control individuals (Bancroft et al., 1982). The presence of a second Y chromosome, as well as other chromosomal abnormalities, can be associated with behavioral difficulties, but no direct evidence linking the Y chromosome to criminality has been found. Small clinical studies of testosterone administration to Klinefelter's patients suggest that self-reported social adjustment at work, concentration, and improvement of mood occurred during the period of therapy (Nielsen et al., 1988).

Male external genitalia generally lead to true hermaphrodites being reared as males (75%). A mutant gene, Y translocations, and/or mosaicism have been offered as explanations for this condition, in which there is presence of both ovarian and testicular tissue. At puberty, evidence of both virilization and feminization may occur (Butler et al., 1969; Simpson, 1976). Surgery to remove organs not concordant with the gender of rearing is indicated. Behavioral data are lacking in this group.

Table 2
Primary Sex Determination Abnormalities

Chromosomal abnormalities	Testicular
Male phenotype and testes	XY gonadal dysgenesis
Klinefelter's 47 XY and variants	Testicular regression syndromes
XYY	(agonadism, micropenis with rudimentary
XX males	testis)
Female phenotype and ovaries	Errors of sexual differentiation
Trisomy X and variants	Male pseudohermaphroditism
Bisexual gonads	Impaired Leydig cell activity
True hermaphrodites	Errors of testosterone biosynthesis
Mosaic/chimeric hermaphrodites	Impaired metabolism of androgens (5α-
Dysgenetic gonads	reductase deficiency)
Turners syndrome 45X and variants	Androgen insensitivity
Gonadal abnormalities	Female pseudohermaphroditism
Ovarian	Virilization by fetal androgens
Dysgenetic ovary, XX dysgenesis	Iatrogenic/maternal androgens
	Teratologic malformations

The suggestion that both gender identity and gender behavior are set by pre- and perinatal hormonal exposure (Money et al., 1957) has undergone much examination since the studies of 5α-reductase deficiency were reported (Walsh et al., 1974; Nowakowski and Lenz, 1961; Imperato-McGinley et al., 1974, 1979). These genetic males who have "pseudovaginal perineoscrotal hypospadias" are for the most part raised as females. During puberty, virilization occurs, with phallic enlargement, testicular descent, deepening of the voice, and increased muscle mass formation. At that time, these individuals change their sex of rearing and assigned gender sex from female to male. Once the male identity is assumed, the gender behavior of these individuals is male, and at least in Dominican society they are accepted as such (Imperato-McGinley et al., 1979).

Testicular feminization, the result of partial or total androgen receptor deficiency or a post-receptor defect, is thought to be the most common form of pseudohermaphroditism (Jagiello and Atwell, 1962; Amrheim et al., 1977; Griffin and Wilson, 1980). In complete testicular feminization, the external genitalia are unambiguously female. This syndrome is a cause of primary amenorrhea. These XY males have serum testosterone concentrations that are normal or higher than normal males. Luteinizing hormone is elevated, with insensitivity to androgen feedback at the hypothalamic level. Both estradiol production by the testis and aromatization of testosterone to estradiol result in the marked feminization at puberty. Due to the risk of testicular neoplasia, gonadectomy should be performed. In cases of incomplete testicular feminization syndrome, since virilization can occur at the time of puberty, the testes should be removed prior to puberty and estrogen therapy instituted. Normal female identity and behavior has been described in these individuals (Griffin and Wilson, 1980).

II. Gender and Sexual Orientation

The syndromes of congenital adrenal hyperplasia, testicular feminization, or 5α-reductase deficiency suggest that we are not necessarily what we secrete. "Hormonal predestination" had classically been used to assign sexual identity, and even the advocates of the role of rearing in determining sexual identity and behavior (Ellis, 1945; Money et al., 1955a, b), have had their viewpoints undergo change with the data on the 5α-reductase deficiency. However, the hormonal role in determining sexual orientation remains inconclusive. Dorner (1976, 1985) has suggested, based on rat models, that high pre- and perinatal exposure to androgens leads to organization of a "male" brain, resulting in mounting, intromission, and ejaculatory behavior; whereas if androgens are low, female sexual behavior (lordosis) would occur. Pre-eminence of a particular center (male or female) would lead to specific sexual orientation. Dorner categorized homosexuality as "central nervous system hermaphroditism." Human data have suggested that altered testosterone concentrations (elevated levels) may be associated with lesbianism (Gartrell et al., 1977; Meyer Bahlburg, 1979). However, other investigators have found no such association to exist, and no difference in testosterone and androstenedione levels between lesbian and heterosexual females (Downey et al., 1987). In fact, even in late-treated women with congenital adrenal hyperplasia, there is not a preponderance of lesbianism, despite the long-term exposure to high androgen levels (Ehrhardt, 1968b). Differences in response to a hormonal challenge (luteinizing hormone response to a single dose of estrogen) between male homosexuals and heterosexuals has been described, with homosexuals showing an increment in LH that was greater than that seen in heterosexual males (Dorner et al., 1975a, b; Gladue, 1984). This increase was felt to result from a "female" neuroendocrine system. Investigators of transsexuality have sought its pathogenesis in terms of a genetic and/or hormonal basis. Eicher et al. (1979) and Spoljar and colleagues (1981) have suggested a concordance between the presence of the H-Y antigen and desired sexual orientation, and discordance with anatomic sex. These data, however, have not been replicated by other groups. Dorner et al. found an increment in LH secretion in response to a single intravenous injection of estrogen in homosexual male to female transsexuals, compared to heterosexuals (Dorner, 1988). However, the response to this same stimulus in lesbian and female-to-male transsexuals was not different from that of heterosexual females (Gooren, 1986). Current concerns suggests that no genetic or hormonal markers exist for a particular sexual orientation.

III. Premenstrual Syndrome

Much has been written on the subject of the physical and behavioral aspects of the menstrual cycle (Green and Dalton, 1953; Coopen and Kessel, 1963; Moos et al., 1969; Reid and Yen, 1981). Disagreement exists not only about the pathogenesis and treatment of this disorder, but also the precise definition of premenstrual syndrome (PMS). Approximately 30% of menstruating women are thought to have PMS (Coopen and Kessel, 1963; Wood et al., 1979), with symptoms occurring primarily during the luteal phase, with improvement in many women occurring during menstrual flow. The luteal phase can be divided into early luteal phase, in which estradiol falls then rises to a second peak, while progesterone rises and peaks (generally recognized as the day after the LH peak until the day of the progesterone peak), and a late luteal phase, with a fall in estradiol and progesterone, which occurs from the day after progesterone peaks until the day before menstrual bleeding.

A variety of symptoms — from moodiness, anger, anxiety, and depression — as well as physical changes, including cramps, bloating, breast tenderness, and headaches, have been described (Logue and Moos, 1986; Rubinow et al., 1986; Mortola et al., 1989; Metcalf et al., 1990; Schecter et al., 1989; Osofsky and Blumenthal, 1985). In some individuals these signs and symptoms are extremely disabling. That "altered states" may arise secondary to PMS has been recognized, and it has been utilized as a defense in legal cases (Benedek, 1988). The pathophysiology of this syndrome has remained elusive, although a hormonal basis has long been sought (Munday et al., 1981; O'Brien et al., 1986). Sexual behavior can also alter throughout the menstrual cycle. Schreiner-Engel (1980), in a review of 32 studies of this area, found 17 of the studies reported increased sexual activity premenstrually, 18 reported increased activity postmentrually, 4 noted increased sexual activity during menstruation, while 8 increased activity at the time of ovulation. Bancroft and colleagues found maximal sexual activity at the midfollicular and late luteal phases of the menstrual cycle (Bancroft et al., 1983). Midcycle testosterone (either total or free) has been associated with an increased frequency of intercourse in some studies (Persky et al., 1978; Morris et al., 1987) but not in others (Bancroft et al., 1983). Schreiner-Engel has found altered vaginal blood flow in response to erotic stimuli, with lowest response occurring in midcycle and highest response on mid- to late luteal phase (1981). These responses positively correlated with testosterone concentrations.

When a GnRH agonist is used to abolish ovarian cycling by down regulating LH and FSH, improvement of symptoms occurs, suggesting a relationship between the reproductive steroids and observed behavioral changes (Muse et al., 1984). Recent data suggest that progesterone, at least when administered in a suppository form, does nothing in terms of altering symptoms (Freeman et al., 1990). Although both estrogens and progestins may change nerve cell electrical/chemical properties, and have behavioral effects, the mechanism(s) by which these steroids or ratios of these steroids produce their effects remains unknown (Pfaff and McEwen, 1983; Rubin et al., 1981).

IV. Aging, Behavior, and Reproductive Hormones

In the perimenstrual years, estrogen secretion diminishes, and estrone replaces estradiol as the major circulating estrogen. Inhibin production decreases, follicle-stimulating hormone (FSH) increases, and eventually, with further decrements in estradiol concentrations, LH rises. Negativism toward menopause has long been promulgated by medicine — as noted by Ballinger (1990); Tilt in 1857 associated menopause with evil effects of hysteria, irritability, and lowness of spirit (depression), concepts that are still fostered by some today. There are no hard data to show that menopause carries with it an increased risk of psychiatric disorders (Barbo, 1987; Dunnel and Cartwright, 1972; Ballinger, 1987). However, increases in complaints of night sweats and hot flashes are common, occurring in 65 to 75% of women who undergo spontaneous menopause (Mishell et al., 1986). These hot flashes can be accompanied by the sensation of pressure in the head, tachycardia, and sleep disturbances. The vasomotor changes that occur seem to relate to alterations in estrogen levels, rather than to any absolute estrogen concentration (Kaiser and Morley, 1990). Repletion with estrogen is the most effective therapy for these symptoms, but progestins, clonidine, and even naloxone have been utilized in the treatment of hot flashes.

Although decreased sexual activity may accompany menopause, this is not clearly linked to the hormonal changes that occur. Loss of partners or altered states of physical health, for example, may diminish sexual activity or interest. Some, but not all, studies suggest a beneficial effect of estrogen on libido, sexual enjoyment, and orgasmic frequency (Dennerstein et al., 1980; Fydor-Freyburgh, 1977; Campbell, 1976; Mazenord et al., 1988). Estrogen/testosterone administration has been shown to result in increased sexual desire, fantasy, and arousal in women, although testosterone levels were markedly above those considered physiologic for women (Sherwin, 1985; Sherwin and Gelfand, 1987). Estrogen plus testosterone therapy resulted in increased pleasure from masturbation compared with all other treatments (Myers et al., 1990).

A double-blind study utilizing estrogen, estrogen plus progesterone, estrogen plus testosterone, or placebo in post-menopausal women noted no change in mood or sexual behavior among the treatment groups (Myers et al., 1990). This would suggest that gonadal steroids do not play a major role in sexual functioning in women. Some studies have, however, suggested that small doses of testosterone may enhance libido in post-menopausal women (Salmon and Geist, 1943). Further studies to conform or disprove these data remain to be performed.

The role of sex steroids in older males is not any more clear than in post-menopausal women. In men, testosterone and bioavailable testosterone (non-SHBG bound) fall with age (Nankin and Calkin, 1986; Tenover et al., 1987; Kaiser et al., 1988). The true incidence of both primary and secondary hypogonadism in elderly males remains unknown; however, in our study, 2.8% of the population studied had primary testicular failure [luteinizing hormone (LH) > 20 mIU/ml, testosterone (T) < 300 ng/dl], 12% had secondary testicular failure (LH < 15 mIU/ml, and T < 300 ng/dl), and 8.3% had compensated testicular failure (LH > 20 mIU/ml, T > 300 ng/dl) (Kaiser et al., 1988). The clinical effects of low steroid levels may include such diverse phenomena as diminished energy level and altered libido (Mooradian et al., 1987). Given the prevalence of hypogonadism among the elderly found in our study, and the changes that low sex steroid levels can produce, hypogonadism may be considered a paradigm of aging in men.

The link between testosterone and erectile capability is less established than that between testosterone and libido. In male castrates sexual function may be retained in as many as 50% — they were capable of responding to erotic films with erections (Eibel, 1977, cited in Heim and Hursch, 1979). With aging, there is little or no decrease in libido (Kaiser et al., 1988; Bretschneider and McCoy, 1988; Seagraves et al., 1981). Despite this, sexual activity does decrease with age and may result from a variety of causes, including loss of a spouse, ill health, and impotence (Morley and Kaiser, 1989). The frequency of intercourse diminishes with aging and Pfeiffer et al. (1968) noted 95% of men ages 46 to 50 had intercourse once a week, while among men aged 66 to 71 only 28% had intercourse once a week and 24% had no intercourse at all. In men over 80 years old, in another study, 29% reported having intercourse weekly (Davidson et al., 1979).

In men diagnosed with hypogonadism (T < 150 ng/dl), treatment with testosterone resulted in both an increased number of erections as well as coitus, both of which were related to testosterone in a dose-dependent manner (Davidson et al., 1979). The relationship of hormones to sexual thoughts and enjoyment seems to involve free testosterone or free T:LH ratios at least in one study (Davidson et al., 1983). Whether these lowered hormone levels and altered hormonal ratios contribute to behavioral change, aging, morbidity or frailty, or mortality remains to studied.

Impotence in older males is usually not associated primarily with changes in gonadal hormones (Table 3) (Morley, 1986). The most common cause of impotence in males over 50 years of age is atherosclerotic vascular disease (Kaiser et al., 1988). Medications, such as thiazide diuretics and all classes of antihypertensives, are also important causes of impotence. Prolactin causes impotence by a mechanism that does not appear to involve its ability to lower testosterone levels. A psychological etiology as the primary cause of impotence occurs in less than 10% of older individuals, while psychological factors may be the primary etiology in 50% of impotent individuals under the age of 50. Treatment of impotence in the majority of older males may include the use of vacuum tumescent devices or penile prostheses. In some younger impotent males, penile intracorporeal injections of papaverine or prostaglandin E_1 may be an alternative therapy. Secondary performance anxiety is often present and requires counseling for both partners.

V. Conclusion

Much mythology exists concerning the role of reproductive hormones and behavior.

Table 3
Major Causes of Impotence

Vascular	Nutritional
Arterial	Obesity
Cavernous sinus leak	Zinc deficiency
Combination of arterial/venous disease	Neurologic
Medications	Multiple sclerosis
Thiazide diuretics	Stroke
Cimetidine	Temporal lobe epilepsy
Antihypertensive agents (all classes)	Spinal cord injury
Psychotropic agents	Autonomic neuropathy
Hormonal	Peripheral neuropathy
Hypogonadism	Systemic disease
Hyperprolactinemia	Liver diseae
Hypothyroidism/hyperthyroidism	Renal failure
Diabetes mellitus	Miscellaneous
	Peyronie's disease

While animal studies have clearly demonstrated effects of sex hormones on diverse behaviors such as singing in birds and aggression in mice, well-conducted studies demonstrating similar effects in humans are lacking. Clearly, environmental and psychological factors can greatly modify the role of hormonal factors in human behavior. The major effect of sex hormones in humans is on libido, and this effect seems to be greater in males than in females. There is a need for careful, unbiased studies in humans to define the role of reproductive hormones in behavior.

References

Amrhein, J. A., Klingensmith, G. J., Walsh, P. C., McKusick, V. A., and Migeon, C. J., Partial androgen insensitivity: the Reifenstein syndrome revisted, *N. Engl. J. Med.*, 297, 350, 1977.

Arnold, A. P. and Gorski, R. A., Gonadal steroid induction of structural sex differences in the central nervous system, *Annu. Rev. Neurosci.*, 7, 413, 1984.

Ballinger, C. B., Psychiatric aspects of the menopause, *Br. J. Psychiatry*, 156, 773, 1990.

Ballinger, C. B., Browning, M. C. K., and Smith, A. H. W., Hormone profiles and psychological symptoms in perimenopausal women, *Maturitas*, 9, 235, 1987.

Bancroft, J., Axworthy, D., and Ratcliffe, S. G., The personality and psycho-sexual development of boys with 47 XXY chromosome constitution, *J. Child Psychol. Psychiatry*, 23, 169, 1982.

Bancroft, J., Sanders, D., Davidson, D., and Warner, R., Mood, sexuality, hormones and the menstrual cycle. III. Sexuality and the role of androgens, *Psychosom. Med.*, 45, 509, 1983.

Barbo, D. M., The physiology of the menopause, *Med. Clin. N. Am.*, 71, 11, 1987.

Benedek, E. P., Premenstrual syndrome: a view from the bench, *J. Clin. Psychiatry*, 49, 498, 1988.

Beyer, C., Morali, G., Naftolin, F., Larsson, K., and Perez-Palacios, G., Effect of some anti-estrogens and aromatase inhibitors on androgen induced sexual behavior in castrated male rats, *Horm. Behav.*, 7, 353, 1976.

Bretschneider, J. G. and McCoy, N. L., Sexual interest in healthy 80 to 102 year olds, *Arch. Sex. Behav.*, 17, 109, 1988.

Butler, L. J., Snodgrass, G. J. A. I., France, N. E., Russell, A., and Swain, V. A. J., True hermaphroditism or gonadal intersexuality, *Arch. Dis. Child.*, 44, 666, 1969.

Campbell, S., Double-blind psychometric studies on the effects of natural estrogens on post-menopausal women, in *The Management of the Menopausal and Post-Menopausal Years*, Campbell, S., Ed., University Park Press, Baltimore, 1976, 149.

Coopen, A. and Kessel, N., Menstruation and personality, *Br. J. Psychiatry*, 109, 711, 1963.

Dalton, K., Antenatal progesterone and intelligence, *Br. J. Psychiatry*, 114, 1377, 1968.

Davidson, J. M., Camargo, C. A., and Smith, E. R., Effects of androgen on sexual behavior in hypogonadal men, *J. Clin. Endocrinol. Metab.*, 48, 955, 1979.

Davidson, J. M., Chen, J. J., Crapo, L., Gray, G. D., Greenleaf, W. J., and Catania, J. A., Hormonal changes and sexual function in aging men, *J. Clin. Endocrinol. Metab.*, 57, 71, 1983.

de Lacoste-Utamsing, C. and Holloway, R. L., Sexual dimorphism in the human corpus callosum, *Science*, 216, 1431, 1982.

Dennerstein, L., Burrows, G. D., Wood, C., and Hyman, G., Hormones and sexuality: effect of estrogen and progestogen, *Obstet. Gynecol.*, 56, 316, 1980.

Dorner, G., *Hormones and Brain Differentiation*, Elsevier, Amsterdam, 1976.

Dorner, G., Specific gonadotrophin secretion, sexual orientation and gender role behavior, *Exp. Clin. Endocrinol.*, 86, 1, 1985.

Dorner, G., Neuroendocrine response to estrogen and brain differentiation in heterosexuals, homosexuals, and transsexuals, *Arch. Sex. Behav.*, 17, 57, 1988.

Dorner, G., Gotz, F., and Rohde, W., On the evocability of a positive oestrogen feedback action on LH secretion in male and female rats, *Endokrinologie*, 66, 369, 1975a.

Dorner, G., Rohde, W., and Schnorr, D., Evocability of a slight positive oestrogen feedback action on LH secretion in castrates and oestrogen-primed men, *Endokrinologie*, 66, 373, 1975b.

Downey, J., Ehrhardt, A. A., Schiffman, M., Dyrenfurth, I., and Becker, J., Sex hormones in lesbian and heterosexual women, *Horm. Behav.*, 21, 347, 1987.

Dunnell, K. and Cartwright, A., *Medicine Takers, Prescribers and Hoarders*, Routledge and Kegan Paul, London and Boston, 1972.

Eaton, G. G., Goy, R. W., and Phoenix, C. H., Effects of testosterone in adulthood on sexual behavior of female hermaphrodite rhesus monkeys, *Nature New Biol.*, 242, 119, 1973.

Ehrhardt, A. A., Epstein, R., and Money, J., Fetal androgens and female gender identity in the early treated adrenogenital syndrome, *Johns Hopkins Med. J.*, 122, 160, 1968a.

Ehrhardt, A. A., Evers, K., and Money, J., Influence of androgen and some aspects of sexual dimorphic behavior in women with the late-treated adrenogenital syndrome, *Johns Hopkins Med. J.*, 123, 115, 1968b.

Eibel, T., Treatment and aftercare of 300 sex offenders, especially with regard to penile plethysmography, in *Proceedings of the German Conference on Treatment Possibilities for Sex Offenders in Eppingen*, Baden-Wurttenberg, J., Ed., Stuttgart, 1977.

Eicher, W., Spoljar, M., Cleve, H., Murken, J. D., Richter, K., and Stangel-Rutkowski, S., H-Y antigen in trans-sexuality, *Lancet*, 2, 1137, 1979.

Ellis, A., The sexual psychology of human hermaphrodites, *Psychosom. Med.*, 7, 108, 1945.

Engel, W., Pfafflin, F., and Wiedeking, C., H-Y antigen in transsexuality and how to explain testis differentiation in H-Y antigen negative males and ovary differentiation in H-Y antigen positive females, *Hum. Genet.*, 55, 315, 1980.

Feder, H. H., Perinatal hormones and their role in the development of sexually dimorphic behaviors, in *Neurology of Reproduction*, Adler, N. T., Ed., Plenum Press, New York, 1981, 127.

Ferguson-Smith, M. A., The prepubertal testicular lesion in chromatin positive Klinefelter's syndrome (primary microorchidism) as seen in mentally handicapped children, *Lancet*, 1, 219, 1959.

Freeman, E., Rickels, K., Sondheiemr, S. J., and Polansky, M., Ineffectiveness of progesterone suppository treatment for premenstrual syndrome, *JAMA*, 264, 349, 1990.

Fydor-Freyburgh, P., The influence of oestrogens on the wellbeing and mental performance of climacteric and postmenopausal women, *Acta Obstet. Gynaecol. Scand. Suppl.* 64, 1, 1977.

Gartrell, N. K., Loriaux, D. L., and Chase, T. N., Plasma testosterone in homosexual and heterosexual women, *Am. J. Psychiatry*, 134, 1117, 1977.

Gladue, B. A. and Clemens, C. G., Androgenic influences in feminine sexual behavior in male and female rats: defeminization blocked by pre-natal anti-androgen treatment, *Endocrinology*, 103, 1702, 1978.

Gladue, B. A., Green, R., and Hellman, R. E., Neuroendocrine response to estrogen and sexual orientation, *Science*, 225, 1496, 1984.

Gooren, L., The neuroendocrine response of luteinizing hormone to estrogen administration in heterosexuals, homosexuals, and transsexual subjects, *J. Clin. Endocrinol. Metab.*, 63, 583, 1986.

Gorski, R., Gordon, J. H., Shryne, J. E., and Southam, A. M., Evidence for a morphological sex difference within the medial preoptic area (MPOA) of the rat, *Brain Res.*, 148, 333, 1978.

Green, R. and Dalton, K., The premenstrual syndrome, *Br. Med. J.*, 1, 1007, 1953.

Griffin, J. E. and Wilson, J. D., The syndrome of androgen resistance, *N. Engl. J. Med.*, 302, 198, 1980.

Heim, N. and Hursch, C. J., Castration for sex offenders: treatment or punishment? A review and critique of recent European literature, *Arch. Sex. Behav.*, 8, 281, 1979.

Imperato-McGinley, J., Guerro, L., Gautier, T., and Peterson, R. E., Steroid 5α-reductase deficiency in man: an inherited form of pseudohermaphroditism, *Science*, 186, 12313, 1974.

Imperato-McGinley, J., Peterson, R. E., Gautier, T., and Sturla, E., Androgens and the evolution of gender identity among male pseudohemaphrodites with 5α-reductase deficiency, *N. Engl. J. Med.*, 300, 1233, 1979.

Jacklin, C. N., Maccoby, E. E., and Doering, C. H., Neonatal sex steroid hormones and timidity in 6–18 month old boys and girls, *Dev. Psychobiol.*, 16, 163, 1983.

Jagiello, G. and Atwell, J. D., Prevalence of testicular feminization, *Lancet*, 1, 329, 1962.

Kaiser, F. E. and Morley, J. E., The menopause and beyond, in *Geriatric Medicine*, Cassel, C. R. and Riesenberg, D., Eds., Springer-Verlag, New York, 1990.

Kaiser, F. E., Viosca, S. P., Morley, J. E., Mooradian, A. D., Stanik Davis, S., and Korenman, S. G., Impotence and aging: clinical and hormonal factors, *J. Am. Geriatr. Soc.*, 36, 511, 1988.

Konishi, M., Birdsong: from behavior to neuron, *Annu. Rev. Neurosci.*, 8, 125, 1985.

Logue, C. M. and Moos, R. H., Perimenstrual symptoms: prevalence and risk factors, *Psychosom. Med.*, 48, 388, 1986.

MacLusky, N. J. and Naftolin, F., Sexual differentiation of the central nervous system, *Science*, 211, 1294, 1981.

Mann, M. A. and Svare, B., Prenatal testosterone exposure elevates maternal aggression in mice, *Physiol. Behav.*, 30, 503, 1983.

Mazenord, B., Pugeat, M., and Forest, M. G., Hormones, sexual function and erotic behavior in women, in *Handbook of Sexology*, Vol. 6, Sitsen, J. M. A., Ed., Elsevier, Amsterdam, 1988, 316.

McEwen, B. S., Neural gonadal steroid actions, *Science*, 211, 1303, 1981.

McEwen, B. S., Gonadal steroid influences on brain development and sexual differentiation, *Int. Rev. Physiol.*, 27, 99, 1983.

Metcalf, M. G., Livesay, J. H., Wells, J. E., and Braiden, V., Physical symptom cyclicity in women with and without premenstrual syndrome, *J. Psychosom. Res.*, 34, 203, 1990.

Meyer Bahlburg, H. F. L., Sex hormones and female homosexuality: a critical examination, *Arch. Sex. Behav.*, 8, 101, 1979.

Mishell, D. R., Jr. and Brenner, P. F., Menopause, in *Infertility, Contraception, and Reproductive Endocrinology*, 2nd ed., Mishell, D. R., Jr. and Davajan, V., Eds., Medical Economics Books, Oradell, NJ, 1986.

Money, J., Hampson, J. G., and Hampson, J. H., Hermaphroditism: recommendations concerning the assignment of sex, change of sex and psychological management, *Bull. Johns Hopkins Hosp.*, 97, 284, 1955a.

Money, J., Hampson, J. G., and Hampson, J. L., The examination of some basic concepts: the evidence of sex, change of sex, and psychological management, *Bull. Johns Hopkins Hosp.*, 97, 301, 1955b.

Money, J., Hampson, J. G., and Hampson, J. H., Imprinting and the establishment of gender role, *Arch. Neurol. Psychiatry*, 77, 333, 1957.

Mooradian, A. D., Morley, J. E., and Korenman, S. G., Biological actions of androgens, *Endocrine Rev.*, 8, 1, 1987.

Moos, R. H., Kopell, B. S., Melges, F. T., Yalom, I. D., Lunde, D. T., Clayton, R. B., and Hamburg, D. A., Fluctuations in symptoms and moods during the menstrual cycle, *J. Psychosom. Res.*, 13, 37, 1969.

Morali, G., Larsson, K., and Beyer, C., Inhibition of testosterone induced sexual behavior in the castrated male rat by aromatase blockers, *Horm. Behav.*, 9, 203, 1977.

Morley, J. E., Impotence, *Am. J. Med.*, 80, 897, 1986.

Morley, J. E. and Kaiser, F. E., Sexual function with advancing age, *Med. Clin. N. Am.*, 73, 1483, 1989.

Morris, N. M., Udry, J. R., Khan-Dawood, F., and Dawood, M. Y., Marital sex frequency and midcycle female testosterone, *Arch. Sex. Behav.,* 16, 27, 1987.

Mortola, J. F., Girton, L., and Yen, S. S. C., Depressive episodes in premenstrual syndrome, *Am. J. Obstet. Gynecol.,* 161, 1682, 1989.

Munday, M. R., Brush, M. G., and Taylor, R. W., Correlations between progesterone, oestradiol and aldosterone levels in the premenstrual syndrome, *Clin. Endocrinol.,* 14, 1, 1981.

Muse, K. N., Cetel, N. S., Futterman, L. A., and Yen, S. S. C., The premenstrual syndrome — effects of "medical ovariectomy," *N. Engl. J. Med.,* 311, 1345, 1984.

Myers, L. S., Dixen, J., Morrissette, D., Carmichael, M., and Davidson, J. M., Effects of estrogen, androgen and progestin on sex psychophysiology and behavior in postmenopausal women, *J. Clin. Endocrinol. Metab.,* 70, 1124, 1990.

Nankin, H. R. and Calkin, J. H., Decreased bioavailable testosterone in aging normal and impotent men, *J. Clin. Endocrinol. Metab.,* 63, 1418, 1986.

Nielsen, J., Pelsen, B., and Sorensen, K., Followup of 30 Klinefelter males treated with testosterone, *Clin. Genet.,* 33, 262, 1988.

Nowakowski, K. H. and Lenz, W., Genetic aspects in male hypogonadism, *Recent Prog. Horm. Res.,* 17, 53, 1961.

O'Brien, P. M. S., Craven, D., Selby, C., and Symonds, E. M., Treatment of premenstrual syndrome with spironolactone, *Br. J. Obstet. Gynaecol.,* 86, 142, 1986.

Olweus, D., Mattsson, A., Schalling, D., and Low, H., Circulating testosterone levels and aggression in adolescent males: a causal analysis, *Psychosom. Med.,* 50, 261, 1988.

Osofsky, H. J. and Blumenthal, S. J., Eds., *Premenstrual Syndrome: Current Findings and Future Directions,* American Psychiatric Press, Washington, D.C., 1985.

Persky, H., Lief, H. I., Strauss, D., Miller, W. R., and O'Brien, C. P., Plasma testosterone level and sexual behavior of couples, *Arch. Sex. Behav.,* 7, 157, 1978.

Pfaff, D. W. and McEwen, B. S., Actions of estrogens and progestins on nerve cells, *Science,* 219, 808, 1983.

Pfeiffer, E., Verwoerdt, A., and Wang, H. S., Sexual behavior in aged men and women, *Arch. Gen. Psychiatry,* 19, 735, 1968.

Phoenix, C. H., Goy, R. W., Gerall, A. A., and Young, W. B., Organizing action of prenatally administered testosterone propionate on the tissues mediating mating behavior in the female guinea pig, *Endocrinology,* 65, 369, 1959.

Phoenix, C. H., Chambers, K. C., Jensen, J. N., and Baughman, W., *Horm. Behav.,* 18, 393, 1984.

Reid, R. L. and Yen, S. S. C., Premenstrual syndrome, *Am. J. Obstet. Gynecol.,* 139, 85, 1981.

Rubin, R. T., Reinisch, J. M., and Haskett, R. F., Postnatal gonadal steroid effects on human behavior, *Science,* 211, 1318, 1981.

Rubinow, D. R., Roy-Byrne, P., Hoban, M. C., Grover, G. N., Stamble, N., and Post, R. M., Premenstrual mood changes: characteristic patterns in women with and without premenstrual syndrome, *J. Affective Disord.,* 10, 85, 1986.

Saal, F. S. Vom, Prenatal exposure to androgen influences morphology and aggressive behavior of male and female mice, *Horm. Behav.,* 12, 1, 1979.

Saal, F. S. Vom and Bronson, F. H., Sexual characteristics of adult female mice are correlated with their blood testosterone levels during prenatal development, *Science,* 208, 597, 1986.

Salmon, T. J. and Geist, S. H., Effect of androgens on libido in women, *J. Clin. Endocrinol. Metab.,* 3, 235, 1943.

Schecter, D., Bachmann, G. A., Vaitukaitus, J., Phillips, D., and Saperstein, D., Preimenstrual syndrome: time course of symptoms in relation to endocrinologically defined segments of the menstrual cycle, *Psychosom. Med.,* 51, 173, 1989.

Schreiner-Engel, P., Female sexual arousability: its relation to gonadal hormones and the menstrual cycle, Ph.D. thesis, New York University, 1980.

Schreiner-Engel, P., Schiavi, R. C., Smith, H., and White, D., Sexual arousability and the menstrual cycle, *Psychosom. Med.,* 43, 199, 1981.

Seagraves, R. T., Schoenberg, H. W., Zarins, C. K., et al., Discrimination of organic versus psychogenic impotence with DSFI: a failure to replicate, *J. Sex. Marital Ther.,* 7, 230, 1981.

Sherwin, B. B., Changes in sexual behavior as a function of plasma sex steroid levels in postmenopausal women, *Maturitas,* 7, 225, 1985.

Sherwin, B. B. and Gelfand, M. M., The role of androgen in the maintenance of sexual functioning in oophorectomized women, *Psychosom. Med.,* 49, 397, 1987.

Simpson, E., Sex reversal and sex determination, *Nature (London),* 300, 404, 1982.

Simpson, J. L., *Disorders of Sexual Differentiation,* Academic Press, New York, 1976.

Spoljar, M., Eicher, W., Eiermann, W., and Cleve, H., H-Y antigen expression in different tissues from transsexuals, *Hum. Genet.,* 57, 52, 1981.

Tenover, J. S., Matsumoto, A. M., Plymate, S. R., and Bremner, W. J., The effects of aging in normal men on bioavailable testosterone and luteinizing hormone secretion: response to clomiphene citrate, *J. Clin. Endocrinol. Metab.,* 65, 1118, 1987.

Toran-Alherand, C. D., Sex steroids and the development of the newborn mouse hypothalamus and preoptic area in vitro. II. Morphological correlates and hormone specificity, *Brain Res.,* 189, 413, 1980.

Wachtel, S. S., Ono, S., Koo, G. C., and Boyse, E. A., Possible role for H-Y antigen in the primary determination of sex, *Nature (London),* 257, 235, 1975.

Wachtel, S., Koo, G., de la Chapelle, A., Kallio, H., Heyman, J. M., and Miller, O. J., H-Y antigen in 46 XY gonadal dysgenesis, *Hum. Genet.,* 54, 25, 1980.

Walsh, P. C., Madden, J. D., Harrod, M. J., Goldstein, J. L., Macdonald, P. C., and Wilson, J. D., Familial incomplete male pseudohermaphroditism type 2, *N. Engl. J. Med.,* 291, 944, 1974.

Walzer, S., Wolff, P. H., Bowen, D., Silbert, A., Bashir, A. S., Gerald, P. S., and Richmond, J. B., A method for the longitudinal study of behavioral development in infants and children: the early development of XXY children, *J. Child Psychol. Psychiatry,* 19, 213, 1978.

Williams, Cl., A re-evaluation of the concept of separable periods of organizational and activational actions of estrogens in development of brain and behavior, *Ann. N.Y. Acad. Sci.,* 474, 282, 1986.

Wood, C., Larsen, L., and Williams, R., Menstrual characteristics of 2343 women attending the Shepard Foundation, *Aust. N.Z. J. Obstet. Gynaecol.,* 19, 107, 1979.

19

Diseases of the Posterior Pituitary

MYRON MILLER

Department of Geriatrics and Adult Development and Division of Geriatric Medicine
Department of Medicine
The Mount Sinai Medical Center
New York, New York

The ability to regulate volume and tonicity of extracellular body water within narrow limits is essential to the maintenance of health and preservation of maximal functional status in humans. The constancy of this important body compartment is maintained by interactions of several hormonal systems along with the integrity of thirst perception and the function of the kidney as an excretory organ. Derangements of any of these elements can lead to marked alteration in extracellular fluid volume status and/or to clinically significant disturbance in tonicity of extracellular fluid, reflected as either hyper- or hyponatremia. The major hormonal regulator of water balance is the antidiuretic hormone (ADH, vasopressin), synthesized and released by the neurohypophysial system, and responsible for the ability of the kidney to reabsorb fluid in a precise fashion. It is through this hormone and effector system that large variations in fluid intake are modulated by the body to maintain constancy of water balance.

I. Biochemistry and Physiology

A. Biosynthesis of ADH

The neurohypophysial system is the site of ADH and oxytocin synthesis, storage, and release and is composed of the cell bodies of the supraoptic and paraventricular neurons of the hypothalamus, their axonal projections through the median eminence and pituitary stalk, and the nerve terminals in the posterior lobe of the pituitary gland (Richter, 1985; North, 1987). The gene for vasopressin has been isolated and its structure determined (Schmale et al., 1983). In humans, the gene is located on chromosome 20 (Riddell et al., 1985). Transcription of the gene results in production of vasopressin mRNA, which is transported into the cell cytoplasm and translated on ribosomes into the hormone precursor molecule, propressophysin, a protein composed of 166 amino acids and which contains not only the hormone but its specific carrier protein, neurophysin, and a glycopeptide. The precursor molecule is packaged by the Golgi complex into secretory granules and through a series of enzymatic cleavages is converted to a vasopressin-neurophysin complex. The secretory granules migrate down the axons and are stored in axon terminals in the posterior pituitary, a process estimated to take 12 to 14 hr. In response to stimuli reaching the neurosecretory neurons, an action potential is initiated that propagates to the axonal terminals and allows an influx of calcium from the extracellular space into the nerve terminal. Through the process of exocytosis, both ADH and its neurophysin are liberated into the bloodstream. Oxytocin and its neurophysin are synthesized in a similar fashion. While ADH is involved in regulation of body water, little is known of the biological role of neurophysin.

In addition to the neural pathways originating in the supraoptic and paraventricular nulcei, there is evidence that ADH is also produced by cells of the suprachiasmatic nucleus. The axons of these cells do not project to the median eminence and posterior pituitary but instead to wide areas of the brain outside the hypothalamus. ADH liberated from these nerve terminals may act as a neuromodulator of neuronal activity in higher central nervous system centers, including those involved in learning, memory, and attention processes (Buijs, 1983).

B. Structure

The released hormone is a nonapeptide made up of a three-amino acid tail attached to six amino acids in a ring structure, in which two cysteine molecules are linked by a disulfide bond (Figure 1). ADH occurs in two forms in mammalian species, with the difference being due to the amino acid in position 8. In most species the hormone contains an arginine residue (arginine vasopressin, AVP), while in the pig, hippopotamus, and peccary lysine occupies this position (lysine vasopressin, LVP). Oxytocin is similar in structure to AVP, differing by the presence of isoleucine in position 3 and leucine in position 8. The neurophysins are larger

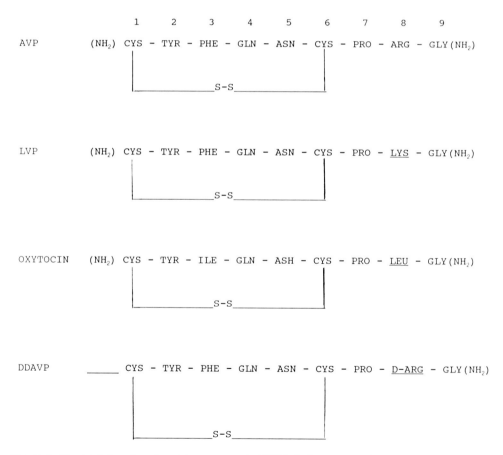

Figure 1. Structural formulas of arginine vasopressin (AVP), lysine vasopressin (LVP), oxytocin, and 1-desamino-8-D-arginine vasopressin (DDAVP).

polypeptides with a molecular weight of approximately 10,000. In humans, there appear to be two forms of neurophysin, one associated with vasopressin and the other with the neurohypophysial hormone oxytocin (North, 1987).

C. Circulation and Metabolism

Following release from the posterior pituitary, vasopressin is quickly distributed into a space approximating the volume of the extracellular fluid compartment. In the bloodstream, vasopressin circulates as the free peptide with a half-life of 3 to 6 min. In normal humans under conditions of *ad libitum* fluid intake, concentration of the hormone in blood ranges from 1 to 8 pg/ml (Miller, 1984). There is some evidence for a diurnal pattern to vasopressin secretion, with maximum values being found late at night and early morning and with lowest values tending to occur in the early afternoon. Inactivation of vasopressin takes place in both the liver and kidney, with the initial event being cleavage of the terminal glycinamide to produce a biologically inactive peptide fragment (Walter and Bowman, 1973). Approximately 10% of secreted hormone is excreted in the urine as intact, biologically active vasopressin in amounts ranging from 27.5 to 140 ng/24 hr (Miller and Moses, 1972a). In addition to its release into the systemic circulation, small amounts of vasopressin in concentrations of approximately 1 to 2 pg/ml are found in the cerebrospinal fluid (Amico et al., 1985).

D. Mechanism of Action and Functions

Numerous studies have established that vasopressin action involves binding of the hormone to specific cell membrane receptors. It appears that there are at least two classes of these receptors, which have been designated V1 and V2, and which differ in their biochemical mechanism of cellular action (Dousa, 1985).

1. V1 Receptors

Vasopressin interaction with V1 receptors, found on myocytes of vascular smooth muscle, glomerular mesangial cells, and hepatocytes, is associated with increased Ca^{2+} cellular flux as mediator of response. This increase in Ca^{2+} movement into the cell leads to rapid hydrolysis of phosphatidylinositol, activation of phospholipase A_2, and release of arachidonic acid from membrane phospholipids (Garg and Kapturczak, 1990). These events culminate in activation of an intracellular contractile system and/or increased synthesis of prostaglandins.

2. V2 Receptors

These receptors are associated with an adenylate cyclase within the contraluminal plasma membrane of cells of the renal collecting tubule. The interaction of vasopressin with the receptor leads to activation of the adenylate cyclase and generation of cAMP as a second messenger. In turn, this leads to activation of protein kinase and phosphorylation of protein substrates, which results in enhanced movement of water across the luminal membrane of the cells of the collecting duct.

The most important physiologic action of vasopressin is on the distal and collecting tubule of the kidney, where it acts to conserve water and concentrate the urine by increasing cell permeability with resultant increase in hydroosmotic flow of water from the luminal fluid to the medullary interstitium (Valtin, 1987). The production of a concentrated urine requires the presence of an intact cortical-medullary concentration gradient for solutes. The main renal medullary solutes are NaCl and urea, and it is their concentration in the medulla that determines the magnitude of the urine-concentrating response to the passive flow of water across the tubular membrane that is induced by ADH. Blood flow in the vasa recti serves to maintain the gradient. Alteration of the blood supply to the medulla or administration of loop diuretics such as furosemide can lead to decline in the gradient with accompanying impaired ability to generate a concentrated urine.

In very high concentrations, through its action on V1 receptors of vascular smooth muscle, vasopressin can cause vasoconstriction. Although this effect of the hormone probably plays little role in normal regulation of blood pressure, levels achieved during acute severe hypotension may be sufficiently high to have a role in maintaining and restoring blood pressure (Zerbe et al., 1982). The pressor effect has been utilized as the basis for intravenous and intra-arterial vasopressin therapy of bleeding esophageal varices (Nusbaum et al., 1974; Rabol et al., 1976).

High concentrations of vasopressin are released into the pituitary portal system, which perfuses the anterior pituitary gland. At this site, vasopressin acts as a potentiator of the corticotropin-releasing hormone and thus plays a role as a regulator of adrenocorticotropic hormone (ACTH) release (Watabe et al., 1988). There is evidence to suggest that vasopressin can also directly stimulate release of ACTH.

Numerous studies have demonstrated that vasopressin is capable of influencing central nervous system function, with effects on learning, memory, behavior, arousal, and emotionality. This subject is extensively reviewed elsewhere in this book.

In recent years, a role for vasopressin has been defined in hemostatic control systems. In concentrations of 20 to 30 pg/ml, levels that can be achieved in response to many stimuli, vasopressin is capable of increasing blood levels of the clotting system components Factor VIIIc and von Willebrand's factor (Grant et al., 1985). These actions can lead to platelet aggregation and promotion of hemostasis. Since 1-desamino-8-D-arginine vasopressin (DDAVP) can produce these effects, it is felt that extrarenal V2 receptors are involved. The magnitude of response is sufficient to be of clinical use in management of patients with hemophilia and von Willebrand's disease and to decrease blood loss during surgical procedures (Kobrinsky et al., 1987).

E. Control Systems

1. Neural Regulation

A number of neurotransmitters and neuromodulators are capable of affecting ADH synthesis and secretion (Figure 2) (Sladek and Armstrong, 1987). There is much evidence to suggest that the final link connecting neural pathways to the magnocellular hypothalamic neurons is mediated by acetylcholine. Other neurotransmitter systems capable of affecting these neurons include dopamine, norepinephrine, glutamate, aspartate, and γ-aminobutyric acid. In addition, neuromodulators including prostaglandins, angiotensin II, and the endogenous opioids (enkephalin, β-endorphin, and dynorphin) have been demonstrated to exert both stimulatory and inhibitory influences on vasopressin secretion (Lightman and Forsling, 1980; Miller, 1980). These actions appear to be due to a presynaptic modulation of neurotransmitter activity. In the case of the endogenous opioids, inhibition of ADH secretion has been associated with κ receptor activity (Leander, 1983).

Atrial natriuretic peptide is found in the hypothalamus and appears capable of inhibiting ADH release that occurs in response to the stimuli of osmolality, dehydration, and hemorrhage (Allen et al., 1988). Other neural factors capable of altering vasopressin secretion include pain and emotional stress, which can affect magnocellular function through direct afferent pathways from the limbic system to the hypothalamus. Emesis is also a potent stimulus for the release of vasopressin and most likely involves activation of neural pathways leading from the area postrema of the medulla (Rowe et al., 1979).

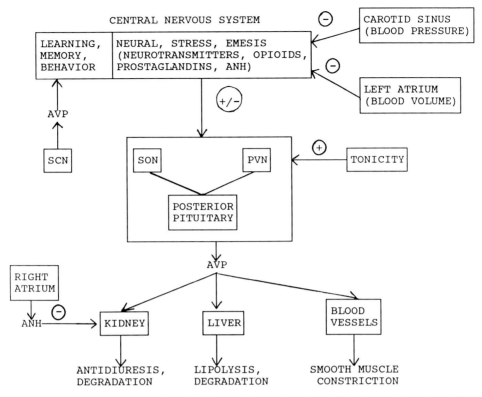

Figure 2. Diagrammatic representation of AVP regulation and actions. SON, Supraoptic nucleus; PVN, paraventricular nucleus; SCN, suprachiasmatic nucleus; ANH, atrial natriuretic hormone. $\oplus$ = stimulatory; $\ominus$ = inhibitory influence. (From Miller, M., in *Endocrine Pathophysiology*, 3rd ed., Hershman, J. M., Ed., Lea & Febiger, Philadelphia, 1988, 299. With permission.)

Table 1
Typical Parameters of Water Regulation in Normal Subjects during Various
Physiological States

Physiological state	Plasma osmolality (mOsm/kg)	Plasma AVP (pg/ml)	Urine osmolality (mOsm/kg)	Urine flow rate (ml/hr)
Overhydration	<282	<1	50–100	600–1200
Initiation of ADH release	282	1	100–200	400–800
Normal hydration	284–292	1–8	500–1200	30–100
Thirst perception	292	3–10	600–1200	12–25
Dehydration (12–24 hr)	>290	5–15	600–1200	15–25

From Miller, M., in *Endocrine Pathophysiology*, 3rd ed., Hershman, J. M., Ed.,
Lea & Febiger, Philadelphia, 1988, 299. With permission.

2. Tonicity

In the normal individual, the amount of hormone release is regulated by the tonicity of the blood through osmoreceptors located in the hypothalamus in or near the cell bodies of the magnocellular nuclei (Figure 2). Serum osmolality in normally hydrated individuals is usually maintained within a narrow range from 284 to 292 mOsm/kg (Robertson et al., 1976). Decrease of serum osmolality to less than 282 mOsm/kg is usually accompanied by inhibition of ADH secretion, with a resultant increase in urine volume and decrease in urine osmolality (Table 1). This hypotonic diuresis can produce urine flow rates as high as 1200 ml/hr and urine concentration to as low as 50 to 60 mOsm/kg (Moses and Streeten, 1967). In response to small increases in blood tonicity, usually due to change in serum sodium concentration, there is a progressive stimulation of ADH release (Figure 3) with an accompanying progressive fall in urine volume and rise in urine osmolality. Initiation of ADH release in normally hydrated subjects occurs when serum osmolality has risen to the range of 282 to 284 mOsm/kg. Maximum urine concentration, in the vicinity of 1200 mOsm/kg, will usually occur when serum osmolality has reached 292 mOsm/kg or greater.

3. Volume

Blood volume is an important determinant of the level of ADH discharge (Robertson and Athar, 1976). Proportionally greater deviations from normality are required to affect hormone release than is needed for osmotic stimulation. Intrathoracic stretch receptors located in the left atrium are responsive to changes in blood volume and by means of alteration in vagal activity can modulate ADH release from the neurohypophysial system. This pathway involves relays in the nucleus of the tractus solitarius in the brainstem, which project to the A1 noradrenergic nucleus and in turn project to the cell bodies of the magnocellular hypothalamic nuclei. A decrease in blood volume of approximately 10% will provoke release of ADH, with progres-

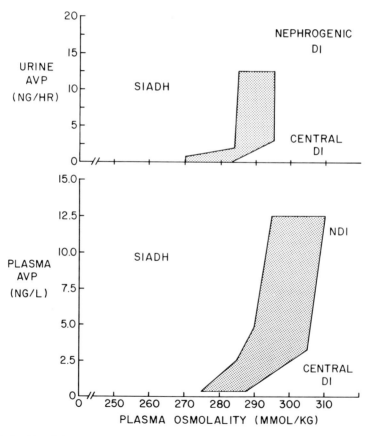

Figure 3. Relationship of plasma and urinary AVP to plasma osmolality in healthy subjects. The shaded areas include values from the water-loaded state, normal hydration, and dehydrated state. Regions shown are those in which values usually occur in patients with diabetes insipidus (DI), nephrogenic diabetes insipidus (NDI), and syndrome of inappropriate ADH secretion (SIADH). (From Miller, M., *Clin. Lab. Med.*, 4, 729, 1984. With permission.)

sively greater increases in hormone level occurring with further fall in blood volume (Dunn et al., 1973). Plasma concentrations of AVP following reduction in blood volume far exceed those that can be achieved by osmotic stimulation. In a similar fashion, expansion of blood volume on the order of 10% results in inhibition of ADH secretion (Moses et al., 1967). There is an interaction between volume and osmotic stimuli for vasopressin release, so that volume depletion results in an enhanced response to an osmotic stimulus while volume expansion necessitates a greater increase in blood osmolality in order to provoke ADH release (Moses and Miller, 1971).

4. Baroreceptor

Changes in blood pressure are capable of affecting vasopressin secretion (Cowley et al., 1980). The receptors mediating change in systemic blood pressure (high-pressure baroreceptors) are located within the carotid body and arch of the aorta. Their afferent impulses are carried by the glossopharyngeal nerve to the brainstem and are subsequently relayed to the hypothalamus by the same pathways that carry information from vagal fibers in the atrium. A decrease in blood pressure of 5 mmHg is usually sufficient to initiate an increase in vasopressin secretion. With larger falls in blood pressure, AVP levels in the circulation can reach concentrations 1000 times those seen in the basal state. These very high concentrations may play a role in maintenance of blood pressure through the vasoconstrictive action of the hormone (Zerbe et al., 1982).

F. Aging Influences

Normal aging is associated with changes both in ADH secretion and in the renal responsiveness to the hormone (Miller, 1985). Plasma AVP concentration undergoes a gradual, progressive increase with advancing age. More significantly, the response of AVP to osmotic stimulation increases with age, so that each increment in plasma osmolality in the older individual results in a greater increase in plasma AVP concentration (Helderman et al., 1978). The basis for this enhanced, osmotically induced AVP release with age is not clearly understood but may be related to the decline in baroreceptor function that also occurs with normal aging (Rowe et al., 1982). Decreased baroreceptor activity would lead to a decline in inhibitory input into the hypothalamic magnocellular neurosecretory neurons.

In parallel with this change in ADH release is an age-related decline in renal concentrating response to the hormone (Lindeman et al., 1966). A decline in maximum achievable urine osmolality is usually present by age 60 years and undergoes progressive fall over the remainder of the life span (Lewis and Alving, 1938; Lindeman et al., 1960; Rowe et al., 1976). It is possible that this acquired impairment in renal responsiveness to ADH is a consequence of down regulation of renal AVP receptors, resulting from exposure to increased circulating levels of hormone. The degree of impaired concentrating ability is rarely of a magnitude sufficient to cause clinically significant disturbance of fluid balance.

Thirst perception is also affected by aging. In normal adults, thirst perception is usually evident when plasma osmolality exceeds 292 to 295 mOsm/kg (Robertson, 1983). Elderly healthy individuals exhibit a diminished sensation of thirst following exposure to water deprivation even though this stress raises plasma osmolality to higher levels than in young subjects and above the osmotic thirst threshold. When access to water is resumed, the elderly consume less water in satisfying their thirst (Phillips et al., 1984). These observations help explain the common clinical finding that older patients with a variety of illnesses often present with features of dehydration yet have poor fluid intake and need encouragement to drink sufficient fluid to correct their deficits.

II. Assessment of Posterior Pituitary Function

A. Clinical Evaluation

When evaluating a patient suspected of having a disorder of posterior pituitary function, initial assessment requires careful attention to the history and physical examination in an attempt to identify features suggestive of altered body water status. Thus, history is obtained of fluid intake, losses from such routes as urinary tract, gastrointestinal tract, or skin in association with fever, thirst perception, presence of known renal, cardiac, hepatic and endocrine disease, and use of drugs that can affect water balance. Physical examination can reveal findings of water depletion such as decreased skin turgor, dry mucous membranes, orthostatic hypotension, and increased heart rate or evidence of water overload such as edema, distended neck veins, and signs of congestive heart failure.

Basic laboratory determinations should include measurement of serum osmolality and the major serum components contributing to total serum solute concentration, including electrolytes, urea, and glucose. Determination of serum calcium and potassium may be of value since elevated calcium or low potassium can lead to reduced renal responsiveness to the action of ADH with resultant polyuria and volume depletion. Urinary measures such as osmolality and sodium concentration are valuable in evaluating the patient suspected of having water-losing or -retaining disorders. Estimation of osmotic excretion and clearance can be made. Free water clearance, which is inversely related to ADH action on the kidney, can be calculated from the formula $C_{H_2O} = V - C_{osm}$. It is often necessary to assess the function of components of the endocrine system by means of suitable tests of thyroid and adrenal function since disturbances of these systems can affect water-handling capacity.

B. AVP Measurement

Diagnosis and treatment of patients with posterior pituitary disorders rarely requires the direct measurement of AVP in the blood or urine. However, the ability to accurately measure AVP has greatly increased knowledge of the physiology of hormone regulation and has improved the understanding of mechanisms underlying pathologic states.

Early approaches to hormone measurements were based on bioassay procedures that reflected the action of AVP on arterial smooth muscle V1 receptors with resultant increase in blood pressure. These procedures were not sufficiently sensitive to quantitate the small amounts of hormone normally present in blood or urine. However, this assay is the basis for measuring the biologic activity of AVP extracted from animal posterior pituitary or manufactured synthetically and is used in establishing reference standards of the hormone. Purified AVP has a potency of 400 pressor units per milligram. Current assay systems often express AVP concentration in biological unitage as well as in units of weight, with the accepted conversion factor relating biological activity and weight being 1 μU = 2.5 pg of AVP.

Sensitive and specific radioimmunoassay (RIA) systems have been developed that are capable of accurately measuring AVP in small volumes of blood and urine (Miller, 1984). Because of the presence of substances in blood or urine that interfere with the assay technique, measurement of the hormone first requires extraction, partial purification, and concentration before RIA can be carried out.

AVP concentration in the serum or plasma of normal subjects is affected by both blood osmolality and the volume status of the individual (Robertson, 1983; Robertson and Athar, 1976). For normally hydrated individuals, whose plasma osmolality ranges from 284 to 292 mOsm/kg, plasma AVP concentration has been found to range from 1 to 8 pg/ml (Figure 3) (Miller, 1984). An increase in plasma osmolality in response to hypertonic saline infusion produces a progressive increase in plasma AVP but rarely exceeds 10 pg/ml (Robertson et al., 1976). Modest dehydration, which produces both an osmotic and volume-mediated stimulus, can increase plasma AVP to approximately 15 pg/ml. A water load sufficient to reduce plasma osmolality to less than 282 mOsm/kg will, in most normal subjects, suppress AVP secretion to levels at or below the detection limit of most assay systems.

Urinary AVP measurement has an advantage over measurement in blood by being an integrated value over a period of time and therefore is less subject to fluctuation from moment to moment in response to changes in physiologic state or environmental influences (Figure 3). In the steady state, urinary AVP excretion represents approximately 15% of AVP secretion. A close relationship between plasma AVP concentration and urine AVP excretion rate has been demonstrated. In healthy normal male subjects, urinary AVP has been reported to range from 27.5 to 140 ng/24 hr (Miller and Moses, 1972a). Healthy women have levels at the lower end of the range reported for men (Merkelbach et al., 1975). Following water deprivation for 14 hr, urine AVP excretion can increase two- to threefold over basal values. Water load suppresses AVP excretion, sometimes to undetectable levels.

III. Functional Measures of AVP Secretion and Action

A. Dehydration Test

Comparison of renal concentrating capacity after dehydration to the subsequent urine concentration achieved following vasopressin administration provides a simple and reliable means of testing the capacity of the neurohypophysial system to release AVP (Table 2). The test is quantitative in that it allows for the detection of subnormal secretion of AVP (Miller et al., 1970). In addition, the test evaluates the capacity of the renal end organ to respond to the hormone. The procedure is based on withholding fluid until the maximal urine concentration due to endogenous vasopressin has been achieved and then administering exogenous vasopressin to determine the maximal capacity of the kidney to concentrate the urine. In normal individuals and in patients with mild degrees of polyuria, the period of fluid deprivation should begin at approximately 6 p.m. and continue over the next 14 to 18 hr. In patients with severe polyuria who have urine volumes of 10 l/day or greater, the period of fluid deprivation is begun at approximately 6 a.m. so that the patient can be carefully monitored and the test terminated if

Table 2
Response to Water Deprivation Test

Clinical condition	Maximum U_{osm} at plateau (mOsm/kg)	Change in U_{osm} after vasopressin (%)	P_{osm} at plateau (mOsm/kg)
Normal	764 ± 212[a]	<5	289 ± 7
Partial DI	438 ± 116	>9	294 ± 4
Severe DI	168 ± 59	>50	306 ± 12
Nephrogenic DI	<150	<45	302–320
Primary polydipsia	696 ± 190	<5	>288
High-set osmoreceptor	>600	<5	>295

[a]Values are mean ± SD.

Adapted from Miller, M., Dalakos, T., Moses, A. M., Fellerman, H., and Streeten, D. H. P., *Ann. Intern. Med.*, 73, 721, 1970.

weight loss exceeds 2 kg or if untoward clinical symptoms occur. Hourly urine samples are obtained starting at 8 a.m. on the morning following initiation of water deprivation and urine osmolality is measured in each sample. Hourly collections are continued until two consecutive samples differ in urine osmolality by less than 30 mOsm/kg. In normal individuals this occurs after 14 to 18 hr of water deprivation, while in patients with severe polyuria a period of 6 to 8 hr is usually sufficient to reach a stable maximum urine osmolality. At this point, five units of aqueous vasopressin is given subcutaneously and urine osmolality is determined 1 hr later. Serum osmolality is measured prior to initiation of the fluid deprivation and again at the time of reaching the plateau in urine osmolality. In normal individuals, fluid deprivation for 18 to 24 hr rarely raises serum osmolality above 292 mOsm/kg. To assure adequacy of dehydration, serum osmolality before injection of vasopressin should be above 288 mOsm/kg. In subjects with normal neurohypophysial function, the maximum urine osmolality that can be reached after water deprivation varies considerably, depending on age, renal medullary solute concentration, and other intrarenal factors. Following injection of vasopressin, urine osmolality rises by less than 5% of the value obtained by fluid deprivation alone, whatever the absolute value of urine osmolality achieved by dehydration. This indicates that sufficient AVP release was induced by water deprivation to achieve a maximal effect on renal concentrating capacity as reflected by urine osmolality and, therefore, the administration of exogenous vasopressin will fail to further raise the urine osmolality to any significant degree.

B. Urine-to-Serum Osmolality Relationship

In normal individuals there is a close relationship between urine osmolality and simultaneously measured serum osmolality (Figure 4). This relationship can be defined for the normal

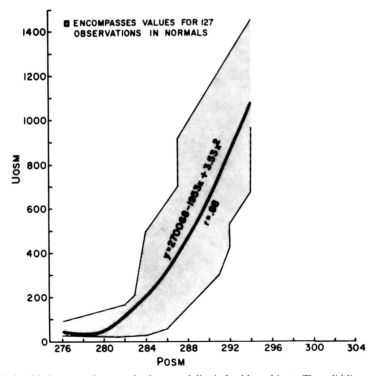

Figure 4. Relationship between plasma and urine osmolality in healthy subjects. The solid line represents the curve of best fit determined from 127 values while the shaded area encompasses the range of values actually observed. (From Miller, M. and Moses, A. M., in *Neurohypophysis,* Moses, A. M. and Share, L., Eds., S. Karger, Basel, 1977, 153. With permission.)

population as a whole so that deviation due to disorders of ADH release or action can be recognized (Miller and Moses, 1977). Measurements of simultaneous serum and urine osmolality are obtained during periods of *ad libitum* fluid intake and during periods of water loading or water deprivation. In these circumstances, serum and urine osmolality should change in parallel and within the normal confidence limits.

C. Hypertonic Saline Infusion

Infusion of hypertonic saline intravenously, in the form of 5% saline solution, will cause a progressive rise in serum osmolality that in healthy subjects will provoke the release of AVP from the neurohypophysial system. In water-loaded normal subects, the serum osmolality at which ADH release is initiated is referred to as the osmotic threshold for ADH release (Aubry et al., 1965). This point is recognized by the abrupt onset of a progressive decrease in urine volume and increase in urine osmolality in response to the released AVP. In a group of normal subjects, this value has been defined as a serum osmolality of 287.3 ± 3.3 mOsm/kg (Moses and Streeten, 1967). Elevation of the serum osmolality to higher levels leads to progressively greater decline in urine volume and increase in urine osmolality until maximum urine-concentrating capacity has been reached, usually when serum osmolality exceeds 292 mOsm/kg. The test is interpreted by calculating changes in free water clearance during the infusion in order to prevent masking of the antidiuretic response by the increase in urine volume which can occur in some patients due to large increase in urinary solute excretion following the saline infusion.

D. Water Load Test

The response to water loading is a useful means of readily and quickly establishing the ability to normally suppress release of AVP (Table 3). Before the water load test is performed, conditions known to affect water handling must be excluded, including the presence of renal, cardiac, or hepatic disease, hypothyroidism, hypoadrenalism, and the use of drugs that may interfere with renal water excretion (Miller and Moses, 1976). In addition, the patient should not be exposed to stimuli that may provoke ADH release even in the presence of a fall in serum osmolality. Such stimuli include severe stress, pain, nausea, hypovolemia, and hypotension. The test is carried out by giving an oral water load of 20 ml/kg body weight over a period of 15 to 20 min (Miller, 1984). Urine is then collected at hourly intervals for the next 5 hr for measurement of volume and osmolality in each specimen. The patient should remain in a recumbent position throughout the test except to void. Blood is obtained for measurement of serum osmolality prior to the administration of the water load. In normal individuals, more

Table 3
Response to Oral Water Load Test[a]

Clinical condition	Minimum U_{Osm} (mOsm/kg)	Water load (%) excreted in 5 hr	P_{Osm} prior to water load (mOsm/kg)
Normal	<100	>80	284–292
SIADH	>100	<80	<284[b]
Low-set osmoreceptor	<100	>80	>284

[a] 20 ml/kg body weight.
[b] P_{Osm} may be normal if treated by fluid restriction prior to test.
From Miller, M., in *Endocrine Pathophysiology,* 3rd ed., Hershman, J. M., Ed., Lea & Febiger, Philadelphia, 1988, 299. With permission.

than 80% of the water load is excreted in 5 hr and urine osmolality will fall to less than 100 mOsm/kg in at least one sample during the test, usually during the second hour. Such a response indicates normal suppressibility of ADH as well as normal capacity of the kidney to generate a dilute urine.

IV. Disorders of Insufficient Vasopressin Secretion or Action

Diabetes insipidus is the polyuric state that results from impaired ability of the kidney to conserve water either as a result of low blood levels of AVP following exposure to normal physiologic stimuli (central or hypothalamic diabetes insipidus) or of inability of the kidney to respond to normal or increased amounts of AVP (nephrogenic diabetes insipidus).

A. Etiology of Central Diabetes Insipidus

Many different disorders can lead to impaired ability to synthesize or release AVP and consequently to central diabetes insipidus (Table 4). In a large series, approximately 25% of the cases were considered to be idiopathic in origin (Moses, 1985). In these individuals diabetes insipidus frequently starts in childhood or in early adult life and appears to be slightly more common in males than in females. A small percentage of patients with idiopathic diabetes insipidus have the disorder as a result of familial disease with a defective AVP gene on chromosome 20 and which is inherited in an autosomal dominant fashion (Braverman et al., 1965; Repaske et al., 1990). A transient form of diabetes insipidus has been noted to occur during pregnancy and may be attributed to high circulating levels of vasopressinase released from the placenta with resultant degradation of vasopressin and reduction in blood levels of the active hormone (Durr et al., 1987; Hime, 1978; Hughes et al., 1989).

Most often, diabetes insipidus is a consequence of damage to the hypothalamus, pituitary stalk, or posterior pituitary gland as a result of tumor, head trauma, or surgery in the area of the hypothalamus or pituitary (Moses, 1985). In these patients, there may be partial or complete loss of anterior pituitary function in addition to the diabetes insipidus. Diabetes insipidus

Table 4

Causes of Hypotonic Polyuria

Hypothalamic diabetes insipidus	Hypercalcemia
Idiopathic and familial	Drug induced
Head trauma	Lithium
Neurosurgical procedures	Demethylchlortetracycline
Tumor (primary and metastatic)	Primary polydipsia
Cerebral anoxia	Psychogenic
Granulomatous disease	Hypothalamic disease
Histiocytosis	Drug induced
Sarcoidosis	Osmotic diuresis
Tuberculosis	Glucose (diabetes mellitus)
Nephrogenic diabetes insipidus	Sodium
Familial	Chronic renal disease
Spontaneous	Diuretic induced
Acquired	Excessive intake
Renal disease	Mannitol
Potassium deficiency	

From Miller, M., in *Endocrine Pathophysiology*, 3rd ed., Hershman, J. M., Ed., Lea & Febiger, Philadelphia, 1988, 299. With permission.

following head trauma or surgery in the region of the hypothalamus and pituitary often is of acute onset, occurring within 12 to 24 hr after the trauma or surgery (Verbalis et al., 1984).

The polyuria in approximately 50 to 60% of cases of post-traumatic or post-operative diabetes insipidus is transient and resolves spontaneously over a period of 3 to 5 days. In approximately 30 to 40% of cases, the diabetes insipidus may persist for many months and is often permanent. The magnitude of the resultant polyuria is variable and is dependent on the severity of the underlying damage to the neurohypophysial system. It is not unusual for the diabetes insipidus to be partial (Miller et al., 1970). In 5 to 10% of patients with post-traumatic or post-operative diabetes insipidus, the course is characterized by a triphasic response (Hollingshead, 1964). These patients exhibit an abrupt onset of polyuria that is followed in several days by the return of a reduced volume of concentrated urine. After a period lasting from several days to several weeks there is a return of the diabetes insipidus, which is then persistent.

Diabetes insipidus can arise as a result of failure of hypothalamic osmoreceptors to trigger ADH release in response to a sufficient osmotic stimulus even though the supraoptic and paraventricular neurons contain adequate amounts of the hormone (de Rubertis et al., 1971). These patients often have accompanying defects in thirst perception, a combination of circumstances that puts the patient at high risk of severe volume depletion and hypernatremia (Halter et al., 1977). Rarely, hypotonic polyuria will develop in patients whose thirst threshold is lower than the osmotic threshold for ADH release. In this circumstance, the presence of thirst perception will result in consumption of fluid before ADH release can be initiated, with consequent development of polyuria. ADH release may be initiated in a normal fashion by nonosmotic stimuli such as hypotension or hypovolemia, so that the severity of fluid loss will be self-limiting.

Disorders of the central nervous system that have accompanying dysfunction of the autonomic nervous system (Shy-Drager syndrome) may have associated impairment in the release of vasopressin (Lockwood, 1976; Zerbe et al., 1983). This defect can be identified by demonstrating absence or marked blunting of the response of plasma vasopressin to postural stimuli such as head-up tilt (Rowe et al., 1982; Zerbe et al., 1983). These patients are characterized by marked orthostatic hypotension. During recumbency, such as while sleeping, marked hypotonic polyuria may develop as a manifestation of ADH deficiency. Both the hypotension and polyuria may respond to vasopressin replacement therapy (Mathias et al., 1986).

B. Pathology

Examination of the hypothalamus of patients who have had long-standing diabetes insipidus reveals loss of most of the neurons in the supraoptic and paraventricular nuclei (Green et al., 1967). The neural loss has been reported in patients with idiopathic diabetes insipidus as well as in patients whose disease was the result of trauma, surgery, or tumor. A loss of greater than 90% of the neurons is required before diabetes insipidus becomes clinically evident.

C. Symptoms and Signs

The major signs and symptoms of ADH deficiency are related to impaired ability of the kidney to conserve water. Thus, polyuria, severe thirst, and polydipsia are the most common presenting symptoms. Often these symptoms are sudden in onset whether due to idiopathic diabetes insipidus or to trauma or injury. The urine is pale in color and the volume increased to amounts as high as 25 l/day. This massive polyuria is accompanied by urinary frequency as often as every 30 to 60 min throughout the day and night. In some patients, however, diabetes insipidus can be mild, with urine volumes of 3 to 4 l and with the patient being unaware of symptoms related to this mild polyuria. Classically, when thirst is present, cold drinks are sought in an attempt to alleviate the thirst (Moses, 1985). Since the thirst center lies in close approximation to the nerve bodies responsible for ADH synthesis, some patients may have diabetes insipidus with impaired thirst perception as well. These individuals are at risk of severe dehydration with all of the accompanying features of severe volume depletion and hypernatremia (de Rubertis et al., 1971; Sridhar et al., 1974). Even when thirst perception is normal, fluid intake rarely is sufficient to compensate for urinary losses. Mild degrees of dehydration, however, are seldom clinically apparent. When access to water is interfered with, severe dehydration with accompanying symptoms of weakness, fever, dry mucous membranes, orthostatic hypotension, and tachycardia may occur.

D. Diagnostic Tests

Measurement of serum osmolality often reveals the presence of an increase in total solute concentration. This is usually accompanied by an increase in serum sodium concentration along with elevations of the serum BUN and creatinine, reflective of the fluid volume-depleted state. At the same time, the urine is inappropriately dilute as indicated by urinary specific gravity and more accurately by the urine osmolality. The magnitude of the urine osmolality is dependent on the severity of the ADH deficiency. In patients with severe diabetes insipidus and very high urine volumes, urine osmolality may be in the range of 50 to 90 mOsm/kg even though plasma osmolality or serum sodium are increased above the normal range. In milder degrees of diabetes insipidus, in which there is a partial deficiency of ADH secretion, urine osmolality may be in the range of 200 to 500 mOsm/kg (Miller et al., 1970).

The diagnosis and severity of the ADH deficiency can be established by means of the dehydration test (Table 2). Patients with deficiency of ADH will respond to the injection of vasopressin with an increase in urine osmolality that exceeds 9% of the osmolality achieved after water deprivation. In patients with severe diabetes insipidus and essentially complete loss of ADH secretory capacity, urine osmolality as a result of water deprivation will remain hypotonic to plasma. Patients with milder degrees of hormone deficiency may increase the urine osmolality to hypertonic levels but still less than the maximum achievable concentration that can be elicited by the injection of exogenous vasopressin (Miller et al., 1970). Serum osmolality measured at the time of the plateau in urine osmolality tends to be higher than in healthy subjects and is raised in proportion to the degree of severity of ADH deficiency. Thus, the dehydration test allows recognition not only of patients with complete hormonal loss and severe polyuria but also of patients with mild degrees of AVP deficiency, who often may not be clinically recognized because their polyuria is mild.

Measurement of osmolality in simultaneously obtained urine and serum samples during the basal state and following a short period of water deprivation can aid in making the diagnosis of diabetes insipidus (Miller and Moses, 1977). When these values are related to those of a normal population, patients with either central or nephrogenic diabetes insipidus will demonstrate urine and serum osmolality values that fall to the right of the normal range (Figure 4). Increasing levels of serum osmolality during water deprivation will be accompanied by little change in urine osmolality. Several variant forms of central diabetes insipidus can be recognized by examining the urine-serum osmolality relationship. Some patients will show a slow rise in urine osmolality with increasing serum osmolality and then have an abrupt increase in urine concentration when serum osmolality reaches high levels (generally over 300 mOsm/kg) in association with plasma volume depletion. These patients can be suspected to have a defective osmoreceptor mechanism as the basis for their polyuria and they retain the ability to release ADH in response to nonosmotic stimuli such as hypovolemia, hypotension, nausea, or drugs. Since thirst is usually perceived when serum osmolality exceeds 292 mOsm/kg, the presence of a normal thirst mechanism in these patients prevents the serum osmolality from being maintained at the high level necessary to stimulate ADH release and thus the patients are usually in a polyuric state. A pattern present in other patients is one in which urine osmolality rises in parallel with an increase in serum osmolality, but the curve is to the right of the normal confidence limits, indicating that these individuals have a normal ADH release mechanism but with a high-set osmoreceptor. Here again, the presence of normal thirst perception results in failure of serum osmolality to rise to a level sufficient to stimulate ADH release. An additional group of patients can be identified who will have urine and serum osmolality values that fall to the right of the normal range and will show a submaximal response of urine osmolality to an increase in serum osmolality. This finding indicates the ability to initiate ADH release in response to an osmotic stimulus but with a subnormal amount of hormone production, that is, partial diabetes insipidus.

The hypertonic saline infusion test is also of value in establishing the diagnosis of diabetes insipidus (Moses and Streeten, 1967). In patients with complete ADH deficiency, saline infusion will not result in a fall of free water clearance even when plasma osmolality is raised well above the normal osmotic threshold to values of 300 mOsm/kg or higher. There is a group of patients with polyuria who will respond to osmotic stimulation with hypertonic saline but only when plasma osmolality is raised far above normal values. These patients can be considered to have a high-set osmoreceptor as the reason for their disturbed water regulation. The test is of particular importance in a small group of patients whose diabetes insipidus is not due to deficiency of ADH synthesis but rather to an inability to release ADH in response to an osmotic stimulus. These patients can be recognized by their ability to develop a concentrated urine when exposed to nonosmotic stimuli for ADH release, such as volume depletion, hypotension, or emesis, and by their failure to develop an antidiuresis following sufficient infusion of hypertonic saline.

Measurement of blood or urine AVP in response to water deprivation or hypertonic saline infusion has been utilized in establishing the diagnosis of diabetes insipidus (Figure 3). Plasma AVP levels have been reported to remain below 0.9 pg/ml following water deprivation sufficient to increase serum osmolality from 288 to 312 mOsm/kg (Zerbe and Robertson, 1981). Patients with mild degrees of polyuria have had plasma AVP levels in the normal range but that were low relative to the simultaneously determined serum osmolality. These patients are considered to have partial degrees of AVP deficiency as the basis for their polyuria. In a similar fashion, urinary AVP excretion has been found to be low or undetectable in many patients with severe polyuria with subnormal response to the stimulus of increase in serum osmolality (Miller and Moses, 1972b). Most patients with diabetes insipidus demonstrate some AVP in the urine in response to water deprivation but these amounts are well below levels seen in normal individuals subjected to the same stimulus. These data further demonstrate that diabetes insipidus is often the result of varying degrees of partial ADH deficiency, rather than a result of complete failure to synthesize and release the hormone.

V. Nephrogenic Diabetes Insipidus

Congenital nephrogenic diabetes insipidus is a rare, usually inherited, form of polyuria, most commonly affecting males, which results from inability of the kidney to respond to the antidiuretic action of ADH (Williams and Henry, 1947). The disease is usually evident shortly after birth and is recognized because of the severe polyuria and accompanying thirst and polydipsia. The signs and symptoms are the same as those in patients with severe forms of ADH deficiency. Much more common is an acquired form of nephrogenic diabetes insipidus that can occur in patients with chronic renal disease, after acute tubular necrosis, in patients with potassium deficiency or hypercalcemia, and after exposure to drugs such as lithium and demethylchlortetracycline (Table 4) (Singer and Forrest, 1976). Common to all of these situations is failure of the renal V2 receptor to respond to ADH. Vascular V1 receptors, however, show unimpaired responsiveness.

The diagnosis of nephrogenic diabetes insipidus is established by demonstrating failure to significantly concentrate the urine following injection of vasopressin or intranasal administration of DDAVP (Table 2). Measurement of plasma or urine AVP will show the hormone to be present in greater than normal amounts in response to the combined stimuli of volume depletion and hypertonicity (Figure 3).

VI. Primary Polydipsia

Primary polydipsia is the condition resulting from chronic overingestion of water, which leads to suppression of ADH and production of hypotonic polyuria (Barlow and de Wardener, 1959). The polydipsia and polyuria in this disorder are usually erratic in contrast to the sustained polydipsia and polyuria of diabetes insipidus. The patients often do not have nocturnal urinary frequency. The disorder is commonly seen in patients with emotional disturbances (Raskind and Barnes, 1984) and occasionally can occur in individuals with central nervous system lesions that produce an increase in thirst perception (Baylis et al., 1981; Kirkland et al., 1983). In patients with underlying psychosis, several disturbances in water-handling capacity have been identified, including defective suppression of AVP by water load, impaired diluting ability, and increased renal sensitivity to AVP (Goldman et al., 1988).

Patients with chronic primary polydipsia may be difficult to distinguish from patients with true diabetes insipidus, but a correct diagnosis can be made following appropriate tests. The diagnosis should be suspected when, in addition to hypotonic polyuria, there is also low plasma osmolality or serum sodium concentration. The dehydration test can establish the diagnosis since a sufficiently long period of water deprivation will result eventually in maximal concentration of the urine (Table 2) (Miller et al., 1970). Measurement of plasma or urine AVP may be low during the period of water ingestion but will reach normal values following prolonged water deprivation (Zerbe and Robertson, 1981).

VII. Other Causes of Polyuria

The excretion of increased amounts of solute in the urine can cause an obligatory water loss with resultant polyuria, increased thirst, and polydipsia (Table 4). The most common circumstance is the osmotic diuresis secondary to glycosuria in patients with poorly controlled diabetes mellitus. Correction of the blood sugar abnormality will lead to resolution of the polyuric state. Polyuria can also occur as a result of increased sodium excretion such as may result from chronic renal disease, increased sodium intake, or the use of diuretic agents. In all of these states, measurement of osmolal excretion and calculation of free water clearance will demonstrate that the increase in urine flow is attributable to the increase in solute excretion rather than to a primary free water diuresis.

VIII. Therapy

The treatment of central diabetes insipidus is based on hormone replacement in order to reduce urinary fluid loss and allow maintenance of normal extracellular fluid volume. This objective can be achieved in several ways, with selection of the agent dependent on whether one is treating acute or chronic polyuria and whether the degree of underlying ADH deficiency is partial or complete. Treatment of the patient with acute onset of diabetes insipidus should be initiated as soon as the diagnosis is established, particularly in those patients with post-traumatic or post-operative polyuria in whom the state of consciousness may be depressed. In this circumstance, aqueous vasopressin can be given subcutaneously in doses of 5 to 10 units every 3 to 6 hr. Because of the short duration of action, the return of endogenous neurohypophysial function can be recognized and vasopressin discontinued, thus avoiding the risk of water overload in patients receiving intravenous fluids. The availability of the AVP analog DDAVP, an agent with markedly enhanced and prolonged antidiuretic activity and devoid of pressor activity, has made this drug the treatment of choice in the acute setting (Cobb et al., 1978; Robinson, 1976). It can be administered intranasally in a dose of 10 to 20 μg (0.1 to 0.2 ml) or subcutaneously in a dose of 2 to 4 μg with a resultant expected antidiuresis lasting for 12 to 24 hr. Careful attention must be paid to the amount and type of fluid being concurrently administered to avoid volume overload and hyponatremia. The monitoring of serum sodium concentration or plasma osmolality serves as a useful guide. Each dose of DDAVP or aqueous vasopressin should be given only after there is evidence of return of polyuria to assure that the diabetes insipidus continues to be present.

The patient with persistent or established diabetes insipidus can be managed by several approaches. In the past, patients were usually treated with intramuscular injections of vasopressin tannate in oil in a dose of 2.5 to 5 units, which would produce an antidiuretic effect lasting from 24 to 72 hr. This hormonal preparation is no longer being manufactured. The present preferred treatment for chronic diabetes insipidus is by means of intranasal DDAVP given in doses of 5 to 20 μg at intervals of 12 or 24 hr. The onset of action is evident within 1 hr after administration and the duration is from 6 to 24 hr. The vast majority of patients are controlled with two daily doses taken at 12-hr intervals. Periodic monitoring of serum sodium is necessary to assure that fluid intake is appropriate. Patients should also monitor body weight on a daily basis to detect possible excessive fluid retention or loss. Disturbances of the ability of the nasal membranes to absorb DDAVP can occur during the course of upper respiratory infections or allergic rhinitis with resultant loss of effectiveness of DDAVP and return of polyuria. In this circumstance, treatment can be provided by subcutaneous DDAVP in doses of 2 to 4 μg every 12 to 24 hr. There have been reports that large oral doses of DDAVP (200 μg) can produce an antidiuresis lasting at least 6 hr (Williams et al., 1986). However, this route of administration is prohibitively expensive.

Patients with diabetes insipidus who have partial deficiency of ADH may respond to oral treatment with several nonhormonal drugs (Miller and Moses, 1976; Moses et al., 1976). Chlorpropamide has been demonstrated both to stimulate ADH release from the neurohypophysial system and to enhance the antidiuretic action of submaximal amounts of ADH on the renal tubule (Miller and Moses, 1970; Moses et al., 1973b). Doses of 200 to 500 mg taken once daily are usually sufficient to produce an antidiuresis in responsive patients. The onset of action is within several hours and usually persists for at least 24 hr. An additional value of chlorpropamide is that it may restore thirst perception in those patients with thirst center defects (Bode et al., 1971; Mahoney and Goodman, 1968). Care must be taken to avoid hypoglycemia, although this is rarely a problem if the patient adheres to a regular schedule of meals and does not have coexisting liver disease. Clofibrate is another drug that is capable of stimulating ADH release and has been useful in doses of 500 mg four times a day (Moses et al., 1973a). In some patients, a combination of low doses of chlorpropamide along with clofibrate may produce a clinically useful level of antidiuresis where either drug alone was unsuccessful. Carbamazepine is another oral agent that appears able to stimulate ADH release but its use has not been widely accepted because of central nervous system, bone marrow, and liver toxicity.

Hormone replacement therapy is not effective in managing the polyuria due to nephrogenic diabetes insipidus. In this disorder, reduction in urine volume can be achieved by producing sodium depletion with resultant reduction in renal medullary gradient and decrease in intravascular volume and glomerular filtration rate. These events lead to increased proximal tubular sodium and water reabsorption and impaired ability to generate a dilute urine (Crawford et al., 1960; Early and Orloff, 1962). The combination of a thiazide diuretic with a sodium-restricted diet has been successful in controlling polyuria. Amiloride in doses of 10 mg twice daily can produce a significant antidiuresis in patients with nephrogenic diabetes insipidus that has developed as a complication of lithium therapy (Batlle et al., 1985). Its value as an effective agent for treatment of hereditary nephrogenic diabetes insipidus has also been suggested (Alon and Chan, 1985). There is evidence that use of prostaglandin synthetase inhibitors such as indomethacin in a dose of 1.5 to 3 mg/kg can produce a clinically useful reduction in urine volume (Libber et al., 1986).

IX. Syndrome of Inappropriate ADH Secretion

The syndrome of inappropriate ADH secretion (SIADH) is a disorder characterized by hyponatremia due to water retention caused by increased ADH. The excessive ADH in the circulation is due to inappropriate nonphysiologic causes such as autonomous release from tumors or response to nonphysiologic stimuli capable of overriding the inhibitory influence of hypoosmolality (Table 5). SIADH is recognized by its cardinal features of dilutional hyponatremia with urine inappropriately concentrated and usually greater than that of plasma, urinary sodium excretion greater than 20 mEq/l, and the absence of edema (Bartter and Schwartz,

Table 5
Causes of SIADH

Malignancy with ectopic hormone production	Drugs
Small cell carcinoma of lung	Chlorpropamide
Pancreatic carcinoma	Vincristine
Thymoma	Vinblastine
Lymphosarcoma, reticulum cell sarcoma,	Cyclophosphamide
Hodgkin's disease	Carbamazepine
Pulmonary disease	Thiazide diuretics
Pneumonia	Narcotics
Lung abscess	General anesthetics
Tuberculosis	Tricyclic and serotonin uptake inhibitor
Central nervous system disorders	antidepressants
Trauma	Oxytocin
Tumor	Other
Infectious	Hypothyroidism
Vascular	Positive pressure breathing
Acute intermittent porphyria	
Lupus erythematosus	

From Miller, M., in *Endocrine Pathophysiology*, 3rd ed., Hershman, J. M., Ed., Lea & Febiger, Philadelphia, 1988, 299. With permission.

1967). Most commonly, SIADH is a disorder affecting elderly persons (Anderson et al., 1985; Miller, 1990).

A. Etiology

In middle-aged individuals, the most common cause of SIADH is the autonomous release of ADH from tumor tissue where it is synthesized, stored, and discharged in the absence of known stimuli (Verbalis, 1986; Vorherr et al., 1974). Of these tumors, small cell or oat cell carcinoma of the lung accounts for 80% of the patients (Vorherr, 1974). Prospective studies of patients with oat cell carcinoma of the lung have shown that more than 50% have impaired water excretion and elevated plasma ADH levels even in the absence of overt hyponatremia (Padfield et al., 1976; Comis et al., 1980). Other malignancies that can be associated with SIADH include pancreatic carcinoma, lymphosarcoma, reticulum cell sarcoma, Hodgkin's disease, and thymoma. In addition to tumors, nontumorous lung tissue can acquire the capacity to synthesize and release ADH autonomously as a result of inflammatory diseases, including tuberculosis and bacterial pneumonia.

A third form of SIADH, especially common in elderly patients, involves release of ADH from the patient's own neurohypophysial system as a result of a wide variety of central nervous system disorders or as a result of drug use (Miller and Moses, 1976). Virtually any disorder of the central nervous system, including inflammatory, neoplastic, infectious, traumatic, or vascular diseases, can result in SIADH (Bartter and Schwartz, 1967). This may be transient, as in the case of inflammatory or infectious diseases, or chronic, as in the case of neoplastic diseases or head trauma. In the community residing elderly, mild hyponatremia with features of SIADH has been observed in approximately 8% of the population. Surveys of patients residing in long-term care facilities have disclosed a prevalence of hyponatremia ranging as high as 18 to 22%, with most of these patients considered to have SIADH as the mechanism of hyponatremia (Miller, 1990).

A number of drugs can stimulate the release of ADH (Miller and Moses, 1976). Chlorpropamide has been the most widely studied and has been shown to be capable not only of stimulating the release of ADH but also of enhancing the antidiuretic action of submaximal concentrations of hormone at the level of the kidney (Moses et al., 1973b). Other drugs capable of stimulating ADH release include the antineoplastic agents vincristine, vinblastine, and cyclophosphamide. Carbamazepine, used in the treatment of tic douloureux, can produce hyponatremia through stimulation of ADH release (Moses et al., 1976). A number of antidepressant agents including the tricyclics and serotonin uptake inhibitors such as fluoxetine can also produce SIADH, most commonly in elderly patients (Cohen et al., 1990). Oxytocin given in large amounts to obstetrical patients can cause water intoxication due to its inherent antidiuretic activity. Exposure to general anesthetics or narcotics can stimulate release of ADH and cause water retention.

B. Pathology

The ADH produced by tumors or by nontumorous lung tissue appears to be identical with native AVP and has the full biological activity of the native hormone (Verbalis, 1986). Because the release of ADH is not suppressible by volume expansion or hypoosmolality, patients with the syndrome are unable to excrete a dilute urine and therefore retain ingested fluid. This results in expansion of the extracellular fluid volume. The expanded extracellular fluid volume is capable of suppressing the renin-angiotensin system with resultant suppression of aldosterone production by the adrenal gland. In addition, the increase in extracellular fluid volume activates the release of the atrial natriuretic hormone from the right atrium (Kamoi et al., 1990). These consequences of volume expansion lead to an increase in urinary sodium excretion and probably accounts for the observation that edema is rarely seen in patients with SIADH. As a result of the action of the increased ADH on the kidney, the urine is concentrated. Thus, the classical finding in SIADH is hyponatremia due to water retention with concomitant urine osmolality in excess of plasma osmolality.

C. Symptoms and Signs

The hyponatremia of SIADH is often mild and asymptomatic. However, patients with SIADH may present with weight gain and with symptoms of hyponatremia including weakness, lethargy, mental confusion, and ultimately in patients with severe hyponatremia, convulsions, and coma (Arieff, 1984). Clinical signs of fluid overload such as edema or hypertension are rare.

D. Diagnostic Evaluation

The establishment of the diagnosis of SIADH requires identification of the underlying cause for which the syndrome serves as a marker and involves exclusion of other causes of hyponatremia such as may occur from renal disease, congestive heart failure, or cirrhosis. Pseudohyponatremia can be seen in patients with very high lipid levels or with severe hyperglycemia. The presence of hypothyroidism and hypoadrenalism must be excluded since these disorders can result in impaired water excretion with dilutional hyponatremia. Careful history and physical examination must be performed to evaluate the patient for the possibility of tumor, inflammatory disease, central nervous system disorder, or drug use that may be the cause of the SIADH.

Evidence of water overload may be manifest in routine laboratory measurements including low levels of serum BUN, creatinine, uric acid, and albumin. The serum osmolality is reduced, as is serum sodium concentration. At the same time, urine is inappropriately concentrated, generally being hypertonic to plasma. Urinary sodium concentration is usually increased to greater than 20 mEq/l and is often much higher.

The diagnosis may be established by means of the water load test (Table 3). Because the test may be dangerous in an already hyponatremic patient, it is not carried out until the serum sodium has been raised to a safe level, generally above 125 mEq/l and the patient is free of symptoms of hyponatremia. In patients with SIADH there will be impaired ability to excrete the water load in the following 5 hr and this will be accompanied by impaired ability to dilute the urine to less than 100 mOsm/kg. Patients who fail to excrete the water load in a normal fashion and who have no other apparent cause for impaired water excretion can be considered to have SIADH.

The test also allows for the recognition of patients with low-set osmoreceptors since these individuals have hyponatremia but are able to excrete the water load normally and dilute the urine when plasma osmolality is further lowered (DeFronzo et al., 1976). When a water load has been given to a patient with SIADH, no further water intake should be permitted until the serum sodium concentration has returned to the pretest value.

Measurement of plasma and urinary AVP has been utilized in the evaluation of patients with hyponatremia (Figure 3) (Miller and Moses, 1972b; Zerbe et al., 1980). Although levels of the hormone may be elevated in patients with SIADH, many such patients have hormone concentrations that fall within the normal range. However, these levels are excessive when related to the plasma osmolality. Some patients with SIADH will show partial suppression of plasma or urine AVP in response to water load, but even in these individuals the levels remain inappropriately elevated. In response to stimulation, such as with hypertonic saline, some patients with SIADH show a progressive increase in plasma AVP that correlates with the induced rise in plasma osmolality, indicating that there is retention of osmotic control of AVP secretion in these patients. In other patients, raising plasma osmolality produces no clearcut relationship between the plasma AVP and corresponding plasma osmolality. In a small group of patients with SIADH, plasma AVP levels appear to be normally suppressed and the possibility is raised that the SIADH may be due to altered renal sensitivity to the hormone or to the production of some other antidiuretic substance.

X. Therapy

Both the rapidity of onset and the severity of symptoms dictate the approach to therapy (Ayus et al., 1987). Acute, severe alterations require prompt intervention while chronic, milder symptoms can be managed by more conservative and gradual measures (Table 6). In general, serum sodium concentrations greater than 125 mEq/l are associated with minimal or mild symptoms that may include fatigue, malaise, and weakness. Although severity of symptoms does not always correlate well with level of serum sodium, concentrations of less than 120 mEq/l may be accompanied by central nervous system alterations ranging from confusion to stupor, coma, convulsions, and death. Even in an apparently asymptomatic individual, a sodium concentration less than 115 mEq/l warrants prompt intervention because of the rapidity with which sudden clinical deterioration can occur (Arieff, 1984).

Symptomatic hyponatremia requires prompt implementation of therapy. In the mildly symptomatic patient who has a serum sodium concentration greater than 125 mEq/l, fluid restriction to 800 to 1000 ml/24 hr is usually sufficient. In patients with more severe symptoms

Table 6
Management of Hyponatremia Due to SIADH

Treatment modality	Mechanism of action	Potential adverse complications
Acute		
Intravenous 3% saline solution, 500 ml over 3–4 hr, followed by 100 ml/hr	Elevation of serum sodium Reduction of cerebral edema	Cerebral pontine myelinolysis Congestive heart failure
Intravenous furosemide, 1 mg/kg body weight	Increased free water excretion in excess of sodium excretion	Hypokalemia, hypomagnesemia
Chronic		
Correction of under lying cause	Removal of stimulus for water retention	—
Water restriction, 800–1000 ml/24 hr	Reduction of extracellular body water	Thirst stimulation
Butorphanol, 4 mg b.i.d.	Inhibition of ADH secretion	CNS effects: confusion, hallucination
Lithium carbonate, 600–1200 mg daily	Inhibition of ADH action via adenylate cyclase-cyclic AMP	CNS effects: confusion, dysarthria
Demeclocycline, 600–1200 mg daily	Inhibition of ADH action via adenylate cyclase-cyclic AMP	Azotemia, photosensitivity Nephrotoxicity in patients with hepatic disease or congestive heart failure
ADH analogs (not yet available)	Competitive antagonism at renal V2 receptor	None known

of hyponatremia, the serum sodium should be increased more rapidly until symptoms begin to improve and the sodium concentration has reached approximately 125 mEq/l. Acute correction beyond this level is not necessary and may be dangerous to the patient (see below). Restoration of serum sodium to normal levels should not be undertaken within the first 48 hr of treatment.

The therapeutic objective is to increase the serum sodium to 125 mEq/l at the rate of approximately 2mEq/l/hr. The amount of sodium required to treat severe hyponatremia usually is from 500 to 800 mEq. This can be delivered through intravenous infusion of approximately 500 ml of 3% saline solution over a period of 3 to 4 hr followed by continued infusion at the rate of 100 ml/hr until serum sodium has reached the mid 120 mEq/l range (Ayus et al., 1982). Laboratory determination of serum sodium concentration at 6-hr intervals is essential in guiding therapy in its initial stages. Patients with very low serum sodium (less than 105 mEq/l) or with symptoms of seizure or coma must be considered as medical emergencies and may benefit from simultaneous administration of intravenous furosemide in a dose of 1 mg/kg body weight to promote a prompt diuresis (Hantman, 1973). These patients may require larger amounts of hypertonic saline to compensate for the enhanced natriuresis that will occur and also require careful monitoring and replacement of serum electrolytes in order to avoid diuresis-induced hypokalemia and hypomagnesemia. The use of furosemide should also be considered for patients in whom there is concern that plasma volume expansion from use of hypertonic saline may lead to precipitation of congestive heart failure. Once the serum sodium has been raised to an appropriate level, any further need for intravenous fluids should be met in the form of 0.9% saline solution to minimize the likelihood of redevelopment of hyponatremia. After initial improvement of the hyponatremia, careful adherence to a regimen of fluid restriction is necessary to avoid recurrence of symptoms. In most patients, maintenance of serum sodium at a level above 125 mEq/l is sufficient to correct the major symptomatic consequences of hyponatremia.

A major concern in the acute therapy of severe hyponatremia is the possibility of inducing central pontine myelinolysis. This serious disorder, which can lead to permanent brain damage or death, appears to be confined to patients with alcoholism and those with severe debilitation or malnutrition in whom serum sodium was rapidly increased by more than 25 mEq/l to levels above 140 mEq/l in less than 48 hr (Arieff, 1984; Ayus et al., 1987). Recent studies indicate that the development of cerebral pontine myelinolysis is not related to the rate of correction of hyponatremia but rather to the rapid increase in serum sodium to normal or greater levels.

Slow correction of symptomatic hyponatremia, that is, at a rate less than 0.7 mEq/l/hr, may be associated with poor outcome. Severe hyponatremia is associated with the development of brain edema that may become progressive and lead to seizures, respiratory arrest, and death if correction is not promptly initiated. Data from a number of studies indicate that rapid initial correction of symptomatic severe hyponatremia so that serum sodium is increased at the rate of 1 to 2 mEq/l/hr results in minimization of risk of the consequence of hyponatremia-induced brain edema.

The chronic management of the hyponatremia due to SIADH is based on identification and correction of the underlying cause whenever possible. When due to drugs, SIADH usually clears following cessation of the offending agent. The SIADH occurring with central nervous system disorders may be corrected with improvement in the disease, that is, as a consequence of effective treatment of infection, evacuation of a subdural hematoma, or recovery from a cerebrovascular accident. However, in many patients with progressive central nervous system disease, SIADH may be chronic and resistant to all attempts at primary treatment.

Moderate to severe hypothyroidism can produce hyponatremia with all of the features of SIADH and is completely correctable following adequate replacement therapy with thyroid hormone. Similarly, hypocortisolism, either primary or due to hypothalamic-pituitary disease, can be associated with impaired water excretion and hyponatremia, which is reversible with glucocorticoid replacement.

In patients with SIADH due to malignancy, especially small cell carcinoma of the lung, successful treatment with surgery, irradiation, or chemotherapy may be accompanied by improvement in features of SIADH. In such patients, the ability to excrete and dilute the urine following an acute oral water load may be an effective means of monitoring response to therapy and of detecting recurrence of disease (Comis et al., 1980).

The mainstay of long-term management of chronic hyponatremia due to SIADH is water restriction, often to a level of 800 to 1000 ml/24 hr. This degree of fluid restriction can be difficult to attain or maintain for long periods of time, especially when thirst is stimulated. For patients in whom this approach is not effective, attempts can be made to increase water excretion without concomitant increase in sodium excretion by the administration of pharmacologic agents capable of either inhibiting antidiuretic hormone release or its renal action.

Both ethanol and phenytoin are capable of inhibiting ADH release under experimental conditions but are rarely effective in clinical application. Peptide opiate agonists, especially those with κ receptor activity, have been demonstrated to be potent inhibitors of ADH release in experimental animals and in normal humans (Leander, 1983; Leander et al., 1987). Although these substances have not yet been tested in patients with SIADH and are not presently licensed for clinical use, they hold promise as agents that may be available in the future. The analgesic agent butorphanol has mixed opiate antagonist-κ receptor agonist activity and has been demonstrated to be capable of inhibiting ADH release in the rat (Miller, 1975) and in humans (Miller, 1980). In a limited number of patients with chronic SIADH of central nervous system cause, butorphanol in a dose of 4 mg b.i.d. has been effective in improving the response to acute water load challenge and in increasing the level of serum sodium under conditions of *ad libitum* fluid intake.

Another experimental approach to management of chronic SIADH has involved drugs capable of inhibiting ADH action on the kidney, thus promoting improved renal water excretion. Both lithium and the tetracycline antibiotic demeclocycline can inhibit ADH function by interfering with ADH-induced activation and post-receptor effects of the adenylate cyclase-cyclic AMP system of cells of the renal distal tubule and collecting system (Forrest et al., 1978). Lithium has been abandoned as a therapeutic agent for SIADH because of the high frequency of toxic side effects, especially those related to central nervous system function. However, demeclocycline has proven to be a useful drug when given in divided doses of 600 to 1200 mg daily (Cherrill et al., 1975; DeTroyer, 1977). This dosage results in impairment of renal concentrating capacity, i.e., acquired nephrogenic diabetes insipidus, with excretion of an isotonic urine of increased volume. In some patients, the increase in urine volume is sufficient to result in normalization of serum sodium even in the absence of fluid restriction. Onset of action usually occurs within 5 to 14 days and is evident by a decrease in urine osmolality. Chronic use of demeclocycline requires that renal function be monitored closely since the drug has been associated with development of azotemia but without evidence of other renal impairment or renal failure and which is reversible on discontinuation of demeclocycline. Patients with hepatic disease and congestive heart failure appear to be more prone to development of nephrotoxicity and therefore demeclocycline must be used with caution in such patients. The drug is expensive and an effective chronic therapeutic regimen may cost between $300 to $400/month.

A number of analogs of vasopressin have been developed that are capable of acting as competitive inhibitors at the renal V2 receptor site (Manning et al., 1987). By blockage of vasopressin action, a state of nephrogenic diabetes insipidus can be induced with resultant increased excretion of free water. While these analogs have not yet been made available for clinical use in patients with SIADH, they represent a future approach to therapy that may be effective in both acute and long-term management of hyponatremia.

References

Allen, M. J., Ang, V. T. Y., Bennett, E. D., and Jenkins, J. S., Atrial natriuretic peptide inhibits osmotically-induced arginine vasopressin release in man, *Clin. Sci.,* 75, 35, 1988.

Alon, U. and Chan, J. C. M., Hydrochlorothiazide-amiloride in the treatment of congenital nephrogenic diabetes insipidus, *Am. J. Nephrol.,* 5, 9, 1985.

Amico, J. A., Tenicela, R., and Robinson, A. G., Neurohypophysial hormones in cerebrospinal fluid of adults: absence of arginine vasotocin and of a diurnal rhythm of arginine vasopressin, *J. Clin. Endocrinol. Metab.,* 61, 794, 1985.

Anderson, R. J., Hsiao-Min, C., Kluge, R., and Schrier, R. W., Hyponatremia: a prospective analysis of its epidemiology and the pathogenetic role of vasopressin, *Ann. Intern. Med.,* 102, 164, 1985.

Arieff, A. I., Central nervous system manifestations of disordered sodium metabolism, *Clin. Endocrinol. Metab.,* 13, 269, 1984.

Aubry, R. H., Nankin, H. R., Moses, A. M., and Streeten, D. H. P., Measurement of osmotic threshold for vasopressin release in human subjects and its modification by cortisol, *J. Clin. Endocrinol. Metab.,* 25, 1481, 1965.

Ayus, J. C., Olivero, J. J., and Frommer, J. P., Rapid correction of severe hyponatremia with intravenous hypertonic saline solution, *Am. J. Med.,* 72, 43, 1982.

Ayus, J. C., Krothapalli, R. K., and Arieff, A. I., Treatment of symptomatic hyponatremia and its relation to brain damage, *N. Engl. J. Med.,* 317, 1190, 1987.

Barlow, E. D. and de Wardener, H. E. D., Compulsive water drinking, *Q. J. Med.,* 28, 235, 1959.

Bartter, F. C. and Schwartz, W. B., The syndrome of inappropriate secretion of antidiuretic hormone, *Am. J. Med.,* 42, 790, 1967.

Batlle, D. C., Von Riotte, A. B., Gaviria, M., and Grupp, M., Amelioration of polyuria by amiloride in patients receiving long-term lithium therapy, *N. Engl. J. Med.,* 312, 408, 1985.

Baylis, P. H., Gaskill, M. B., and Robertson, G. L., Vasopressin function in polyuric patients, *Q. J. Med.,* 50, 345, 1981.

Bode, H. N., Harey, B. M., and Crawford, J. D., Restoration of normal drinking behavior by chlorpropamide in patients with hypodipsia and diabetes insipidus, *Am. J. Med.,* 51, 304, 1971.

Braverman, L. E., Mancini, J. P., and McGoldrick, D. M., Hereditary idiopathic diabetes insipidus, *Ann. Intern. Med.,* 63, 503, 1965.

Buijs, R. M., Vasopressin and oxytocin — their role in neurotransmission, *Pharmacol. Ther.,* 22, 127, 1983.

Cherrill, D. A., Stote, R. M., Birge, J. R., and Singer, I., Demeclocycline treatment in the syndrome of inappropriate antidiuretic hormone secretion, *Ann. Intern. Med.,* 83, 654, 1975.

Cobb, W. E., Spare, S., and Reichlin, S., Neurogenic diabetes insipidus: management with dDAVP (1-desamino-8-D-arginine vasopressin), *Ann. Intern. Med.,* 88, 183, 1978.

Cohen, B. J., Mahelsky, M., and Adler, L., More cases of SIADH with fluoxetine, *Am. J. Psychiatry,* 147, 948, 1990.

Comis, R. L., Miller, M., and Ginsberg, S. J., Abnormalities in water homeostasis in small cell anaplastic lung cancer, *Cancer,* 45, 2414, 1980.

Cowley, A. W., Jr., Switzer, S. J., and Guinn, M. M., Evidence and quantification of the vasopressin arterial pressure control system in the dog, *Circ. Res.,* 46, 58, 1980.

Crawford, J. D., Kennedy, G. C., and Hill, L. E., Clinical results of treatment of diabetes insipidus with drugs of the chlorothiazide series, *N. Engl. J. Med.,* 262, 737, 1960.

DeFronzo, R. A., Goldberg, M., and Agus, Z. S., Normal diluting capacity in hyponatremic patients. Reset osmostat or a variant of the syndrome of inappropriate antidiuretic hormone secretion, *Ann. Intern. Med.,* 84, 538, 1976.

de Rubertis, F. R., Michelis, M. F., Beck, N., Field, J. B., and Davis, B. B., Essential hypernatremia due to ineffective osmotic and intact volume regulation of vasopressin secretion, *J. Clin. Invest.*, 50, 97, 1971.

DeTroyer, A., Demeclocycline: treatment for syndrome of inappropriate antidiuretic hormone secretion, *JAMA*, 237, 2723, 1977.

Dousa, T. P., Renal actions of vasopressin, in *The Posterior Pituitary: Hormone Secretion in Health and Disease*, Baylis, P. H. and Padfield, P. L., Eds., Marcel Dekker, New York, 1985, 141.

Dunn, F. L., Brennan, T. J., Nelson, A. E., and Robertson, G. L., The role of blood osmolality and volume in regulating vasopressin secretion in the rat, *J. Clin. Invest.*, 52, 3212, 1973.

Durr, J. A., Hoggard, J. G., Hunt, J. M., and Schrier, R. W., Diabetes insipidus in pregnancy associated with abnormally high circulating vasopressinase activity, *N. Engl. J. Med.*, 316, 1070, 1987.

Earley, L. E. and Orloff, J., The mechanism of antidiuresis associated with administration of hydrochlorothiazide to patients with vasopressin resistant diabetes insipidus, *J. Clin. Invest.*, 41, 1988, 1962.

Forrest, J. N., Cox, M., Hong, C., Morrison, G., Bia, M., and Singer, I., Superiority of demeclocycline over lithium in the treatment of chronic syndrome of inappropriate secretion of antidiuretic hormone, *N. Engl. J. Med.*, 298, 173, 1978.

Garg, L. C. and Kapturczak, E., Stimulation of phosphoinositide hydrolysis in renal medulla by vasopressin, *Endocrinology*, 127, 1022, 1990.

Goldman, M. B., Luchins, D. J., and Robertson, G. L., Mechanisms of altered water metabolism in psychotic patients with polydipsia and hyponatremia, *N. Engl. J. Med.*, 318, 397, 1988.

Grant, P. J., Davies, J. A., Tate, G. M., Boothby, M., and Prentice, C. R. M., Effects of physiological concentrations of vasopressin on haemostatic function in man, *Clin. Sci.*, 69, 471, 1985.

Green, J. R., Buchan, G. C., Alvord, E. C., and Swanson, A. G., Hereditary and idiopathic types of diabetes insipidus, *Brain*, 90, 707, 1967.

Halter, J. B., Goldberg, A. P., Robertson, G. L., and Porte, D., Selective osmoreceptor dysfunction in the syndrome of chronic hypernatremia, *J. Clin. Endocrinol. Metab.*, 44, 609, 1977.

Hantman, D., Rossier, B., Zohlman, R., and Schrier, R. W., Rapid correction of hyponatremia in the syndrome of inappropriate secretion of antidiuretic hormone. An alternative treatment to hypertonic saline, *Ann. Intern. Med.*, 78, 870, 1973.

Helderman, J. H., Vestal, R. E., Rowe, J. W., Tobin, J. D., Andres, R., and Robertson, G. L., The response of arginine vasopressin to intravenous ethanol and hypertonic saline in man: the impact of aging, *J. Gerontol.*, 33, 39, 1978.

Hime, M. C., Diabetes insipidus in pregnancy. Case report, incidence and review of literature, *Obstet. Gynecol. Surv.*, 33, 375, 1978.

Hollingshead, W. H., The interphase of diabetes insipidus, *Mayo Clin. Proc.*, 39, 92, 1964.

Hughes, J. M., Barron, W. M., and Vance, M. L., Recurrent diabetes insipidus associated with pregnancy: pathophysiology and therapy, *Obstet. Gynecol.*, 73, 462, 1989.

Kamoi, K., Ebe, T., Kobayashi, O., Ishida, M., Sato, F., Arai, O., Tamura, T., Takogi, A., Yamada, A., Ishibashi, M., and Yamaji, T., Atrial natriuretic peptide in patients with the syndrome of inappropriate antidiuretic hormone secretion and with diabetes insipidus, *J. Clin. Endocrinol. Metab.*, 70, 1385, 1990.

Kirkland, J. L., Pearson, D. J., Goddard, C., and Davies, I., Polyuria and inappropriate secretion of arginine vasopressin in hypothalamic sarcoidosis, *J. Clin. Endocrinol. Metab.*, 56, 269, 1983.

Kobrinsky, N. L., Letts, R. M., Patel, L. R., Israels, E. D., Monson, R. C., Schwetz, N., and Cheang, M. S., 1-Desamino-8-D-arginine vasopressin (desmopressin) decreases operative blood loss in patients having Harrington rod spinal fusion surgery, *Ann. Intern. Med.*, 107, 446, 1987.

Leander, J. D., A kappa opioid effect: increased urination in the rat, *J. Pharmacol. Exp. Therap.*, 224, 89, 1983.

Leander, J. D., Hart, J. C., and Zerbe, R. L., Kappa agonist-induced diuresis: evidence for stereoselectivity, strain differences, independence of hydration variables and a result of decreased plasma vasopressin levels, *J. Pharm. Exp. Ther.*, 292, 33, 1987.

Lewis, W. H., Jr. and Alving, A. S., Changes with age in the renal function in adult men, *Am. J. Physiol.*, 123, 500, 1938.

Libber, S., Harrison, H., and Spector, D., Treatment of nephrogenic diabetes insipidus with prostaglandin synthesis inhibitors, *J. Pediatr.,* 108, 305, 1986.

Lightman, S. L. and Forsling, M. L., Evidence for endogenous opioid control of vasopressin release in man, *J. Clin. Endocrinol. Metab.,* 50, 569, 1980.

Lindeman, R. D., Van Buren, H. C., and Raisz, L. G., Osmolar renal concentrating ability in healthy young men and hospitalized patients without renal disease, *N. Engl. J. Med.,* 262, 1306, 1960.

Lindeman, R. D., Lee, T. D., Jr., Yiengst, M. J., and Shock, N. W., Influence of age, renal disease, hypertension, diuretics, and calcium on the antidiuretic responses to suboptimal infusions of vasopressin, *J. Lab. Clin. Med.,* 68, 206, 1966.

Lockwood, A. H., Shy-Drager syndrome with abnormal respirations and antidiuretic hormone release, *Arch. Neurol.,* 33, 292, 1976.

Mahoney, J. H. and Goodman, A. D., Hypernatremia due to hypodipsia and elevated threshold for vasopressin release. Effects of treatment with hydrochlorothiazide, chlorpropamide and tolbutamide, *N. Engl. J. Med.,* 279, 1191, 1968.

Manning, M., Bankowski, K., and Sawyer, W. H., Selective agonists and antagonists of vasopressin, in *Vasopressin: Principles and Properties,* Gash, D. M. and Boer, G. J., Eds., Plenum Press, New York, 1987, 335.

Mathias, C. J., Fosbraey, P., da Costa, D. F., Thornley, A., and Bannister, R., The effect of desmopressin on nocturnal polyuria, overnight weight loss, and morning postural hypotension in patients with autonomic failure, *Br. Med. J.,* 293, 353, 1986.

Merkelbach, U., Czernichow, P., Gaillard, R. C., and Vallotton, M. B., Radioimmunoassay of [8-arginine]-vasopressin. II. Application to determination of antidiuretic hormone in urine, *Acta Endocrinol.,* 80, 453, 1975.

Miller, J. H. and Shock, N. W., Age differences in the renal tubular response to antidiuretic hormone, *J. Gerontol.,* 8, 446, 1953.

Miller, M., Inhibition of ADH release in the rat by narcotic antagonists, *Neuroendocrinology,* 19, 241, 1975.

Miller, M., Role of endogenous opioids in neurohypophysial function of man, *J. Clin. Endocrinol. Metab.,* 50, 1016, 1980.

Miller, M., Assessment of hormonal disorders of water metabolism, *Clin. Lab. Med.,* 4, 729, 1984.

Miller, M., Influence of aging on vasopressin secretion and water regulation, in *Vasopressin,* Schrier, R. W., Ed., Raven Press, New York, 1985, 249.

Miller, M., Disorders of water metabolism, in *Endocrine Pathophysiology,* 3rd Ed., Hershman, J. M., Ed., Lea & Febiger, Philadelphia, 1988, 299.

Miller, M., Disorders of water and sodium balance, in *The Merck Manual of Geriatrics,* Abrams, W. B. and Berkow, R., Eds., Merck, Sharp & Dohme Research Laboratories, Rahway, NJ, 1990, 24.

Miller, M., Dalakos, T., Moses, A. M., Fellerman, H., and Streeten, D. H. P., Recognition of partial defects in antidiuretic hormone secretion, *Ann. Intern. Med.,* 73, 721, 1970.

Miller, M. and Moses, A. M., Mechanism of chlorpropamide action in diabetes insipidus, *J. Clin. Endocrinol. Metab.,* 30, 488, 1970.

Miller, M. and Moses, A. M., Radioimmunoassay of urinary antidiuretic hormone in man: response to water load and dehydration in normal subjects, *J. Clin. Endocrinol. Metab.,* 34, 537, 1972a.

Miller, M. and Moses, A. M., Urinary antidiuretic hormone in polyuric disorders and in inappropriate ADH syndrome, *Ann. Intern. Med.,* 77, 715, 1972b.

Miller, M. and Moses, A. M., Drug-induced states of impaired water excretion, *Kidney Int.,* 10, 96, 1976.

Miller, M. and Moses, A. M., Clinical states due to alterations of ADH release and action, in *Neurohypophysis,* Moses, A. M. and Share, L., Eds., S. Karger, Basel, 1977, 153.

Moses, A. M., Clinical and laboratory observations in the adult with diabetes insipidus and related syndromes, *Frontiers Horm. Res.,* 13, 156, 1985.

Moses, A. M. and Miller, M., Osmotic threshold for vasopressin release as determined by saline infusion and by dehydration, *Neuroendocrinology,* 7, 219, 1971.

Moses, A. M. and Miller, M., Drug-induced dilutional hyponatremia, *N. Engl. J. Med.,* 291, 1234, 1974.

Moses, A. M. and Streeten, D. H. P., Differentiation of polyuric states by measurement of responses to changes in plasma osmolality induced by hypertonic saline infusions, *Am. J. Med.,* 42, 368, 1967.

Moses, A. M., Miller, M., and Streeten, D. H. P., Quantitative influence of blood volume expansion on the osmotic threshold for vasopressin release, *J. Clin. Endocrinol. Metab.,* 27, 655, 1967.

Moses, A. M., Howanitz, J., Van Gemert, M., and Miller, M., Clofibrate-induced antidiuresis, *J. Clin. Invest.,* 52, 535, 1973a.

Moses, A. M., Numann, P., and Miller, M., Mechanism of chlorpropamide-induced antidiuresis in man: evidence for release of ADH and enhancement of peripheral action, *Metabolism,* 22, 59, 1973b.

Moses, A. M., Miller, M., and Streeten, D. H. P., Pathophysiologic and pharmacologic alterations in the release and action of ADH, *Metabolism,* 25, 697, 1976.

North, W. G., Biosynthesis of vasopressin and neurophysins, in *Vasopressin: Principles and Properties,* Gash, D. M. and Boer, G. J., Eds., Plenum Press, New York, 1987, 175.

Nusbaum, M., Younis, M. T., Baum, S., and Blakemore, W. S., Control of portal hypertension. Selective mesenteric arterial infusion of vasopressin, *Arch. Surg.,* 108, 342, 1974.

Padfield, P. L., Morton, J. J., Brown, J. J., Lever, A. F., Robertson, J. I. S., Wood, M., and Fox, R., Plasma arginine vasopressin in the syndrome of antidiuretic hormone excess associated with bronchogenic carcinoma, *Am. J. Med.,* 61, 825, 1976.

Phillips, P. A., Rolls, B. J., Ledingham, J. G. G., Forsling, M. L., Morton, J. J., Gowe, M. J., and Wollner, L., Reduced thirst after water deprivation in healthy elderly men, *N. Engl. J. Med.,* 311, 753, 1984.

Rabol, A., Juhl, E., Schmidt, A., and Winkle, K., The effect of vasopressin and triglycyl lysine vasopressin on splanchnic circulation in cirrhotic patients with portal hypertension, *Digestion,* 14, 285, 1976.

Raskind, M. and Barnes, R. F., Water metabolism in psychiatric disorders, *Semin. Nephrol.,* 4, 316, 1984.

Repaske, D. R., Phillips, J. A., III, Kirby, L. T., Tze, W. J., D'Ercole, A. J., and Battey, J., Molecular analysis of autosomal dominant neurohypophyseal diabetes insipidus, *J. Clin. Endocrinol. Metab.,* 70, 752, 1990.

Richter, D., The neurohypophysial hormones vasopressin and oxytocin: gene structure, biosynthesis and processing, in *The Posterior Pituitary: Hormone Secretion in Health and Disease,* Baylis, P. H. and Padfield, P. L., Eds., Marcel Dekker, New York, 1985.

Riddell, D. C., Mallonee, R., Phillips, J. A., III, Parks, J. S., Sexton, L. A., and Hamerton, J. L., Chromosomal assignment of human sequences encoding arginine vasopressin — neurophysin II and growth hormone releasing factor, *Somat. Cell Mol. Genet.,* 11, 189, 1985.

Robertson, G. L., Thirst and vasopressin function in normal and disordered states of water balance, *J. Lab. Clin. Med.,* 101, 351, 1983.

Robertson, G. L. and Athar, S., The interaction of blood osmolality and blood volume in regulating plasma vasopressin in man, *J. Clin. Endocrinol. Metab.,* 42, 613, 1976.

Robertson, G. L., Shelton, R. L., and Athar, S., The osmoregulation of vasopressin, *Kidney Int.,* 10, 25, 1976.

Robinson, A. G., dDAVP in the treatment of central diabetes insipidus, *N. Engl. J. Med.,* 294, 507, 1976.

Rowe, J. W., Shock, N. W., and De Fronzo, R., The influence of age on the renal response to water deprivation in man, *Nephron,* 17, 270, 1976.

Rowe, J. W., Shelton, R. L., Helderman, J. H., Vestal, R. E., and Robertson, G. L., Influence of the emetic reflex on vasopressin release in man, *Kidney Int.,* 16, 729, 1979.

Rowe, J. W., Minaker, K. L., Sparrow, D., and Robertson, G. L., Age-related failure of volume-pressure-mediated vasopressin release, *J. Clin. Endocrinol. Metab.,* 54, 661, 1982.

Schmale, H., Heinsohn, S., and Richter, D., Structural organization of the rat gene for the arginine vasopressin-neurophysin precursor, *EMBO J.,* 2, 763, 1983.

Singer, I. and Forrest, J. N., Jr., Drug-induced states of nephrogenic diabetes insipidus, *Kidney Int.,* 10, 82, 1976.

Sladek, C. D. and Armstrong, W. E., Effect of neurotransmitters and neuropeptides on vasopressin release, in *Vasopressin: Principles and Properties,* Gash, D. M. and Boer, G. J., Eds., Plenum Press, New York, 1987, 275.

Sridhar, C. B., Calvert, G. D., and Ibbertson, H. K., Syndrome of hypernatremia, hypodipsia and partial diabetes insipidus: a new interpretation, *J. Clin. Endocrinol. Metab.*, 38, 890, 1974.

Valtin, H., Physiological effects of vasopressin on the kidney, in *Vasopressin: Principles and Properties,* Gash, D. M. and Boer, G. J., Eds., Plenum Press, New York, 1987, 369.

Verbalis, J. G., Tumoral hyponatremia, *Arch. Intern. Med.,* 146, 1686, 1986.

Verbalis, J. G., Robinson, A. G., and Moses, A. M., Postoperative and post-traumatic diabetes insipidus, in *Diabetes Insipidus,* Czernichow, P. and Robinson, A. G., Eds., S. Karger, Basel, 1984, 247.

Vorherr, H., Para-endocrine tumor activity with emphasis on ectopic ADH secretion, *Oncology,* 29, 382, 1974.

Vorherr, H., Vorherr, U. F., McConnell, T. S., Goldberg, N. M., Kornfeld, M., and Jordan, S. W., Localization and origin of antidiuretic principle in para-endocrine active malignant tumors, *Oncology,* 29, 201, 1974.

Walter, R. and Bowman, R. H., Mechanism of inactivation of vasopressin and oxytocin by the isolated perfused rat kidney, *Endocrinology,* 92, 189, 1973.

Watabe, T., Tanaka, K., Kumagae, M., Itoh, S., Kogure, M., Hasegawa, M., Horiuchi, T., Morio, K., Takeda, F., Ubukata, E., Miyabe, S., and Shimizu, N., Role of endogenous arginine vasopressin in potentiating corticotrophin-releasing hormone-stimulated corticotrophin secretion in man, *J. Clin. Endocrinol. Metab.,* 66, 1132, 1988.

Williams, R. H. and Henry, C., Nephrogenic diabetes insipidus: transmitted by females and appearing during infancy in males, *Ann. Intern. Med.,* 27, 84, 1947.

Williams, T. D. M., Dunger, D. B., Lyon, C. C., Lewis, R. J., Taylor, F., and Lightman, S. L., Antidiuretic effect and pharmacokinetics of oral 1-desamino-8-D-arginine vasopressin. I. Studies in adults and children, *J. Clin. Endocrinol. Metab.,* 63, 129, 1986.

Zerbe, R. L. and Robertson, G. L., A comparison of plasma vasopressin measurements with a standard indirect test in the differential diagnosis of polyuria, *N. Engl. J. Med.,* 305, 1539, 1981.

Zerbe, R. L., Stropes, L., and Robertson, G. L., Vasopressin function in the syndrome of inappropriate antidiuresis, *Annu. Rev. Med.,* 31, 315, 1980.

Zerbe, R. L., Bayorh, M. A., and Feuerstein, G., Vasopressin: an essential pressor factor for blood pressure recovery following hemorrhage, *Peptides,* 3, 509, 1982.

Zerbe, R. L., Henry, D. P., and Robertson, G. L., Vasopressin response to orthostatic hypotension: etiological and clinical implications, *Am. J. Med.,* 74, 265, 1983.

20

Geriatric Neuroendocrinology

ARSHAG D. MOORADIAN
St. Louis University Medical School
St. Louis, Missouri

I. Introduction

The recent changes in the demographics of developed countries have led to the emergence of the geriatric imperative. In 1980 the Census Bureau estimated that almost 11% of Americans are above the age of 65 years, and by the year 2030 this segment of the population will account for 21.1% of all Americans. The fastest growing segment of the population is that of the very old (over 85 years of age). Thus the increase in average life span is not totally attributable to decreased infant mortality rates, but is also related to true prolongation of life in adults secondary to improved medical care, nutritional status, and a variety of hitherto unidentified factors.

Because of this change in demographics, the importance of studying the aging process has become widely acknowledged. The interaction of aging and a variety of disease states is of particular interest. Not only is there an age-related decrease in homeostatic reserve, but also organ dysfunction is common in the elderly and the distinction between health and disease becomes more difficult to make. The interaction of aging with the neuroendocrine system is characterized by substantial reciprocity. Whereas aging can alter the neuroendocrine function, changes in the neuroendocrine system in turn can probably alter the rate of aging, at least for some tissues. Whether the neuroendocrine system has a central role in senescence is still not known. However, one of the popular theories of aging is the neuroendocrine theory (Mooradian, 1991; Hart and Turturro, 1983). It is suggested that a "pacemaker" of aging, possibly located in the hypothalamus, pituitary, or pineal gland, times the onset of senescence. The experimental evidence so far does not prove or disprove this hypothesis. This facet of the interaction between aging and the neuroendocrine system is beyond the scope of this chapter. The focus instead is on the various neuroendocrine changes that have been described in aged humans or animals. The impact of these changes on the metabolic milieu, cognitive function, and overall well-being of the individual will be discussed. Since Alzheimer's disease is the prototype of age-related degenerative diseases of the brain, the neuroendocrine changes found in patients with Alzheimer's disease will also be reviewed. The common neuroendocrine changes seen in the elderly are summarized in Table 1.

II. Principles of Geriatric Neuroendocrinology

The general principles of geriatric medicine also apply to geriatric neuroendocrinology (Mooradian et al., 1988). The coexistence of multiple endocrine diseases as part of polyglandular failure syndrome should be kept in mind. The clinical manifestations of various neuroendo-

Table 1
Common Neuroendocrine Changes with Aging

Hormone	Basal level	Stimulated level
Anterior pituitary		
Growth hormone	N or ↓	↓
Prolactin	N	
	↑ in men	
	↓ in women	
Thyrotropin (TSH)	N or ↑	N (↓ in men)
Luteinizing hormone (LH)	↑	↓
Follicle-stimulating hormone (FSH)	↑	↓
Adrenocorticotropic hormone (ACTH)	N	N
β-Endorphin	N	N
Posterior pituitary		
Arginine vasopressin	↑	↓ (volume-receptor mediated)
		↑ (osmoreceptor mediated)

crine diseases can be atypical and some are often attributed to the aging process. This will delay the seeking of medical attention and prompt institution of therapy. For example, in young women, irregularity of the menstrual cycle is often an early sign of pituitary disease. This relatively sensitive clinical index of pituitary dysfunction is not helpful in elderly women. In elderly men, sexual dysfunction or loss of libido is often mistakenly attributed to aging and an underlying neuroendocrine dysfunction is often missed.

Coexisting diseases and use of multiple drugs in the elderly interfere with the clinical picture, alter laboratory tests, and may complicate management. Increased body adiposity, loss of muscle mass, and glucose intolerance are common changes in aging and yet they may well be the harbinger of Cushing's disease. Depression or acute illness, common problems in elderly patients, are known to have a profound effect on laboratory workups of neuroendocrinologic disease. Commonly prescribed drugs in the elderly, such as antidepressants, can elevate serum prolactin concentrations to levels that are consistent with the diagnosis of pituitary prolactinoma. Chlorpropamide in diabetic patients can cause water intoxication, simulating the syndrome of inappropriate antidiuretic hormone secretion (SIADH).

The high prevalence of health food consumption in the elderly is also a potential confounding factor. Chronic use of ginseng tea will activate the hypothalamic pituitary adrenal axis and cause hypertension. Ingestion of large amounts of β-carotene will lead to yellow discoloration of the skin similar to that seen in hypothyroidism.

The interpretation of endocrine tests in elderly patients is also complicated by the fact that the normal range of values is usually determined in younger populations. The altered values in the elderly can be looked on as either "normal" for age or considered abnormal. This important issue still remains unanswered. The effect of drugs on serum hormone measurements should be kept in mind when interpreting the laboratory test results.

One of the neuroendocrine problems more commonly seen in the elderly is ectopic hormone production from neoplasms. Elderly patients presenting with Cushing's syndrome, inappropriate ADH secretion (SIADH), or hypercalcemia should be thoroughly evaluated for underlying malignancy. Awareness of this possibility may result in early detection of cancer and avoid unnecessary work-up for endocrine disease. The possibility of ectopic hormone production should be suspected when the elevated serum hormone concentrations are out of proportion to the clinical manifestations seen in those with ectopic hormone hypersecretion.

With aging, a variety of changes in receptor or post-receptor activity have been described. These alterations result in decreased hormone responsiveness. Although adequate experimental data are lacking, it is possible that age-related changes in hormone responsiveness underlie some of the neuroendocrine changes seen in the elderly. For example, decreased adrenergic responsiveness in the central nervous system may contribute to increased prevalence of hypogonadotropic hypogonadism in this patient population.

The management of endocrine disease in the elderly is generally similar to that in younger patients. Some differences, however, should be acknowledged. Surgical procedures such as adrenalectomy or hypophysectomy are associated with a higher rate of morbidity and mortality in the elderly. Life expectancy of the patient should be considered when recommending pituitary irradiation, a therapeutic modality that may require a prolonged period of time to result in clinical response. Nevertheless, age alone should not be the sole criterion for denying a given therapy for the patient. The functional status of the patient, coexisting diseases, and "biological" age of the individual should be taken into account when making a decision on the form of therapy. Finally, when it comes to hormone replacement therapy, it is prudent to start with small doses and gradually increase the dose, along with close monitoring for a possible untoward side effect.

III. Histologic Alterations in the Pituitary Gland

There is little information on the effects of aging on the pituitary gland. The gland reaches its maximal size during middle age and then gradually may decrease in size (Everitt, 1980). Autopsy studies, however, have indicated that there is no change in pituitary weight with advancing age (Andres and Tobin, 1977). In women, pituitary weight is reduced with the onset of menopause. Histologic changes of the pituitary seen in old age include reduced vascularity, increased fibrosis, and altered distribution of cell types. The proportion of eosinophilic cells is decreased, while the proportion of basophilic and chromophobic cells is increased. There is also increased vacuolation of basophilic cells with aging. Studies using the immunoperoxidase staining technique have found a marked increase in pituitary content of folliculotropin (FSH) and luteotropin (LH) in post-menopausal women and an increase in LH in elderly men (Gregerman and Bielman, 1981). The pituitary content of growth hormone (GH), thyrotropin (TSH), and prolactin is not altered with age (Calderon et al., 1978; Kovacs et al., 1977). The corticotropin (ACTH) content may be slightly reduced in the pituitary with age.

Small adenomas or areas of hyperplasia are common in the pituitary of people over the age of 40 (Burrow et al., 1981). The reported prevalence of pituitary adenomas in autopsy studies is highly variable. McKeown (1965) reported 39 adenomas in 1500 pituitaries studied in patients over 70 years. Costello (1936) reported a 22.5% prevalence of adenomas in 1000 unselected cases. In another study, 20 pituitary adenomas were found out of 152 examined (Kovacs et al., 1980). All adenomas were chromophobic, and 53% stained positively for prolactin. None of the adenomas was positive for FSH, LH, TSH, or ACTH, and only one adenoma was positive for GH.

The increased prevalence of incidental pituitary adenomas is further confounded with the fact that aging is associated with alterations in the appearance of the sella turcica, such as demineralization and increase in size. Thus in patients over 75 years, who do not have any clinical or biochemical evidence of pituitary disease, up to 65% may have complete or partial empty sella (Andres and Tobin, 1977). Awareness of this fact will help physicians avoid unnecessary diagnostic work-ups and inappropriate management.

IV. Physiologic Alterations with Age

A. Hypothalamus

Most age-related hormonal changes are modulated either directly or indirectly by the changes in neurotransmitter function. A host of alterations in the aging CNS have been reported, the most crucial of which are those related to the hypothalamus, perhaps because of its central role in pituitary hormone secretion. The best studied neurotransmitter change is the catecholaminergic system. Aged male rodents have been consistently found to have reduced hypothalamic catecholamine levels and reduced turnover (Finch and Landfield, 1985; Rogers and Bloom, 1985). The studies in female rodents are complicated by the fact that hormonal changes associated with aging modulate hypothalamic neurotransmitter physiology. Overall it appears that in aged female rats the hypothalamic norepinephrine levels and turnover are reduced, while serotonin levels are increased (Walker et al., 1980). Drugs that may alter serotonin metabolism, such as p-chlorophenylalanine, with 5-hydroxytryptophan or progesterone may restore LH secretion in old rats (Walker, 1982; Franks et al., 1980). Other important changes observed in aged female rats include partially blunted post-castration rise in hypothalamic catecholamine at 2 years of age (Wilkes and Yen, 1981), and reduced dopamine levels in the median eminence of the hypothalamus (Demarest et al., 1982) and in hypophysial portal blood (Gudelsky et al., 1981; Reymond and Porter, 1981). The latter changes are also observed in aged male rats with elevated plasma prolactin levels. Since prolactin is known to stimulate hypothalamic dopamine turnover and increases dopamine levels in hypophysial portal blood (Gudelsky et al., 1981; Reymond and Porter, 1981), it is suggested that dopaminergic neurons in aged rats have reduced sensitivity to prolactin (Finch and Landfield, 1985). Other important changes in neurotransmitter content of the hypothalamus with age include reduced β-endorphin and vasopressin levels and increases in met-enkephalin levels (Rogers and Bloom, 1985). Although the precise biochemical consequences of these changes are still unknown, it is likely that they are involved in the age-related changes of the endocrine system.

B. Anterior Pituitary

1. Growth Hormone

Age-related alterations in the physiology of GH secretion and action have received considerable attention (Table 2). It has been suggested that some of the muscle wastage commonly seen in the elderly may be related to reduced GH effects. Most of these effects are mediated by somatomedins or insulin-like growth factors (IGFs) (Mooradian and Morley, 1987). This family of peptides is responsible for the GH effect in promoting protein synthesis in muscle, glucose oxidation in adipose tissue, and cell replication. The two major somatomedins are types A (IGF-II) and C (IGF-I). Aging does not appear to alter serum IGF-II levels, but numerous studies have shown that serum IGF-I concentrations decrease with age (Rudman et al., 1981; Sara et al., 1982; Johanson and Blizzard, 1981; Clemmons and Van Wyk, 1984; Florini et al., 1985; Vermeulen, 1987; Bennett et al., 1986; Ho et al., 1987). Very low levels are found in frail, elderly nursing home patients with poor nutritional status (Rudman et al., 1986). Factors that modulate somatomedin release and that are more likely to be found in the elderly include malnutrition, alcoholic liver disease, diabetes mellitus, hypothyroidism, and use of glucocorticoids (Table 3).

The effect of aging on GH secretion is more controversial. GH release from the pituitary gland is governed by the interacting effects of three major factors: GH-releasing hormone stimulates GH release; somatostatin, a 14-amino acid hypothalamic peptide, inhibits GH release, and so do the somatomedins by direct effect on the pituitary and indirectly through

Table 2
Age-Related Alterations in Growth Hormone Secretion
and Action

	Change
Hormone level	
Basal	N or ↓
24-hr integrated level	N
Nocturnal peak amplitude	↓
Induced GH secretion by	
Sleep	↓
Dopa	↓
Insulin-induced hypoglycemia	N or ↓
Arginine infusion	N or ↓
Hormone action	
IGF-I level (somatomedin-C)	↓
Receptor binding to IGF-I in fibroblasts	N
Fibroblast proliferative response to IGF-I	N

Table 3
Factors that Reduce Somatomedin
Release and Are Commonly Found in
the Elderly

Malnutrition
Alcoholic liver disease
Diabetes mellitus
Hypothyroidism
Relative estrogen excess in elderly men
Use of glucocorticoids

stimulation of hypothalamic somatostatin release. The effect of age on GH secretion is clearly age dependent. In women basal GH levels fall with advancing age (Vidalon et al., 1973), while in men they remain unchanged or increase slightly (Prinz and Weitzman, 1983; Davis, 1979). This change may be related to loss of estrogen in post-menopausal women and relatively high estrogen levels in elderly men compared to young men. Estrogen administration increases both resting (Wiedemann et al., 1976) and stimulated GH secretion (Frantz and Rabkin, 1965). Even physiologic doses of estrogen increase the 24-hr integrated GH secretion or GH secretory response to exercise and to GH-releasing hormone (GHRH) (Dawson-Hughes et al., 1986). The effect of estrogen could be the result of both a direct effect on hypothalamic-pituitary unit and an indirect one via lowering of serum IGF-I levels.

The 24-hr integrated GH levels do not decline with age (Florini et al., 1985). Vermeulen (1987), however, found that both the size of the total GH peak at night and the amplitude of the peaks were less in older subjects compared to younger controls. The basal GH levels in this study were not different among the groups studied. The serum peak IGF-I level correlated with both the total GH area and the total integrated GH levels. Thus the decreased IGF-I level with aging is probably related to decreased GH peaks (Vermeulen, 1987).

The GH response to physiologic or pharmacologic stimuli can also be altered. Sleep-induced GH secretion declines with age (Prinz and Weitzman, 1983; Davis, 1979; Carlson et al., 1972). Sixty-five percent of the inpatients over the age of 75 had decreased GH response to dopa stimulation (Impallomeni et al., 1987). The GH response to insulin-induced hypoglycemia or arginine infusion is either slightly decreased or unchanged with aging (Laron et al., 1967; Muggeo et al., 1975; Dudl et al., 1973).

The variability in GH response is probably related to the inclusion of subjects with intercurrent disease or use of medications known to alter GH secretory response. In addition, age-related increase in adiposity may explain the apparent reduction in pituitary hormonal reserve. Obese subjects are known to have blunted GH response to various provocative stimuli (Williams et al., 1984). It is not clear at the present whether the age-related changes in GH level are regulated at the level of gene expression. Of interest are the studies in mice that found decreased steady state levels of GH mRNA in its pituitary gland, although in that particular strain of mice aging is not associated with changes in GH levels (Crew et al., 1987).

The age-related changes in tissue response to IGF-I do not appear to be significant. The mitogenic response of fibroblasts from aged subjects to IGF-I and the receptor binding to IGF-I are normal (Conover et al., 1985).

The biological significance of the age-related changes in GH and IGF-I concentrations is not known. It has been suggested that GH deficiency simulates many features that are common in the elderly (Rudman, 1985). These include decline in muscle and bone mass with preferential accumulation of fat, and decline in the size of viscera such as the kidney, liver, and spleen. Whether these changes in the elderly can be reversed with GH replacement remains to be seen. In a study of seven post-menopausal women aged 52 to 70 years, GH administration for 1 year failed to increase appendicular bone density, bone formation, or resorption (Aloia et al., 1976). When GH was administered with calcitonin, however, there was a modest increase in appendicular bone density (Aloia et al., 1977). Although calcitonin alone could have improved the bone density, the authors suggested that GH had a contributing effect in bone remodeling.

In a limited study of three frail elderly men aged 75 to 85 years, Root and Oskie found that daily growth hormone injections for 10 days resulted in the expected net nitrogen retention and increased free fatty acids, but they failed to show an increase in urinary hydroxyproline levels and the red blood cells of these patients had partial resistance to the *in vitro* inhibition of glucose uptake induced by GH (Root and Oskie, 1969). These limited observations have led some to believe that certain metabolic responses to GH are blunted in the elderly.

Supportive evidence for biologic significance of age-related alterations in GH secretion must be based on controlled studies demonstrating the efficacy of GH replacement in reversing the reduced bone and muscle mass in the elderly.

2. Prolactin

Prolactin is the only pituitary hormone under predominantly inhibitory control. Dopamine is the main inhibitory factor released from the hypothalamus. Thyrotropin-releasing hormone (TRH) and estrogens are stimulators of prolactin release. More recently, various hypothalamic peptides have been found to modulate prolactin secretion but their physiologic role has not been conclusively demonstrated (Adelman et al., 1986). If dysregulation is a common concomitant of aging, then one would expect increased serum prolactin levels in the elderly, secondary to a release from the inhibitory stimuli, the main regulatory factors in prolactin secretion. The age-related decrease in brain tyrosine hydroxylase and catecholamines (Semorajski et al., 1971) may indeed suggest that decreased dopaminergic activity with age should manifest itself with increased prolactin secretion, unless other factors commonly altered with age will influence the prolactin secretion. The basal prolactin levels are slightly increased in men, while in elderly women they tend to decrease (Davis, 1979; Vekemann and Robin, 1975). These changes are probably related to the alterations in serum estrogen levels with aging. The circadian rhythm of prolactin secretion is maintained with aging. In animal models, the basal prolactin levels may be increased (Gudelsky et al., 1981; Reymond and Porter, 1981) or remain unaltered despite a decrease in pituitary content of prolactin mRNA levels (Crew et al., 1987). In rats, pituitary prolactinomas and hyperprolactinemia are common with aging. This may be in part secondary to decreased dopaminergic inhibition of prolactin secretion. In aging male and female rats with elevated prolactin levels the dopamine levels in the pituitary stalk are significantly reduced compared to younger rats (Gudelsky et al., 1981; Reymond and Porter, 1981).

The prolactin response to TRH is also blunted in the elderly, suggesting decreased pituitary prolactin reserve (Jacques et al., 1987). Although the nocturnal rise in prolactin secretion may be absent in some elderly men, the circadian rhythmicity of prolactin secretion appears to be unaltered with age (Touitou et al., 1981; Marruma et al., 1982). The biological significance of these changes is totally unknown, since there is no known physiologic role of prolactin in the elderly.

3. Thyrotropin and Thyrotropin-Releasing Hormone

Pituitary TSH secretion is under the tight control of two opposing factors: the hypothalamic TRH and the circulating thyroid hormones. Aging usually does not alter serum levels of thyroid hormones, although free triiodothyronine (T_3) level may be slightly reduced in a subgroup of the elderly (Robuschi et al., 1987). Animal studies have suggested that there is an age-related decrease in hypothalamic TRH content and secretion (Pekary et al., 1984, 1987). This was associated with a twofold increase in pituitary TRH receptor number (Pekary et al., 1985). The effect of these changes on TSH secretory pattern is complex. These changes are summarized in Table 4.

There are substantial inconsistencies in the reported changes in basal TSH levels with age. High (Harman et al., 1984; Ohara et al., 1974; Cuttelod et al., 1974), low (Montermini et al., 1985; Bermudez et al., 1975), or unaltered (Bermudez et al., 1975; Snyder and Utiger, 1972a, b; Wenzel et al., 1974) basal TSH levels have been found in the elderly. Some studies have reported the changes only in elderly men or only in elderly women. Overall the basal serum concentration of TSH increases modestly with age, especially in women, but does not exceed the upper limit of normal. A TSH value of above 10 μU/ml on more than one occasion is usually diagnostic for primary thyroidal failure (Sawin et al., 1985). Using this criterion it was found that 4.4% of an unselected population older than 60 years in the original cohort of the Framingham study had primary thyroidal failure. It is possible that some of these patients had an alteration in the set point of pituitary TSH secretion rather than a true tissue hypothyroid state. TSH sensitivity to thyroid hormones is decreased in the elderly, suggesting an age-related alteration in the set-point of TSH secretion (Ordene et al., 1983). In older subjects the TSH response to TRH was not enhanced following the small decrease in serum thyroid hormone concentrations induced by iodide administration (Ordene et al., 1983). The circadian

Table 4

Age-Related Changes in TSH Secretion and Action

	Change
TSH secretion	
Basal level	N or slightly ↑
Circadian variation	Blunted
Response to TRH	N (women)
	↓ (men)
	Anomalous GH secretion
Response to thyroid hormones	↓
TSH action	
Thyroid response to TSH	↓
Thyroxine (T_4) level	N
T_3 resin uptake	N
Triiodothyronine (T_3) level	N or slightly ↓

variation of TSH secretion is also blunted in the elderly. In addition, serum GH rises following TRH administration in the elderly (Chiodera et al., 1986). These observations collectively support the notion that aging is associated with altered neuroendocrine regulation of pituitary function. The studies on TSH response to variable doses of TRH have suggested that the pituitary thyrotropin of elderly men may have reduced sensitivity to TRH. In women, however, TSH response to TRH is unaltered with age. In earlier studies a decreased TSH response to TRH was observed in women as well (Cuttelod et al., 1974; Wenzel et al., 1974; Wenzel and Horn, 1976). Although TSH response to TRH usually correlates with basal TSH levels, in the elderly with elevated basal TSH levels, TRH infusion at 0.4 μg/min for 4 hr did not result in the expected level of TSH secretion (Harman et al., 1984). These observations suggest that hypothalamic pituitary regulation of thyroid hormone secretion is altered in the elderly. The precise biochemical basis of age-related alterations in pituitary TSH secretion is not clear. It may be related to altered biologic activity of TRH secondary to hitherto unidentified changes in TRH processing, or can be related to altered thyroid hormone transport to their receptor sites in the thyrotropin. Alternatively, since TSH secretion is also influenced by a variety of neural and neurochemical modulators such as dopamine, somatostatin, and norepinephrine (Morley, 1981), it is possible that an age-related change in these modulators may affect the TSH secretory pattern.

It appears that the resetting of the hypothalamic-pituitary-thyroid axis in the elderly is an adaptive process and does not cause hypothyroidism.

4. Adrenocorticotrophic Hormone

The interaction of glucocorticoids and the central nervous system has been the focus of gerontologic research for five decades. As early as 1949 Findlay noted the features of premature aging in patients with Cushing's syndrome (Findlay, 1949). Accelerated aging observed in some breeder rats has been attributed to stress-induced hyperadrenocorticism (Wexler, 1976). Landfield (1928) hypothesized that aging changes in the brain, particularly in the hippocampus, are modulated by glucocorticoids (Landfield, 1978). In rats aging is associated with selective loss of corticosterone-binding neurons in the CA3 hippocampal zone (Sapolsky et al., 1984), suggesting a causal role, albeit partial, of glucocorticoids in brain aging.

Adrenalectomy would retard the aging changes in the hippocampus, partly because of increased ACTH stimulatory effects on biochemical and electrophysiological parameters of the brain (Finch and Landfield, 1985). It is noteworthy that administration of ACTH analog (ORG2766) decelerated brain aging in rats (Landfield, 1981).

The effect of glucocorticoids on the rate of aging in the brain is reciprocated by the effect of aging brain on glucocorticoid production. With the onset of aging changes in the brain, hippocampal inhibition of ACTH release is attenuated. Whether this will result in increased ACTH or glucocorticoid production is controversial. Overall it appears that ACTH release and resultant adrenal production of glucocorticoids increase with age beginning in midlife, with a decrease in glucocorticoid production with further senescence (Finch and Landfield, 1985). In vitro studies have shown that adrenocortical cells from aged rats secrete less glucocorticoids, compared to adrenal cells obtained from young rats (Malamed and Carsia, 1983).

The studies in human subjects are also inconclusive. The age-related changes in pituitary adrenal axis are summarized in Table 5. The weight of evidence favors an age-related decline in both the cortisol production and clearance rate (Morley, 1987; Wolfsen, 1982). The age-related decrease in lean body mass partially offsets the decrease in cortisol secretion. Thus aging changes balance out and plasma cortisol tends to remain stable with aging. The circadian rhythm of cortisol secretion is not altered with aging (Jensen and Blichert-Toft, 1971; Blichert-

Table 5
Age-Related Changes in Hypothalamic-Pituitary-Adrenal Axis

	Change
Hypothalamic pituitary unit	
Basal ACTH level	N
Sensitivity to negative feedback by glucocorticoids	↓
ACTH response to	
CRF (corticotropin-releasing hormone)	N
Insulin-induced hypoglycemia	N
Intravenous metyrapone	N
Adrenal gland	
Glucocorticoids	
Cortisol response to ACTH	N or prolonged
Basal cortisol level	N
Cortisol levels in response to perioperative stress	↑
Circadian rhythm of cortisol secretion	Phase advance
Androgens	
Dehydroepiandrosterone	↓
Androstenedione	↓
Mineralocorticoids	
Aldosterone[a]	↓

[a]The decrease is mostly secondary to decreased renin activity
with age.

Toft, 1975), although the peak and nadir of plasma cortisol levels in men over 40 occur approximately 3 hr earlier (Sherman et al., 1985). This phase advance in cortisol secretion suggests that there might be subtle age-related changes in the biological clock regulating circadian rhythms.

In older men ACTH response to corticotropin-releasing hormone (CRH) is normal despite increased cortisol response, suggesting a diminished sensitivity of ACTH to negative feedback by glucocorticoids (Parlor et al., 1986). The cortisol response to insulin-induced hypoglycemia (Cartlidge et al., 1970; Muggeo et al., 1975) or intravenous metyrapone test (Blichert-Toft et al., 1970; Blichert-Toft and Hummer, 1977) are similar in healthy elderly and the young. The cortisol response to ACTH stimulation of the adrenal glands is usually normal (Blichert-Toft et al., 1970; West et al., 1961) or is slightly prolonged (Blichert-Toft et al., 1967) in healthy elderly subjects. The elderly, however, have higher plasma cortisol levels when depressed (Greden et al., 1986; Asnis et al., 1981) and in response to perioperative stress (Blichert-Toft, 1975).

The age-related attenuation of the pituitary ACTH sensitivity to glucocorticoid suppressive effects is also demonstrated by Oxenkrug et al. (1983), who found that the older individual has higher post-dexamethasone plasma cortisol levels. This age-related difference in cortisol response to dexamethasone was confirmed in subsequent studies (Davis et al., 1984; Nelson et al., 1984). It is noteworthy that depression and dementia are common in the elderly and both these conditions are associated with blunted dexamethasone suppression of cortisol secretion.

Of interest is that circadian secretory pattern of β-endorphin, a fragment sharing with ACTH the parent molecule, is unaltered with age (Rolandi et al., 1987). The β-endorphin response to exercise is also normal in the elderly. Unlike the peripheral plasma levels, cerebrospinal fluid concentrations of β-endorphin decrease with age (Hatfield et al., 1987).

It appears therefore that aging is associated with significant alterations in hypothalamic pituitary adrenal axis and that this system in turn may modulate certain aging phenomena in the brain.

5. Gonadotropins

The age-related changes in gonadotropin secretion and reproductive hormone physiology have been the focus of gerontologic research since 1889, when Brown-Sequard injected himself with a testicular extract and reported a feeling of rejuvenation. In women, reproductive senescence is heralded by dramatic changes such as menopause and hot flushes. The changes in men are more subtle and often may go unnoticed. Careful assessment of biochemical and hormonal profile shows that significant changes in reproductive hormones occur in both aging men and women. The reproductive hormonal changes that may occur with aging in men are summarized in Table 6. Generally the reduced serum testosterone and bioavailable testosterone with age are accompanied by increase in mean LH and FSH levels (Deslypere and Vermeulen, 1986). The diurnal rhythm of testosterone secretion is blunted in elderly men. Compared to young men, the LH pulse frequency may be reduced in elderly men but pulse amplitude is retained (Deslypere et al., 1982). This is not, however, a universally observed phenomenon. Kaiser et al. (1988) found decreased LH pulse amplitude in elderly men while the change in pulse frequency was not significant. In these subjects, gonadal dysfunction appears to be the primary modulator of reproductive senescence. In a subgroup of elderly men, however, hypothalamic/pituitary dysfunction appears to be the predominant age-related change. The hormonal profile in these subjects is consistent with hypogonadotropic hypogonadism (Korenman et al., 1987). In women, on the other hand, gonadal hypofunction has the key role in reproductive senescence and the changes in gonadotropin secretion are secondary phenomena. By 4 years after menopause the direct ovarian secretion of estrogen practically disappears and the plasma estradiol (E_2) and estrone (E_1) are derived from the aromatization of adrenal androstenedione in fat, muscle, skin, liver, and the hypothalamus (Siiteri and MacDonald, 1973; Judd et al., 1982). The E_1 levels are higher than E_2 levels after menopause. The changes in the levels of these hormones with further aging are usually insignificant.

The relative importance of gonadal hypofunction as compared to hypothalamic reproductive senescence is clearly species dependent. In rodents, the hypothalamus has a central role in pacing the ovulatory cycles and "rejuvenation" of reproductive function in old rats could be transiently achieved with a variety of pharmacologic and electrophysiologic manipulations such as administration of tyrosine, L-dopa, iproniazid or lergotrile (adrenergic agonists), progesterone, or electrical stimulation of the hypothalamus (Finch, 1978; Wise, 1983). The ovary in rodents is not an innocent bystander in reproductive senescence. A key role of the ovarian factors, particularly estrogen, in hypothalamic aging is indicated by the finding that

Table 6
Reproductive Hormone Changes with Aging

In men
  Reduced total serum testosterone
  Reduced bioavailable testosterone
  Increased testosterone binding
  Blunted diurnal rhythm of testosterone secretion
  Increased mean LH and FSH levels
  Reduced LH response to GnRH
  Decreased LH pulse frequency and amplitude
  Decreased tissue 5 α-reductase activity
  High prevalence of hypogonadotropic and hypergonadotropic hypogonadism
In women
  Direct ovarian secretion of estrogens markedly reduced
  Estradiol and estrones are derived from peripheral aromatization of adrenal androgens
  Estrone levels are higher than estradiol levels
  Markedly increased LH and FSH levels

chronically ovariectomized rodents of 16 to 28 months of age can resume normal estrous cycles when grafted with young ovaries (Aschheim, 1976; Felicio et al., 1983; Nelson et al., 1980). In rats with recent cessation of ovulatory cycles, the pituitary response to gonadotropin-releasing hormone (GnRH) is normal. With further senescence the pituitary response to GnRH is variable, but it appears that the impairment correlates with the hormonal status of the animal (Cooper et al., 1984), or perhaps with the presence of pituitary tumors, particularly prolactinomas (Felicio et al., 1980).

The hyperprolactinemia in aged rats may explain their lack of serum LH elevation with aging in this species. In mice, however, where plasma prolactin is not elevated, spontaneous LH elevations with aging are documented (Parkening et al., 1982; Finch et al., 1977).

Despite the differences and inconsistencies in the reported studies, the reproductive senescence occurs both at the gonadal and the hypothalamic level. The contribution of each change, however, varies among the species.

C. Posterior Pituitary

Arginine vasopressin (AVP) and oxytocin are the two main hormones secreted by the posterior pituitary (Mooradian and Morley, 1987). Both these hormones have distinct carrier proteins known as neurophysins. These carrier proteins are involved in axonal transport and storage of AVP and oxytocin at the axonal terminals in the posterior lobe of the pituitary gland. The physiologic roles of oxytocin other than those involved in lactation and parturition are not known. The age-related changes in oxytocin secretion have not been studied either. In contrast, the age-related changes in AVP secretion and action have been extensively evaluated. This hormone has been shown to have important effects not only in water homeostasis but also in diverse processes controlled by the central nervous system such as thermoregulation (Kasting et al., 1980) and memory retention (deWeid and Van Ree, 1982). When plasma concentrations are very high, a distinct effect on smooth muscles of the vasculature and the gut is noted (Mooradian and Morley, 1987).

Normally the pituitary gland is the only source of AVP. Certain malignancies, however, notably oat cell carcinomas of the lung, are capable of secreting AVP or AVP-like peptides. In elderly patients with the syndrome of inappropriate ADH secretion (SIADH), an underlying malignancy should always be excluded. Of various physiologic and pharmacologic stimuli of vasopressin (Table 7), the AVP secretion is most sensitive to changes in plasma osmolality (Anderson, 1978; Robertson, 1977; Schrier et al., 1979). The osmal threshold for AVP secretion and the rate of increase in plasma AVP per unit increase in plasma osmolality (AVP/OSM) are modulated by other factors, notably the blood volume status. Interdependence of volume receptor-mediated and osmoreceptor-mediated secretion is not surprising in view of the fact that they share a common final pathway at the level of AVP-producing neuronal cells.

Aging has a profound effect on AVP secretion and action. The basal serum levels of AVP are usually elevated with age. Volume receptor-mediated release of AVP is reduced in the elderly (Rowe et al., 1982), presumably secondary to reduced baroreceptor sensitivity. On the other hand, in a subgroup of elderly patients with borderline counterregulatory reflexes, upright posture may result in larger changes in effective blood volume, resulting in excess AVP secretion. In contrast to the decreased AVP response to volume receptors, AVP response to osmotic stimuli is enhanced (Miller, 1985; Helderman et al., 1978). The lowest level of plasma osmolality that will initiate AVP secretion (osmotic threshold) is reduced in the elderly and AVP/OSM is increased with age. The elderly are less sensitive to the AVP-suppressive effects of ethanol infusion. Whereas continuous ethanol infusion causes a prolonged inhibition of AVP secretion in the young, in older subjects a breakthrough secretion of AVP occurs

Table 7
Effect of Age on Arginine Vasopressin Secretion by
Various Stimuli

Stimuli of AVP secretion	Effect of age
Osmoreceptor	↑
Baroreceptor	↓
Volume receptor	↓
Nociceptive center	?
Emetic center	?
Glucopenia	N
Hypercapnea	?
Angiotensin II	↓
Drugs[a]: inhibitory effect of ethanol	↓

[a]The effect of age on drug-induced inhibition or potentiation of AVP secretion is not known.

(Helderman et al., 1978). It appears that the CNS drive for AVP secretion is increased with age. Aging per se does not alter the AVP plasma clearance rate or volume of distribution (Robertson and Rowe, 1980). The target organ resistance to AVP action in aged animals with normal renal function appears to be secondary to elevated plasma AVP levels, possibly down regulating AVP receptors (Miller, 1987). Obviously, in older animals with impaired renal function the apparent sensitivity to AVP is reduced.

Another important physiologic stimulus of AVP secretion is angiotensin II. With aging, plasma renin activity is reduced (Tsundo et al., 1986) along with a decrease in angiotensin-converting enzyme activity (Lieberman, 1975). Thus the elderly tend to have reduced capacity for generating angiotensin II, a potent stimulator of AVP secretion and thirst. Hypoangiotensinemia was implicated as the pathogenetic mechanism of dehydration in a group of hypernatremic elderly patients (Yamamoto et al., 1988).

Although various age-related changes in neurotransmitter metabolism have been described, and some of these neurotransmitters are known modulators of AVP secretion, the available experimental data are not sufficient to allow the establishment of a causal link between the various physiological changes in AVP secretion and the changes in neurotransmitter activity with age.

D. Pituitary Dynamic Testing

The enthusiasm for dynamic testing of pituitary function in clinical practice has faded over the years. The initial expectations that such testing would differentiate pituitary disease from hypothalamic dysfunction were not fulfilled because of a substantial degree of overlap in the pituitary response to various releasing hormones when patients with pituitary disease were compared to those with hypothalamic pathology. TSH response to TRH, a relatively common pituitary test, is now becoming obsolete with the advent of the new immunoradiometric TSH assays capable of differentiating low levels of TSH from the normal levels. Nevertheless, the occasional patient may be seen who may require pituitary dynamic testing. The alterations in the response of pituitary to releasing hormones that are commonly seen in the elderly are summarized in Table 8. The GH response to GHRH (growth hormone-releasing hormone) may be normal or attenuated with age (Mooradian et al., 1988). The response of GH to other provocative stimuli may also be blunted, particularly in obese elderly or in the presence of intercurrent illness. The LH and FSH response to GnRH (gonadotropin hormone-releasing hormone) in elderly men tends to be reduced and delayed (Harman et al., 1982), especially in the presence of critical illness (Woolf et al., 1985; Quint and Kaiser, 1985). The TSH response to TRH is either normal or reduced, especially in elderly men. Depression, uremia, malnutri-

Table 8
Effect of Age on Pituitary Dynamic Testing

The stimulus	Hormone measured	Change
GnRH	LH	↓
	FSH	↓
TRH	TSH	N or ↓ (in men)
	Prolactin	↓
CRF	ACTH	N
Metyrapone stimulation	Cortisol	N
Dexamethasone suppression	Cortisol	↓
GHRH	GH	N or ↓
Insulin-induced	Cortisol	N
hypoglycemia	GH	↓
Arginine infusion	GH	↓

tion, or nonthyroidal illness and steroid therapy are additional factors commonly associated with blunted TSH response to TRH. The prolactin response to TRH may also be blunted in the elderly (Jacques et al., 1987). The ACTH response to CRF (corticotropin-releasing factor) is unaltered with age (Pavlov et al., 1986).

Overall healthy aging does not seem to alter pituitary response to various releasing hormones. In the presence of intercurrent disease, however, and when the patient is taking certain medications, the pituitary response to these releasing hormones can be blunted. Thus when the pituitary test results are abnormal in frail elderly patients, caution should be exercised to avoid misinterpretation.

V. Hypopituitarism

The literature on the clinical presentation of hypopituitarism in the elderly is very limited. It is likely that the clinical diagnosis of pituitary insufficiency in the elderly is difficult to suspect, since the classical features of hypopituitarism such as fatigue, anemia, postural hypotension, weight loss, hypoglycemia, and hypogonadism are common problems in the elderly. In a study of five patients between 70 and 90 years of age with idiopathic hypopituitarism, Belchetz (1985) found that extreme pallor, hyponatremia, and postural hypotension are common features in the clinical presentation. All patients had low TSH, GH, gonadotropin, cortisol, and prolactin levels and blunted pituitary response to GnRH and adrenal response to ACTH. These patients had normal skull roentgenograms although in two cases pituitary atrophy was found on post-mortem examination. A similar case was reported in a 67-year-old diabetic man, who presented with loss of gonadotropin and ACTH response while thyroid function appeared to be intact (Fiatarone, 1988). Diabetes, a common disease in the elderly, may have contributed to the pathogenesis of pituitary insufficiency in this patient. Other causes of hypopituitarism that are more likely to be found in the elderly are tuberculosis and amyloidosis. Transient depression of pituitary function is common with acute illness and should not be confused with hypopituitarism.

VI. Neuroendocrine Changes in Azheimer's Disease

Aging is associated with a variety of changes in brain content of neurotransmitters (Rogers and Bloom, 1985) (Table 9). Some of these changes may contribute to age-related change in cognitive function. Although the exact cause of memory disturbance in Alzheimer's disease is still unknown, there appears to be a host of changes in neurotransmitter and neuropeptide levels in the central nervous system that may be crucial in the pathogenesis of dementia (Table 10). The reduced levels of neurotransmitters such as acetylcholine or norepinephrine and of neuropeptides such as CRF, somatostatin, and neuropeptide Y will result in profound hormonal changes (Mooradian et al., 1988). It is noteworthy that the degenerative changes in Alzheimer's disease extend beyond the cerebral cortex to involve subcortical structures, including the hypothalamus. The reduction in hypothalamic content of acetylcholine, norepinephrine, and somatostatin plays a key role in altered pituitary function in those patients. There is ample evidence to suggest that the hypothalamic-pituitary adrenal axis may be overactive in at least 50% of those patients with Alzheimer's disease (Davis et al., 1986). This may be related to reduced inhibitory tone of norepinephrine on this axis. Thus the afternoon and evening concentrations of plasma cortisol following dexamethasone suppression tests are significantly elevated (Davis et al., 1986) in about half of the patients. These changes do not appear to be mediated by CRF, since post-mortem tissue studies of cerebrospinal fluid measurement have found mildly reduced levels of CRF (Fine, 1986). In the cerebral cortex of Alzheimer's patients the reduced concentrations of CRF-like immunoreactivity were associated with reciprocal increase in CRF receptors. This suggests that CRF-receptive cells may be preserved in the cortex of these patients (DeSouza et al., 1986).

Table 9
Common Changes in Neurotransmitter Content of Aged Brains

Decreased levels	Increased levels
Cortex	Hypothalamus
Aspartate	Met-enkephalin
Taurine	Serotonin
Glutamate	
GABA	
VIP (temporal lobe)	
Serotonin (hippocampus)	
Subcortical structures	
Dopamine ⎫	
GABA ⎬ (basal ganglia)	
Glutamate ⎭	
Beta endorphin ⎫ (hypothalamus)	
Vasopressin ⎭	
Substance P (putamen)	
Neurotensin (substantia nigra)	

Table 10
Neuroendocrine Changes in Alzheimer's Disease

Central nervous system content of neurotransmitters
    Decreased acetylcholine
    Decreased norepinephrine
Central nervous system content of neuropeptides
    Decreased corticotrophin-releasing factor (CRF)
    Decreased somatostatin
    Decreased neuropeptide Y
Hormonal changes
    Increased plasma cortisol levels following dexamethasone suppression
    Increased serum TSH concentration
    Increased serum GH concentration
    Increased serum insulin concentrations
    Reduced fasting serum glucose concentration
    Decreased estrogen-stimulated neurophysin secretion

The plasma TSH and GH concentrations are elevated in Alzheimer's disease, possibly because of reduced somatostatin activity (Christie et al., 1987). The elevated GH concentrations are often associated with increased somatomedin levels in the serum and cerebrospinal fluid (Sara et al., 1982). This suggests that the GH secreted in these patients is biologically active. Another common feature is increased serum insulin levels with decreasing fasting serum glucose concentrations (Bucht et al., 1983). This may be due to reduced somatostatin concentrations or more likely is secondary to malnutrition that is common in patients with Alzheimer's disease. It remains to be seen if chronic "hypoglycemia" contributes to the neuronal loss in this disease (Reubi and Palacios, 1986).

A hormonal change that could be due to reduced cholinergic activity is the decreased estrogen-stimulated neurophysin level (Christie et al., 1987). The clinical significance of this observation is not clear.

Although there is some overlap between the hormonal changes seen with aging with those seen in patients with Alzheimer's disease, distinct differences, particularly in GH physiology, are noted.

VII. Neuroendocrine Changes in Late-Life Depression

Although significant progress in our understanding of the biologic basis of depression has been made, the rate of age-related neuroendocrine and neurotransmitter changes in late-life depression is still unknown (Fitten et al., 1989). The evidence available so far suggests that the age-related neurochemical changes may have a protective role against depression. Thus the changes in neurotransmitter activity seen with normal aging are often reversed in patients with depression (Table 11). Whereas elderly subjects have increased norepinephrine and 5-hydroxyindoleacetic acid (5-HIAA) levels in the cerebrospinal fluid (CSF), in depression the

Table 11

A Comparison of the Neuroendocrine Changes Seen in Depression and with Normal Aging[a]

	Change in depression	Change with aging
Neurotransmitters		
Cholinergic activity	↑	↓
Norepinephrine	↓	↑
β-Adrenergic receptors	↑	↓
α$_2$-Adrenergic receptors	± ↓	?
Serotonin metabolites	↓	↑
Serotonin receptors	↑	↓
Somatostatin	↓	↑
Corticotropin-releasing factor	↑	↑
Neuroendocrine changes		
TSH response to TRH	↓	↓
Dexamethasone suppression of cortisol	↓	↓
Clonidine stimulation of growth hormone	↓	↓

[a]TSH, Thyroid-stimulating hormone; TRH, thyrotropin-releasing hormone; ↑, increase; ↓, decrease; ?, unknown.

Adapted from Fritten, L. J., Morley, J. E., Gross, P. L., Petry, S. D., and Cole, K. D., *J. Am. Geriatr. Soc.*, 37, 459, 1989.

brain content of these neurotransmitters may be depleted (Veith and Raskind, 1988; Raskind et al., 1988; Mann et al., 1985, 1986; Wong et al., 1984). Increased cholinergic activity has been suggested as another factor involved in depression (Janowsky et al., 1972). Aging, on the other hand, is associated with decreased cholinergic activity in various areas of the brain. A discordance between aging and depression is also seen in various neuroendocrinologic parameters. Aging is associated with increased somatostatin levels along with a decrease in growth hormone (GH) secretion (Mooradian et al., 1988). Depressed patients, on the other hand, have reduced somatostatin levels in the CSF and increased nocturnal GH secretion (Mendlewicz et al., 1985; Garner and Yamada, 1982). The altered pituitary-thyroid or pituitary-adrenal axis with aging simulates the changes seen in depressed patients. Thus, in both depression and aging, TSH response to TRH may be blunted (Mooradian et al., 1988; Fitten et al., 1989). The pituitary-adrenal axis is hyperactive in depressed patients as well as in nondepressed elderly subjects. This is probably secondary to increased secretion of CRF (Mooradian et al., 1988; Fitten et al., 1989). It is noteworthy that CRF may have an important role in producing the vegetative symptoms associated with depression such as anorexia, psychomotor retardation, decreased rapid eye movement (REM) sleep, slow gastrointestinal transit time, and decreased sexual activity (Gold and Rubinow, 1987). It appears that the age-related changes in neurotransmitter levels may mitigate against development of depression, and the increased incidence of vegetative symptoms in the elderly depressed patients may be related to increased CRF levels with age.

Conclusions

Significant changes in brain neurotransmitter levels and various neuroendocrine parameters occur with age. Some of these changes may be involved in the pathogenesis of neurodegenerative diseases of aging. At present, however, there is no evidence to implicate any one factor in age-related changes in cognitive function or late-life depression. It is more likely that a constellation of interrelated changes are involved in these diseases. It appears that not all the changes seen with aging have deleterious implications in the evolution of common diseases in the elderly. This is especially true in the pathogenesis of depression, in which some of the age-related changes in neurotransmitter activity may have a protective role.

References

Adelman, J. P., Mason, A. J., Hayflick, J. S., and Seeburg, P. H., Isolation of the gene and hypothalamic cDNA for the common precursor of gonadotropin-releasing hormone and prolactin release-inhibiting factor in human and rat, *Proc. Natl. Acad. Sci. U.S.A.,* 83, 179, 1986.

Aloia, J. F., Zanzi, I., Ellis, K., et al., Effects of growth hormone in osteoporosis, *J. Clin. Endocrinol. Metab.,* 43, 992, 1976.

Aloia, J. F., Zanzi, I., Vaswani, A., et al., Combination therapy for osteoporosis, *Metabolism,* 26, 787, 1977.

Anderson, B., Regulation of water intake, *Physiol. Rev.,* 58, 582, 1978.

Andres, R. and Tobin, J. D., Endocrine systems, in *Handbook of the Biology of Aging,* Finch, C. E. and Hayflick, L., Eds., Van Nostrand Reinhold, New York, 1977, 367.

Aschheim, P., Aging in the hypothalamic-hypophyseal-ovarian axis in the rat, in *Hypothalamus, Pituitary and Aging,* Everitt, A. V. and Burgess, J. A., Eds., Charles C Thomas, Springfield, IL, 1976, 376.

Asnis, G. M., Sachar, E. J., Helbreich, U., et al., Cortisol secretion in relation to age in major depression, *Psychosomat. Med.,* 43, 235, 1981.

Belchetz, P. E., Idiopathic hypopituitarism in the elderly, *Br. Med. J.*, 291, 241, 1985.

Bennett, A. E., Wahner, H. W., Riggs, B. L., and Hintz, R. L., Insulin-like growth factors I and II: aging and bone density in women, *J. Clin. Endocrinol. Metab.*, 59, 701, 1986.

Bermudez, F., Surks, M. I., and Oppenheimer, J. H., High incidence of decreased serum triiodothyronine concentration in patients with nonthyroidal disease, *J. Clin. Endocrinol. Metab.*, 41, 27, 1975.

Blichert-Toft, M., Secretion of corticotropin and somatotropin by the senescent adenohypophysis in man, *Acta Endocrinol. (Copenhagen)*, 78 (Suppl. 195), 115, 1975.

Blichert-Toft, M. and Hummer, L., Serum immunoreactive corticotropin and response to metyrapone in old age in man, *Gerontology*, 23, 236, 1977.

Blichert-Toft, M., Hippe, E., and Jensen, H. K., Adrenal cortical function as reflected by the plasma hydrocortisone and urinary 17-ketogenic steroids in relation to surgery in elderly patients, *Acta Chir. Scand.*, 133, 591, 1967.

Blichert-Toft, M., Blichert-Toft, B., and Jensen, H. K., Pituitary-adrenocortical stimulation in the aged as reflected in levels of plasma cortisol and compound S, *Acta Chir. Scand.*, 136, 665, 1970.

Bucht, G., Adolfsson, R., Lithner, F., et al., Changes in blood, glucose and insulin secretion in patients with senile dementia of Alzheimer type, *Acta Med. Scand.*, 213, 387, 1983.

Burrow, G. N., Wortzman, G., Rewcastle, N. B., Holgate, R. C., and Kovacs, K., Microadenomas of the pituitary and abnormal sellar tomograms in an unselected autopsy series, *N. Engl. J. Med.*, 304, 156, 1981.

Calderon, L., Ryan, N., and Kovacs, K., Human pituitary growth hormone cells in old age, *Gerontology*, 24, 441, 1978.

Carlson, H. E., Gillin, J. C., Gordon, P., et al., Absence of sleep-related growth hormone peaks in aged normal subjects and in acromegaly, *J. Clin. Endocrinol. Metab.*, 34, 1102, 1972.

Cartlidge, N. E. F., Black, M. M., Hall, M. R. P., et al., Pituitary function in the elderly, *Gerontol. Clin.*, 12, 65, 1970.

Chiodera, P., Gundi, A., Delsignore, R., et al., Growth hormone response to thyrotropin-releasing hormone in healthy old men, *Neuroendocrinol. Lett.*, 8, 211, 1986.

Christie, J. E., Whalley, L. J., Bennie, J., et al., Characteristic plasma hormone changes in Alzheimer's disease, *Br. J. Psychiatry*, 150, 674, 1987.

Clemmons, D. R. and Van Wyk, J. J., Factors controlling blood concentration of somatomedin-C, *Clin. Endocrinol. Metab.*, 13, 113, 1984.

Conover, C. A., Dollar, L. A., Rosenfeld, R. G., et al., Somatomedin-C binding and actions in fibroblasts from aged and progeric subjects, *J. Clin. Endocrinol. Metab.*, 60, 685, 1985.

Cooper, R. L., Roberts, B., Rogers, D. C., Seay, S. G., and Conn, P. M., Endocrine status versus chronologic age as predictors of altered luteinizing hormone secretion in aging rat, *Endocrinology*, 114, 391, 1984.

Costello, T. Y., Subclinical adenoma of the pituitary gland, *Am. J. Pathol.*, 12, 205, 1936.

Crew, M. D., Spindler, S. R., Walford, R. L., and Koizumi, A., Age-related decrease of growth hormone and prolactin gene expression in the mouse pituitary, *Endocrinolology*, 121, 1251, 1987.

Cuttelod, S., Lemarchand-Beraud, T., Magnenat, P., Perret, C., Poli, S., and Vannotti, A., Effect of age and role of kidneys and liver on thyrotropin turnover in man, *Metabolism*, 23, 101, 1974.

Davis, K. L., Davis, B. M., Mathe, A. A., et al., Age and the dexamethasone suppression test in depression, *Am. J. Psychiatry*, 141, 872, 1984.

Davis, K. L., Davis, B. L., Greenwald, B. S., et al., Cortisol and Alzheimer's disease. I. Basal studies, *Am. J. Psychiatry*, 143, 300, 1986.

Davis, P. J., Aging and endocrine function, *Clin. Endocrinol. Metab.*, 8, 603, 1979.

Dawson-Hughes, B., Stern, D., Goldman, J., et al., Regulation of growth hormone and somatomedin-C secretion in postmenopausal women: effect of physiological estrogen replacement, *J. Clin. Endocrinol. Metab.*, 63, 424, 1986.

Demarest, K. T., Moore, K. E., and Riegle, G. D., Dopaminergic neuronal function, anterior pituitary dopamine content and serum concentrations of prolactin, luteinizing hormone, and progesterone in the aged female rat, *Brain Res.*, 247, 347, 1982.

Deslypere, J. P. and Vermeulen, A., Leydig cell function in normal men: effect of age, lifestyle, residence, diet and activity, *J. Clin. Endocrinol. Metab.*, 59, 955, 1986.

Deslypere, J. P., Kaufman, J. M., Vermeulen, T., et al., Influence of age on the pulsatile luteinizing hormone release and responsiveness of the gonadotropins to sex hormone feedback in men, *J. Clin. Endocrinol. Metab.*, 64, 68, 1982.

DeSouza, E. B., Whitehouse, P. J., Kuhar, M. J., Price, D. C., and Vale, W. W., Reciprocal changes in corticotropin-releasing factor (CRF)-like immunoreactivity and CRF receptors in cerebral cortex of Alzheimer's disease, *Nature (London)*, 319, 593, 1986.

deWeid, D. and Van Ree, J. M., Neuropeptides, mental performance and aging, *Life Sci.*, 31, 709, 1982.

Dudl, R. J., Ensinck, J. W., Palmer, J. E., and Williams, R. H., Effect of age on growth hormone secretion in man, *J. Clin. Endocrinol. Metab.*, 37, 11, 1973.

Everitt, A. V., Neuroendocrine function and aging, *Adv. Exp. Med. Biol.*, 129, 233, 1980.

Felicio, L. S., Nelson, J. F., and Finch, C. E. Spontaneous pituitary tumorigenesis and plasma estradiol in aging female C57BCL/6J mice, *Exp. Gerontol.*, 115, 139, 1980.

Felicio, L. S., Nelson, J. F., Gosden, R. G., and Finch, C. E., Long-term ovariectomy delays the loss of ovulating cycling potential in aging mice, *Proc. Natl. Acad. Sci. U.S.A.*, 80, 6076, 1983.

Fiatarone, M., Pituitary function in the elderly diabetic, *Ger. Med. Today*, 7(2), 76, 1988.

Finch, C. E., Reproductive senescence in rodents: factors in the decline of fertility and loss of regular estrous cycle, in *Aging and Reproduction*, Schneider, E. L., Ed., Raven Press, New York, 1978, 193.

Finch, C. E. and Landfield, P. W., Neuroendocrine and autonomic functions in aging mammals, in *Handbook of the Biology of Aging*, 2nd ed., Finch, C. E. and Schneider, E. L., Eds., Van Nostrand Reinhold, New York, 1985, 567.

Finch, C. E., Jone, C. V., Wisner, J. R., Jr., Sinha, Y. N., deVellis, J. S., and Swerdloff, R. S., Hormone production by the pituitary and testes of male C57BL/6J mice during aging, *Endocrinology*, 101, 1310, 1977.

Findlay, T., Role of the neurohypophysis in the pathogenesis of hypertension and some allied disorders associated with aging, *Am. J. Med.*, 7, 70, 1949.

Fine, A., Peptides and Alzheimer's disease, *Nature (London)*, 319, 537, 1986.

Fitten, L. J., Morley, J. E., Gross, P. L., Petry, S. D., and Cole, K. D., Depression. UCLA geriatric grand rounds, *J. Am. Geriatr. Soc.*, 37, 459, 1989.

Florini, J., Prinz, P. N., Vitiello, M. V., et al., Somatomedin-C levels in healthy young and old men: relationship to peak and 24-hour integrated levels of growth hormone, *J. Gerontol.*, 40, 2, 1985.

Franks, S., McElhone, J., Young, S. N., Kraulis, I., and Ruf, R. B., Factors determining the diurnal variation in progesterone-induced gonadotropin release in the ovariectomized rat, *Endocrinology*, 107, 353, 1980.

Frantz, A. G. and Rabkin, M. T., Effects of estrogen and sex difference on secretion of human growth hormone, *J. Clin. Endocrinol. Metab.*, 25, 1470, 1965.

Garner, R. M. and Yamada, T., Altered neuropeptide concentrations in cerebrospinal fluid of psychiatric patients, *Brain Res.*, 238, 298, 1982.

Gold, P. N. and Rubinow, D. R., Neuropeptide function in affective illness: corticotropin-releasing hormone and somatostatin as model systems, in *Psychopharmacology: The Third Generation of Progress*, Meltzer, H. Y., Ed., Raven Press, New York, 1987, 617.

Greden, J. F., Flegel, P., Haskett, R., et al., Age effects in serial hypothalamic-pituitary-adrenal monitoring, *Psychoneuroendocrinology*, 11, 195, 1986.

Gregerman, R. I. and Bielman, E. L., Aging and hormones, in *Textbook of Endocrinology*, 6th ed., Williams, R. M., Ed., W. B. Saunders, Philadelphia, 1981, 1192.

Gudelsky, G. A., Nansel, D. D., and Porter, J. C., Dopamine control of prolactin secretion in the aging male rat, *Brain Res.*, 204, 446, 1981.

Harman, S. M., Tsitouras, P. D., Costa, P. T., et al., Reproductive hormones in aging men: basal pituitary gonadotropins and gonadotropin responses to luteinizing hormone-releasing hormone, *J. Clin. Endocrinol. Metab.*, 54, 547, 1982.

Harman, S. M., Wehmann, R. E., and Blackman, M. R., Pituitary-thyroid hormone economy in healthy aging men: basal indices of thyroid function and thyrotropin responses to constant infusion of thyrotropin-releasing hormone, *J. Clin. Endocrinol. Metab.*, 58, 320, 1984.

Hart, R. W. and Turturro, A., Theories of aging, *Rev. Biol. Res. Aging*, 1, 5, 1983.

Hatfield, B. D., Goldfarb, A. H., Sforzo, G. A., et al., Serum beta endorphin and affective responses to graded exercise in young and elderly men, *J. Gerontol.*, 42, 429, 1987.

Helderman, J. H., Vestal, R. E., Rowe, J. W., et al., The response of arginine vasopressin to intravenous ethanol and hypertonic saline in man: the impact of aging, *J. Gerontol.*, 33, 39, 1978.

Ho, Ky., Evans, W. S., Blizzard, R. M., et al., Effects of sex and age on the 24-hour profile of growth hormone secretion in man: importance of endogenous estrogen, *J. Clin. Endocrinol. Metab.*, 64, 51, 1987.

Impallomeni, M., Yeo, T., Rudd, A., et al., Investigation of anterior pituitary function in elderly inpatients over the age of 75, *Q. J. Med.*, 63, 505, 1987.

Jacques, C., Schlienger, J. L., Kissell, C., et al., TRH-induced TSH and prolactin responses in the elderly, *Age Aging*, 16, 181, 1987.

Janowsky, D. S., El-Youself, M. K., Davis, J. M., and Serkerke, J. H., A cholinergic-adrenergic hypothesis of mania and depression, *Lancet*, 2, 632, 1972.

Jensen, H. K. and Blichert-Toft, M., Serum corticotropin, plasma cortisol and urinary secretion of 17-ketogenic steroids in the elderly (age group: 66—94 years), *Acta Endocrinol. (Copenhagen)*, 66, 25, 1971.

Johanson, A. J. and Blizzard, R. M., Low somatomedin-C levels in older men rise in response to growth hormone administration, *Johns Hopkins Med. J.*, 149, 115, 1981.

Judd, H. L., Shamonki, I. M., Frumar, A. M., et al., Origin of serum estradiol in postmenopausal women, *Obstet. Gynecol.*, 59, 680, 1982.

Kaiser, F. E., Viosca, S. P., Mooradian, A. D., Morley, J. E., and Korenman, S. G., Impotence and aging: alterations in hormonal secretory patterns with age, *Clin. Res.*, 36, 96A, 1988.

Kasting, N. W., Veale, W. L., and Cooper, R. E., Convulsive and hypothalamic effects of vasopressin in the brain of the rat, *Can. J. Physiol. Pharmacol.*, 58, 316, 1980.

Korenman, S. G., Stanik-Davis, S., Mooradian, A. D., et al., Evidence for a high prevalence of hypogonadotropic hypogonadism in sexually dysfunctional older men, *Clin. Res.*, 35, 186A, 1987.

Kovacs, K., Ryan, N., Horvath, E., Penz, G., and Ezrin, C., Prolactin cells of the human pituitary gland in old age, *J. Gerontol.*, 32, 534, 1977.

Kovacs, K., Ryan, N., Horvath, E., et al., Pituitary adenomas in old age, *J. Gerontol.*, 35, 16, 1980.

Landfield, P. W., An endocrine hypothesis of brain aging and studies in brain-endocrine correlations and monosynaptic neurophysiology during aging, in *Parkinson's Disease*, Vol. 2, Aging and neuroendocrine relationships, Finch, C. E., Ed., Plenum Press, New York, 1978, 179.

Landfield, P. W., Adrenocortical hypothesis of brain and somatic aging, in *Biological Mechanisms of Aging*, Conference proceedings, Schimke, R. T., Ed., National Institutes of Health Publ. No. 81, 1981, 658.

Laron, Z., Doron, M., and Amikam, B., Plasma growth hormone in old age, *Harefuah*, 73, 375, 1967.

Lieberman, J., Elevation of serum angiotensin-converting enzyme (ACE), level in sarcoidosis, *Am. J. Med.*, 59, 365, 1975.

Malamed, S. and Carsia, R. V., Aging of the rat adrenocortical cell response to ACTH and cyclic AMP in vitro, *J. Gerontol.*, 38, 130, 1983.

Mann, J. J., Petito, C., Stanley, M., et al., Amine receptor binding and monoamine oxidase activity in post-mortem human brain tissue: effect of age, gender, and post-mortem delay, in *Clinical and Pharmacological Studies in Psychiatric Disorders*, Burrows, G. D., Norman, T. R., and Dennesteen, L., Eds., John Libey, London, 1985, 37.

Mann, J. J., Stanley, M., McBride, P. A., et al., Increased serotonin and beta adrenergic receptor binding in the frontal cortices of suicide victims, *Arch. Gen. Psychiatry*, 43, 954, 1986.

Marruma, P., Carcani, C., Baraghini, G. F., et al., Circadian rhythm of testosterone and prolactin in aging, *Maturitas*, 4, 131, 1982.

McKeown, F., *Pathology of the Aged*, Butterworths, London, 1965.

Mendlewicz, J., Linkowski, P., Kerkhofs, M., et al., Diurnal hypersecretion of growth hormone in depression, *J. Clin. Endocrinol. Metab.*, 60, 505, 1985.

Miller, M., Influence of aging on vasopressin secretion and water regulation, in *Vasopressin*, Schrier, R. W., Ed., Raven Press, New York, 1985.

Miller, M., Increased vasopressin secretion. An early manifestation of aging in the rat, *J. Gerontol.*, 42, 3, 1987.

Montermini, M., Borciani, E., d'Amato, L., et al., Funzionalita tiroidea in eta senile (abstract), *Atti delle Terze Giornale Italiane della Tiroide*, Torino, Italy, 1985, 114.

Mooradian, A. D., Molecular theories of aging, in *Frontiers in Geriatric Nutrition*, Morley, J. E., Glick, Z., and Rubenstein, L. Z., Eds., Raven Press, New York, in press.

Mooradian, A. D. and Morley, J. E., The hypothalamus and the pituitary glands, in *Diagnosis and Pathology of Endocrine Diseases*, Mendelsohn, G., Ed., Lippincott, Philadelphia, 1987, 351.

Mooradian, A. D., Morley, J. E., and Korenman, S. G., Endocrinology in aging, *Disease-a-Month*, 7, 398, 1988.

Morley, J. E., Neuroendocrine control of thyrotropin secretion, *Endocrine Rev.*, 2, 396, 1981.

Morley, J. E., Geriatric endocrinology, in *Diagnosis and Pathology of Endocrine Disease*, Mendelsohn, G., Ed., Lippincott, Philadelphia, 1987, 603.

Muggeo, M., Fedele, D., Tiengo, A., et al., Human growth hormone and cortisol response to insulin stimulation in aging, *J. Gerontol.*, 30, 546, 1975.

Nelson, J. F., Felicio, L. S., and Finch, C. E., Ovarian hormones and the etiology of reproductive aging in mice, in *Aging — Its Chemistry*, Deitz, A. A., Ed., American Association of Clinical Research, Washington, D.C., 1980, 64.

Nelson, W. H., Orr, W. W., Jr., Shane, S. R., et al., Hypothalamic-pituitary-adrenal axis activity and age in major depression, *J. Clin. Psychiatry*, 45, 120, 1984.

Ohara, H., Kobayashi, T., Shiraishi, M., and Wada, T., Thyroid function of the aged as viewed from the pituitary-thyroid system, *Endocrinol. Jpn.*, 21, 377, 1974.

Ordene, K. W., Pan, C., Barzel, U. S., and Surks, M. I., Variable thyrotropin response to thyrotropin-releasing hormone after small decreases in plasma thyroid hormone concentrations in patients of advanced age, *Metabolism*, 32, 881, 1983.

Oxenkrug, G. F., Pomara, N., McIntyre, I. M., et al., Aging and cortisol resistance to suppression by dexamethasone: a possible correlation, *Psychiatry Res.*, 10, 125, 1983.

Parkening, T. A., Collins, T. J., and Smith, E. R., Plasma and pituitary concentrations of LH, FSH, and prolactin in aging C57BL/6 mice at various times in the estrous cycle, *Neurobiol. Aging*, 3, 31, 1982.

Pavlov, E. P., Harman, S. M., Chrousos, G. P., et al., Responses of plasma adrenocorticotropin, cortisol, and dehydroepiandrosterone to ovine corticotropin-releasing hormone in healthy aging men, *J. Clin. Endocrinol. Metab.*, 62, 767, 1986.

Pekary, A. E., Carlson, H. E., Yamada, T., Sharp, B., Walfish, P. G., and Hershman, J. M., Thyrotropin-releasing hormone levels decrease in hypothalamus of aging rats, *Neurobiol. Aging*, 5, 221, 1984.

Pekary, A. E., Turner, L., Mirell, C., Walfish, P. G., and Hershman, J. M., Effect of aging on TRH receptors, T_4 to T_3 conversion and liver enzyme levels in Long-Evans rats, *Clin. Res.*, 33, 29A, 1985.

Pekary, A. E., Mirell, C. J., Turner, L. F., Jr., Walfish, P. G., and Hershman, J. M., Hypothalamic secretion of thyrotropin-releasing hormone declines in aging rats, *J. Gerontol.*, 42, 447, 1987.

Prinz, P. N., Weitzman, E. D., Cunningham, G. R., et al., Plasma growth hormone during sleep in young and aged men, *J. Gerontol.*, 38, 519, 1983.

Quint, A. R. and Kaiser, F. E., Gonadotropin determinations and thyrotropin-releasing hormone and luteinizing hormone-releasing hormone testing in critically ill postmenopausal women with hypothyroxinemia, *J. Clin. Endocrinol. Metab.*, 60, 464, 1985.

Raskind, M. A., Preskind, E. R., Veith, R. C., et al., Increased plasma and cerebrospinal fluid norepinephrine in older men: differential suppression by clonidine, *J. Clin. Endocrinol. Metab.*, 66, 438, 1988.

Reubi, J. C. and Palacios, J., Somatostatin and Alzheimer's disease: a hypothesis, *J. Neurol.*, 233, 370, 1986.

Reymond, M. J. and Porter, J. C., Secretion of hypothalamic dopamine into pituitary stalk blood of aged female rats, *Brain Res. Bull.*, 7, 69, 1981.

Robertson, G. L., The regulatio of vasopressin function in health and disease, *Recent Prog. Horm. Res.*, 23, 333, 1977.

Robertson, G. L. and Rowe, J. W., The effect of aging on neurohypophyseal function, *Peptides,* 1 (Suppl.), 159, 1980.

Robuschi, G., Safron, M., Braverman, L. E., et al., Hypothyroidism in the elderly, *Endocrine Rev.,* 8, 142, 1987.

Rogers, J. and Bloom, F. E., Neurotransmitter metabolism and function in the aging central nervous system, in *Handbook of the Biology of Aging,* 2nd ed., Finch, C. E. and Schneider, E. L., Eds., Van Nostrand Reinhold, New York, 1985, 645.

Rolandi, E., Franceschini, R., Marabini, A., et al., Twenty-four-hour beta endorphin secretory pattern in the elderly, *Acta Endocrinol.,* 115, 441, 1987.

Root, A. W. and Oskie, F. A., Effects of human growth hormone in elderly males, *J. Gerontol.,* 24, 97, 1969.

Rowe, J. W., Minaker, K. L., Sparrow, D., and Robertson, G. L., Age-related failure of volume-pressure-mediated vasopressin release, *J. Clin. Endocrinol. Metab.,* 54, 661, 1982.

Rudman, D., Growth hormone, body composition and aging, *J. Am. Geriatr. Soc.,* 33, 800, 1985.

Rudman, D., Kutner, M. H., Rogers, C. M., et al., Impaired growth hormone secretion in the adult population, *J. Clin. Invest.,* 67, 1361, 1981.

Rudman, D., Nagraji, H. S., Mattson, D. E., et al., Hyposomatomedinemia in the nursing home patient, *J. Am. Geriatr. Soc.,* 34, 427, 1986.

Sapolsky, R. M., Krey, L. C., McEwen, B. S., and Rainbow, T. C., Do vasopressin-related peptides induce hippocampal corticosterone receptors? Implications for aging, *J. Neurosci.,* 4, 1479, 1984.

Sara, V. R., Hall, K., Enzell, K., et al., Somatomedins in aging and dementia disorders of the Alzheimer type, *Neurobiol. Aging,* 3, 117, 1982.

Sawin, C. T., Castelli, W. P., Hershman, J. M., McNamara, P., and Bacharach, P., The aging thyroid: thyroid deficiency in the Framingham study, *Arch. Intern. Med.,* 145, 1386, 1985.

Schrier, R. W., Bert, T., and Anderson, R. J., Osmotic and nonosmotic control of vasopressin release, *Am. J. Physiol.,* 236, F321, 1979.

Semorajski, T., Rolsten, C., and Ordy, J. M., Changes in behavior, brain and neuroendocrine chemistry with age and stress in C57BL-10 male mice, *J. Gerontol.,* 26, 168, 1971.

Sherman, B., Wysham, C., and Pfohl, B., Age-related changes in the circadiam rhythm of plasma cortisol in man, *J. Clin. Endocrinol. Metab.,* 61, 439, 1985.

Siiteri, P. K. and MacDonald, P. C., Role of extraglandular estrogen in human endocrinology, in *Handbook of Physiology-Endocrinology,* Vol. 2, Griep, R. O. and Astwood, E., Eds., American Physiological Society, Washington, D.C., 1973.

Snyder, P. J. and Utiger, R. D., Thyrotropin response to thyrotropin-releasing hormone in normal females over forty, *J. Clin. Endocrinol. Metab.,* 34, 1096, 1972a.

Snyder, P. J. and Utiger, R. D., Response to thyrotropin-releasing hormone (TRH) in normal man, *J. Clin. Endocrinol. Metab.,* 34, 380, 1972b.

Touitou, Y., Febre, M., Lagoguey, M., et al., Age- and mental health-related circadian rhythms of melatonin, prolactin, luteinizing hormone and follicle-stimulating hormone in man, *J. Endocrinol.,* 91, 467, 1981.

Tsundo, K., Abe, K., Goto, T., et al., Effect of age on the renin-angiotensin-aldosterone system in normal subjects: simultaneous measurement of active and inactive renin, renin substrate and aldosterone in plasma, *J. Clin. Endocrinol. Metab.,* 62, 384, 1986.

Veith, R. C. and Raskind, M. A., The neurobiology of aging: does it predispose to depression?, *Neurobiol. Aging,* 9, 101, 1988.

Vekemann, M. and Robin, C., Influence of age on serum prolactin levels in men and women, *Br. J. Med.,* 4, 738, 1975.

Vermeulen, A., Nyctohemeral growth hormone profiles in young and aged men: correlation with somatomedin-C levels, *J. Clin. Endocrinol. Metab.,* 64, 884, 1987.

Vidalon, C., Khurana, R. C., Chae, S., et al., Age-related changes in growth hormone in non-diabetic women, *J. Am. Geriatr. Soc.,* 21, 253, 1973.

Walker, R. F., Reinstatement of LH surges by serotonin neuroleptics in aging, constant estrous rats, *Neurobiol. Aging,* 3, 253, 1982.

Walker, R. F., Cooper, R. L., and Timiras, P. S., Constant estrous: role of rostral hypothalamic monoamines in development of reproductive dysfunction in aging rats, *Endocrinology,* 107, 209, 1980.

Wenzel, K. W. and Horn, W. R., Triiodothyranine (T3) and thyroxine (T4) kinetics in aged men, in *Thyroid Research Excerpts Medica,* Robbins, J. and Utiger, R. D., Eds., Elsevier, Amsterdam, 1976, 270.

Wenzel, K. W., Meinhold, H., Herpich, M., Adlkofer, F., and Schleusener, H., TRH-stimulationstest mit alters-und geschlechtsabhangigem TSH-anstieg bei normalpersonen, *Klin. Wochenschr.,* 52, 722, 1974.

West, C. D., Brown, H., Simons, E. L., et al., Adrenocortical function and cortisol metabolism in old age, *J. Clin. Endocrinol. Metab.,* 21, 1197, 1961.

Wexler, B. C., Comparative aspects of hyperadrenocorticism and aging, in *Hypothalamus, Pituitary and Aging,* Everitt, A. F. and Burgess, J. A., Eds., Charles C Thomas, Springfield, IL, 1976, 333.

Wiedemann, E., Schwartz, E., and Frantz, A. G., Acute and chronic estrogen effects upon serum somatomedin activity, growth hormone, and prolactin in man, *J. Clin. Endocrinol. Metab.,* 42, 942, 1976.

Wilkes, M. M. and Yen, S. S. C., Attenuation during aging of the post-ovariectomy rise in median eminence catecholamines, *Neuroendocrinology,* 33, 144, 1981.

Williams, T., Berelowitz, M., Joffe, S. N., et al., Impaired growth hormone responses to growth hormone-releasing factor in obesity, *N. Engl. J. Med.,* 311, 1403, 1984.

Wise, P. M., Aging of the female reproductive system, *Rev. Biol. Res. Aging,* 1, 195, 1983.

Wolfsen, A. R., Aging and the adrenals, in *Endocrine Aspects of Aging,* Korenman, S. G., Ed., Elsevier-North Holland, New York, 1982, 55.

Wong, D. F., Wagner, N. N., Jr., Dannals, R. F., et al., Effects of age on dopamine and serotonin receptors measured by positron tomography in the living human brain, *Science,* 226, 1393, 1984.

Woolf, P. D., Harnell, R. W., McDonald, J. V., et al., Transient hypogonadotrophic hypogonadism caused by critical illness, *J. Clin. Endocrinol. Metab.,* 60, 444, 1985.

Yamamoto, T., Harada, H., Fukuyama, J., Hayashi, T., and Mori, I., Impaired arginine vasopressin secretion associated with hypoangiotensinemia in hypernatremic dehydrated elderly patients, *JAMA,* 259, 1039, 1988.

21

Psychoneuroimmunology

MARGARET E. KEMENY
Department of Psychiatry and Biobehavioral Sciences
School of Medicine
University of California, Los Angeles
Los Angeles, California

GEORGE F. SOLOMON
Department of Psychiatry and Biobehavioral Sciences
School of Medicine
University of California, Los Angeles
Los Angeles, California
and
Department of Psychiatry
Veterans Administration Medical Center
Sepulveda, California

JOHN E. MORLEY
Division of Geriatric Medicine
St. Louis University School of Medicine
St. Louis, Missouri

and

TRACY L. HERBERT
Department of Psychology
University of California, Los Angeles
Los Angeles, California

I. Introduction

The nervous system is known to have the capacity to regulate almost all the organ systems in the body, including the cardiovascular, gastrointestinal, and endocrine systems. In contrast, it has been believed that the immune system is relatively autonomous, stimulated by foreign antigenic substances and regulated internally by cytokines produced from immunologic cells. While this premise is at odds with much of the clinical wisdom of centuries (Shukla et al., 1981), it was only relatively recently that accumulating evidence from diverse fields began to indicate that the nervous system and the immune system can communicate in a bidirectional fashion (Ader, 1981; Locke et al., 1984). Moreover, it is currently proposed that this communication may be essential to the functioning of the immune system, and possibly the nervous system as well. The field of psychoneuroimmunology is concerned with this bidirectional communication and with its clinical and bioregulatory implications. Two forms of evidence support a nervous-immune system interaction, and these will be reviewed in this chapter: (1) direct anatomical and physiological evidence indicating linkages between the nervous and immune systems, and (2) indirect evidence indicating that during psychological disturbance, the immune system is altered, as are the likelihood and course of immunologically mediated or resisted diseases.

II. Communication from the Nervous System to the Immune System

A. Central Nervous System Lesions and Stimulation

Electrolytic lesions of the hypothalamus have been shown to be associated with a variety of immune alterations, including *in vivo* measures such as lethal anaphylaxis, delayed cutaneous hypersensitivity, and antibody production and graft rejection (Luparello et al., 1964; Macris et al., 1970). More recently, other short-lived changes in immune functions tested *in vitro* have also been observed. For example, Roszman and colleagues (see Roszman et al., 1985) have demonstrated that anterior hypothalamic (AHT) lesions in rats result in a marked decrease in the number of nucleated spleen cells and thymocytes, a reduction in responsiveness of spleen cells to stimulation with the mitogen concanavalin A (ConA), and impaired natural killer (NK) cell activity. In studies attempting to determine the mechanisms explaining the effects on mitogen responsiveness, Roszman and colleagues have shown that the macrophages of animals with AHT lesions were more suppressive than those of control animals.

Evidence also exists that suggests that immune enhancement occurs following lesioning of particular brain regions. For example, Brooks and colleagues (1982) found that hippocampal lesions resulted in an increase in nucleated splenic cell numbers, while lesions in other brain regions resulted in a decrease in cell numbers. An increase in proliferative response to ConA was also observed following hippocampal lesions. These data suggest that these effects may be due to changes in levels of hormones, since removal of the pituitary abrogates some of the effects seen (Roszman et al., 1985). In contrast, stimulation of hypothalamic areas has enhancing effects on certain immune parameters, including antibody production and graft rejection (Korneva, 1967).

The immune system also appears to be affected by lesions in extrahypothalamic areas of the brain. For example, neurotoxic lesions of the lateral septal area of rats, which have been shown to alter female sexual behavior, feeding behavior, and ovarian function (King and Nance, 1986), have also been shown to reduce antibody levels following immunization with ovalbumin (Nance et al., 1987).

Finally, there is some evidence for laterality in the relationship between brain regions and immunity. In one set of studies, lesioning of the left cerebral neocortex depressed certain T cell-mediated responses but lesions on the right did not (see Biziere et al., 1985). Furthermore, lesions of the left neocortex have been shown to result in a decrease in the number of plaque-forming cells to sheep red blood cell administration, while this T-dependent response has been shown to be enhanced in mice with a right cortical lesion. In addition, left-sided lesions can depress the proliferative response of spleen lymphocytes to mitogens and lower NK cell activity, while the same effects are not seen following right-sided lesions.

B. Autonomic Innervation of Immune Organs

Research is accumulating that autonomic nerve fibers are present in immune organs (see reviews by Bulloch, 1985; Felten et al., 1987). Innervation appears to be primarily sympathetic, involving neurons containing norepinephrine (NE), in addition to other neuropeptides such as vasoactive intestinal peptide, cholecystokinin, and neuropeptide Y (Felten et al., 1985,

1987). Parasympathetic innervation of the thymus has also been suggested on the basis of macroscopic, microscopic, and ultrastructural studies (e.g., Bulloch and Moore, 1981).

Both primary (bone marrow, thymus) and secondary (spleen, lymph nodes, gut-associated lymphoid tissue) immune organs are sympathetically innervated via small, unmyelinated postganglionic noradrenergic (NA) fibers. Nerve fibers have been visualized using a number of techniques, and their distribution appears to be directed more toward compartments of T lymphocytes and macrophages than B lymphocytes. The nerve fibers have been shown to enter the primary and secondary immune organs along blood vessels (but also apart from blood vessels), and to distribute widely throughout the organs, associating with lymphocytes and monocytes. Association between nerve terminals and lymphocytes can involve either local paracrine secretion of NE, or direct contact via what appear to be synapses. The purpose of the innervation remains unclear, but it has been suggested that innervation of the thymus, for example, may influence the development of the thymus, the distribution of cells within it, and possibly the differentiation of cells, migration of cells, or secretion of endocrine products of the organ.

Felten and colleagues (1987) have summarized evidence that the NE in the spleen, and potentially in other lymphoid organs, satisfies four criteria for neurotransmission. First, nerve fibers are present in lymphoid organs and compartmentalized in functionally similar regions of the organs. NA fibers have been shown to be capable of synthesizing NE in immune organs on the basis of fluorescence, histochemical, neurochemical, and denervation studies. Second, NE has been shown to be released in immune organs. For example, using an *in vivo* dialysis technique, NE has been shown to be released in the spleen from a neural compartment (S. V. Felten et al., 1986). Third, adrenoreceptors have been found to be present on lymphocytes (e.g., Staehelin et al., 1985), macrophages (Abrass et al., 1985), and neutrophils (Davies and Lefkowitz, 1980). Fourth, NE has been demonstrated to play a functional role in the immune response on the basis of chemical sympathectomy studies. That is, if chemical sympathectomy occurred in the neonatal period, antibody responses in adulthood were found to be augmented (Besedovsky et al., 1979; Williams et al., 1981). However, chemical sympathectomy of the adult mouse resulted in reduced (Livnat et al., 1985, 1987) or unaltered (Miles et al., 1981) cell-mediated immune responses.

C. Neuroendocrine and Neuropeptide Influences on Immune Processes

A variety of hormones and neuropeptides have been shown to alter immune processes both *in vivo* and *in vitro* (see Ahlqvist, 1981), although *in vivo* and *in vitro* effects are not and would not necessarily be expected to be similar. Pharmacologic levels of a given neurohormone/peptide may have quite different immunologic effects than would physiologic levels. Within physiologic ranges, an inverted U-shaped dose-response curve is common, in which small increments in level enhance immune effects and high levels suppress them (Moore, 1978). On a clinical level, both Addison's disease (hypoadrenal-cortisolism) and Cushing's disease (hypercortisolism) are associated with states of moderate immune deficiency. In addition, the net effect of a peptide *in vitro* appears to depend on the dose, time of incubation, culture medium, and source of lymphocytes, and may also be cell cycle dependent (Stead et al., 1987). The hormones and neuropeptides that have been most extensively studied with reference to immune parameters will be discussed below.

1. Corticosteroids

The corticosteroids have been known to influence immune processes since the 1940s, when their anti-inflammatory effects were discovered (Table 1). There are glucocorticoid receptors on virtually all nucleated cells in the body, including leukocytes (Munck and Leung, 1977). The primary effects of the glucocorticoids appear to be the inhibition of both the production and action of intercellular mediators, including lymphokines (Fahey et al., 1981). Specifically, glucocorticoids can decrease the *in vitro* production of γ-interferon, colony-stimulating factor, interleukin-2 (IL-2), and interleukin-1 (IL-1) (see Fauci, 1979; Munck et al., 1984). The effects of glucocorticoids on NK cell activity and the proliferative response of lymphocytes in response to mitogens may be the result of the inhibition of various lymphokines that stimulate NK cells or T cells. In addition, *in vivo* levels of corticosteroids in peripheral blood over the course of a day have been shown to be inversely related to the number of circulating lymphocytes (Miyawaki et al., 1984; Ritchie et al., 1983), consistent with research indicating that corticosteroids cause redistribution of lymphocytes out of the circulation and into immune organs such as the bone marrow (Cohen, 1972; Cohen and Crnic, 1984). The proliferative response of lymphocytes to mitogen and antigen has also been shown to vary directly with the cortisol rhythm (Tavadia et al., 1975).

2. Growth Hormone

Based on studies of the restoration of T cell function in aged rats, growth hormone (GH) is believed to exert a regulatory effect on the immune system. Specifically, GH administration results in an increase in T cell function and NK activity in aged rats, and these increases reach the levels seen in younger rats. These effects, however, are not found when very old rats are used (Davila et al., 1987; Kelley et al., 1986).

3. Prolactin

In rodents, inhibition of prolactin (PRL) secretion suppresses the function of T and B cells, and treatment with PRL or drugs that stimulate PRL secretion increases cell-mediated immune responses, such as proliferation to mitogens (see Bernton, 1989, for review). Interestingly, treatment with prolactin or drugs that stimulate PRL secretion antagonizes glucocorticoid-mediated immune suppression as seen in chronic stress (Bernton et al., 1988). The effects of PRL on human immune functioning are not yet understood.

4. Opioid Peptides and Adrenocorticotropic

There are an increasing number of studies aimed at determining the influence of the opioid peptide β-endorphin (BE) and adrenocorticotropic hormone (ACTH), both derived from the

Table 1
Effects of Glucocorticoids on the Immune System[a]

Inhibitory effects
    Decreases peripheral blood lymphocytes, eosinophils, basophils, monocytes, and neutrophils
    Inhibits production of IL-1, IL-2, IL-2 receptor, γ-interferon
    Inhibits F_c receptor expression
    Inhibits *in vitro* and *in vivo* proliferation of T lymphocytes to antigens and mitogens
    Inhibits many monocyte functions, including antigen presentation, lymphokine production,
        differentiation, and phagocytosis
    Inhibits immunoglobulin production *in vivo*
    Inhibits T suppressor cell function *in vivo* and *in vitro*
Enhancing effects
    Enhances PWM plaque-forming cell responses *in vitro*
    Enhances immunoglobulin production *in vitro*
    Enhances antibody-dependent cellular cytotoxicity *in vivo*

[a]See Claman (1988) and Munck and Leung (1977) for review.

precursor molecule pro-opiomelanocortin (POMC), on *in vitro* measured of immune function. Studies of the effects of the opioid peptides have shown conflicting results. For example, chemotaxis in neutrophils and monocytes appears to be enhanced by BE (van Epps and Salan, 1984; Simpkins et al., 1984). BE has also been shown to enhance NK cell activity (Kay et al., 1984), but more recent studies suggest that it may inhibit NK activity (Prete et al., 1986) or have a variable effect (Chiappelli et al., 1991). The direction of the effect may be due to the concentration of the peptide (Williamson et al., 1987).

Conflicting evidence also exists for the relationship between BE and the proliferative response to mitogens, with some studies showing an enhancing effect (Gilman et al., 1982) and others showing an inhibitory effect (McCain et al., 1982). Recently, Heijnen and colleagues (1987) showed that ACTH and BE, at physiological concentrations, can both enhance and inhibit the proliferative response of human lymphocytes, depending on concentration and donor. While BE can enhance the primary antibody response (Heijnen and Ballieux, 1986), α-endorphin inhibits this response (Heijnen et al., 1985). Leu- and Met-enkephalins have also been shown to enhance NK activity (Wybran, 1985). In addition, evidence suggests that BE may be capable of both enhancing (Brown and van Epps, 1986) and suppressing (Peterson et al., 1987) mitogen-stimulated production of γ-interferon (IFN). Donor variability appears to play a role in the divergent findings regarding the effects of BE on γ-IFN production (Brummitt et al., 1988), lymphocyte proliferation (Heijnen et al., 1987), and NK cell activity (De Sanctis et al., 1986). Donor differences may be due to differences in the number or affinity of BE receptors, the number or responsiveness of responding immune cells, the composition or activation of other cells in the sample, or the hormonal milieu (Brummitt et al., 1988).

The presence of specific receptors on lymphocytes for ACTH and the nonopiate part of the BE molecule supports the possibility of an effect of these peptides on immune processes (Bost et al., 1987). There is conflicting support, however, for the presence of an opiate receptor on lymphocytes (Mehrishi and Mills, 1983; Mendelsohn et al., 1985).

5. Vasoactive Intestinal Peptide, Somatostatin, and Substance P

Vasoactive intestinal peptide (VIP) has been shown to modulate immunoglobulin production, T cell proliferative response (Stanisz et al., 1986; Payan et al., 1984), and NK activity. In addition, it has been shown to inhibit the production of IL-2 following stimulation with ConA. Vasoactive intestinal peptide has also been shown to influence lymphocyte trafficking (Ottaway, 1984).

Somatostatin (SOM) inhibits lymphocyte proliferation and immunoglobulin synthesis *in vitro* (Stanisz et al., 1986). However, when SOM is administered *in vivo,* proliferation and immunoglobulin (Ig) synthesis are enhanced, possibly as a result of its effects on other cell types. SOM has also been shown to stimulate histamine release from mast cells and inhibit its release from basophils.

Substance P (SP) has been shown to enhance DNA synthesis following stimulation with ConA of murine Peyer's patch and splenic lymphocytes, as well as increase immunoglobulin synthesis (Stanisz et al., 1986). *In vivo* infusion of SP results in a similar increase in proliferation and immunoglobulin production by these cells. SP has also caused histamine release from mast cells isolated from intestinal lamina propria (Shanahan et al., 1985).

6. Gonadal Hormones

The notion that gonadal steroids influence immune function is supported by four lines of evidence (see Grossman, 1985). First, there are sex differences in immune functioning. For example, immunoglobulin production is greater in females than males (e.g., Eidinger and Garrett, 1972). Second, gonadectomy and sex steroid hormone replacement influence the immune system. Estrogens can depress various cell-mediated immune responses, whereas castration can increase resistance to infection and shorten skin graft rejection time. In addition, exposure to diethylstilbestrol (DES) *in utero* is associated with immune changes in both rats (Blair, 1981) and humans (Hines et al., 1990). Third, the immune response is altered during pregnancy. In most women, cellular immunity is depressed during pregnancy (Finn et al., 1972), with some evidence suggesting that these effects are due to progesterone levels. Fourth, immune cells bear receptors for gonadal steroids. Receptors for estrogen, androgen, and progesterone have been found in the reticuloepithelial matrix of the thymus and, in some studies, on T cells. In addition, *in vitro* studies support an effect of gonadal steroids on immune functioning.

III. Communication from the Immune System to the Nervous System

Numerous studies indicate that the brain can respond to immunologic changes. Besedovsky et al. (1977) showed that inoculation of rats with sheep red blood cells resulted in large increases in activity in individual hypothalamic cells after 5 days. Korneva and Climenko (Korneva and Shkinek, 1988) have demonstrated, both temporally and spatially, a sequence of firing rates of hypothalamic neurons following immunization. Specifically, electrical stimulation in synchrony with natural firing enhanced aspects of the immune response, whereas stimulation out of synchrony suppressed them.

Various researchers have investigated the effects of IL-1 on production of hypothalamic and anterior pituitary hormones. Bernton and colleagues (1987) found that IL-1 added *in vitro* to rat anterior pituitary cells leads to increased secretion of ACTH and other hormones. However, Sapolsky and colleagues (1987) and Berkenbosch and colleagues (1987) did not find this effect in similar studies. Sapolsky and colleagues (1987) did find that rats injected via jugular catheters with IL-1 showed increased levels of ACTH and corticosterone in the blood in a dose-dependent manner. Rats exposed to IL-1 via the femoral vein showed a rise in CRF in the portal blood. Berkenbosch and colleagues (1987) found that intraperitoneal injections of IL-1 resulted in elevated ACTH blood levels. Thus, IL-1 may have effects both at the level of the hypothalamus and the pituitary.

Blalock and colleagues (1985) have demonstrated that lymphocytes stimulated with antigen produce small amounts of ACTH and BE, with the amount of ACTH produced being sufficient to activate the adrenal cortex. Smith and colleagues (1982) have demonstrated that Newcastle disease virus (NDV) stimulated the release of plasma corticosterone in hypophysectomized mice. Dunn and colleagues (1987), however, argue that these results may have been due to incomplete hypophysectomy, since they were unable to replicate the findings when hypophysectomy was verified. In the work of Blalock, different peptides are produced following stimulation with different antigens, which suggested to Blalock (1984) that the immune system may serve a sensory function alerting the brain that the body is being stimulated by a particular foreign organism. Conceivably, then, the brain could initiate responses, such as changes in blood flow, which would facilitate the immune response.

The thymus gland is believed to influence the neuroendocrine system and is, in turn, influenced by the neuroendocrine system, particularly thyroid hormone (Fabrise and Mocchegiani, 1985). Products of the thymus, thymopentin and thymopoietin, can enhance *in vitro* production by rat pituitary cells of ACTH, BE, and β-lipotropin, in a time- and dose-dependent fashion (Malaise et al., 1987). Thymectomy has been shown to delay puberty (Besedovsky and Sorkin, 1974). The thymic products also appear to influence hormone-related behaviors. For example, perinatal thymectomy impairs the ability of adult female rats to perform normal sexual behavior. Such animals show decreased behavioral sensitivity to estrogen (Gorsky, personal communication).

Research is accumulating that indicates that factors derived from immune cells have effects on cells in the brain, such as glial cells (see Benveniste et al., 1988, for review). For example, Merrill and colleagues (1984) have shown that supernatants from activated human T cells can cause rat astrocytes and oligodendrocytes to proliferate. The effects of immune products appear to be quite specific, however. For instance, IL-2 has been shown to cause the proliferation and differentiation of oligodendrocytes, but to have no effect on astrocytes (Benveniste and Merrill, 1986). In another study, IL-1 stimulated astrocyte but not oligodendroglia growth (Giulian and Lachman, 1985). Overall, a variety of immune cytokines (such as IL-2, IL-1, γ-IFN, B cell growth factor) appear to be able to exert modulatory effects on specific brain cells. In addition, brain cells have been shown to secrete soluble factors that regulate immune cells (Fontana et al., 1982).

IV. Experiential Effects on Immune Processes in Animals

A. Conditioning and Immune Processes

One of the earliest observations implying a role for the CNS in immune function was the crude demonstration in 1926 of classical conditioning of leukocyte responses to antigen (Metal'nikov and Chorine, 1926). More recently, Ader and Cohen (1981) conducted an elegant series of experiments confirming conditioning of immune processes. In the majority of these experiments, cyclophosphamide, an immunosuppressive drug that causes gastric upset, was used as the unconditioned stimulus (UCS). Saccharin-flavored water was used as the conditioned stimulus (CS). The UCS and CS were paired, that is, cyclophosphamide (CY) and saccharin-flavored water were administered to a group of rodents simultaneously. Then the CS, saccharin-flavored water, was administered alone to some of the rodents. Rodents exposed to the UCS-CS pairing and then CS alone demonstrated a reduced antibody response to sheep red blood cells, for example, in comparison to the animals who received only the CS-UCS pairing or neither. Thus, the immunosuppressive effects of CY were induced in response to the saccharin-flavored water alone, indicating classical conditioning of the immune response. These experiments have been replicated by other investigators (e.g., Rogers et al., 1979; Wayner et al., 1978). Ader and Cohen (1982) have also demonstrated that the conditioned immune suppressive effect is clinically significant. Specifically, conditioned immune suppression in NZB × NZW mice retarded age-dependent onset of, and survival from, systemic lupus erythematosus (SLE) in these mice who are susceptible to SLE. Results also suggest that the conditioning effect is not dependent on a change in corticosteroid levels (see Ader and Cohen, 1985, for a review of the conditioning research). More recent studies suggest that aspects of the immune system (e.g., NK cell activity) can also be enhanced through classical conditioning (Solvason et al., 1988).

B. Stressor Exposure and Immune Processes

A number of studies have assessed the relationship between exposure to stressors and the etiology and progression of immunologically related diseases, such as viral infections, cancer, and autoimmunity, in various animal models. For example, early studies showed that exposure to a variety of forms of stress (e.g., shock, confinement, loud noise) was associated with severity of, and survival from, viral infections (e.g., Johnsson and Rasmussen, 1965). Stress exposure has also been associated with the onset but particularly the course of cancer (spontaneous, chemically induced, or induced by a virus) (see Justice, 1985, for a review), and the course of adjuvant-induced arthritis in the rat (Amkraut et al., 1971). These earlier studies have formed the basis for suspecting that stress exposure may have an impact on immune processes.

The effects of stressors on immune processes have been studied in rodents, primates, and other species. Stressors include those that involve both physical and emotional components (e.g., foot shock, cold water swim, maternal separation), and those that result in emotional distress only (e.g., conditioned fear). In both models, stress exposure has been associated with alterations in a variety of immune parameters, including involution of the thymus, diminished proliferative response to mitogens, decreased lymphocyte cytotoxicity, altered numbers of T lymphocyte subsets, and decreased antibody response. Gisler and colleagues (Gisler, 1974; Gisler et al., 1971; Gisler and Schenkel-Hullinger, 1971) have conducted a number of studies with various stressors (acceleration, ether anesthesia, restraint, overcrowding) and have shown a variety of immunologic effects, including a reduction in plaque-forming cell response in tissue culture to sheep red cells, and changes in the number of T and B lymphocytes in the spleen, liver, and bone marrow. In early work on stress and the antibody response, Solomon (1969) found that immune effects of different stressors vary in the same species. Specifically, in inbred rats, apprehension of electric shock resulted in no change in primary or secondary antibody response, overcrowding stress suppressed both primary and secondary response, and rapid eye movement (REM) deprivation suppressed the primary response.

The functional ability of the macrophage/monocyte cell following stress exposure has been studied only rarely. Recently, Coe and colleagues (1988) found that infant squirrel monkeys separated from their mothers for 24 hr showed an increase in one measure of macrophage function, chemiluminescence, that persisted for at least 2 weeks and returned to normal following reunion. A similar stressor in infant bonnet monkeys resulted in a suppression of proliferative response to mitogen (Laudenslager et al., 1982).

Whether or not an *in vitro* or *in vivo* immune test is used may be a critical factor in determining the effects of stress exposure. Laudenslager and colleagues (1988) have found that certain stress procedures, for example, tail shock, produce small, unreliable effects on *in vitro* mitogen stimulation tests, but robust and consistent effects when an *in vivo* measure of antibody production to a novel antigen is studied. These researchers conclude that stress exposure may alter the "integrated outcome of the immune response to an antigen, not just a single component which might be compensated for by some other aspect of the process" (Laudenslager et al., 1988, p. 100).

The association between stress exposure and immune processes may also depend on the compartment of the immune system from which lymphocytes are obtained. For example, using rats, Lysle et al. (1987) found that exposure to 16 brief electric shocks suppressed responsiveness to the mitogen, concanavalin A (ConA) for lymphocytes obtained from the peripheral blood and spleen, but not for those obtained from lymph nodes. On the other hand, Shavit and colleagues (1987) found a similar suppression of NK cell activity in cells derived from the rat spleen, bone marrow, and peripheral blood following morphine administration.

C. Stress Moderators and Immune Processes

The nature and extent of the relationship between stress exposure and immune parameters may depend on certain host or environmental factors that "moderate" the stress-immunity relationship. A number of moderators of the stressor-immunity relationship in animals have been tested, including factors associated with (1) the nature of the stressor (such as duration, intensity, and controllability), (2) the stressor context (such as social relationships), (3) individual differences in the host prior to the stressor (such as early experience, gender, and aggressiveness), and (4) individual differences in the response to the stressor (such as defeat).

1. Nature of the Stressor

The duration, intensity, and timing of stressor exposure have been studied in relationship to immune processes. In an often-quoted study of stressor *duration,* which has yet to be replicated, Monjan and Collector (1977) demonstrated that 2 weeks of auditory stress exposure decreased the proliferative response to the mitogens ConA and phytohemagglutinin (PHA), but 2 months of stress exposure increased the proliferative response. In a study of different numbers of shocks, Lysle and colleagues (1987) found that increasing the number of foot shocks per session over one, three, or five daily sessions in male rats progressively decreased the proliferative response to the mitogen ConA in a whole-blood assay. Using splenic lymphocytes, decreasing proliferation was seen with increasing numbers of shocks, but this effect was attenuated over time. In another study of chronic stressor exposure, Lysle and colleagues (1987) found that daily shock sessions for 1 hr for 5 days did not suppress the proliferative response as did more acute stress, suggesting possible habituation rather than enhancement following chronic stress exposure.

With respect to the *intensity* of the stressor, graded increases in the intensity have been found to be associated with increasing levels of suppression of lymphocyte proliferation to stimulation with PHA (Keller et al., 1981). The same stressor may have immunoenhancing vs. immunosuppressing effects, depending on its intensity (Korneva and Shkinek, 1988).

The continuous vs. intermittent nature of the stress exposure has also been studied. Shavit and colleagues (1985) have found that prolonged, intermittent foot shock over 4 days suppresses NK cell activity in the rat, while brief and continuous foot shock for the same total time does not. Since the intermittent foot shock results in an analgesia mediated by endogenous opioids, they suggest that the NK cell activity changes are influenced by the increase in opioid production. More recently, these investigators have shown that a single exposure to the opioid form of foot shock can suppress splenic NK cell activity (Shavit et al., 1987).

The time relationship between antigenic challenge and stress administration may also be important. For example, Okimura and Nigo (1986) found that restraint stress on each of the 2 days following inoculation with sheep red blood cells had no effect on plaque formation in the mouse. However, if the stress was applied for the 2 days prior to the inoculation, a dramatic decrease in plaque formation was seen. Zalcman and colleagues (1988) have found a critical period for stress administration, 72 hr following antigenic challenge, during which plaque formation is reduced. Stress at other time points after inoculation, however, did not result in any immune reduction (Croiset et al., 1989).

Overall, then, the nature and extent of certain immune changes appear to depend on the duration, intensity, and timing of stress exposure. However, there are a variety of inconsistencies in the data and there remains insufficient evidence to answer key questions, including the conditions under which habituation or immune enhancement can occur following stress exposure.

2. Stressor Context

Coe and colleagues (1987) have found that the presence of peers moderates the effects of stress on immune parameters in squirrel monkeys. Infant squirrel monkeys were separated from their mothers and then placed in cages alone. This separation led to a protest reaction and agitation, as well as to increases in corticosteroid levels and decreases in antibody levels. If, however, the infant monkeys were placed with juvenile monkeys immediately following the separation, then smaller increases in corticosteroids and smaller decreases in antibody levels were seen, and these factors returned to baseline faster.

There is also some evidence that the extent of an immune response following stress exposure depends on whether the animal is exposed to antigen during the light or dark phase of the circadian cycle. Laudenslager and colleagues (1988) found that, in both control and shock conditions, rats immunized during the dark or active part of their cycle produced more antibody to a novel antigen than rats immunized in the light phase. These results may be due to corticosteroid effects on lymphocytes during the dark phase when corticosteroid levels are highest.

3. Individual Differences Prior to the Stressor

The effect of certain environmental conditions on immune processes appears to differ in male and female mice. For example, male mice housed in groups of five per cage had lower numbers of B lymphocytes producing antibody following injection with sheep erythrocytes than male mice housed alone (Rabin et al., 1988). These differences were not apparent when female mice were studied.

Early experience may also alter adult immune response to challenge. Solomon et al. (1968) has shown that handling in the first 21 days of life in Fisher rats was associated with a more vigorous primary and secondary antibody response to a novel antigen injected at 9 weeks of age. Lown and Dutka (1987) found that early postnatal, preweaning handling in mice enhanced B and T cell proliferative responses measured in adulthood. In contrast, Raymond and colleagues (1986) found a decreased level of plaque-forming cells following handling in certain strains of mice and no effects in others. Early experience may not only influence baseline levels of adult immunity but may also influence the effects of stress on immunity in adult animals. For example, adult rats that had been stressed by immobilization during the first 2 weeks of life showed greater suppression of antibody response following exposure to a similar stress than controls.

Individual differences in behavior or "temperament" may also be associated with differences in immune responsiveness or health. Amkraut and Solomon (1972) discovered that inbred BALB/C female mice that spontaneously develop fighting behavior are more resistant to murine virus sarcomas than nonfighting females. Temoshok and colleagues (1987) found that a behavioral factor (inactivity/dominance) was associated with higher NK cell activity in female hamsters with induced melanoma.

There have been a few studies that compare the effects of stress on immune parameters in animals of different ages. For example, chronic stress was found to have a greater effect on the proliferative response of lymphocytes in younger (12- and 18-month-old) rats than in older (25-month-old) rats, in which this aspect of immune responsiveness was already significantly decreased (Odio et al., 1987). In another study, no difference was found in rejection of virus-induced tumors in 3-month-old group-housed male mice in comparison to individually housed mice; however, there was a decrease in tumor rejection in 6-month-old, and more markedly in 9-month-old, mice (Amkraut and Solomon, 1972).

4. Individual Differences in Response to the Stressor

There has been interest in the role of "controllability" of the stressor on immune processes, since controllability can be viewed as an analog for aspects of the coping process in humans. Laudenslager and Ryan (1983) found that proliferative responses to the mitogens, ConA and PHA, were reduced in rats exposed to inescapable shock, but not in rats who received the same amount of shock but could terminate (or control) it. Inescapable, but not escapable, shock has also been shown to reduce NK cell activity (Shavit et al., 1983). However, these findings have not as yet been replicated by these investigators or by other laboratories (Laudenslager et al., 1988). Moreover, a recent study (Zalcman et al., 1988) found no effect of controllability of shock on plaque formation in mice.

Croiset, Ballieux, Heijnen, and colleagues (Croiset et al., 1987, 1989) have studied the effects of a particular behavioral response to a stressor, passive-avoidance, on immune parameters in rats. Passive-avoidance is defined as the "avoidance of entering a dark cage, despite a preference for the dark, due to prior exposure to a mild electric shock in the dark cage". Passive-avoidance was shown to be associated with elevated corticosterone levels and an increased number of splenic antibody-secreting cells (Croiset et al., 1987). The initially elevated number of cells was decreased in rats who later showed the maximal passive-avoidant behavior. In a second study (Croiset et al., 1989), rats in the passive-avoidance trial again showed an immediate increase in antibody-secreting cells, which was found to be decreased below control values 24 hr later if the rats showed passive-avoidant behavior when tested for retention.

Dominance hierarchies have been correlated with immune parameters in various animal species. For example, in Tilapia fish, dominant fish have higher levels of NK cell activity and proliferative response than do submissive fish (Cooper et al., in press; Ghoneum et al., 1986). The immune suppression in the submissive fish appears to be due to the endogenous opioid system since the NK response can be blocked by naltrexone (Faisal et al., 1989a, b). "Defeat" in response to aggressive encounters has also been studied. Miczek and colleagues (1982) found an opioid-mediated analgesia that manifested only after behavioral display of a posture of defeat in intruders to an established colony. In a study of immune response, intruder rats showed a diminished antibody response to a novel antigen, particularly among those rats who assumed submissive postures to the aggressive encounters (Fleshner et al., 1989).

V. Experiential Effects on Immune Processes in Humans

A. Conditioning and Immune Processes

In a recent study, the first evidence for conditioning of the immune response in humans was found (Bovbjerg et al., 1990). In this study, 20 female ovarian cancer patients receiving cyclic chemotherapy were assessed several days before treatment, as well as on the day of treatment. Results suggest that nausea was higher and proliferative responses to PHA, ConA, and *Staphylococcus aureus* (SPA) were lower on the treatment day than several days prior to treatment. These effects were not accounted for by the patients' levels of anxiety, but support the notion that the immune response may have been conditioned due to the repeated pairings of treatment environment and the immunosuppressive effects of chemotherapy.

B. Stressor Exposure and Immune Processes

While the relationship of stressful life experiences to the etiology and progression of infectious, autoimmune, and neoplastic disease in humans has been observed for centuries (see Zegans, 1984), there has been an increase in the number and sophistication of research studies in this area over the past 20 years (see Cohen and Williamson, in press; Weiner, in press). For example, following the development of the Schedule of Recent Experiences by Holmes and Rahe (1967), a checklist of major life change events, a number of studies found that individuals with a large number of recent major life events were likely to develop an illness (including those that are immunologically mediated or resisted), over the upcoming months or years (see Brown and Harris, 1978; Mechanic, 1974; Cohen, 1981 for a critique of this research). Other studies have evaluated the relationship between particular stressful events and the etiology and progression of disease. For example, the death of a spouse has been found to be associated with an increased morbidity and mortality rate in the subsequent year period (Parkes and Brown, 1972). However, other studies have failed to find such associations (Clayton, 1974), or have found them only in subpopulations of bereaved individuals.

Exposure to certain stressful life experiences has been shown to be associated with changes in the immune system in humans (Table 2). Studies of major life change events, more commonplace events, chronic events, and truly acute events have been conducted. The major life event of bereavement has been found to be followed by a decrease in the proliferative capacity of lymphocytes in response to the mitogen PHA in both a cross-sectional study, in which bereaved individuals were compared to matched controls (Bartrop et al., 1977), and in a longitudinal study, in which blood samples drawn following the spouse's death were compared to blood samples drawn prior to the death (Schleifer et al., 1983). Other studies indicating a relationship between the experience of bereavement and changes in immune parameters, including NK cell activity, have been conducted as well (Irwin et al., 1987a).

The major life change of marital separation has also been found to be associated with the immune system. In one study that compared separated or divorced women to a matched group of married women, it was found that those women who were separated or divorced had higher levels of antibody to the latent Epstein-Barr virus (EBV), indicating lower cellular immune control of viral latency, a lower percentage of NK cells, and lower lymphocyte proliferative response to PHA (Kiecolt-Glaser et al., 1987a). In addition, higher antibody levels to EBV and herpes simplex type 1 (HSV1) were found in separated or divorced men when they were compared to a matched group of married men (Kiecolt-Glaser et al., 1988).

The more commonplace distressing experience of examinations has been studied extensively in relationship to immune processes. Kiecolt-Glaser, Glaser, and colleagues (Kiecolt-Glaser et al., 1984a–c; Glaser et al., 1985a,b, 1986) have shown that a variety of immune parameters are altered in medical students on the day their examinations begin when compared to parameters measured 1 month before examinations. Immune processes that appear to be sensitive to the stress of exams include NK cell activity; the number of NK cells, T cells, and helper/inducer T cells; lymphocyte proliferative response to mitogen; and γ-IFN production. In each case, the immune parameter is decreased at the time of examination. In addition, these investigators have found that the level of antibody to latent herpesviruses (such as EBV, HSV) is increased at the time of examination. These changes appear to be independent of the nutritional status of the students, sleep loss, and other health behaviors that might confound an association between examination stress and immune processes. Other studies of examinations have also been conducted, and they too indicate decreases in specific immune parameters at the time of examination (e.g., Dorian et al., 1981, 1982).

There have been no human studies comparing the effects of acute and chronic stressors in the same individuals. However, the long-term effects of chronic stressors and the immediate effects of acute stressors have been evaluated in separate studies. These reports suggest that chronic stressors may "depress" certain immune processes while there may be an immediate enhancement to acute stressors. For example, in a study of chronic stress, individuals who cared for a spouse with Alzheimer's disease (AD) were compared to matched individuals who did not (Kiecolt-Glaser et al., 1987b). Caregivers of AD patients were more distressed and showed decrements in the number of T cells and helper/inducer T cells, as well as increases in antibody titers to EBV in comparison to controls. These differences did not appear to be a result of differences in nutritional status, alcohol consumption, or caffeine intake. In a small study of another form of chronic stress, individuals who resided near the Three Mile Island nuclear power plant during and following the power plant disaster were found 6 years later to have more neutrophils, fewer B cells, NK cells, and suppressor/cytotoxic T cells, and higher antibody titers to HSV and cytomegalovirus (CMV) than matched controls (McKinnon et al.,

Table 2
Naturalistic Stressors

Stressor	Refs.	Effects[a]	Special subject characteristics
Multiple recent major life events			
	Locke and Heisel, 1977	[Ab levels to swine flu vaccine]	
	Greene, 1978	(–) Lymphocyte cytotoxicity [Nasal wash IFN] [Nasal virus shed] [Lymphocyte transformation]	
	McClelland and Jemmott, 1980	(–) salivary IgA	High need for power
	Kiecolt-Glaser et al., 1984a	(–) NK activity [Serum IgA, IgG, IgM] [Salivary IgA]	
	Kiecolt-Glaser et al., 1984d	[NK activity] [Response to mitogens]	Psychiatric inpatients
	Locke et al., 1984	(–) NK activity (+) NK activity	High distress Low distress
	Irwin, 1986a	(–) NK activity	
	Irwin, 1986b	[% CD4, CD8]	
	Irwin et al., 1987b	(–) NK activity [% CD4, CD8] [CD4/CD8 ratio]	
	Kemeny et al., 1989a	[% CD4, CD8]	Genital herpes patients
	Zautra, 1989	(–) CD4/CD8 ratio [% CD3, CD20]	Rheumatoid arthritis patients
	Cohen et al., 1990	[NK activity] [% CD4, CD8] [CD8$^+$CD11b$^+$CD11b$^-$]	
	Jemmott et al., 1991	(–) NK activity	
Multiple recent minor life events			
	McClelland, 1982	(–) Salivary IgA	Prisoners
	Kemeny et al., 1989a	(–) % CD8 [% CD4]	Genital herpes patients
	Levy, 1989	(–) NK activity	
	Moss, 1989	[NK activity]	
	Zautra, 1989	(+) % CD20 [% CD3, CD4/CD8 ratio]	Rheumatoid arthritis patients
	Cohen et al., 1990	(–) NK activity (–) % CD4 (–) CD8$^+$CD11b$^-$ (+) % CD8 [CD8$^+$CD11b$^+$]	
Anticipated life stress			
	Kemeny et al., 1989a	(–) % CD4 [% CD8]	Genital herpes patients
Bereavement			
	Bartrop et al., 1977	(–) response to mitogens [B, T rosettes] [Serum IgA, IgG, IgM] [Autoantibodies] [Delayed hypersensitivity]	
	Schleifer et al., 1983	(–) Response to mitogens [B, T rosettes]	

Table 2 (continued)

Stressor	Refs.	Effects[a]	Special subject characteristics
	Linn et al., 1984	[Serum IgG, IgA, IgM]	
		[Response to mitogens]	
		[Delayed hypersensitivity]	
	Irwin, 1986a	[NK activity]	
	Irwin, 1986b	[% CD4, CD8]	
	Irwin et al., 1987a; study 1	(−) NK activity	
		[Number of lymphocytes]	
	Irwin et al., 1987a; study 2	[NK activity]	
		[Number of lymphocytes]	
	Kemeny et al., 1991a	[Response to mitogens]	HIV+ and HIV− gay men
		[% and number of CD4, CD16, activated CD8]	
		[Serum neopterin]	
Examination			
	Dorian et al., 1981	(−) Response to mitogens	
		(+) % late rosettes	
	Dorian et al., 1982	(+) Number of B, T rosettes	High distress
		(−) *In vitro* Ab synthesis	
		(−) Response to mitogens	
		[Ag-specific T_s cell activity]	
		[NK activity]	
	Jemmott et al., 1983	(−) Salivary IgA	
	Kiecolt-Glaser et al., 1984a	(−) NK activity	
		(+) Serum IgA	
		[Serum IgG, IgM]	
		[Salivary IgA]	
	Kiecolt-Glaser et al., 1984c	(−) NK activity	
		(−) % CD4	
		(−) CD4/CD8 ratio	
		[% CD8]	
	Kiecolt-Glaser et al., 1984b	(−) Transformation of B lymphocytes by EBV	
	Glaser et al., 1985a	(+) Ab titers to EBV, HSV1, CMV	
	Glaser et al., 1985b	(−) % CD3, CD4, CD8	
		(−) Response to mitogens	
		[CD4/CD8 ratio]	
	McClelland, 1985	(−) Salivary IgA	
	Glaser et al., 1986	(−) NK activity	
		(−) % CD57	
		(−) IFN production	
	Glaser et al., 1987	(−) Ag-specific T cell killing	
		(−) Activity of leukocyte migration inhibition factor	
		(−) IFN production	
		(+) Ab to EBV	
	Jemmott and Magloire, 1988	(−) Salivary IgA	
Separation/divorce			
	Kiecolt-Glaser et al., 1987a	(−) Response to mitogens	Women
		(−) % CD16	
		(+) Ab titers to EBV	
		[% CD4, CD8]	
		[CD4/CD8 ratio]	

Table 2 (continued)

Stressor	Refs.	Effects[a]	Special subject characteristics
	Kiecolt-Glaser et al., 1988	(+) Ab titers to EBV, HSV1 [% CD4, CD8] [CD4/CD8 ratio]	Men
Caregiving for chronic illness			
	Kiecolt-Glaser et al., 1987b	(−) % CD3, CD4 (−) CD4/CD8 ratio (+) Ab titers to EBV [% CD8, CD16]	
Unemployment			
	Arnetz et al., 1987	(−) Response to mitogens [Number of monocytes] [Number of CD20, CD57, CD3, CD4, CD8]	
Proximity to nuclear disaster			
	Schaeffer, 1985	(−) Salivary IgA (−) % CD20, CD3, CD4, CD8 [CD4/CD8 ratio]	
	McKinnon et al., 1989	(−) Number of CD20, CD8, CD57 (+) Number of neutrophils (+) Ab titers to HSV, CMV [Number of CD4] [Number of eosinophils, monocytes] [Serum IgG, IgM] [Ab titers to rubella]	
Earthquake			
	Kemeny, 1991b	(+) % CD56, CD16, CD8 (+) % $CD8^+CD11B^+$ [Response to mitogens] [CD4] [$CD4^+CD45RA^+$, $CD4^+CD45RA^-$] [$CD8^+HLA^-DR^+$]	
Spaceflight			
	Fischer, 1972	(+) Lymphocyte counts [Response to mitogens]	Astronauts
	Kimzey, 1975	(−) Response to mitogens (−) % T (+) WBC (+) Number of PMN granulocytes	Astronauts
Experimental Stressors Battle task vigilance			
	Palmblad et al., 1976	(−) Phagocytosis (+) IFN production	
Sleep deprivation			
	Palmblad et al., 1979	(−) Response to mitogens [Granulocyte function]	

Table 2 (continued)

Stressor	Refs.	Effects[a]	Special subject characteristics
Mental arithmetic			
	Naliboff et al., 1990	(–) % CD4	
		(+) % CD8, CD57, CD56,	
		CD16	
		[% CD3]	
		[NK activity]	
		[Response to mitogens]	

[a]All immune parameters reported in these articles are listed. Significant effects on specific immune parameters are indicated, with the direction of the relationship between stress and the immune parameter indicated in parentheses. Immune parameters tested but that showed no significant effects are listed in brackets.

1989). These individuals also had higher levels of urinary epinephrine and norepinephrine, and higher blood pressure and heart rates (Baum et al., 1983; Davidson and Baum, 1986). Finally, in a study of the chronic stress of unemployment, Arnetz and colleagues (1987) found that over a 1-year period following unemployment there was a decrease in lymphocyte response to PHA when compared to employed controls.

A few studies have been conducted on the immediate effects of acute stress exposure. In an experimental study of stress exposure, Palmblad and colleagues (1976) found a heightened ability of lymphocytes to produce interferon in response to viral challenge following a 77-hr vigil involving the performance of a simulated battle task. Phagocytosis was reduced, but returned to a level higher than baseline after the stressor exposure. In another experimental study, the stress of examiner-pressured mental arithmetic in young, but not old, subjects resulted in a prompt increase in NK cell numbers and activity (Naliboff et al., 1990). Kemeny and colleagues (1991b) found the number of NK cells and CD8 suppressor/cytotoxic T cells to be increased in individuals 2 to 4 hr after a major earthquake in Los Angeles when compared to samples drawn 6 weeks and 1 year later. It is interesting that in the Palmblad et al. and Naliboff et al. studies an increase in a measure of immune function was found, and in the Kemeny et al. and Naliboff et al. studies an increase in the number of NK cells was found. The direction of these changes is opposite to those found in studies of more prolonged distress, but consistent with those found in studies of acute *physical* stress. For example, Fiatarone et al. (1989) have shown that strenuous exercise for a short period of time increases NK cell activity in both young and old subjects. These studies support the notion that the immediate effects (within minutes to hours) of acute stress may be the opposite of the effects seen if the stressor is prolonged for days (e.g., anticipating examinations) or weeks (e.g., bereavement) (Table 2).

It is important to recognize that the majority of studies of stressor exposure and immune parameters in humans have not controlled for the behaviors that distressed individuals engage in that are known to have effects on the immune system (e.g., alcohol consumption, drug use, nutritional deficits, lack of exercise, sleep loss; see studies by Kiecolt-Glaser and colleagues for exceptions). Thus, it cannot be determined whether the immune changes found in these studies are actually a result of distress or due to distress-related behavior change (see Kiecolt-Glaser and Glaser, 1988b, for a discussion of these methodological issues).

C. Stress Moderators and Immune Processes

As in animal experiments, several moderators of the stressor-immunity relationship have been studied, including (1) the stressor context (such as social relationships), (2) individual differences prior to the stressor (such as personality, gender, and age), and (3) individual differences in the response to the stressor (such as affective state). In some cases these constructs have actually been studied independently of exposure to stress.

1. Stressor Context

As in the animal studies, the nature of social relationships at the time of stressor exposure influences the extent of subsequent immune change. For example, Kiecolt-Glaser and colleagues (1984a) have shown that the effects of examinations on NK cell activity was strongest in medical students who reported the highest level of loneliness. The effect of loneliness in medical students undergoing examination was also seen in relationship to the ability of B cells to transform in response to EBV. In addition, they have shown that lonelier psychiatric patients had lower NK cell activity and proliferative responses than less lonely patients (Kiecolt-Glaser et al., 1984d). The extent to which separation or divorce is associated with changes in immunity in women appears to depend on the nature of the ongoing social relationship as measured by degree of attachment to the ex-husband (Kiecolt-Glaser and colleagues, 1987a). These investigators have also found that the quality of marriage is related to specific immune parameters in both men and women (Kiecolt-Glaser et al., 1987a, 1988).

2. Individual Differences Prior to the Stressor

In contrast to the relationship between personality and predisposition to disease, the relationship between personality and immune processes has been studied only rarely. Power motivation, or the desire for prestige or having an impact on others, has been studied in relationship to salivary IgA levels in diverse populations (college students, prisoners, dental students) by one group of investigators (McClelland et al., 1980; Jemmott et al., 1983). The results indicate that those who inhibit the expression of their power motivation, and who also experience power-related stressors, show decrements in salivary IgA levels. However, there is a great deal of debate concerning the validity of salivary IgA measures (see Stone et al., 1987), so these data must be viewed with caution. More recently, these investigators have reported data indicating that stressed power motivation is also associated with relatively lower NK cell activity (Jemmott et al., in press).

A recent study of personality suggests that a tendency to consistently respond to stressful experiences with dysphoric affect (negative affectivity) was associated with greater variability in the number and function of NK cells over a 1-year period in patients with malignant melanoma (Kemeny et al., 1991c).

In one study of differences between younger and older individuals in the association between stressors and immune parameters, Solomon and colleagues (1991) found that a certain type of anticipated life stress was associated with lower NK cell activity in old but not young persons. Naliboff et al. (1990), in an experimental study of the differential effects of psychological stress on young (21 to 41 years) and old (65 to 85 years) subjects, found that NK activity was enhanced in young but not old subjects. In contrast, following the physical stress of exercise, young (21 to 39 years) and old subjects (65 years or older) showed the same immune changes (Fiatarone et al., 1989). These studies suggest, then, that under some environmental demands there may be age-related differences in immune parameters.

3. Individual Differences in Response to the Stressor

The primary response to stress exposure that has been examined in studies of immune parameters is affective state. For example, *depressed mood* has been shown to be associated with changes in a variety of immune parameters, for example, decreased proliferative response to the mitogen PHA in a group of men, half of whom had experienced a serious family illness or death (Linn et al., 1984); decreased NK cell activity in a group of women, the majority of whom had a husband with cancer or who had died of cancer (Irwin et al., 1987b); and lower NK cell activity in bereaved women (Irwin et al., 1987a). Depression in psychiatric inpatients (as measured by the MMPI) has also been shown to be associated with impaired DNA repair capacities in lymphocytes following X-irradiation. *Anxiety* ratings, in a sample of men undergoing the stress of hospitalization, were found to be correlated with a lower proliferative response to the mitogens PHA and ConA, and a higher number of delayed-type hypersensitivity skin test reactions (Linn et al., 1981). Finally, in a longitudinal study of dental students, daily fluctuations in negative and positive mood were associated with fluctuations in specific secretory IgA antibody levels to orally administered rabbit albumin (Stone et al., 1987). In summary, however, very little is yet known about the relationship between specific normal affective states, and immune processes.

Numerous studies of affective disorders and immune response have been conducted; however, many of these studies have evaluated patients on psychiatric medications, which may have direct effects on the immune response, or they have failed to include adequately matched control subjects. Examples of carefully controlled studies of unmedicated patients with a diagnosis of major depression have been conducted by Schleifer and colleagues. In the first (Schleifer et al., 1984), 18 hospitalized patients with a major depressive disorder (MDD) were found to have a significantly lower number of T and B cells, as well as a significantly lower proliferative response to the mitogens PHA, ConA, and PWM. No immunologic differences were found in outpatient MDD patients (Schleifer et al., 1985). In a larger study of 91 hospitalized and outpatient MDD patients and matched controls, no immunologic differences were found between patients and controls (Schleifer et al., 1989). However, they found significant differences between groups when age was considered. In the older patients, the proliferative response to PHA and the percent of CD4 (helper/inducer) T cells was lower than in controls, while the reverse was true for the younger patients. In addition, among the depressed patients, more severe depression was associated with lower proliferative responses. Thus, it appears that the relationship between major depression and immune processes is quite complex, and may depend on age, severity of depression, and hospitalization status.

There have also been studies attempting to experimentally manipulate response to stressors and to determine the effects of these interventions on immune processes in healthy individuals. Kiecolt-Glaser and colleagues (1984c) found that frequency of relaxation practice following relaxation training was associated with an increase in CD4 T lymphocytes in medical students undergoing examination. They have also found that a relaxation intervention, when compared to a "social contact only" control group, was associated with an increase in NK cell activity and a decrease in antibody levels to HSV in geriatric residents of independent living facilities (Kiecolt-Glaser et al., 1985). These effects returned to baseline at a follow-up point 1 month after the intervention period. In a study of a self-help type of psychosocial intervention for women who were unemployed, no intervention effects were seen on proliferative response to PHA or lymphocyte subsets (Arnetz et al., 1987). Finally, an interesting study was conducted to assess whether the process of writing about and presumably "working through" feelings about a traumatic situation could have an impact on immune processes. College students were asked to write about a traumatic experience for 20 min a day for 4 days (Pennebaker et al., 1988). The investigators found that proliferative response to PHA was enhanced in these students following the experiment when compared to those who were asked to write about trivial topics. In summary, while the effect of psychosocial interventions on immune processes is an important area of investigation, there is only limited knowledge about this area currently.

VI. Clinical Implications

The extent of immune change found in the majority of studies of psychosocial factors and immune processes is small and rarely falls outside the normal range. These modest effects, however, do not preclude an influence on the health of the organism. In fact, a few studies have attempted to assess the relationship between psychological factors and immune processes in individuals at risk for a disease or diagnosed with a disease. For example, Kemeny and colleagues (1989a) found that depressed mood was associated with a higher number of genital herpes recurrences experienced by a group of individuals with chronic recurrent herpes simplex. In addition, depressed mood was associated with a decrease in the level of CD8 (suppressor/cytotoxic) T cells, which for some individuals appeared to precede herpes outbreaks. In a larger follow-up study, specific mood states (e.g., anxiety/fear) were found to predict when herpes recurrences would take place (Cohen et al., 1990).

Stressor exposure and psychological factors have also been studied in relationship to immune parameters in human immunodeficiency virus (HIV) seropositive individuals (see Solomon et al., 1991, for review). For example, HIV-seropositive individuals repeatedly bereaved of close friends (Kemeny et al., 1991a) did not show immune alterations when compared to matched HIV-positive controls; however, individuals bereaved of an intimate partner did show immune changes (Kemeny et al., 1991d). In both studies depressed mood in individuals who were *not* bereaved was significantly associated with immune markers of HIV progression (e.g., a lower level of CD4 T cells, evidence of immune activation, and a lower proliferative response to PHA). These investigators have also found that chronic depression over a 2-year period in HIV-seropositive men predicted a more rapid decline in CD4 T cells over a 5-year period when compared to nondepressed HIV-positive matched controls (Kemeny et al., 1990). However, Coates and colleagues (1989) found no effect of a stress management intervention conducted over an 8-week period with HIV-positive individuals on NK cell activity, lymphocyte proliferative response to ConA, *Candida,* and CMV, serum IgA, or lymphocyte subsets.

In a study of persons with acquired immunodeficiency syndrome (AIDS), a variety of measures of dysphoria were associated with lower numbers of several T cell subsets, while positive emotions and coping (e.g., the ability to say "no" to an unwanted favor) has the reverse correlations (Temoshok et al., 1987). However, in apparent contradiction, in persons with AIDS-related complex (ARC) dysphoria was associated with higher numbers of CD4 cells and control of emotions with higher suppressor/inducer cells and NK activity as well (Temoshok et al., 1987). These confusing findings may be related to the nature of the immunopathology of HIV infection, which has features both of immune activation and immune deficiency at different phases of illness.

Psychological factors and immune processes in cancer patients have also been studied. Fawzy and colleagues (1990) found that a psychosocial group intervention conducted over a 6-week period aimed at enhancing coping skills in malignant melanoma patients was associated with an increase in interferon-augmented NK cell activity and the number of NK cells relative to a control group at a 6-month follow-up point. These changes were seen particularly in those patients who reported decreased levels of anxiety and depression and increased levels of anger over the 6-month period. Levy and colleagues (1985) found that breast cancer patients who were rated as more adjusted had *lower* levels of NK cell activity than those who were rated as less adjusted. High scores on a measure of social support and functional level and on a measure of fatigue were also associated with lower NK cell activity (Levy et al., 1985). These final two measures were also predictive of NK cell activity at a 3-month follow-up point (Levy et al., 1987).

VII. Future Directions

In the relatively new field of psychoneuroimmunology, there are a number of important issues that need to be addressed. Among these questions are: (1) Does the CNS serve an essential regulatory role in the normal functioning of the immune system? Or does the CNS, when disturbed, distort the normal processes autonomously regulated by the immune system? (2) What specific aspects of the immune system does the CNS regulate or influence? Cohn (1985) has suggested that the immune system may be autonomous in its antigen-dependent functions, such as self-nonself discrimination, but regulated by the CNS in its antigen-independent processes, such as ontogeny, rate of cell turnover, migration, and sensitivity to signals. Studies in psychoneuroimmunology have failed to investigate several of these important aspects of the immune system. (3) What is the level of specificity in communication between the nervous and immune system? There is a fine degree of specificity in communication both within the nervous system and within the immune system, mediated by particular communication substances and receptors. It remains unclear, however, whether specific neuropeptides or hormones have specific rather than more general effects on particular types of immune cells, and whether specific immune cells are more responsive to nervous system signals. In addition, it is not yet clear whether specific forms of psychological disturbance, for example, depression vs. anxiety, have different immunological consequences, or whether arousal or general distress alters immune processes irrespective of the specific nature of the affective state. (4) To what extent is sleep alteration a mediator of the relationship between psychological disturbance and immune alteration? Sleep patterns are altered in many of the conditions described above, such as major depression, bereavement, and during examinations. Sleep deprivation has been shown to alter various immune parameters (Palmblad et al., 1979). More recently, changes in immune parameters such as the production of IL-1 have been shown to change during various sleep stages (Moldofsky et al., 1986). For example, IL-1 has been shown to be produced during slow-wave sleep. In addition, recombinant tumor necrosis factor and IL-1 enhance slow-wave sleep (Shoham et al., 1987). Thus, sleep alteration may be an essential condition through which psychologic disturbance can alter immune processes.

VIII. Conclusion

Jerne (1985) has stated that the nervous and immune systems are phenotypically similar, with each able to respond by enhancement and suppression to a nearly infinite variety of external and internal stimuli to maintain homeostatic competence. Memory and experience promote adaptive behavior that is sustained by reinforcement and plasticity in both systems, and adaptive behavior can be viewed as the goal of the organism as a whole. One approach to viewing the interaction of behavior, the nervous system, and the immune system, is to recognize that adaptive behavior is promoted by the fact that behavior and physiology are inextricably intertwined (Weiner, 1989). As Weiner has pointed out, the organism regulates its actions in response to signals from others and changes in the environment, and coordinates actions with patterned physiological changes. In this view, physiological changes are intrinsic to behavior and not a consequence of it. Specific environmental signals release or set off coordinated patterns of behaviors and physiological responses. For example, in some species ovulation is promoted during mating for the purposes of reproduction. Health can be viewed as the capacity of the organism to regulate its own behavior and physiology, and produce appropriate coordinated response patterns to a challenge. When an individual cannot regulate his/her own behavior and physiology, regulatory disturbances may take place that, in turn, may lead to disease under certain conditions.

It now appears that the two systems mediating interaction with the environment, the central nervous and immune systems, communicate with each other and perhaps can be thought of as an integrated mechanism for regulating defense and adaptation. The rapidly developing field of psychoneuroimmunology offers hope of understanding these complex interrelationships and for providing new approaches to health maintenance and to treatment of illness.

References

Abrass, C. K., O'Connor, S. W., Scarpace, P. J., and Abrass, I. B., Characterization of the beta-adrenergic receptor of the rat peritoneal macrophage, *J. Immunol.*, 135, 1338, 1985.

Ader, R. and Cohen, N., Conditioned immunopharmacologic response, in *Psychoneuroimmunology*, Ader, R., Eds., Academic Press, New York, 1981, 281.

Ader, R. and Cohen, N., Behaviorally conditioned immunosuppression and murine systemic lupus erythematosus, *Science*, 215, 1534, 1982.

Ader, R. and Cohen, N., CNS-immune system interactions: conditioning phenomena, *Behav. Brain Sci.*, 8, 379, 1985.

Ahlqvist, J., Hormonal influences on immunological and related phenomena, in *Psychoneuroimmunology*, Ader, R., Eds., Academic Press, New York, 1981, 355.

Amkraut, A. and Solomon, G. F., Stress and murine sarcoma virus (Moloney)-induced tumors, *Cancer Res.*, 32, 1428, 1972.

Amkraut, A., Solomon, G. F., and Kraemer, H. C., Stress, early experience and adjuvant-induced arthritis in the rat, *Psychosom. Med.*, 3, 203, 1971.

Arnetz, B. B., Wasserman, J., Petrini, B., Brenner, S. O., Levi, L., Eneroth, P., Salovaara, H., Hjelm, R., Salovaara, L., Theorell, T., and Petterson, I. L., Immune function in unemployed women, *Psychosom. Med.*, 49, 3, 1987.

Bartrop, R. W., Luckhurst, E., Lazarus, L., Kiloh, L. G., and Penny, R., Depressed lymphocyte function after bereavement, *Lancet*, 1, 834, 1977.

Baum, A., Gatchel, R. J., and Schaeffer, M. A., Emotional, behavioral, and physiological effects of chronic stress at Three Mile Island, *J. Consult. Clin. Psychol.*, 5, 565, 1983.

Benveniste, E. N. and Merrill, J. E., Interleukin-2 stimulation of oligodendroglial proliferation and maturation, *Nature (London)*, 321, 610, 1986.

Benveniste, E., Butler, J., Gibbs, D., Chen, A., and Whitaker, J., Rat astrocyte proliferation by human B-cell growth factors, *Ann. N.Y. Acad. Sci.*, 540, 392, 1988.

Berkenbosch, G., Van Oers, J., de Rey, A., Tilders, F., and Besedofsky, H., Corticotropin-releasing factor-producing neurons in the rat activated by interleukin-1, *Science*, 238, 524, 1987.

Bernton, E. W., Prolactin and immune host defenses, *Prog. Neuroendocrinimmunol.*, 2, 21, 1989.

Bernton, E. W., Beach, J. E., Holaday, J. W., Smallridge, R. C., and Fein, H. G., Release of multiple hormones by a direct action of interleukin-1 on pituitary cells, *Science*, 238, 519, 1987.

Bernton, E., Bryant, H., Woldeyesus, J., and Holaday, J., Suppression of lymphocyte and adrenal cortical function by corticosterone: in vivo antagonism by prolactin, *Pharmacologist*, 30, A123, 1988.

Besedovsky, H. O. and Sorkin, E., Thymic involvement in female sexual maturation, *Nature (London)*, 249, 356, 1974.

Besedovsky, H., Sorkin, E., Felix, D., and Haas, H., Hypothalamic changes during the immune response, *Eur. J. Immunol.*, 7, 323, 1977.

Besedovsky, H. O., Del Rey, A., Sorkin, E., Da Prada, M., and Keller, H. H., Immunoregulation mediated by the sympathetic nervous system, *Cell Immunol.*, 48, 346, 1979.

Biziere, K., Guillaumin, J. M., Degenne, D., Bardos, P., Renoux, M., and Renoux, G., Lateralized neocortical modulation of the T-cell lineage, in *Neural Modulation of Immunity,* Guillemin, R., Cohn, M., and Melnechuk, T., Eds., Raven Press, New York, 1985, 81.

Blair, P. B., Immunologic consequences of early exposure of experimental rodents to diethylstilbestrol and steroid hormones, in *Developmental Effects of Diethylstilbestrol in Pregnancy,* Herbst, A. L. and Bern, H. A., Eds., Thieme-Stratton, New York, 1981, 167.

Blalock, J. E., The immune system as a sensory organ, *J. Immunol.,* 132, 1067, 1984.

Blalock, J., Smith, E. M., and Meyer, W. J., Corticotropin-releasing activity of monokines, *Science,* 230, 1035, 1985.

Bost, K. L., Smith, E. M., Wear, L. B., and Blalock, J. E., Presence of ACTH and its receptor on a beta-lymphocytic cell line: a possible autocrine function for a neuroendocrine hormone, *J. Biol. Regul. Homeost. Agents,* 1, 23, 1987.

Bovbjerg, D. H., Redd, W. H., Maier, L. A., Hollard, J. C., Lesko, L. M., Niedzwiecki, D., Rubin, S. C., and Hakes, T. B., Anticipatory immune suppression and nausea in women receiving cyclic chemotherapy for ovarian cancer, *J. Consult. Clin. Psychol.,* 58, 153, 1990.

Brooks, W. H., Cross, R. J., Roszman, T. L., and Markesbery, W. R., Neuroimmunomodulation: neural anatomical basis for impairment and facilitation, *Ann. Neurol.,* 12, 56, 1982.

Brown, G. W. and Harris, R., *Social Origins of Depression: A Study of Psychiatric Disorder in Women,* The Free Press, New York, 1978.

Brown, S. L. and van Epps, D. E., Opioids peptides modulate production of interferon-gamma by human mononuclear cells, *Cell Immunol.,* 103, 19, 1986.

Brummitt, C. F., Sharp, B. M., Gekker, G., Keane, W. F., and Peterson, P. K., Modulatory effects of beta-endorphin on interferon-gamma production by cultured peripheral blood mononuclear cells: heterogeneity among donors and the influence of culture medium, *Brain Behav. Immun.,* 2, 187, 1988.

Bulloch, K., Neuroanatomy of lymphoid tissue: a review, in *Neural Modulation of Immunity,* Guillemin, R., Cohn, M., and Melnechuk, T., Eds., Raven Press, New York, 1985, 111.

Bulloch, K. and Moore, R. Y., Innervation of the thymus gland by brain stem and spinal cord in mouse and rat, *Am. J. Anat.,* 162, 157, 1981.

Chiappelli, F., Yamashita, N., Faisal, M., Kemeny, M., Bullington, R., Nguyen, L., Clement, L. T., and Fahey, J. L., Differential effect of beta-endorphin on three human cytotoxic cell populations, *Int. J. Immunopharmacol.,* 13, 291—297, 1991.

Claman, H. N., Corticosteroids and the immune response, *Adv. Exp. Med. Biol.,* 245, 203, 1988.

Clayton, P. J., Mortality and morbidity in the first year of widowhood, *Arch. Gen. Psychiatry,* 30, 747, 1974.

Coates, T. J., McKusick, L., Kuno, R., and Stites, D. P., Stress reduction training changed number of sexual partners but not immune function in men with HIV, *Am. J. Public Health,* 79, 885, 1989.

Coe, C. L., Rosenberg, L. T., Fischer, M., and Levine, S., Psychological factors capable of preventing the inhibition of the antibody response in separated infant monkeys, *Child Dev.,* 58, 1420, 1987.

Coe, C. L., Rosenberg, L. T., and Levine, S., Prolonged effect of psychological disturbance on macrophage chemiluminescence in the squirrel monkey, *Brain Behav. Immun.,* 2, 151, 1988.

Cohen, F., Stress and bodily disease, *Psychiatr. Clin. N. Am.,* 4, 269, 1981.

Cohen, F., Kemeny, M., Kearney, K., Zegans, L., Neuhaus, J., Conant, M., and Stites, D., Psychological states, immunity, and genital herpes recurrence: stress, mood and personality as predictors, in preparation, 1990.

Cohen, J. J., Thymus-derived lymphocytes sequestered in the bone marrow of hydrocortisone-treated mice, *J. Immunol.,* 108, 841, 1972.

Cohen, J. J. and Crnic, L. S., Behavior, stress, and lymphocyte recirculation, in *Stress, Aging, and Immunity,* Cooper, E. L., Ed., Marcel Dekker, New York, 1984, 73.

Cohen, S. and Williamson, G. M., Stress and infectious disease in human, *Psychol. Bull.,* in press.

Cohn, M., What are the "must" elements of immune responsiveness, in *Neural Modulation of Immunity,* Guillemin, R., et al., Eds., Raven Press, New York, 1985, 3.

Cooper, E. L., Peters, G., Ahmed, I. I., Faisal, M., and Ghoneum, M., Aggression in Tilapia affects immunocompetent leukocytes, *Agg. Behav.,* in press.

Croiset, G., Veldhuis, H. D., Ballieux, R. E., De Wied, D., and Heijnen, C. J., The impact of mild emotional stress induced by the passive avoidance procedure on immune reactivity, *Ann. N.Y. Acad. Sci.,* 496, 477, 1987.

Croiset, G., Ballieux, R. E., De Wied, D., and Heijnen, C. J., Effects of environmental stimuli on immunoreactivity: further studies on passive avoidance behavior, *Brain Behav. Immunol.,* 2, 138, 1989.

Davidson, L. M. and Baum, A., Chronic stress and post-traumatic stress disorders, *J. Consult. Clin. Psychol.,* 54, 303, 1986.

Davies, A. O. and Lefkowitz, R. J., Corticosteroid-induced differential regulation of beta adrenergic receptors circulating human polymorphonuclear leukocytes and mononuclear leukocytes, *Endocrinology,* 51, 599, 1980.

Davila, D. R., Brief, S., Simon, J., Hammer, R. E., Brinster, R. L., and Kelley, K. W., Role of growth hormone in regulating T-dependent immune events in aged, nude, and transgenic rodents, *J. Neurosci. Res.,* 18, 106, 1987.

De Sanctis, G., De Carolis, C., Moretti, C., Perricone, R., Fabbri, A., Gnessi, L., Fraioli, F., and Fontana, L., Endogenous opioids and the immune system: demonstration of inhibiting as well as enhancing effects of beta-endorphin on natural killer activity, *Rivista di Immunologia ed Immunofarmacologia,* 6, 13, 1986.

Dorian, B. J., Keystone, E., Garfinkel, P. E., and Brown, G. M., Immune mechanisms in acute psychological stress, *Psychosom. Med.,* 43, 84, 1981.

Dorian, B. J., Garfinkel, P., Brown, G., Shore, A., Gladman, D., and Keystone, E., Aberrations in lymphocyte subpopulations and function during psychological stress, *Clin. Exp. Immunol.,* 50, 132, 1982.

Dunn, A. J. and Hall, N. R., Thymic extracts and lymphokine-containing supernatant fluids stimulate the pituitary-adrenal axis but not cerebral catecholamine or indolamine metabolism, *Brain Behav. Immun.,* 1, 113, 1987.

Eidinger, D. and Garrett, T. J., Studies of the regulatory effects of the sex hormones on antibody formation and stem cell differentiation, *J. Exp. Med.,* 136, 1098, 1972.

Fabrise, N. and Mocchegiani, E., Endocrine control of thymic factor production in young adults and old mice, *Cell Immunol.,* 91, 325, 1985.

Fahey, J. L., Guyre, P. M., and Munck, A., Mechanisms of anti-inflammatory actions of glucocorticoids, *Adv. Inflammation Res.,* 2, 21, 1981.

Faisal, M., Chiappelli, F., Ahmed, I. I., Cooper, E. L., and Wiener, H., Social confrontation "stress" in aggressive fish is associated with an endogenous opioid-mediated suppression of proliferative response to mitogens and nonspecific cytotoxicity, *Brain Behav. Immun.,* 3, 214, 1989a.

Faisal, M., Chiappelli, F., Cooper, E., and Weiner, H., Social confrontation in Tilapia suppresses cell-mediated immunity: evidence for the role of endogenous opioids, *Psychosom. Med.,* 51, 247, 1989b.

Fauci, A. S., Mechanisms of the immunosuppressive and anti-inflammatory effects of glucocorticosteroids, *J. Immunopharmacol.,* 1, 1, 1979.

Fawzy, F. I., Kemeny, M. E., Fawzy, N. W., Elashoff, R., Morton, D., Cousins, N., and Fahey, J. L., A structured psychiatric intervention for cancer patients. II. Changes over time in immunological parameters, *Arch. Gen. Psychiatry,* 47, 729, in press.

Felten, D. L., Felten, S. Y., Carlson, S. L., Olschowka, J. A., and Livnat, S., Noradrenergic and peptidergic innervation of lymphoid tissue, *J. Immunol.,* 135, 755, 1985.

Felten, D. L., Felten, S. Y., Bellinger, D. L., Carlson, S. L., Ackerman, K. D., Madden, K. S., Olschowka, J. A., and Livnat, S., Noradrenergic sympathetic interactions with the immune system structure and function, *Immunol. Rev.,* 100, 225, 1987.

Felten, S. Y., Housel, J., and Felten, D. L., Use of in vivo dialysis for evaluation of splenic norepinephrine and serotonin, *Soc. Neurosa Abstr.,* 12, 1065, 1986.

Fiatarone, M. A., Morley, J. E., Bloom, E. T., Benton, D., Solomon, G. F., and Makinodan, T., The effects of exercise on natural killer cell activity in young and old subjects, *J. Gerontol.,* 44, 37, 1989.

Finn, R., St. Hill, C. A., Govan, A. J., Ralfs, I. G., and Gurney, F. J., Immunological responses in pregnancy and survival of fetal homograft, *Br. J. Med.,* 3, 150, 1972.

Fleshner, M., Laudenslager, M. L., Simons, L., and Maier, S. F., Reduced serum antibodies associated with social defeat in rats, *Physiol. Behav.*, 45, 1, 1989.

Fontana, A., Kristensen, F., Dubs, R., Gemsa, D., and Weber, E., Production of prostaglandin E and an interleukin 1-like factor by cultured astrocytes and C6 glioma cells, *J. Immunol.*, 129, 2413, 1982.

Ghoneum, M., Faisal, M., Peters, G., Ahned, I. I., and Cooper, E. L., Suppression of natural cytotoxic cell activity by social aggressiveness of Tilapia, *Dev. Comp. Immunol.*, 12, 595, 1986.

Gilman, S. C., Schwarz, J. M., Milner, R. J., Bloom, F. E., and Feldman, J. D., Beta-endorphin enhances lymphocyte proliferative responses, *Proc. Natl. Acad. Sci. U.S.A.*, 79, 4226, 1982.

Gisler, R. H., *Psychother. Psychosom.*, 23, 197, 1974.

Gisler, R. H. and Schenkel-Hullinger, L., Hormonal regulation of the immune response. II. Influence of pituitary and adrenal activity on immune responsiveness in vitro, *Cell Immunol.*, 2, 646, 1971.

Gisler, R. H., Bussard, A. E., Mazie, J. C., and Hess, R., Hormonal regulation of the immune response. I. Induction of an immune response in vitro with lymphoid cells from mice exposed to acute systemic stress, *Cell Immunol.*, 2, 634, 1971.

Giulian, D. and Lachman, L. B., Interleukin-1 stimulation of astroglial proliferation after brain injury, *Science*, 228, 497, 1985.

Glaser, R., Kiecolt-Glaser, J. K., Speicher, C. E., and Holliday, J. E., Stress, loneliness, and changes in herpesvirus latency, *J. Behav. Med.*, 8, 249, 1985a.

Glaser, R., Kiecolt-Glaser, J. K., Stout, J. C., Tarr, K. L., Speicher, C. E., and Holliday, J. E., Stress-related impairments in cellular immunity, *Psychiatry Res.*, 16, 233, 1985b.

Glaser, R., Rice, J., Speicher, C. E., Stout, J. C., and Kiecolt-Glaser, J. K., Stress depresses interferon production by leukocytes concomitant with a decrease in natural killer cell activity, *Behav. Neurosci.*, 100, 675, 1986.

Glaser, R., Rice, J., Sheridan, J., Fertel, R., Stout, J., Speicher, C. E., Pinsky, D., Kotur, M., Post, A., Beck, M., and Kiecolt-Glaser, J. K., Stress-related immune suppression: health implications, *Brain Behav. Immunol.*, 1, 7, 1987.

Gorsky, R. A., Immune involvement in reproductive behavior and fertility during development and aging, personal communication.

Grossman, C. J., Interaction between the gonadal steroids and the immune system, *Science*, 227, 257, 1985.

Heijnen, C. J. and Ballieux, R. E., Influence of opioid peptides on the immune system, *Adv. J. Inst. Adv. Health*, 3, 114, 1986.

Heijnen, C. J., Bevers, C., Kavelaars, A., and Ballieux, R. E., Effect of alpha-endorphin on the antigen-induced primary antibody response of human blood B cells in vitro, *J. Immunol.*, 136, 213, 1985.

Heijnen, C. J., Zijlstra, J., Kavelaars, A., Croiset, G., and Ballieux, R. E., Modulation of the immune response by POMC-deprived peptides, *Brain Behav. Immunol.*, 1, 284, 1987.

Hines, M., Kemeny, M., Weiner, H., and Fahey, J., Estrogen and immunological development: immunological characteristics in women exposed to diethylstilbestrol (DES) prenatally, paper presented at the First International Congress ISNIM (International Society of Neuroimmunomodulation), Florence, Italy, May, 1990.

Holmes, T. H. and Rahe, R. H., The Social Readjustment Rating Scale, *J. Psychosom. Med.*, 11, 213, 1967.

Irwin, M., Daniels, M., Bloom, E. T., and Weiner, H., Life events, depression, and natural killer cell activity, *Psychopharmacol. Bull.*, 22, 1093, 1986a.

Irwin, M., Daniels, M., Weiner, H., and Bloom, E. T., Depression and changes in T-cell subpopulations, *Psychosom. Med.*, 48, 303, 1986b.

Irwin, M., Daniels, M., Smith, T., Bloom, E., and Weiner, H., Impaired natural killer cell activity during bereavement, *Brain Behav. Immunol.*, 1, 98, 1987a.

Irwin, M., Daniels, M., Bloom, E., Smith, T. L., and Weiner, H., Life events, depressive symptoms, and immune function, *Am. J. Psychiatry*, 144, 437, 1987b.

Jemmott, J. B., III, Borysenko, J. Z., Borysenko, M., McClelland, D. C., Chapman, R., Meyer, D., and Benson, H., Academic stress, power motivation, and decrease in secretion rate of salivary secretory immunoglobulin A, *Lancet*, 1, 1400, 1983.

Jemmott, J. B., III, Hellman, C., McClelland, D. C., Locke, S. E., Kraus, L., Williams, R. M., and Valeri, C. R., Motivational syndromes associated with natural killer cell activity, *J. Behav. Med.*, in press.

Jerne, N. K., *Science*, 229, 1057, 1985.

Johnsson, T. and Rasmussen, A. F., Jr., *Arch. Ges. Virusforsch.*, 18, 393, 1965.

Justice, A., Review of the effects of stress on cancer in laboratory aniamls: importance of time of stress application and type of tumor, *Psychol. Bull.*, 98, 108, 1985.

Kay, N., Allen, J., and Morley, J. E., Endorphins stimulate normal human peripheral blood lymphocyte natural killer activity, *Life Sci.*, 35, 53, 1984.

Keller, S. E., Weiss, J., Schleifer, S. J., Miller, M. D., and Stein, M., Suppression of immunity by stress: effect of a graded series of stressor on lymphocyte stimulation in the rat, *Science*, 213, 1397, 1981.

Kelley, K. W., Brief, S., Westly, H. J., Novakofsky, J., Bechtel, P. J., Simon, J., and Waller, E. B., GH-3 pituitary adenoma cells can reverse thymic aging in rats, *Proc. Natl. Acad. Sci. U.S.A.*, 8344, 5663, 1986.

Kemeny, M. E., Cohen, F., Zegans, L. S., and Conant, M. A., Psychological and immunological predictors of genital herpes recurrence, *Psychosom. Med.*, 51, 195, 1989a.

Kemeny, M., Duran, R., Weiner, H., Taylor, S., Visscher, B., and Fahey, J. L., Bereavement of partner and immune processes in HIV positive and negative homosexual men, paper presented at the Seventh International Conference on AIDS, Florence, Italy, June, 1991b.

Kemeny, M., Duran, R., Taylor, S., Weiner, H., Visscher, B., and Fahey, J., Chronic depression predicts CD4 decline over a five year period in HIV seropositive men, paper presented at the Sixth International Conference on AIDS, San Francisco, June, 1990.

Kemeny, M. E. Weiner, H., Taylor, S. E., Schneider, S., Visscher, B., and Fahey, J. L., Repeated bereavement, depressed mood, and immune response in HIV seropositive and seronegative homosexual men, submitted.

Kemeny, M., Chiappelli, F., and Fahey, J., Immunological effects of an acute, naturalistic stressor: changes in lymphocyte function and phenotype immediately following the October 1, 1987, earthquake in Los Angeles, submitted.

Kemeny, M. E., Herbert, T., Fawzy, F. J., and Fawzy, N. W., and Fahey, J. L., Negative affectivity marital status, and immunologic functioning in melanomic patients, submitted.

Kiecolt-Glaser, J. K. and Glaser, R., Psychological influences on immunity: implications for AIDS, *Am. Psychol.*, 43, 892, 1988b.

Kiecolt-Glaser, J. K., Garner, W., Speicher, C., Penn, G. M., Holliday, J., and Glaser, R., Psychosocial modifiers of immunocompetence in medical students, *Psychosom. Med.*, 46, 7, 1984a.

Kiecolt-Glaser, J. K., Speicher, C. E., Holliday, J. E., and Glaser, R., Stress and the transformation of lymphocytes by Epstein-Barr virus, *J. Behav. Med.*, 7, 1, 1984b.

Kiecolt-Glaser, J. K., Glaser, R., Strain, e. C., Stout, J. C., Tarr, K. L., Holliday, J. E., and Speicher, C. E., Modulation of cellular immunity in medical students, *J. Behav. Med.*, 9, 5, 1984c.

Kiecolt-Glaser, J. K., Ricker, D., George, J., Messick, G., Speicher, C. E., Garner, W., and Glaser, R., Urinary cortisol levels, cellular immunocompetency, and loneliness in psychiatric inpatients, *Psychosom. Med.*, 46, 15, 1984d.

Kiecolt-Glaser, J. K., Glaser, R., Williger, D., Stout, J., Messick, G., Sheppard, S., Ricker, D., Romisher, S. C., Briner, W., Bonnell, G., and Donnerberg, R., Psychosocial enhancement of immunocompetence in a geriatric population, *Health Psychol.*, 4, 25, 1985.

Kiecolt-Glaser, J. K., Fisher, L. D., Ogrocki, P., Stout, J. C., Speicher, C. E., and Glaser, R., Marital quality, marital disruption, and immune function, *Psychosom. Med.*, 49, 13, 1987a.

Kiecolt-Glaser, J. K., Glaser, R., Shuttleworth, E. C., Dyer, C. S., Ogrocki, P., and Speicher, C. E., Chronic stress and immunity in family caregivers of Alzheimer's disease victims, *Psychosom. Med.*, 49, 523, 1987b.

Kiecolt-Glaser, J. K., Kennedy, S., Malkoff, S., Fisher, L., Speicher, C. E., and Glaser, R., Marital discord and immunity in males, *Psychosom. Med.*, 50, 213, 1988.

King, T. R., Neuroestrogenic control of feeding behavior and body weight in rats with kainic acid lesions of the lateral septal area, *Physiol. Behav.*, 3, 475, 1986.

Korneva, E. A., The effect of stimulating different mesencephalic structures on protective immune response patterns, *Secherov Physiol. J. USSR*, 53, 42, 1967.

Korneva, E. A. and Shkinek, E. K., *Hormones and the Immune System*, Hayka, Moscow, 1988.

Laudenslager, M. L., The psychobiology of loss: lessons from human and nonhuman primates, *J. Soc. Issues*, 44, 19, 1988.

Laudenslager, M. L. and Ryan, S. M., Coping and immunosuppression: inescapable but not escapable shock suppresses lymphocyte proliferation, *Science*, 221, 568, 1983.

Laudenslager, M. L., Reite, M. L., and Harbeck, R. J., Suppressed immune response in infant monkeys associated with maternal separation, *Behav. Neural Biol.*, 36, 40, 1982.

Laudenslager, M. L., Fleshner, M., Hofstadter, P., Held, P. E., Simons, L., and Maier, S. F., Suppression of specific antibody production by inescapable shock: stability under varying conditions, *Brain Behav. Immunol.*, 2, 92, 1988.

Levy, S. M., Herberman, R. B., Maluish, A. M., Schlien, B., and Lippman, M., Prognostic risk assessment in primary breast cancer by behavioral and immunological paramters, *Health Psychol.*, 4, 99, 1985.

Levy, S., Herberman, R., Lippman, M., and d'Angelo, T., Correlation of stress factors with sustained depression of natural killer cell activity and predicted prognosis in patients with breast cancer, *J. Clin. Oncol.*, 5, 348, 1987.

Linn, B. S., Linn, M. W., and Jensen, J., Anxiety and immune responsiveness, *Psychol. Rep.*, 49, 969, 1981.

Linn, M. W., Linn, B. S., and Jensen, J., Stressful events, dysphoric mood, and immune responsiveness, *Psychol. Rep.*, 54, 219, 1984.

Livnat, S., Felten, S. Y., Carlson, S. K., Bellinger, D. L., and Felten, D. L., Involvement of peripheral and central catecholamine systems in neural-immune interactions, *J. Neuroimmunol.*, 10, 5, 1985.

Livnat, S., Madden, K. S., Felten, D. L., and Felten, S. Y., Regulation of the immune system by sympathetic neural mechanisms, *Prog. Neuropsychopharmacol. Biol. Psychiatry*, 11, 143, 1987.

Locke, S. E. and Heisel, J. S., The influence of stress and emotions on the human immune response, *Biofeedback Self Regul.*, 2, 320, 1977.

Locke, S. E., Kraus, L., Leserman, J., Hurst, M. W., Heisel, J. S., and Williams, R. M., Life change stress, psychiatric symptoms, and natural killer cell activity, *Psychosom. Med.*, 46, 441, 1984.

Lown, B. A. and Dutka, M. E., Early handling enhances mitogen responses of splenic cells in adult C3H mice, *Brain, Behavior, and Immunity*, 1, 356, 1987.

Luparello, T. J., Stein, M., and Park, C. D., Effect of hypothalamic lesions on rat anaphylaxis, *Am. J. Physiol.*, 207, 911, 1964.

Lysle, D. T., Lyte, M., Fowles, H., and Rabin, B. S., Shock induced modulation of lymphocyte reactivity: suppression, habituation, and recovery, *Life Sci.*, 41, 1805, 1987.

Macris, N. T., Schiavi, R. C., Camerino, M. S., and Stein, M., Effect of hypothalamic lesions on immune processes in the guinea pig, *Am. J. Physiol.*, 219, 1205, 1970.

Malaise, M. G., Hazee-Hagelstein, M. T., Reuter, A. M., Vrinds-Gavaert, Y., Goldstein, G., and Franchimont, P., Thymopoetin and thymopentin enhance the levels of ACTH, BE, and beta-lipoprotein from rat pituitary cells in vitro, *Acta Endocrinol.*, 114, 455, 1987.

McCain, H. W., Lamster, I. B., Bozzone, J. M., and Grbic, J. T., Beta-endorphin modulates human immune activity via non-opiate receptor mechanisms, *Life Sci.*, 31, 1619, 1982.

McClelland, D. C. and Jemmott, J. B., III, Power motivation, stress and physical illness, *J. Hum. Stress*, 6, 6, 1980.

McKinnon, W., Weisse, C. S., Reynolds, C. P., Bowles, C. A., and Baum, A., Chronic stress, leukocyte subpopulations and humoral response to latent viruses, *Health Psychol.*, 8, 389, 1989.

Mechanic, D., Discussion of research programs on relations between stressful life events and episodes of physical illness, in *Stressful Life Events: Their Nature and Effects*, Dohrenwend, B. S. and Dohrenwend, B. P., Eds., John Wiley & Sons, New York, 1974, 87.

Mehrishi, J. N. and Mills, I. H., Opiate receptors on lymphocytes and platelets in man, *Clin. Immunol. Immunopathol.*, 27, 240, 1983.

Mendelsohn, L. G., Kerchner, G. A., Culwell, M., and Ades, E. W., Immunoregulation by opioid peptides, *J. Clin. Lab. Immunol.*, 16, 125, 1985.

Merrill, J. E., Kutsunai, S., Mohlstrom, C., Hofman, F., Groopman, J., and Golde, D. W., Proliferation of astroglia and oligodendroglia in response to human T-cell derived factors, *Science*, 224, 1428, 1984.

Metal'nikov, S. and Chorine, V., The role of conditioned reflexes in immunity, *Ann. Inst. Pasteur*, 40, 893, 1926.

Miczek, K. A., Thompson, M. L., and Schefter, L., Opioid-like analgesia in defeated mice, *Science*, 215, 1520, 1982.

Miles, K., Quintans, E., Chelmicka-Schorr, E., and Earnason, B. G. W., The sympathetic nervous system modulates antibody response to thymus-independent antigens, *J. Neuroimmunol.*, 101, 1981.

Miyawaki, T., Taga, K., Nagaoki, T., Seki, H., Suzuki, Y., and Taniguchi, N., Circadian changes of T lymphocyte subsets in human peripheral blood, *Clin. Exp. Immunol.*, 55, 618, 1984.

Moldofsky, H., Lue, F. A., Eisen, J., Keystone, E., and Gorczynski, R. M., The relationship of interleukin-1 and immune functions to sleep in humans, *Psychosom. Med.*, 48, 309, 1986.

Monjan, A. A. and Collector, M. J., Stress induced modulation of the immune response, *Science*, 196, 307, 1977.

Moore, R. Y., Central neural control of circadian rhythms, in *Frontiers in Neuroendocrinology*, Ganong, W. and Martini, L., Eds., Raven Press, New York, 1978, 185.

Munck, A. and Leung, K., Glucocorticoid receptors and mechanisms of action, in *Receptors and Mechanism of Action of Steroid Hormones*, Part II, Pasqualini, J. R., Eds., Marcel Dekker, New York, 1977, 311.

Munck, A., Guyre, P. M., and Holbrook, N. J., Physiological functions of glucocorticoids in stress and their relation to pharmacological actions, *Endocrine Rev.*, 5, 25, 1984.

Naliboff, B. D., Benton, D., Solomon, G. F., Morley, J. E., Fahey, J. L., Bloom, E. T., Makinodan, T., and Gilmore, S. L., Immunological changes in young and old subjects during brief laboratory stress, (manuscript submitted for publication).

Nance, D. M., Rayson, D., and Carr, R. I., The effects of lesions in the lateral septal and hippocampal areas on the humoral immune response of adult female rats, *Brain Behav. Immunol.*, 1, 292, 1987.

Odio, N., Brodish, A., and Ricardo, M. J., Effects on immune responses by chronic stress are modulated by aging, *Brain Behav. Immunol.*, 1, 204, 1987.

Okimura, T. and Nigo, Y., Stress and immune responses. I. Suppression of T cell function in restraint-stressed mice, *Jpn. J. Pharmacol.*, 40, 505, 1986.

Ottaway, C. A., In vitro alteration of receptors for vasoactive intestinal peptide changes the in vivo localization of mouse T cells, *J. Exp. Med.*, 160, 1054, 1984.

Palmblad, J., Cantell, K., Strander, H., Froberg, J., Karlsson, C., Levi, L., Gronstrom, M., and Unger, P., Stressor exposure and immunological response in man: interferon-producing capacity and phagocytosis, *J. Psychosom. Res.*, 20, 193, 1976.

Palmblad, J., Petrini, B., Wasserman, J., and Akerstedt, T., Lymphocyte and granulocyte reactions during sleep deprivation, *Psychosom. Med.*, 41, 273, 1979.

Parkes, C. M. and Brown, R. J., Health after bereavement, *Psychosom. Med.*, 34, 449, 1972.

Payan, D. A., Levine, J. D., and Goetzl, E. J., Modulation of immunity and hypersensitivity by sensory neuropeptides, *J. Immunol.*, 132, 1601, 1984.

Pennebaker, J. W., Kiecolt-Glaser, J. K., and Glaser, R., Disclosure of traumas and immune function: health implications for psychotherapy, *J. Consult. Clin. Psychol.*, 56, 239, 1988.

Peterson, P. K., Sharp, B., Gekker, G., Brummitt, C., and Keane, W. F., Opioid-mediated suppression of interferon-gamma production by cultured peripheral blood mononuclear cells, *J. Clin. Invest.*, 80, 824, 1987.

Prete, P., Levin, E. R., and Pedram, A., The in vitro effects of endogenous opiates on natural killer cells, antigen-specific cytolytic T cells and T-cell subsets, *Exp. Neurol.*, 92, 349, 1986.

Rabin, B. S., Ganguli, R., Cunnick, J. E., and Lysle, D. T., The central nervous system-immune system relationship, *Clin. Lab. Med.*, 8, 253, 1988.

Raymond, L. N., Reyes, E., Tokuda, S., and Jones, B. C., Differential immune response in two handled inbred strains of mice, *Physiol. Behav.*, 37, 295, 1986.

Ritchie, A. W., Oswald, I., Micklem, H. S., Boyd, J. E., Elton, R. A., Jazwinska, E., and James, K., Circadian variation of lymphocyte sub-populations: a study with monoclonal antibodies, *Br. Med. J.*, 286, 1773, 1983.

Rogers, M. P., Dubey, D., and Reich, P., The influence of the psyche and the brain on immunity and disease susceptibility: a critical review, *Psychosom. Med.*, 41, 147, 1979.

Roszman, T. L., Cross, R. J., Brooks, W. H., and Markesbery, W. R., Neuroimmunomodulation: effects of neural lesions on cellular immunity, in *Neural Modulation of Immunity*, Guillemin, R., Cohn, M., and Melnechuk, T., Eds., Raven Press, New York, 1985, 95.

Sapolsky, R., Rivier, C., Yamamoto, G., Plotsky, P., and Vale, W., Interleukin-1 stimulates the secretion hypothalamic corticotropin-releasing factor, *Science*, 238, 522, 1987.

Schleifer, S. J., Keller, S. E., Camerino, M., Thornton, J. C., and Stein, M., Suppression of lymphocyte stimulation following bereavement, *JAMA*, 250, 374, 1983.

Schleifer, S. J., Keller, S. E., Meyerson, A. T., Raskin, M. J., Davis, K. L., and Stein, M., Lymphocyte function in major depressive disorder, *Arch. Gen. Psychiatry*, 41, 484, 1984.

Schleifer, S. J., Keller, S. E., Samuel, S. G., Kenneth, L. D., and Stein, M., Depression and immunity: lymphocyte function in ambulatory depressed patients, hospitalized schizophrenic patients, and patients hospitalized for herniorrhaphy, *Arch. Gen. Psychiatry*, 42, 129, 1985.

Schleifer, S. J., Keller, S. E., Bond, R. N., Cohen, J., and Stein, M., Major depressive disorder and immunity: role of age, sex, severity, and hospitalization, *Arch. Gen. Psychiatry*, 46, 81, 1989.

Shanahan, F., Denburg, J. A., Fox, J., Bienestock, J., and Befus, D., Mast cell heterogeneity: effects of neuroenteric peptides on histamine release, *J. Immunol.*, 135, 1331, 1985.

Shavit, Y., Ryan, S. M., Lewis, J. W., Laudenslager, M. L., Terman, G. W., Maier, S. F., Gale, R. P., and Liebeskind, J. C., Inescapable but not escapable stress alters immune function, *Physiologist*, 26, A-64, 1983.

Shavit, Y., Terman, G. W., Martin, F. C., Lewis, J. W., Liebeskind, J. C., and Gale, R. P., Stress, opiod peptides, the immune system, and cancer, *J. Immunol.*, 135, 834, 1985.

Shavit, Y., Martin, F. C., Yirmiya, R., Ben-Eliyahu, S., Terman, G. W., Weiner, H., Gale, R. P., and Liebeskind, J. C., Effects of a single administration of morphine or footshock stress on natural killer cell cytotoxicity, *Brain Behav. Immunol.*, 1, 318, 1987.

Shoham, S., Davenne, D., Dinarello, C. A., and Kruger, J. M., Recombinant tumor necrosis factor and interleukin-1 enhance slow-wave sleep, *Am. J. Physiol.*, 253, R142, 1987.

Shukla, H. C., Solomon, G. F., and Doshi, R. S., The relevance of some Ayurvedic (traditional Indian medical) concepts to modern holistic health, *J. Holistic Health*, 4, 25, 1981.

Simpkins, C. O., Dickey, C. A., and Fink, M. P., Human neurtrophil migration is enhanced by beta-endorphin, *Life Sci.*, 34, 2251, 1984.

Smith, E. M., Meyer, W. J., and Blalock, J. E., Virus-induced corticosterone in hypophysectomized mice: a possible lymphoid adrenal axis, *Science*, 218, 1311, 1982.

Solomon, G. F., Stress and antibody response in rats, *Int. J. Neuropharmacol.*, 20, 97, 1969.

Solomon, G. F., Levine, S., and Kraft, J. K., Early experience and immunity, *Nature (London)*, 220, 821, 1968.

Solomon, G. F., Kemeny, M. E., and Temoshok, L., Psychoneuroimmunologic aspects of human immunodeficiency virus infection, in *Psychoneuroimmunology II*, Ader, R., Felten, D. L., and Cohen, N., Eds., Academic Press, Orlando, 1991.

Solomon, G. F., Benton, D., Morley, J. E., Fiatarone, M. A., Bloom, E. T., Fahey, J. L., and Makinodan, T., Anticipated life stress, distress, and immune function in healthy old people, submitted.

Solvason, H. B., Ghanta, V. K., and Hiramoto, R. N., Conditioned augmentation of natural killer cell activity: independence from nociceptive effects and dependence on interferon-beta, *J. Immunol.*, 140, 661, 1988.

Staehelin, M., Muller, P., Portenier, M., and Harris, A. W., Beta adrenergic receptors and adenylate cyclase activity in murine lymphoid cell lines, *J. Cyc. Nucl. Prot. Phosphoryl. Res.*, 10, 55, 1985.

Stanisz, A. M., Befus, A. D., and Bienenstock, J., Differential effects of vasoactive intestinal peptide, substance P and somatostatin on immunoglobulin synthesis and proliferation by lymphocytes from Peyer's patches, mesenteric lymph nodes, and spleen, *J. Immunol.*, 136, 152, 1986.

Stead, R. H., Bienenstock, J., and Stanisz, A. M., Neuropeptide regulation of mucosal immunity, *Immunol. Rev.,* 100, 333, 1987.

Stone, A. A., Cox, D. S., Valdimarsdottir, H., and Neale, J. M., Secretory IgA as a measure of immunocompetence, *J. Human Stress,* 13, 136, 1987.

Tavadia, H. B., Fleming, K. A., Hume, P. D., and Simpson, H. W., Circadian rhythmicity of human plasma cortisol and PHA-induced lymphocyte transformation, *Clin. Exp. Immunol.,* 22, 190, 1975.

Temoshok, L., Zich, J., Solomon, G. F., and Stites, D., An intensive psychoimmunologic study of long-surviving persons with AIDS, paper presented at the Third International Conference on AIDS in Washington, June, 1987.

van Epps, D. E. and Saland, L., Beta-Endorphin and Met-enkephalin stimulate human peripheral blood mononuclear cell chemotaxis, *J. Immunol.,* 132, 3046, 1984.

Wayner, E. R., Flannery, G. R., and Singer, G., Effects of taste aversion conditioning on the primary antibody response to sheep red blood cells and *Brocella abortus* in the albino rat, *Physiol. Behav.,* 21, 995, 1978.

Weiner, H., The dynamics of the organism: implications of recent biological thought for psychosomatic theory and research, *Psychosom. Med.,* 51, 608, 1989.

Weiner, H., The dynamics of the organism: implications of recent biological thought for psychosomatic theory and research, in *Psychoneuroimmunology II,* Ader, R., Felten, D. L., and Cohen, N., Eds., Academic Press, New York, in press.

Williams, J. M., Peterson, R. G., Shea, P. A., Schmedthe, J. F., Bauer, D. C., and Felten, D. L., Sympathetic innervation of murine thymus and spleen: evidence for a functional link between the nervous and immune systems, *Brain Res. Bull.,* 6, 83, 1981.

Williamson, S. A., Knight, R. A., Lightman, S. L., and Hobbs, J. R., Differential effects of beta-endorphin fragments on human natural killing, *Brain Behav. Immunol.,* 1, 329, 1987.

Wybran, J., Enkephalins and endorphins as modifiers of the immune system: present and future, *Fed. Proc.,* 44, 90, 1985.

Zalcman, S., Minkiewicz-Janda, A., Richter, M., and Anisman, H., Critical periods associated with stressor effects on antibody titers and on the plaque-forming cell response to sheep red blood cells, *Brain Behav. Immunol.,* 2, 254, 1988.

Zautra, A. J., Okun, M. A., Robinson, S. E., Lee, D., Roth, S. H., and Emmanuel, J., Life stress and lympholyte alterations among patients with rheumatoid arthritis, *Health Psychol.,* 8, 1, 1989.

Zegans, L. S., An attempt at integration, in *Emotions in Health and Illness,* Grune & Stratton, Orlando, 1984, 235.

Index

INDEX

A

A13 cell groups, colocalization of with somatostatin, 238

A cells, glucagon-containing, 233

Acceptors, 65

Acetylcholine
in ADH regulation, 516
in control of growth hormone secretion, 259—260

Acquired immunodeficiency syndrome (AIDS), psychosocial factors in, 581

Acromegaly, 459
biochemical findings in, 460—461
clinical features of, 459—460
discovery of, 1
facial appearance of patient with, 460
with growth hormone excess, 485
treatment of, 461—462

Activity-sleep cycles, adrenal steroids coordinating, 345—347

Adaptation, 129
damaging effects of adrenal steroids on, 347—349

Addictive drugs, tolerance to dependence on, 391—392

Addison's disease
hypothyroidism in, 456
immune deficiency in, 565

Adenohypophysis
factors affecting responsiveness of to releasing and inhibiting hormones, 9—11
influence on hormone-producing cell types of, 106

Adenylate cyclase, 63
activation of, 515
inhibition of, 9

Adiposigenital dystrophy, 1

Adrenal cortex
hypertrophy of, 420—421
role of hormones of in adaptation, 129—130

Adrenal glands
insufficiency of with destruction of hypothalamic CRF neuronal system, 167
steroidogenesis defects of, 491
tumors of, 491

Adrenal medulla
enlargement of, 420—421
hormones of in adaptation mechanisms, 129

Adrenal steroids
as coordinators of activity-sleep cycles and ingestive behaviors, 345—347
pathological aspects of action of, 347—349

Adrenalectomy, for Cushing's disease, 466

Adrenalin release, 129

Adrenarche, 486
premature, 490, 493

Adrenergic afferents, in control of growth hormone secretion, 259

Adrenocortical carcinoma, short stature with, 479

Adrenocorticotropic hormone (ACTH)
abnormal secretion of in Cushing's disease, 463—465
actions of, 378
in adaptation mechanisms, 130
age-related change in secretion and action of, 548—549
amino acid sequence of, 382
behavioral neuroendocrinology of, 378—384
"big", 30
bioassay methods for, 21, 27—30
biosynthesis of "big", 30
and cortisol regulation, 418
CRF-41 effects on, 165
CRF-induced secretion of, 151
deficiency of in hypothalamic disease, 446
early studies on hypothalamic control of secretion of, 130—131
ectopic secretion of, 465
effects of lymphokines on, 568
enhanced secretion of, 2
evaluation of, 447
factors in release of, 8
half-life *in vivo* of, 30
hypersecretion of with Cushing's syndrome, 406
in immune processes, 566—567
immunoactive, 28—30
inhibition of release of, 153
integrated neuroendocrine control of secretion of, 161
interleukin-1 effects on release of, 163
localization of in brain, 11
mechanisms of action of, 383
mechanisms shutting off secretion of after stress, 348
neurotransmitter-induced secretion of, 151—152
neurotropic effects of, 379—382
noradrenergic control over release of, 13
profiles for over time for plasma cortisol, 28
response of to stress, 418—419
short-look feedback of, 14
stimulation of release and function of, 353
stress-induced secretion of, 2—3
structure-activity studies of, 382—383
synthesis and structure of, 378—379
in TRH-tuberoinfundibular neuron regulation, 298
vasopressin in regulation of, 3—4, 516
vasopressin receptors mediating release of, 367

Adrenocorticotropic hormone (ACTH)/cortisol response, in hypothalamic disorder, 448

Adrenocorticotropic hormone (ACTH)-secreting pituitary tumors, 462—467

Adrenocorticotropic hormone-related peptides
mechanisms of action of, 383
selected effects of, 381
structure-activity relationships of, 383

595

E

M